RECENT DEVELOPMENTS IN

ALCOHOLISM

VOLUME 14

THE CONSEQUENCES OF ALCOHOLISM

RECENT DEVELOPMENTS IN

Edited by

MARC GALANTER

New York University School of Medicine
New York, New York

Associate Editors

HENRI BEGLEITER, RICHARD DEITRICH,
RICHARD FULLER, DONALD GALLANT,
DONALD GOODWIN, EDWARD GOTTHEIL,
ALFONSO PAREDES, MARCUS ROTHSCHILD,
and DAVID VAN THIEL

Assistant Editors

DEIRDRE WINCZEWSKI
MAUREEN CARUSO

An Official Publication of the American Society of Addiction Medicine and the Research Society on Alcoholism.
This series was founded by the National Council on Alcoholism.

ALCOHOLISM

VOLUME 14
THE CONSEQUENCES OF ALCOHOLISM

Medical
Neuropsychiatric
Economic
Cross-Cultural

PLENUM PRESS • NEW YORK AND LONDON

The Library of Congress has catalogued this work as follows:

Recent developments in alcoholism: an official publication of the American Medical Society on Alcoholism, and the Research Society on Alcoholism, and the National Council on Alcoholism—Vol. 1– —New York: Plenum Press, c1983–
v.: ill.; 25 cm.
Cataloging in publication.
Editor: Marc Galanter.
ISSN 0738-422X = Recent developments in alcoholism.

1. Alcoholism—Periodicals. I. Galanter, Marc. II. American Medical Society on Alcoholism. III. Research Society on Alcohol (U.S.) IV. National Council on Alcoholism. [DNLM: 1. Alcoholism—periodicals. W1 RE106AH(P)]

HV5001.R4 616.86'1'05—dc19 83-643791

Library of Congress [8311] AACR 2 MARC-S

ISBN 0-306-45747-4

A Division of Plenum Publishing Corporation
233 Spring Street, New York, N.Y. 10013

http://www.plenum.com

10 9 8 7 6 5 4 3 2 1

Printed in the United States of America

Contributors

Tiina Arppe, Department of Sociology, The University of Helsinki, 00200 Helsinki, Finland

Enrique Baraona, Department of Medicine, Mount Sinai School of Medicine, New York, New York; and Bronx VA Medical Center, Bronx, New York 10468

Mary F. Brunette, Psychiatric Research Center, Dartmouth Medical School, Lebanon, New Hampshire 03766

Jordi Camí, Institut Municipal d'Investigació Mèdica and Universitat Pompeu Fabra, Barcelona, Spain

Carlos Campillo, Instituto Mexicano de Psiquiatría, Tlalpan, 14370 México, DF

Silvia Carreño, Instituto Mexicano de Psiquiatría, Calzada, CP 14370 México, DF

Ricardo Castaneda, Department of Psychiatry, New York University School of Medicine, Bellevue Hospital Medical Center, New York, New York 10016

Frank J. Chaloupka, Department of Economics, University of Illinois at Chicago, Chicago, Illinois 60607; and Health Economics Program, National Bureau of Economic Research, New York, New York 10017-5405

Juan Ramon De la Fuente, Instituto Mexicano de Psiquiatría, Calzada, CP 14370 México, DF

Robert E. Drake, Psychiatric Research Center, Dartmouth Medical School, Lebanon, New Hampshire 03766

Magi Farré, Universitat Pompeu Fabra and Universitat Autónoma de Barcelona, Barcelona, Spain

Douglas Fountain, The Lewin Group, Fairfax, Virginia 22031

Howard S. Friedman, Department of Medicine, Long Island College Hospital, Brooklyn, New York; and Department of Medicine, SUNY Health Sciences Center at Brooklyn, Brooklyn, New York 11201

Richard K. Fuller, Division of Clinical and Prevention Research, National Institute on Alcohol Abuse and Alcoholism, Bethesda, Maryland 20892-7003

Peter R. Giancola, Western Psychiatric Institute and Clinic, Department of Psychiatry, University of Pittsburgh School of Medicine, Pittsburgh, Pennsylvania 15213

Maria Luisa González, Institut Municipal d'Investigació and Universitat Autónoma de Barcelona, Barcelona, Spain

David A. Gorelick, Intramural Research Program, National Institute on Drug Abuse, National Institutes of Health, Baltimore, Maryland 21224

Edward Gottheil, Department of Psychiatry, Jefferson Medical College, Thomas Jefferson University, Philadelphia, Pennsylvania 19107

Ellen F. Gottheil, Department of Psychiatry and Behavioral Sciences, University of Washington Medical School, Seattle, Washington 98195

Michael Grossman, Department of Economics, City University of New York Graduate School, New York, New York, 10036, and Health Economics Program, National Bureau of Economic Research, New York, New York 10017-5405

Henrick J. Harwood, The Lewin Group, Fairfax, Virginia 22031

Harold D. Holder, Prevention Research Center, Berkeley, California 94704

Margaretha Jarvinen, Institute of Sociology, University of Copenhagen, 1361 Copenhagen, Denmark

Takenobu Kamada, Department of Gastroenterology, Osaka Rosai Hospital, Osaka 591, Japan

Maria A. Leo, Department of Medicine, Mount Sinai School of Medicine, New York, New York; and Bronx VA Medical Center, Bronx, New York 10468

Robert Levy, Department of Psychiatry, New York University School of Medicine, Bellevue Hospital Medical Center, New York, New York 10016

Charles S. Lieber, Departments of Medicine and Pathology, Mount Sinai School of Medicine, New York, New York; and Alcohol Dependence Treatment Program and Section of Liver Disease and Nutrition, Bronx VA Medical Center, Bronx, New York 10468

Gina Livermore, The Lewin Group, Fairfax, Virginia 22031

David Lyons, Department of Physiology and Pharmacology, Wake Forest University School of Medicine, Winston-Salem, North Carolina 27157

Elena Medina-Mora, Instituto Mexicano de Psiquiatría, Calzada, CP 14370 México, DF

Ruth Montalvo, Department of Medicine, Division of Gastroenterology and Nutrition, The University of Texas Health Science Center at San Antonio, San Antonio, Texas 78284-7878

Howard B. Moss, Western Psychiatric Institute and Clinic, Department of Psychiatry, University of Pittsburgh School of Medicine, Pittsburgh, Pennsylvania 15213

John Mullahy, Department of Preventive Medicine, Bradley Memorial, University of Wisconsin, Madison, Wisconsin 53706

Katsuhisa Noda, Department of Gastroenterology, Osaka Rosai Hospital, Osaka 591, Japan

Mary O'Malley, Department of Psychiatry, New York University School of Medicine, Bellevue Hospital Medical Center, New York, New York 10016

Alfonso Paredes, Laboratory for the Study of the Addictions, West Los Angeles, VA Medical Center, Los Angeles, California 90073

Linda J. Porrino, Department of Physiology and Pharmacology, Wake Forest University School of Medicine, Winston-Salem, North Carolina 27157

Gudrun Pöschl, Laboratory of Alcohol Research, Liver Disease and Nutrition, and Department of Medicine, Salem Medical Center, D-69121 Heidelberg, Germany

Luciana Ramos, Instituto Mexicano de Psiquiatría, Tlalpan, 14370 México, DF

Martha Romero, Instituto Mexicano de Psiquiatría, Tlalpan, 14370 México, DF

Henry Saffer, Department of Economics, Kean University, Union, New Jersey 07083; and Health Economics Program, National Bureau of Economic Research, New York, New York 10017-5405

Gabriela Saldivar, Instituto Mexicano de Psiquiatría, Tlalpan, 14370 México, DF

Steven Schenker, Department of Medicine, Division of Gastroenterology and Nutrition, The University of Texas Health Science Center at San Antonio, San Antonio, Texas 78284-7878

Jordi Segura, Institut Municipal d'Investigació and Universitat Autónoma de Barcelona, Barcelona, Spain

Helmut K. Seitz, Laboratory of Alcohol Research, Liver Disease and Nutrition, and Department of Medicine, Salem Medical Center, D-69121 Heidelberg, Germany

Ulrich A. Simanowski, Laboratory of Alcohol Research, Liver Disease and Nutrition, and Department of Medicine, Salem Medical Center, D-69121 Heidelberg, Germany

Jody L. Sindelar, Department of Epidemiology and Public Health, Yale University School of Medicine, New Haven, Connecticut 06520

Edward G. Singleton, Behavior Therapy Treatment Research Center, Johns Hopkins University School of Medicine, Baltimore, Maryland 21224

Hilary R. Smith, Department of Physiology and Pharmacology, Wake Forest University School of Medicine, Winston-Salem, North Carolina 27157

Norman Sussman, Department of Psychiatry, New York University School of Medicine, Bellevue Hospital Medical Center, New York, New York 10016

Rafael de la Torre, Institut Municipal d'Investigació and Universitat Autónoma de Barcelona, Barcelona, Spain

Laurence Westreich, Department of Psychiatry, New York University School of Medicine, Bellevue Hospital Medical Center, New York, New York 10016

Christopher T. Whitlow, Department of Physiology and Pharmacology, Wake Forest University School of Medicine, Winston-Salem, North Carolina 27157

Harumasa Yoshihara, Department of Gastroenterology, Osaka Rosai Hospital, Osaka 591, Japan

Preface

From the President of the Research Society on Alcoholism

On behalf of the Research Society on Alcoholism, I am pleased to introduce this 14th volume of *Recent Developments in Alcoholism* about the consequences of alcoholism. Current concepts are presented in well-organized sections that focus on the medical, neuropsychiatric, economic, and biobehavioral consequences of alcoholism. This volume contains up-to-date discussions of these issues. The editors and associate editors should be congratulated for bringing together such important information. This volume will be a valuable resource for investigators and therapists alike.

Ivan Diamond M.D., Ph.D.
President, Research Society on Alcoholism

From the President of the American Society of Addiction Medicine

On behalf of the American Society of Addiction Medicine, I am pleased to announce that our society once again will cosponsor *Recent Developments in Alcoholism.* This volume addresses the issues of age, gender, socioeconomy, and behaviors as they relate to alcohol research and the disease of alcoholism. The medical consequences of alcoholism are ably edited by Dr. Charles Lieber, while the neuropsychiatric consequences of alcoholism are addressed by Drs. Gottheil. This volume is rounded out with the in-depth discussion of the economic consequences of alcoholism, edited by Dr. Fuller, and an international perspective on the behavioral consequences of alcoholism, edited by Dr. Paredes.

G. Douglas Talbott, M.D., President
American Society of Addiction Medicine

Contents

I. Medical Consequences of Alcoholism

Charles S. Lieber, Section Editor

Chapter 2

Alcohol and the Pancreas
Steven Schenker and Ruth Montalvo

Chapter 3

Alcohol and Cancer
Helmut K. Seitz, Gudrun Pöschl, and Ulrich A. Simanowski

Chapter 4

Alcohol and Lipids
Enrique Baraona and Charles S. Lieber

Chapter 5

Cardiovascular Effects of Alcohol
Howard S. Friedman

II. Neuropsychiatric Consequences of Alcoholism

Edward Gottheil and Ellen F. Gottheil, Section Editors

Chapter 12

The Effects of Price on the Consequences of Alcohol Use and Abuse
Frank J. Chaloupka, Michael Grossman, and Henry Saffer

Chapter 13

Drinking, Problem Drinking, and Productivity
John Mullahy and Jody L. Sindelar

Chapter 14

The Cost Offsets of Alcoholism Treatment
Harold D. Holder

IV. An International Perspective of the Biobehavioral Consequences of Alcoholism

Alfonso Paredes, Section Editor

Overview
Alfonso Paredes

Chapter 15

Experience with the Alcohol Use Disorders Identification Test (AUDIT) in Mexico
Elena Medina-Mora, Silvia Carreño, and Juan Ramon De la Fuente

Chapter 16

Problems Associated with Hazardous and Harmful Alcohol Consumption in Mexico
Carlos Campillo, Martha Romero, Gabriela Saldivar, and Luciana Ramos

Chapter 17

Sanctification of "The Accursed": Drinking Habits of the French Existentialists in the 1940s
Tiina Arppe

Chapter 18

Cocaine Metabolism in Humans after Use of Alcohol: Clinical and Research Implications
Jordi Camí, Magi Farré, Maria Luisa González, Jordi Segura, and Rafael de la Torre

Chapter 19

Interrelationship between Alcohol Intake, Hepatitis C, Liver Cirrhosis, and Hepatocellular Carcinoma
Harumasa Yoshihara, Katsuhisa Noda, and Takenobu Kamada

RECENT DEVELOPMENTS IN

ALCOHOLISM

VOLUME 14

THE CONSEQUENCES OF ALCOHOLISM

I

Medical Consequences of Alcoholism

Charles S. Lieber, Section Editor

Overview

Charles S. Lieber

The purpose of the five review chapters in this section is to focus on the medical consequences of the metabolism of ethanol in the body and how, as a result, alcoholics differ from nonalcoholics biochemically and pathologically.

A few decades ago, the medical issues relating to the disease of chronic alcoholism were not widely studied, because the intrinsic toxicity of alcohol was not fully appreciated and alcoholism was considered to be primarily a social or behavioral problem. However, the prevalence of just one medical problem, cirrhosis of the liver, has now reached such a magnitude that this complication of alcoholism represents, in and of itself, a major public health problem. We now recognize that 75% of all medical deaths attributable to alcoholism are the result of cirrhosis of the liver; in large urban areas, it has become a leading cause of death in the age group of 25 to 65 years. Although not all cirrhotic subjects are alcoholics, it is now generally recognized that a majority of patients with cirrhosis do admit to excessive alcohol consumption. Other tissues can also be severely affected, including, as reviewed here, effects on the cardiovascular system and the pancreas, as well as several more general detrimental actions of ethanol in terms of lipid metabolism and carcinogenesis.

The question often raised is "in what way does an alcoholic differ from a nonalcoholic?" Inquiries have focused on psychological makeup, behavioral differences, and socioeconomic factors. More recently, however, physical, including genetic, differences have been delineated, and prior to development of various disease entities, chronic ethanol exposure results in profound

Charles S. Lieber • Departments of Medicine and Pathology, Mount Sinai School of Medicine, New York, New York; and Alcohol Dependence Treatment Program and Section of Liver Disease and Nutrition, Bronx VA Medical Center, Bronx, New York 10468.

Recent Developments in Alcoholism, Volume 14: The Consequences of Alcoholism, edited by Galanter. Plenum Press, New York, 1998.

biochemical and morphological changes. Consequently, an alcoholic does not respond normally to alcohol, other drugs, or even other toxic agents. Some of these persistent changes are consequences of the injurious effects of ethanol and associated nutritional disorders, whereas others may represent adaptive responses to the profound changes in intermediary metabolism that are a direct and immediate consequence of the oxidation of ethanol itself.

Chapter 1, by Drs. Lieber and Leo, deals with ethanol metabolism and some of its effects on the liver and stomach. The bulk of ethanol metabolism occurs in the liver, which also suffers from the brunt of its toxicity. One focus of Chapter 1 is on the microsomal ethanol oxidizing system (MEOS), discovered three decades ago and which is now finally recognized as a pathway of major significance for ethanol-related pathology. It involves a specific cytochrome P450, now called 2E1, which has been fully characterized and has the unique property of activating many xenobiotics to highly toxic metabolites, thereby explaining the increased vulnerability of the heavy drinker to a variety of drugs and environmental compounds. New treatments of alcoholic liver disease are now evolving, based either on the attenuation of the oxidative stress induced by P4502E1-mediated ethanol metabolism or to some associated abnormality in the phosphatidylcholine backbone of the membranes.

Some ethanol metabolism also occurs in the stomach. Although it is quantitatively much lower than in the liver, it may nevertheless be of importance to explain some adverse alcohol–drug interactions. The metabolism in the stomach involves a form of alcohol dehydrogenase (ADH) not present in the liver, namely σ-ADH, which has now been fully characterized and its gene cloned. The acute gastritis seen in heavy drinkers has been clearly attributed to direct alcohol toxicity. The pathogenesis and treatment of chronic gastritis has been more elusive, but a significant role for *Helicobacter pylori* (HP) is now emerging, with ethanol either favoring its implantation and/or interacting with and potentiating the effects of the caustic ammonia (NH_3) produced by HP. Some previous as well as recent studies document the responsiveness of alcoholic gastritis to antibiotic therapy, which was reported, already four decades ago, to effectively eliminate gastric NH_3 production.

Chapter 2, by Dr. Schenker, deals with another gastrointestinal organ sometimes severely affected by ethanol, namely the pancreas. Alcoholic pancreatitis is considered a "chronic" form of pancreatitis because it is associated with irreversible changes in function and structure, ultimately resulting from the autodigestion of the pancreas. Various theories proposed to explain alcohol-induced pancreatitis are discussed, including oxidative damage mediated by free radicals, but the results are still inconclusive, mainly because of the difficulties in studying this organ because of the inaccessibility of the pancreas in humans and the lack of experimental models in animals. Heretofore, most cases of alcoholic pancreatitits have come to the attention of the clinician at a relatively advanced and late stage, with severe organ damage refractory to treatment. Recognition of early stages and better understanding of their pathogenesis may ultimately provide hope for more effective therapy.

Chapter 3, "Alcohol and Cancer," by Dr. Seitz and co-workers, summarizes evidence linking alcohol consumption to an array of cancers. New insights on pathogenesis are provided, especially the recognition that carcinogenesis can already be stimulated at relatively low levels of alcohol consumption. This is an important observation relative to the increasingly prevailing concept that low levels of consumption are not harmful but may be beneficial. This important issue is addressed further in Chapter 4, by Baraona and Lieber, on "Alcohol and Lipids." It addresses the many interactions between alcohol and lipid metabolism, especially the pathogenesis and treatment of alcoholic fatty liver and hyperlipemia, with emphasis on the relationship between alcohol and atherosclerosis. The various mechanisms whereby moderate alcohol consumption may decrease the incidence of coronary complications are reviewed in detail. This analysis comprises not only alcohol-induced changes in lipids but also those that may be related to congeners in alcoholic beverages.

The issue of coronary heart disease and stroke and their relationship to moderate and heavy alcohol intake are also reviewed from a cardiologist's point of view in Chapter 5, by Dr. Friedman. He points out that the development of hypertension, for which alcohol abuse is a leading risk factor, could explain most of the increased incidence of cardiovascular disease in alcoholics, whereas the favorable effects of moderate alcohol use on atherogenesis could account for most of the reduction in coronary heart disease and ischemic stroke. He also points out that, on the one hand, the protective effect of moderate alcohol use on the risk of developing stable angina pectoris is comparable to that for myocardial infarction. On the other hand, alcohol use also adversely affects the mortality rate of an acute myocardial infarction with established cardiovascular disease. This is consistent with the finding of an increased incidence of sudden death in alcohol abusers with coronary heart disease. He also notes that alcohol use enhances the antiplatelet actions of aspirin which may increase the risk of hemorrhage in individuals receiving aspirin for cardiovascular disease. In addition, he stresses the diametrically opposite effects of alcohol consumption on ischemic and hemorrhagic stroke. From a thorough analysis of all of the facts and views, Dr. Friedman concludes that "the body of evidence argues against any recommendation that alcohol use be encouraged for its cardiovascular medicinal value."

As a cardiologist, Dr. Friedman's view reinforces the more general consideration that the introduction of moderate drinking into the life of an abstainer involves the unpredictable risk of loss of control, with the potential for social and medical disintegration. By contrast, in a moderate drinker who has demonstrated the capacity to maintain intake at an acceptable level, there is no compelling reason to change his or her lifestyle and eliminate a pleasurable and possibly beneficial habit, provided there is no underlying cardiovascular disease and that there is no occupational or other special hazard involved, such as pregnancy.

In their aggregate, these five chapters provide a comprehensive, yet succinct review of the body of evidence produced on a worldwide basis concerning both beneficial and adverse effects associated with alcohol consumption, emphasizing the importance and variability of the dose–effect relationship and the resulting sometimes opposite effects. Better understanding of the pathogenesis involved will allow for a more rational and practical application of these findings to patient care, both in terms of their immediate implementation and for some possible future therapeutic approaches.

1

Metabolism of Ethanol and Some Associated Adverse Effects on the Liver and the Stomach

Charles S. Lieber and Maria A. Leo

Abstract. Current knowledge of alcohol oxidation and its effects on hepatic metabolism and its toxicity are summarized. This includes an evaluation of the relationship of the level of consumption to its interaction with nutrients (especially retinoids, carotenoids, and folate) and the development of various stages of liver disease. Ethanol metabolism in the stomach and its link to pathology and *Helicobacter pylori* is reviewed. Promising therapeutic approaches evolving from newly gained insight in the pathogenesis of medical complications of alcoholism are outlined. At present, the established approach for the prevention and treatment of alcoholic liver injury is to control alcohol abuse, with the judicial application of selective antioxidant therapy, instituted at early stages, prior to the social or medical disintegration of the patient, and associated with anti-inflammatory agents at the acute phase of alcoholic hepatitis. In addition, effective antifibrotic therapy may soon become available.

1. Magnitude of the Problem

The most severe functional and structural alcohol-induced alterations occur in the liver, and cirrhosis of the liver (usually as a complication of alcoholism) is a common cause of death. In a prospective survey of US veterans, it was found that, within 48 months, more than half of those with cirrhosis, and two

Charles S. Lieber • Departments of Medicine and Pathology, Mount Sinai School of Medicine, New York, New York; and Alcohol Dependence Treatment Program and Section of Liver Disease and Nutrition, Bronx VA Medical Center, Bronx, New York 10468. **Maria A. Leo** • Department of Medicine, Mount Sinai School of Medicine, New York, New York; and Bronx VA Medical Center, Bronx, New York 10468.

Recent Developments in Alcoholism, Volume 14: The Consequences of Alcoholism, edited by Galanter. Plenum Press, New York, 1998.

thirds of those with cirrhosis plus alcoholic hepatitis, had died.[1] This outcome is more severe than that of many cancers, yet it is attracting much less concern, both among the public and the medical profession. This may be due, at least in part, to the prevailing, pervasive and pernicious perception that not much can be done about this major public health issue. However, new insights in the pathophysiology of the alcohol-induced disorders now allow for the prospects of earlier recognition and more successful prevention and treatment, prior to the medical and social disintegration of the patient. This chapter updates previous reviews on this topic.[2–4]

2. Metabolism of Ethanol and Resulting Toxicity

Alcohol is a small molecule, both water and lipid soluble. It therefore readily permeates all organs of the body and affects most of their vital functions, usually as a consequence of its metabolism, primarily in the liver (Fig. 1).

2.1. *Metabolic Disorders Associated with Alcohol Oxidation by Alcohol Dehydrogenase*

The oxidation of ethanol via the alcohol dehydrogenase pathway results in the production of acetaldehyde with loss of H, which reduces NAD to NADH and produces a number of cellular disorders.

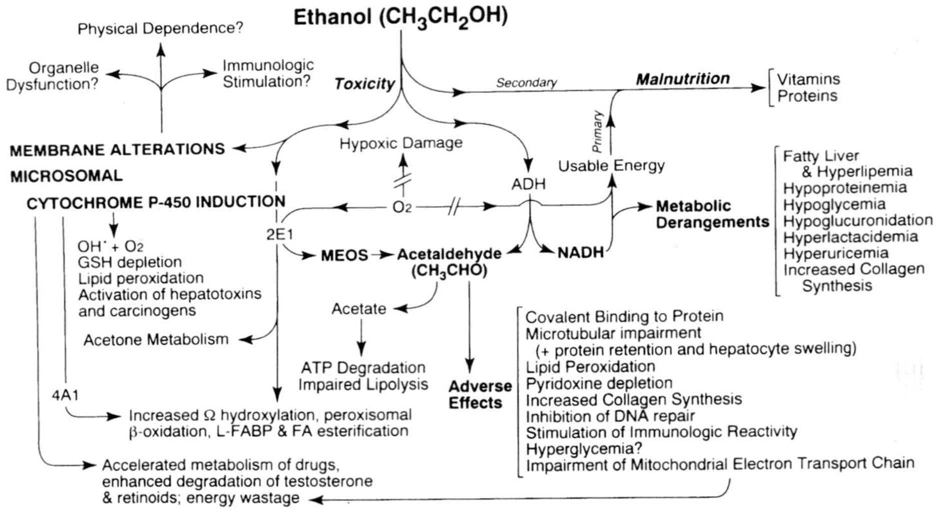

Figure 1. Hepatic, nutritional, and metabolic abnormalities after ethanol abuse. Malnutrition, whether primary or secondary, can be differentiated from metabolic derangements or direct toxicity, resulting partly from redox changes or effects secondary to microsomal induction, including increased acetaldehyde production. (From Lieber.[5])

2.1.1. Hepatic ADH. The large amounts of reducing equivalents generated overwhelm the hepatocyte's ability to maintain redox homeostasis and a number of metabolic disorders ensue[5] (Fig. 1), including hyperlactacidemia, which contributes to the acidosis and also reduces the capacity of the kidney to excrete uric acid, leading to secondary hyperuricemia. The latter is aggravated by the alcohol-induced ketosis and acetate-mediated enhanced ATP breakdown and purine generation.[6] Hyperuricemia explains, at least in part, the common clinical observation that excessive consumption of alcoholic beverages frequently aggravates or precipitates gouty attacks. The increased NADH also opposes gluconeogenesis, thereby promoting a cause of hypoglycemia, and raises the concentration of α-glycerophosphate, which favors lipogenesis by trapping fatty acids. In addition, excess NADH may promote fatty acid synthesis directly. The net result is fat accumulation with enlargement of the liver, resulting in fatty liver, the first stage of alcoholic liver disease.

Women differ from men in terms of ethanol metabolism, gastric (see Section 2.1.2), and hepatic. Hepatic ADH activity is suppressed by testosterone and its derivatives,[7] and indeed ADH activity in the livers of women is significantly higher than in men; however, after the age of 53 in men and 50 in women, the sex difference is no longer apparent.[8] Of course ADH activity, measured *in vitro*, is only one of the determinants of ethanol metabolism *in vivo* and discrepancies between the two are not uncommon.[9]

2.1.2. Gastric ADH

2.1.2a. Ethnic and Gender Differences; Effects of Drugs. The human gastric mucosa possesses several ADH isoenzymes, one of which[10] (class IV ADH or σ-ADH) is not present in the liver. It is also absent or markedly decreased in activity in a large percentage of Japanese subjects.[11] Moreno and Parés[12] isolated the σ-ADH. Its full-length cDNA has now been obtained and the complete amino acid sequence deduced[13,14]; its gene has been cloned and localized to chromosome 4.[15] Gastric ADH is responsible for a large portion of ethanol metabolism found in cultured human gastric cells.[16] Its *in vivo* counterpart is reflected by the first-pass metabolism (FPM) of ethanol, namely, the fact that for a given dose of ethanol, blood levels are usually higher after intravenous (IV) than after oral administration.

Since peripheral blood levels of alcohol represent the difference between the amount of ethanol that reaches the circulation and the amount metabolized, if the rate of entry is close to the rate of oxidation, even moderate differences in the bioavailability of ethanol may result in striking blood level changes, with substantial effects on the brain and other tissues. The lower rate of FPM in normal women as compared to normal men[17] and the even lower rate in alcoholic women as compared to normal women,[17] or in alcoholic men as compared to nonalcoholic men,[17,18] all paralleled changes in gastric ADH. These findings are consistent with a role for gastric ethanol oxidation, as are also the inhibition of gastric ADH and the increased blood ethanol levels by aspirin[19] as well as the differential effects of H_2-blockers on FPM.[20,21] The H_2-blockers that inhibit gastric ADH activity *in vitro*[20,22–24] also do so in cultured gastric cells[16,25] and result in increased blood alcohol levels *in vivo*.[26] Although questioned at first, such increases in blood level have now been confirmed[23,27] for a low alcohol dose of 0.15 g/kg, and are particularly striking after repetitive consumption of small doses,[28] a pattern common in social drinkers (Fig. 2). The H_2-blocker effect on blood alcohol levels also has been shown with higher doses of ethanol,[21,29–31] with an associated increase in intoxication score,[32] but these effects at higher ethanol dosage are still the subject of controversy. It must be pointed out, however, that some of the negative investigations used dilute concentrations of alcohol,[33] at which gastric FPM is minimal.[34]

As mentioned, for a given dose of alcohol, blood levels achieved are higher in women than in men. This effect is particularly striking in alcoholic women, but it is also of great significance for social drinking in normal women. Indeed, normal women develop higher blood levels than men because women are usually smaller than men, whereas the amounts of alcohol offered to them in social settings does not take this gender difference into account. Furthermore, the alcohol consumed is distributed in a 12% smaller water space,[17] because of a difference in body composition (more fat and less water in women). Moreover, less of the alcohol will be broken down in the stomach

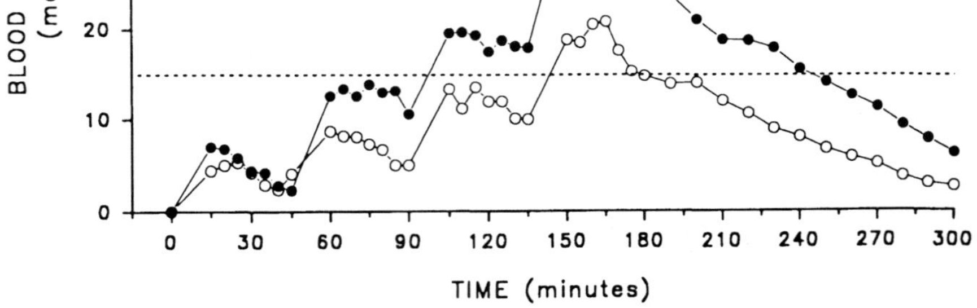

Figure 2. Effects of cimetidine (400 mg bid for 7 days) on blood alcohol levels after oral consumption of repeated small doses of ethanol in subjects with substantial first-pass metabolism prior to the administration of cimetidine. In nine months, four small doses of ethanol (150 mg/kg) were imbibed at 45-min intervals. Cimetidine resulted in a persistent increase of blood alcohol levels. ○, Before cimetidine; ●, after cimetidine. (From Gupta *et al.*[28])

and more will reach the peripheral blood because women also have lower gastric ADH activity than men,[17] at least below the age of 50 years,[35] an effect much more striking in alcoholic than in nonalcoholic women. These gender differences, however, are obvious already at levels of social drinking. Thus, what is considered a moderate dose for men is not necessarily moderate for women. Moderate drinking is now defined as not more than two drinks per day in men, but only one drink per day in women,[36] a drink being defined as 12 ounces of regular beer, 5 ounces of wine, or 1½ ounces of distilled spirits (80 proof).

In contemporary social settings, women are commonly served amounts of alcohol comparable to those given to men. Making women, aware of their increased vulnerability, may strengthen their resolve to resist the social pressures that may lead to inappropriate levels of consumption, possibly resulting in impairment of the ability to drive and to perform other similar tasks. Increased bioavailability secondary to a low level of gastric ADH may thus influence the severity of medical problems related to drinking. Taken together, the observations described above suggest that the differences in gastric ADH activity between men and women do, at least in part, explain the difference in blood ethanol levels. In addition, gastric emptying plays a role. Indeed, the menstrual cycle is important for women's metabolism of alcohol, in part through its effects on gastric emptying.[37] Gastric emptying is delayed during the luteal phase of the menstrual cycle, which is characterized by high estradiol and progesterone. Gastric emptying is one of the factors that determines the time of exposure of ethanol to gastric ADH metabolism, as well as speed of intestinal absorption. Thus, blood alcohol levels and related effects of alcohol intake vary somewhat over the menstrual cycle. Acceleration of gastric emptying may also contribute to the increase in blood alcohol after some H_2 blockers, such as ranitidine.[38]

2.1.2b. "Alcoholic" Gastritis. Acute and chronic gastritis, common in the alcoholic, is discussed elsewhere.[39] Since a substantial amount of alcohol can be metabolized by human gastric cells,[16] the resulting toxic acetaldehyde could play a pathological role. In addition, *Helicobacter pylori* (HP) infection is more common in alcoholics than in nonalcoholics,[40] raising the question of the relative role of alcohol and HP in the pathogenesis of gastritis in the alcoholic. HP could adversely affect the gastric mucosa in several ways. HP contains alcohol dehydrogenase activity.[41] Thus, in the presence of alcohol, this can again promote production of the toxic acetaldehyde. However, in human antral gastric mucosa, HP infection is associated with a significant decrease in mucosal alcohol dehydrogenase activity[42]; the net effect on gastric ethanol metabolism and acetaldehyde production had not been clarified, but this was studied in 18 alcoholics with dyspepsia.[43] HP was found in 14 and was associated with chronic antral gastritis. In the four HP-negative alcoholics, gastric biopsy specimens were normal. Studies were repeated 3 to 4 weeks after controlled alcohol abstinence during hospitalization. There was no change in histological findings during this period, indicating that alcohol itself was not the major causative agent. HP was then eliminated in 10 subjects by giving them triple therapy (bismuth subsalicylate, amoxicillin, and metronidazole). This treatment for HP was associated with almost complete normalization of histological findings. By contrast, four control subjects who received antacids alone showed no improvement in histology. Dyspeptic symptoms included epigastric pain, nausea, vomiting, heartburn, halitosis, burping, postprandial bloating, and flatulence, which were used to calculate a "total dyspepsia score" for each patient. The HP-positive patients significantly improved after antibiotic treatment and elimination of HP, whereas there was no change with antacid treatment (Fig. 3). Thus, this study demonstrated that clearance of HP and the associated histological gastritis strongly correlate with resolution of dyspeptic symptoms in alcoholics and that HP is the predominant pathogenic agent of chronic gastritis in the patients. In view of evidence gathered, antibiotic treatment should now be contemplated for routine therapy of gastritis in the alcoholic.

2.2. *Adverse Effects Resulting from Microsomal Ethanol Oxidation, Its Induction, and Interactions with Other Chemicals*

2.2.1. The 2E1-Containing Microsomal Ethanol Oxidizing System. Four decades ago, a new pathway for alcohol metabolism was discovered, namely the microsomal ethanol oxidizing system (MEOS).[44,45] Unlike ADH, the MEOS is strikingly inducible by chronic ethanol consumption. The key enzyme of the MEOS is the ethanol-inducible cytochrome P4502E1 (2E1), which is increased five- to tenfold in liver biopsies of recently drinking subjects,[46] with a corresponding rise in mRNA.[47] Other cytochrome P450 (1A2, 3A4) may also be

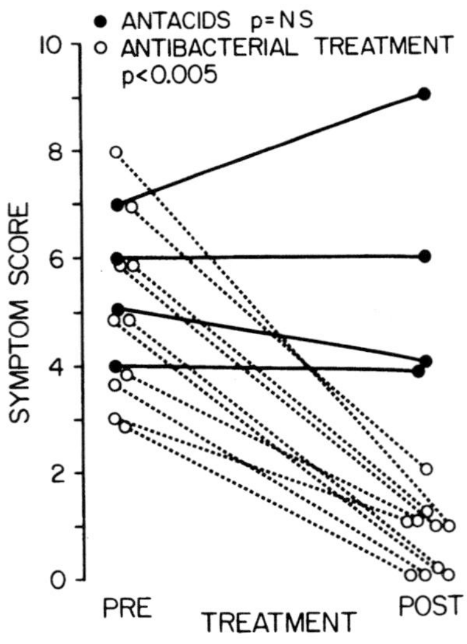

Figure 3. Effect of treatment of symptom scores in *Helicobacter pylori*-positive alcoholics. ●, Antacid treatment; ○, antibacterial treatment; $p < 0.005$ for scores before and after antibacterial treatment; not significant for scores before and after antacid treatment. (From Uppal *et al.*[43])

involved.[48] The presence of 2E1 was also shown in extrahepatic tissues[49] and in nonparenchymal cells of the liver, including Kupffer cells.[50] In rats, ethanol treatment caused a sevenfold increase in cytochrome P4502E1 (CYP2E1) content in Kupffer cells.

2.2.2. Interaction with Other Drugs. The 2E1 induction contributes to the ethanol tolerance that develops in the alcoholic and spills over to other drugs that are microsomal substrates. The tolerance of the alcoholic to various psychoactive drugs generally has been attributed to central nervous system adaptation, but in addition, metabolic adaptation must be considered, because the clearance rate of many drugs from the blood is enhanced in alcoholics.[51] The metabolic drug tolerance persists for several days to weeks after the cessation of alcohol abuse, and the duration of recovery varies with each drug.[52] During that period, the dosage of these drugs has to be increased to offset the accelerated breakdown.

In contrast with the inductive effect of long-term ethanol consumption, after short-term administration, inhibition of hepatic drug metabolism is seen, primarily because of its direct competition for a common metabolic process involving cytochrome P450.[51] Methadone exemplifies this dual interaction: whereas long-term ethanol consumption leads to increased hepatic microsomal metabolism of methadone and decreased levels in the brain and liver, short-term administration has the opposite effect—it inhibits microsomal demethylation of methadone and enhances brain and liver concentrations of the drug.[53] These effects are of clinical relevance: approximately 50% of the patients taking methadone are alcohol abusers. The combination of ethanol with tranquilizers and barbiturates also results in increased drug concentrations in the blood, sometimes to dangerously high levels, commonly observed in successful suicides.

2.2.3. Activation of Xenobiotics. In addition to the oxidation of ethanol, 2E1 also has an extraordinary capacity to activate many xenobiotics to highly toxic metabolites. This includes industrial solvents such as bromobenzene[54] and vinylidene chloride,[55] as well as anesthetics such as enflurane[56,57] and halothane,[58] commonly used medications such as isoniazid and phenylbutazone,[59] illicit drugs (i.e., cocaine), and over-the-counter analgesics, such as acetaminophen, paracetamol, and N-acetyl-*p*-aminophenol, which have been shown to be a good substrate for human 2E1.[60] The induction of 2E1 explains the increased vulnerability of the heavy drinker to the toxicity of these substances. Among alcoholic patients, hepatic injury associated with acetaminophen has been described following repetitive intake for headaches (including those associated with withdrawal symptoms), dental pain, or the pain of pancreatitis. Amounts well within the accepted tolerable rate (2.5–4 g) have been incriminated as the cause of hepatic injury in alcoholic patients.[61,62] It is likely that the enhanced hepatotoxicity of acetaminophen after chronic ethanol consumption is caused, at least in part, by an increased microsomal production of reactive metabolite(s) of acetaminophen. Consistent with this view is the observation that, in animals fed ethanol chronically, the potentiation of acetaminophen hepatotoxicity occurred after ethanol withdrawal,[63] at which time production of the toxic metabolite may be at its peak, since at that time competition by ethanol for a common microsomal pathway has been withdrawn. Thus, maximal vulnerability to the toxicity of acetaminophen occurs immediately after cessation of drinking, when there is also the greatest need for analgesia, because of the headaches and other symptoms associated with withdrawal. This also explains the synergistic effect between acetaminophen, ethanol, and fasting,[64] since all three deplete reduced glutathione (GSH), thereby contributing to the toxicity of each compound because GSH provides one of the cell's fundamental mechanisms for the scavenging of toxic free radicals (Fig. 4) (see Section 2.4).

The 2E1 promotes the generation of active oxygen species, which are toxic and may overwhelm the antioxidant system of the liver and other tissues with striking consequences. A similar effect may also be produced by the free hydroxyethyl radical generated from ethanol by 2E1. A depletion in the steady-state levels of hepatocellular GSH, in synergy with other conditions, leads to hepatocellular necrosis and liver injury. GSH is selectively depleted in the mitochondria[65] and may contribute to the striking alcohol-induced alterations of that organelle. Alpha-tocopherol, the major antioxidant in the membranes, is depleted in patients with cirrhosis[66] (Fig. 5). This deficiency in the defense systems, coupled with increased acetaldehyde (see Section 2.4), oxygen, and other free radical generation (by the ethanol-induced microsomes), may contribute to liver damage via lipid peroxidation and also via enzyme inactivation.[67] Replenishment of GSH can be achieved by administration of GSH precursors such as acetylcysteine or *S*-adenosyl-L-methionine (SAMe)[68] (Fig. 4) (see Section 5.2.1.2).

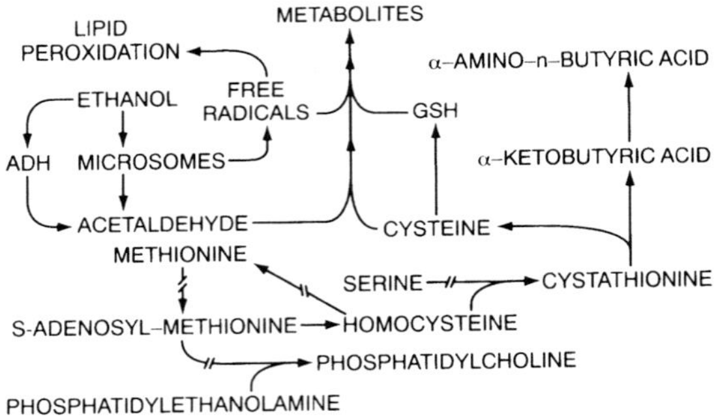

Figure 4. Link between accelerated acetaldehyde production and increased free radical generation by the induced microsomes, resulting in enhanced lipid peroxidation, with metabolic blocks (see text) due to alcohol, folate deficiency, and/or alcoholic liver disease, illustrating possible beneficial effects of GSH, its precursors (including *S*-adenosylmethionine) as well as phosphatidylcholine. (From Lieber.[245])

Alcohol influences carcinogenesis in many ways and at different sites, as reviewed by Seitz in Chapter 3. One pathogenic factor is the effect of ethanol on enzyme systems participating in the cytochrome P450-dependent activation of carcinogens. Alcoholics are commonly heavy smokers, and there is a synergistic effect of alcohol consumption and smoking on cancer development, with long-term ethanol consumption enhancing the mutagenicity of tobacco-derived products.[69]

2.2.4. Ethanol and Vitamin A. Ethanol consumption depresses hepatic levels of vitamin A in animals and in man,[70] even when given with diets containing large amounts of vitamin A,[71] reflecting, in part, accelerated microsomal degradation of the vitamin via pathways of microsomal retinol metabolism, inducible by either ethanol or drug administration.[72,73] Deficiency of vitamin A, which plays a key role in the maintenance of the integrity of normal mucosal linings, has been invoked in the pathogenesis of cancerous lesions. Supplementation of the alcoholic with vitamin A, however, is complicated by the fact that excess vitamin A is hepatotoxic.[74] Long-term ethanol consumption en-

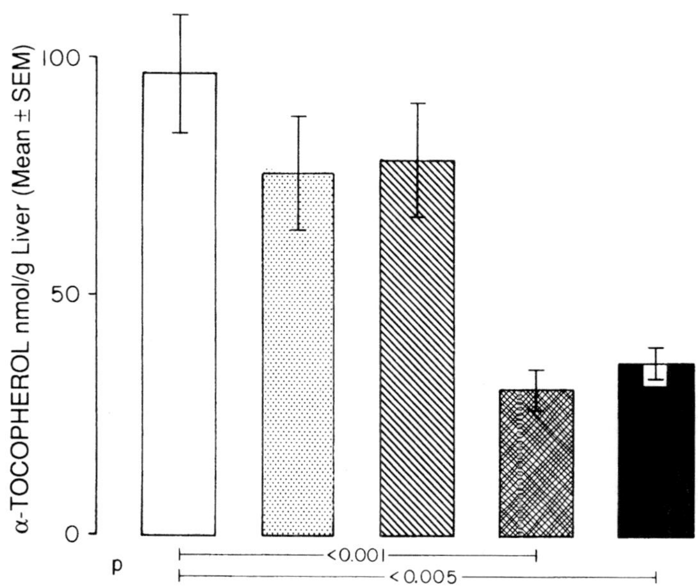

Figure 5. Effects of various liver diseases on total hepatic tocopherol levels. Only the two cirrhotic groups had significantly lower α-tocopherol levels. □, Controls (n = 13); ⬚, nonalcoholic liver disease (n = 13); ▧, alcoholics without cirrhosis (n = 14); ▩, alcoholic cirrhosis (n = 10); ■, alcoholic cirrhosis (transplant recipients; n = 8). (From Leo *et al.*[66])

hances the latter effect, resulting in striking morphological and functional alterations of the mitochondria,[75] along with hepatic necrosis and fibrosis.[76] Thus, in heavy drinkers there is a narrowed therapeutic window for vitamin A.

2.3. *Role of Catalase*

Catalase is capable of oxidizing alcohol *in vitro* in the presence of an H_2O_2-generating system[77] and its interaction with H_2O_2 in the intact liver was demonstrated.[78] However, its role is limited by the small amount of H_2O_2 generated,[79] and under physiological conditions, catalase thus appears to play no major role in ethanol oxidation.

The catalase contribution might be enhanced if significant amounts of H_2O_2 become available through β-oxidation of fatty acids in peroxisomes.[80] However, peroxisomal β-oxidation was observed only in the absence of ADH activity. In its presence the rate of ethanol metabolism is reduced by adding fatty acids,[81] and, conversely, β-oxidation of fatty acids is inhibited by NADH produced from ethanol metabolism via ADH.[81] Similarly, generation of reducing equivalents from ethanol by ADH in the cytosol inhibits H_2O_2 generation, leading to significantly diminished rates of peroxidation of alcohols via catalase.[82] Various other results also indicated that peroxisomal fatty acid oxidation does not play a major role in alcohol metabolism.[83]

Furthermore, when fatty acids were used by Handler and Thurman[80] to stimulate ethanol oxidation, this effect was very sensitive to inhibition by aminotriazole, a catalase inhibitor. Therefore, if this mechanism were to play an important role *in vivo,* one would expect a significant inhibition of ethanol metabolism after aminothiazole administration *in vivo,* when physiological amounts of fatty acids and other substrates for H_2O_2 generation are present. A number of studies, however, have shown that aminotriazole treatment has little, if any, effect on alcohol oxidation *in vivo,* as reviewed by Takagi *et al.*[84] and Kato *et al.*[85,86] The principal contenders have agreed that catalase cannot account for microsomal ethanol oxidation.[87,88] However, catalase could contribute to fatty acid oxidation. Indeed, long-term ethanol consumption is associated with increases in the content of a specific cytochrome (P4504A1) that promotes microsomal ω-hydroxylation of fatty acids, which may be followed by ω-oxidation; this could compensate, at least in part, for the deficit in fatty acid oxidation due to the ethanol-induced injury of the mitochondria.[39] Products of ω-oxidation also increase liver cytosolic fatty acid-binding protein (L-FABPc) content and peroxisomal β-oxidation,[89] an alternate but modest pathway for fatty acid disposition (see Section 3.1).

2.4. *Toxicity of Acetaldehyde*

Ethanol oxidation produces acetaldehyde (Fig. 1), a highly toxic metabolite with extraordinary reactivity. Acetaldehyde is rapidly metabolized to acetate, mainly by a mitochondrial high-affinity aldehyde dehydrogenase

(ALDH), the activity of which is congenitally low in many Orientals. This results in exaggerated blood acetaldehyde levels in Orientals and the associated flushing. ALDH activity is also significantly reduced by chronic ethanol consumption.[90] The decreased capacity of mitochondria of alcohol-abusing subjects to oxidize acetaldehyde, associated with unaltered or even enhanced rates of ethanol oxidation (and therefore acetaldehyde generation because of MEOS induction) (see Section 2.2.1), results in an imbalance between production and disposition of acetaldehyde. This generates in the elevated acetaldehyde levels observed after chronic ethanol consumption in man[91] and in baboons[92,93]; the latter revealed a tremendous increase of acetaldehyde in hepatic venous blood,[92] reflecting high tissue levels. Acetaldehyde's toxicity is due, in part, to its capacity to form protein adducts. In turn, acetaldehyde–protein adduct formation interferes with the activity of many key enzymes and repair systems, and thus becomes an important cause of direct toxicity at the tissue level, eventually resulting in cell necrosis. Indeed, minute concentrations of acetaldehyde (as low as 0.05 μmole/liter) were found to impair the repair of alkylated nucleoproteins.[94] The toxicity is associated with a significant reduction in the capacity of the liver to utilize oxygen,[93] and there is uncoupling of oxidation with phosphorylation in mitochondria damaged by chronic ethanol consumption.[95] Moreover, acetaldehyde promotes GSH depletion, free radical-mediated toxicity, and lipid peroxidation. By binding to the tubulin of the microtubules, acetaldehyde seriously impairs the secretion of proteins from the liver into the plasma, with a corresponding hepatic retention.[96] The increases in lipid, protein, water,[97] and electrolytes result in enlargement of the hepatocytes—the experimental counterpart of the ballooning of the hepatocyte seen in the alcoholic. Acetaldehyde adducts promote collagen production (see Section 5.1) and may also serve as neoantigens, generating an immune response in mice[98] and in humans.[99–101]

Acetaldehyde was shown to be capable of causing lipid peroxidation in isolated perfused livers.[102] *In vitro,* metabolism of acetaldehyde via xanthine oxidase or aldehyde oxidase may generate free radicals, but the concentration of acetaldehyde required is much too high for this mechanism to be of significance *in vivo.* However, another mechanism to promote lipid peroxidation is via GSH depletion. One of the three amino acids of this tripeptide is cysteine. Binding of acetaldehyde with cysteine and/or glutathione (GSH) (Fig. 4) may contribute to a depression of liver GSH.[103] Acute ethanol administration inhibits GSH synthesis and produces an increased loss from the liver.[104] GSH is selectively depleted in the mitochondria[65] and may contribute to the striking alcohol-induced alterations of that organelle. GSH offers one of the mechanisms for the scavenging of toxic free radicals, as shown in Fig. 4, which also illustrates how the ensuing enhanced GSH utilization (and thus turnover) results in a significant increase in α-amino-*n*-butyric acid.[105] Although GSH depletion per se may not be sufficient to cause lipid peroxidation, it is generally agreed upon that it may favor the peroxidation produced by other factors. GSH has been shown to spare and potentiate vitamin E[106]; it is important in the protection of cells against electrophilic drug injury in general, and against reactive oxygen species in particular, especially in primates, which are more vulnerable to GSH depletion than rodents.[107] Iron overload may play a contributory role, since chronic alcohol consumption results in increased iron uptake by hepatocytes[108] and since iron exposure accentuates the changes of lipid peroxidation and in the glutathione status of the liver cell induced by acute ethanol intoxication.[109] Lipid peroxidation is not only a reflection of tissue damage, it may also play a pathogenic role, for instance, by promoting collagen production.[110]

3. Effect of Gender and Interactions with Age, Hormones, and Heredity

3.1. Ethanol, Gender, and Heredity

The effect of gender on ADH-mediated gastric and hepatic ethanol metabolism are discussed in Section 2.1.1. In addition, chronic ethanol consumption has a profound interaction with testosterone metabolism, resulting in a castrationlike effect in males,[39] whereas there is evidence that the progression to more severe liver injury is accelerated in women[111] and the incidence of chronic advanced liver disease is higher among women than among men for a similar history of alcohol abuse.[112] A daily intake of alcohol of 40 g in men (3 drinks)[113,114] but only 20 g in women[113,114] resulted in a statistically significant increase in the incidence of cirrhosis in a well-nourished population.

The mechanism whereby the female gender potentiates alcohol-induced liver damage is not known. It could relate to the hormonal status. Indeed, both endogenous and exogenous (i.e., contraceptive) female hormones have been shown to result in some impairment of liver function in a significant number of women. Elevated acetaldehyde levels in women compared to men may also explain why ethanol causes tissue damage more rapidly in women than men.[115] A sex-specific cytochrome P450 has been invoked as a cause of sex- and species-related differences in drug toxicity in rats.[116] Similarly, as already mentioned, long-term ethanol consumption was associated with increases in the content of a specific cytochrome (P4504A1); and more so in male than in female rats,[117] the microsomal ω-hydroxylation of lauric acid was significantly greater and the rise in males (89%) was significantly higher than in females (4%). In turn, products of ω-oxidation increase liver cytosolic fatty acid-binding protein (L-FABPc) content and peroxisomal β-oxidation.[89] Furthermore, L-FABP is a major contributor to the ethanol-induced increase in liver cytosolic proteins[118] and plays a role in protecting the liver against the excess accumulation of free fatty acids by binding them and thereby making them less reactive. Whereas the ethanol-induced increase in fatty acid-binding capacity provided an excess of binding sites for the fatty acids in males, the increase in females was barely sufficient.[119] Moreover, the difference in fatty acid accumulation was compounded by a lesser compensatory increase in ω-oxidation after chronic alcohol consumption in females compared to males (see Section 2.3). Under these circumstances the risk for development of a deleterious accumulation of fatty acids in the liver is increased, thereby potentially contributing to the enhanced vulnerability of females to alcohol-induced hepatotoxicity. Increased vulnerability due to gender differences in gastric ethanol metabolism are discussed in Section 2.1.

In summary, gender differences in response to alcohol, suspected for centuries, are now objectively documented, with one of the most striking differences being the increased bioavailability of alcohol in women. Thus, sex must be recognized as one of the determinants of alcohol metabolism, and hence of the severity of alcoholic liver injury. This is a factor of increasing significance, because male–female differences in drinking are smaller than they were a generation ago, especially in terms of drinking by young women.[120]

3.2. *Age*

The elderly may drink less alcohol, but this is offset by age-related decreases in body fluids, which result in a lower volume of distribution for ethanol, and thus higher blood alcohol levels for a given level of consumption. Prognosis is age-related. One-year mortality was found to be 50% among cirrhotics over the age of 60 but only 7% in the younger ones.[121] Many other organs are also differentially affected. There is an effect of social drinking on intellectual capacities as a function of age. Linnoila *et al.*[122] found that, with increased blood alcohol levels, tests of perception and attention decrease progressively, and that the older subjects perform less well than the younger ones at all blood alcohol levels.

3.3. *Heredity*

The role of heredity in the development of alcoholism in men is well established[123] and has now been shown to play a major role in the etiology of alcoholism in women as well.[124] The dopamine D_2 gene has been incriminated,[125,126] but this is now questioned.[127,128] Individual differences in rates of ethanol metabolism also appear, in part, to be genetically controlled, and it is suspected that genetic factors influence the severity of alcohol-induced liver disease.[123] Indeed, preliminary results[129] indicated different *ADH3* allele frequencies in patients with alcohol-related end-organ damage compared to controls, suggesting that genetically determined differences in alcohol metabolism may, in part, explain differences in susceptibility to disease (possibly through enhanced generation of toxic metabolites), but this has been questioned.[130] Similarly, a significant association of a particular *RFLP* haplotype of the *COL1A2* locus and alcoholic cirrhosis has been reported[131] but disputed by others.[132] That susceptibility to alcoholic liver disease is, in part, genetically determined has been shown by twin studies,[133] and recently a significant association was found between the occurrence of the glutathione-*S*-transferase null genotype and that of alcoholic liver cirrhosis.[134]

4. Alcohol and Nutrition

Ethanol is not only a psychoactive drug; besides its pharmacological action, it has a substantial energy value (7.1 kcal/g). It is almost as energy-dense as fat and more energy-dense than carbohydrates or proteins. In many societies, alcoholic beverages are considered part of the food supply, whereas in others, alcohol is consumed mainly for its mood-altering effects. In the alcoholic, alcohol represents on the average 50% of the total dietary energy intake; as a consequence, alcohol displaces many normal nutrients in the diets, resulting in primary malnutrition and associated symptomatology, foremost that of folate, thiamine, and other vitamin B deficiencies. Alcohol also impairs the activation and utilization of nutrients (Fig. 1), and secondary malnutrition may result from either maldigestion or malabsorption caused by gastrointestinal complications associated with alcoholism, mainly pancreatic insufficiency; it also promotes nutrient degradation (see Section 2.2.4). At the tissue level, alcohol replaces various normal substrates; the most seriously affected organ is the liver, which contains the bulk of the body's enzymes that are capable of sustaining ethanol metabolism. Ethanol acts as a preferred substrate and displaces up to 90% of the liver's normal fuel, which is fat.[39] Consequently, the latter accumulates, resulting in a fatty liver, the first stage of alcoholic liver disease.

Originally, it was believed that liver disease in the alcoholic is due exclusively to malnutrition. Subsequently, as reviewed elsewhere,[39,135] the hepatotoxicity of ethanol has been established by the demonstration that, in the absence of dietary deficiencies and even in the presence of protein-, vitamin-, and mineral-enriched diets, ethanol produces fatty liver with striking ultrastructural lesions,[136] both in rats and in human volunteers, and fibrosis with cirrhosis in nonhuman primates.[137,138]

Although ethanol is rich in energy (7.1 kcal/g), chronic consumption of substantial amounts of alcohol is not associated with the expected effect on body weight.[139] In addition to mitochondrial inefficiency secondary to chronic ethanol abuse and acetaldehyde toxicity, some of the energy deficit could be attributed to induction of the microsomal ethanol oxidizing system (a metabolic pathway that oxidizes ethanol without associated chemical energy production) (see Section 2.2.1).

5. Alcoholic Liver Disease

5.1. *Clinical and Pathological Presentations, Pathogenesis*

Because of its intrinsic toxicity, alcohol can injure the liver even in the absence of dietary deficiencies.[39] Fatty liver, the first manifestation of alcoholic liver disease, can begin within days of heavy drinking. This is followed by early fibrosis, which in turn can be associated with alcoholic hepatitis. Eventually, there is irreversible damage leading to severe fibrosis and subsequently to cirrhosis. The various clinical manifestations of alcoholic liver disease are well documented[39] and will not be reviewed here.

Fibrosis as a result of necrosis and inflammation is thought to be the underlying mechanism of alcoholic cirrhosis. However, cirrhosis commonly develops without an apparent intermediate stage of alcoholic hepatitis, both in alcoholics[140,141] and in baboons given alcohol.[142–145] Indeed, independently of necrosis and inflammation, alcohol directly affects stellate cells in the liver (also called lipocytes, Ito, or fat-storing cells), causing the deposition of collagen, the characteristic protein of the fibrous tissues. Long-term alcohol consumption transforms stellate cells into collagen-producing myofibroblast-like cells.[146,147] *In vitro,* these cells respond to acetaldehyde with a further increase in collagen[148] and its messenger mRNA.[149]

Phospholipids, the backbone of all cellular membranes, are the primary targets of peroxidation, and membranes can be strikingly altered by ethanol.[150] In baboons given alcohol, phosphatidylcholine is generally depleted in the liver[145] and especially in liver mitochondria,[151] causing a marked decrease in cytochrome oxidase activity and oxygen consumption. This deficiency was corrected by replenishing phospholipids *in vitro,*[152] and in rats, *in vivo.*[153] Similarly, when alcohol-fed baboons were given polyenylphosphatidylcholine, a polyunsaturated phospholipid mixture extracted from soybeans, the concentrations of hepatic phosphatidylcholine and the activity of phosphatidylethanolamine methyltransferase were restored,[145] the number of transformed stellate cells was reduced, and septal fibrosis ($p < 0.001$) as well as cirrhosis was fully prevented.[143,144]

Cirrhosis, which results from an imbalance between the degradation and production of collagen, may represent the failure of degradation to keep pace with synthesis. Indeed, in transformed stellate cells, polyenylphosphatidylcholine[154] and its active phospholipid species dilinoleoylphosphatidylcholine (DLPC)[144] suppresses the acetaldehyde-mediated increase in collagen accumulation, most likely by stimulating collagenase activity. The role of collagenase has also been shown indirectly in humans by the correlation between the severity of alcoholic fibrosis and the activity of a circulating collagenase inhibitor, the tissue inhibitor of metalloproteinase.[155]

Cytokines such as transforming growth factor-β and tumor necrosis factor-α also stimulate fibrogenesis (see Section 5.2.3). Tumor necrosis factor-α may contribute to the anorexia and muscle wasting associated with severe liver disease.[156]

Derangements of the immune system occur in alcoholic liver disease,[157] but whether they are a consequence or a cause of the liver injury remains debatable. Viral hepatitis due to hepatitis B or C virus commonly accompanies chronic hepatitis in alcoholics. Even in the absence of risk factors such as intravenous drug abuse, portal or lobular inflammation is strongly associated with the hepatitis C virus in alcoholics,[158] suggesting that alcohol may favor the acquisition, replication, or persistence of the virus, which can potentiate associated liver disorders.

5.2. *Treatment and Prevention of Liver Disease*

The traditional approach toward alcoholism is based on addressing underlying psychological and behavioral problems (discussed in other chapters), coupled with treatment of late-stage medical complications. The latter efforts focus on the management of the consequences of cirrhosis, such as ascites and bleeding. These traditional approaches, though helpful, have not impacted on the prevalence of the disease and come too late to revert the liver to normal. Better understanding of how alcohol affects the liver allows for earlier and more direct avenues to prevent or counteract alcohol's effects, with focus on early detection of alcoholism, utilizing in part biochemical markers of heavy drinking, such as carbohydrate-deficient transferrin (CDT), screening, among heavy consumers for signs of medical complications (for instance, through the use of traditional "liver" tests), and reducing the task of treatment to manageable size by focusing major therapeutic efforts on susceptible subgroups (see Section 5.2.4).

Contrasting with retinoids, the toxicity of which is well established, this is not been settled for β-carotene. Heretofore, there was a consensus that no obvious β-carotene toxicity exists. It must be noted, however, that in nonhuman primates, enhanced toxicity of β-carotene in the presence of ethanol has been observed.[159]

5.2.1. Antioxidant Therapy

5.2.1a. Carotenoids. Retinol is an antioxidant but it is a weak one, and, as noted above, its use is complicated by its intrinsic hepatotoxicity, which is exacerbated by ethanol. Unlike retinol, its precursor β-carotene is considered to lack toxicity. Furthermore, in addition to acting as a retinol precursor, β-carotene is an efficient quencher of singlet oxygen and can function as a radical-trapping antioxidant; it also has been shown to have the potential of acting as a more efficient antioxidant than retinol. Carotenoids inhibit free radical-induced lipid peroxidation[160–162] and arachidonic acid oxidation.[163] They may prevent lipid peroxidation by acting through specific enzyme inhibition. Indeed, as shown by Lomnitski *et al.*,[164] β-carotene inhibits the activity of lipoxygenase toward linoleate. Administration of β-carotene reduces the level of circulating lipid peroxides.[165] However, in a study in rats, Alam and Alam[166] reported no change in either blood or tissue lipid peroxides following ingestion of 180 mg/kg per day of β-carotene for a period of 11 weeks and carotenoids did not protect against peroxidation in choline-deficient rats,[167] whereas a study in guinea pigs noted a protective effect against *in vivo* lipid peroxidation when animals were pretreated with β-carotene.[168] Furthermore, Palozza and Krinsky[169] reported that β-carotene inhibited malondialdehyde production in a concentration-dependent manner and delayed the radical-initiated destruction of endogenous α- and γ-tocopherol in the rat, and Kim-Jun[170] reported inhibitory effects of β-carotene on lipid peroxidation in mouse epidermis. At present, possible interactions of β-carotene with liver disease and/or alcohol are virtually uncharted but cannot be excluded, since enhanced hepatic toxicity of β-carotene in the presence of ethanol has been observed, with a defect in utilization and/or excretion associated with liver injury and/or alcohol abuse.[66,159] Furthermore, in men, heavy drinking was associated with a relative increase in serum β-carotene[171] and relatively moderate drinking in women was also shown to have such an effect.[172] It is noteworthy that epidemiological studies revealed that β-carotene supplementation may increase the incidence of pulmonary cancer and cardiovascular complications in smokers,[173] an effect related to an interaction between β-carotene and alcohol.[174] Thus, β-carotene supplementation must be used cautiously in alcoholics.

5.2.1b. Methionine and S-Adenosyl Methionine. As previously discussed, one major antioxidant agent is the reduced form of glutathione (GSH). However, therapeutic use of GSH itself is complicated by the fact that its replenishment through supplementation is hampered by its lack of penetration into the hepatocytes, except for its ethyl derivative, which is obviously unsuitable for the treatment of alcoholic liver injury. Cysteine is one of the three amino acids of GSH, and the ultimate precursor of cysteine is methionine (Fig. 4); its deficiency in alcoholics has been incriminated and its supplementation has been considered for the treatment of alcoholic liver injury, but some difficulties have been encountered. Indeed, excess methionine was shown to have some adverse effects,[175] including a decrease in hepatic ATP. Horowitz *et al.*[176] reported that the blood clearance of methionine after an oral load of this amino acid was slowed in patients with cirrhosis. Since about half the methionine is metabolized by the liver, the above observations suggest impaired hepatic metabolism of this amino acid in patients with alcoholic liver disease. To be utilized, methionine has to be activated to *S*-adenosylmethionine (SAMe) (Fig. 4). However, Duce *et al.*[177] found a decrease in SAMe synthetase activity in cirrhotic livers. As a consequence, SAMe depletion ensues after chronic ethanol consumption.[68] Potentially, such SAMe depletion may have a number of adverse effects. SAMe is the principal methylating agent in various transmethylation reactions important for nucleic acid and protein synthesis, as well as membrane fluidity and functions, including the transport of metabolites and transmission of signals across membranes and maintenance of membranes. Thus, depletion of SAMe may promote the membrane injury documented in alcohol-induced liver damage.[150] SAMe is not only the methyl donor in almost all transmethylation reactions, but it plays a key role in the synthesis of polyamines.

Compared to methionine, administration of SAMe has the advantage of bypassing the deficit in SAMe synthesis (from methionine) referred to above (Fig. 4). The usefulness of SAMe administration has been demonstrated in the baboon[68] and in various clinical studies, some of which are still ongoing, as reviewed elsewhere.[178]

5.2.1c. Vitamin E and Miscellaneous Other Antioxidants. Bjørneboe *et al.*[179] reported a reduced hepatic α-tocopherol content after chronic ethanol feeding in rats receiving adequate amounts of vitamin E, as well as in the blood of alcoholics. Hepatic lipid peroxidation was significantly increased after chronic ethanol feeding in rats receiving a low vitamin E diet,[180] indicating that dietary vitamin E is an important determinant of hepatic lipid peroxidation induced by chronic ethanol feeding. The lowest hepatic α-tocopherol was found in rats receiving a combination of low vitamin E and ethanol; both low dietary vitamin E and ethanol feeding significantly decreased hepatic α-tocopherol content, the latter in part because of increased conversion of α-tocopherol to α-tocopherylquinone.[180] In patients with cirrhosis, diminished hepatic vitamin E levels have been observed[66] (Fig. 5), as also shown by von Herbay *et al.*[181] These deficient antioxidant defense systems, coupled with increased generation of acetaldehyde and oxygen radical by the ethanol-induced microsomes (Fig. 4), may contribute to liver damage. Effectiveness of vitamin E supplementation in alcoholic cirrhosis recently has been evaluated: 500 mg daily of α-topheryl acetate during 1 year did not influence hepatic laboratory parameters, mortality, or hospitalization rates of decompensated alcoholic cirrhotics, although serum levels of the vitamin significantly increased.[182]

Other antioxidant medications that have been proposed include (+)-cyanidanol-3, selenium, and thioctic acid, but their beneficial effects still need confirmation.[183] As reviewed below, polyunsaturated phosphatidylcholine provides a new, unexpected but potent antioxidant therapy.[184–186]

5.2.1d. Polyenyl- and Dilinoleoyl-Phosphatidylcholine. It is generally believed that polyunsaturated lipids favor peroxidation. Indeed, because of their multiple double-bond configuration, polyunsaturated fats are much more susceptible than saturated or monounsaturated ones to free radical peroxidation.[187] Surprisingly, however, some reports suggest that the opposite may occur. Effects of high monounsaturated and polyunsaturated fat diets on plasma lipoproteins and lipid peroxidation were studied in type II diabetes mellitus.[188] All indices of plasma lipid peroxidation in the diabetic group and lipid peroxides in the controls were significantly lower on these than on the baseline diet. It was postulated that since both high monounsaturated and polyunsaturated fat diets increase hepatic metabolism of low-density lipoproteins and shorten their circulating half-life, they may reduce lipid peroxidation, compared to high saturated fat diets. By such a mechanism, polyunsaturated fat diets may offset any increased susceptibility of polyunsaturated-enriched low-density lipoprotein to peroxidation. Similarly, whereas malondialdehyde concentration in plasma increased with a rise in blood lipids, it was inversely correlated to the proportion of linoleic acid in serum lipoprotein phospholipids, suggesting that oxidants and lipoprotein metabolism may be of greater importance for intravascular lipid peroxidation than the proportion of polyunsaturated fatty acids in the lipoprotein lipids. Furthermore, experimentally, studies in newborn rats demonstrated that lipid nutrition containing high concentrations of polyunsaturated fatty acids (PUFA) confers protection against pulmonary oxygen toxicity.[189,190] Specifically, newborn rat offspring of dams fed diets high in PUFA had elevated concentrations of PUFA in their lung lipids, with significantly improved survival in hyperoxia compared with offspring of dams fed regular rat chow. Conversely, in newborn offspring of dams fed low PUFA, high saturated fatty acid diets were found to convey greater susceptibility to pulmonary oxygen toxicity. In addition, when Intralipid, derived from soybean oil and containing a high percentage of *n*-6 family PUFA, and also linolenic acid, an *n*-3 family PUFA, were given for 3 weeks before and then throughout pregnancy and lactation, 1- and 5-day-old offspring of Intralipid diet-fed dams demonstrated significant increases in lung lipid *n*-6 family PUFA compared to regular diet-fed offspring. Associated with these fatty acid changes were significantly improved survival rates in hyperoxic animals. These findings supported the hypothesis that increasing lung PUFA content may provide increased O_2 free radical scavenging capacity.[191] Similar results have been found with *in vitro* studies.[192] However, there are also opposite results: cultured hamster fibroblast cells enriched with PUFA had increased susceptibility to the lethal effects of 95% oxygen.[193]

In addition, evidence gathered in rodents and in nonhuman primates revealed striking antioxidant effects of a soybean extract rich in polyunsaturated lecithin, namely polyenylphosphatidylcholine (PPC), about half of which consists of dilinoleoylphosphatidylcholine (DLPC).[144] Indeed, it was found that PPC prevents hepatic lipid peroxidation and attenuates associated injury induced by CCl_4 in rats.[185] Furthermore, PPC also decreased oxidant stress in the baboon,[194] a species in which protection against alcohol-induced liver injury (including fibrosis and cirrhosis) had been previously demonstrated[144] (see Section 5.1). Using gas chromatography/mass spectrometry (GC/MS), hepatic OH-nonemal and F_2-isoprostanes (F_2-IP), parameters of lipid peroxidation, were determined in liver needle biopsies. Whereas alcohol increased both, PPC administration resulted in their significant reduction.

Alcohol-feeding also significantly decreased GSH, an effect that was attenuated by PPC. As the phospholipid species of PPC are highly bioavailable (see Section 5.1) and readily integrated in the liver membranes, they could act as scavengers of the excess O_2 free radicals and thereby prevent their toxic interaction with critical membrane polyunsaturated fatty acids. In a sense, they could act as some kind of radical "trap" or "sink."

In addition to the radical sink hypothesis, linoleic acid in DLPC could also act in some way as a more direct antioxidant, by analogy with conjugated dienoic derivatives of linoleic acid. Similarly to DLPC, these positional and geometric isomers of linoleic acid, particularly the 9 *cis*, 11 *trans* variety, are selectively incorporated into membrane phospholipids[195] and, as for DLPC, they exert striking antioxidant effects[195,196]; they also suppressed peroxide formation from unsaturated fatty acid in a test-tube model.[195]

5.2.2. Steroid Therapy. Several investigators[197-200] have reported significant improvement in survival rates of encephalopathic patients treated with steroids, but not in those with milder illness. Some other studies did not confirm these findings; More recently, however, in patients who had either spontaneous hepatic encephalopathy or a high hepatic discriminant function (based on elevated prothrombin time and bilirubin concentration), prednisolone (40 mg/day for 28 days) improved survival by 2 months.[201] Survival was still improved at 1 year, but not at 2.[202] Oxandrolone therapy was associated with a beneficial effect in moderately malnourished patients.[203]

5.2.3. Antifibrotic and Other Therapies under Study. Polyunsaturated phosphatidylcholine (PPC)[143] or virtually pure PPC[144] was found, in the nonhuman primate, to fully prevent alcohol-induced fibrosis and cirrhosis (see Section 5.1). PPC contains choline, but it was found that choline in amounts present in PPC has no protective action against the fibrogenic effects of ethanol in the baboon.[204]

As already mentioned, alcohol is also known to produce striking changes in membranes,[150] with significant alterations in the membrane phospholipids[152]; the phospholipid supplementation may act, in part, by correcting some of the phospholipid abnormalities. Phosphatidylcholine can be synthesized *de novo* by two pathways. The major route for synthesis in most cells is via the cytidyldiphosphocholine pathway. However, in the liver, an alternate pathway, namely phosphatidylethanolamine *N*-methylation, is responsible, by some estimates, for 15–30% of the synthesis.[205] Phosphatidylethanolamine *N*-methyltransferase (PEMT) (Enzyme Commission number [EC] 2.1.1.17) plays a key role in that pathway for the synthesis of membrane phosphatidylcholine. Its activity was reported to be decreased in patients with alcoholic cirrhosis,[176] but it was not known whether this is a consequence of the cirrhosis or whether it precedes it. However, a recent study revealed that the PEMT decrease occurred prior to the development of the cirrhosis, and that it reversed upon alcohol withdrawal while fibrosis still persisted, indicating that the reduction in PEMT activity is not simply a consequence of the fibrosis.[145] In any event, the decrease in PEMT activity after alcohol may be responsible, at least in part, for the associated decrease in phospholipids.[144,145] Conversely, restoration of PEMT activity with PPC supplementation may contribute to the correction of this defect. Thus, on the one hand, PEMT depletion after alcohol may exacerbate the hepatic phospholipid depletion and the associated membrane abnormalities, which may play a role in triggering fibrosis, whereas PPC, by repleting hepatic phospholipids and normalizing PEMT activity, may contribute to the protection against alcoholic cirrhosis provided by PPC supplementation.[143,144] PPC is especially suited to correct hepatic phospholipid depletion. Indeed, phospholipids rich in essential fatty acids have a high bioavailability. More than 50% of orally administered PPC is made biologically available for the organism either by intact absorption (lesser extent) or by reacylation of absorbed lysophosphatidylcholine (greater extent).[206] Pharmacokinetic studies in humans using $^{3}H/^{14}C$-labeled phosphatidylcholine showed the absorption to exceed 90%.[207] Similar observations were made in animals.[208–210] Furthermore, although much of the PPC in the diet is degraded by pancreatic phospholipase A_2,[211] the products (*l*-acyl-lysophosphatidyl-choline and fatty acids) are absorbed in the jejunum.[212] Animal studies show that phosphatidylcholines recovered in intestinal lymph after feeding fat enriched with single fatty acids are highly enriched in both *sn*-1 and *sn*-2 positions with the same acyl groups that were fed.[213] Thus, it can be anticipated that during absorption of a diet enriched with 18:2 fatty acids, new phosphatidylcholines will be formed from dietary 18:2-lysophosphatidylcholine that will have an 18:2–18:2 composition. Various authors[214–216] reported PPC accumulation in the liver during the first 24 to 48 hr after administration. It was also found in our baboon studies that, although the baseline value of DLPC was low, there was a significant increase of DLPC in the liver of the supplemented baboons.[144] Thus, PPC supplementation results in increased hepatic DLPC, which, as discussed before, may be the active compound. Activity may require the presence of both 18:2 fatty acids, or alternatively only one 18:2 may suffice *in vivo*. Indeed, all 18:2 phosphatidylcholines were present in the liver in significantly increased amounts in baboons fed PPC rich in DLPC.[144]

Since peroxidation products are fibrogenic,[110] their decrease after PPC (see Section 5.2.1.4) could also explain, at least in part, the antifibrogenic property of the phospholipids. We have obtained preliminary results indicating that acetaldehyde, by forming adducts with procollagen peptides, may decrease their feedback inhibition of collagen synthesis, thereby increasing collagen production.[217] Furthermore, other aldehydes (such as malonaldehyde) are produced from lipid peroxidation and they may also stimulate collagen production (see Section 2.4). However, PPC also prevented liver fibrosis and cirrhosis induced by heterologous albumin[218] and hepatic levels of 4-HNE did not differ significantly in rats receiving albumin injections from those supplemented with PPC, nor were these levels significantly above those of controls (S. Aleynik *et al.*, 1996, unpublished data). Thus, lipid peroxidation does not seem to be causally implicated in the liver injury induced by heterologous albumin or in its alteration by PPC. Therefore, in the case of heterologous albumin-induced fibrosis, it would be reasonable to assume that PPC protects against liver fibrosis by some additional mechanism, for instance, thorough increased collagenase activity demonstrated in cultured stellate cells.[154] Consistent with this, the hepatoprotective effect of PPC was not only for the prevention, but also for the attenuation of preexisting liver fibrosis and cirrhosis.[218] Furthermore, PPC acts at prefibrotic steps: it attenuated hepatomegaly, fatty liver, and hyperlipemia in alcohol fed rats[153] and it restored activation of key mitochondrial enzymes such as cytochrome oxidase. The effectiveness of PPC for the prevention and/or treatment of liver cirrhosis is now being tested in a multicenter randomized trial in man (VA Cooperative Study 391).

Colchicine, which inhibits collagen synthesis and procollagen secretion in embryonic tissue,[219] may also provide a useful approach for the treatment of alcoholic liver disease.[220,221] However, these studies have raised questions regarding differences in severity between colchicine-treated and placebo-treated groups and the high dropout rate.[222] Additional controlled trials are presently ongoing.

In a placebo-controlled, crossover study, administration of ursodeoxycholic acid for 4 weeks reduced both bilirubin and liver enzyme levels in patients with alcoholic cirrhosis who were actively drinking.[223] Longer studies with corresponding follow-up are now needed.

Experimentally, silymarin exerts hepatoprotective actions through free-radical scavenging and immunomodulatory effects. In clinical trials, it appears to improve liver function test results and to decrease immunologic abnormalities in patients with alcoholic liver disease. However, both positive and negative effects on survival have been reported, and the role of silymarin in the treatment of alcoholic liver disease remains to be determined.[224,225]

In experimental models, malotilate reduced acute toxic liver damage and ethanol's inhibition of hepatocyte regeneration—a key factor in determining patient survival.[226] It is therefore hoped that it might improve survival in patients with alcoholic liver disease.

After long-term alcohol administration, there is a strong positive correlation between plasma endotoxin levels and severity of liver injury.[227] Whereas short-term administration of alcohol was reported to enhance endotoxin hepatotoxicity when the dose of endotoxin was small, the effect of alcohol was masked when larger doses of endotoxin were given.[228] It has been proposed that tumor necrosis factor (TNF), a mediator of endotoxic shock and sepsis, also plays a role in alcoholic hepatitis. Circulating levels of TNF-α and interleukin-1 remained elevated for up to 6 months after the diagnosis of alcoholic hepatitis, whereas interleukin-6 normalized in parallel with clinical recovery.[229] Concentrations of all three cytokines correlated with biochemical parameters of liver injury. Sheron *et al.*[230] also found that plasma interleukin-6 is increased in severe alcoholic hepatitis and postulated that this may mediate hepatic or extrahepatic tissue damage. On the one hand, TNF levels appear to be elevated in multiple types of experimental injury and in alcoholic liver disease, as are the levels of some other cytokines.[156] On the other hand, low physiological amounts of cytokines appear to be important for liver regeneration (and perhaps are beneficial to the organism as a whole). The task at hand is to acquire further knowledge on how cytokines and ethanol interact and to conserve the positive growth-enhancing effects of cytokines while attenuating their cytotoxic effects. In experimental models of carbon tetrachloride-induced liver injury, elevated TNF-α levels appear to contribute to hepatocellular damage. Administering soluble TNF receptors reduced the degree of experimental injury and lowered mortality.[231] Moreover, a TNF receptor fusion protein provides protection against death in animal models of gram-positive and gram-negative bacterial sepsis.[232] However, in patients with septic shock, treatment with the TNF receptor fusion protein did not reduce mortality, and higher doses appeared to be associated with increased mortality.[233] The relevance of these findings to the treatment of severe alcoholic liver diseases is not yet clear; how soluble TNF receptor therapy can be made to benefit patients with severe alcoholic hepatitis remains to be determined.

A multitude of other antifibrotic agents have been proposed, as reviewed elsewhere.[234,235] Generally, they are either disappointing or not yet fully validated in humans.

Finally, liver transplantation, originally not applied to alcoholic cirrhosis, is now increasingly being considered for individuals who have stopped drinking,[236] although it is still being questioned. Furthermore, the required duration of abstinence as well as the relapse rate are still the subject of debate. Unfortunately, because of donor shortage, transplantation cannot be provided to the vast majority of patients with severe alcoholic liver disease for whom control of alcohol consumption and medical treatment still represent the main therapeutic approaches. Fortunately, the advances made in elucidating the pathophysiology of alcohol-induced liver injury now yield new prospects for more successful medical treatments.

5.2.4. Timing of Therapy. It is obvious that among the alcohol users there is a subpopulation of very heavy drinkers who are particularly at risk for developing alcoholism and its complication. Screening for heavy drinkers is now facilitated by biological markers of excessive alcohol consumption.[237,238] Of the various markers studied, carbohydrate-deficient transferrin is particularly useful.[239,240] Because major complications (such as cirrhosis) do not develop in all heavy drinkers, there is a need for early detection of those susceptible individuals before their social or medical disintegration in order to prevent, rather than simply treat, their major somatic complications. Indeed, treatment at late stages comes too late to restore the liver. Among these individuals at risk, namely the heavy drinkers, the physician can now recognize lesions in the liver that, already at a very early stage, allow the physician to predict which subjects are prone to undergo rapid progression to the cirrhotic stage upon continuation of drinking.

Traditionally, antifibrotic therapy is considered in patients with alcoholic hepatitis and/or complications of established cirrhosis. Indeed, alcoholic hepatitis is characterized by the appearance of necrosis with an inflammatory reaction, including polymorphonuclear cells, capable of triggering a fibrotic reaction. The long-term incidence of cirrhosis in patients with alcoholic hepatitis is nine times higher than in those with fatty liver.[241] Thus, alcoholic hepatitis has been viewed as the precursor lesion of alcoholic cirrhosis, but alcoholic cirrhosis can also develop in the absence of alcoholic hepatitis. Although it can occur anywhere in the hepatic acinus, the earliest deposition of fibrous tissue is generally seen around the central veins and venules now called *terminal hepatic venules*.[242] Such perivenular fibrosis has been described in alcoholic hepatitis, but it is important to note that perivenular fibrosis can also be seen in the absence of widespread inflammation and necrosis, in association with what most pathologists would label as "simple" fatty liver. Thus, cirrhosis commonly develops without an apparent intermediate stage of alcoholic hepatitis, both in alcoholics[243] and in baboons given alcohol.[68,138,144] Once perivenular fibrosis has developed, it indicates that the patient has already entered the fibrotic process and that, upon continuation of drinking, he or she will rapidly develop more severe stages, including cirrhosis.[243] This lesion must not be considered as a marker of vulnerability to the development of subsequent cirrhosis, and therefore can be used as an indication for active intervention. Perivenular fibrosis is commonly associated with perisinusoidal and pericellular fibrosis and correlates with collagenization of the Disse space, but these other changes are more difficult to quantify on routine light microscopy. Independently of necrosis and inflammation, alcohol (via acetaldehyde) directly affects stellate cells in the liver. Long-term alcohol consumption transforms stellate cells into collagen-producing myofibroblastlike cells,[146,147,244] and acetaldehyde stimulates collage synthesis in these cells (see Section 5.1), causing the deposition of collagen, the characteristic protein of the fibrous tissue. It is at this early fibrotic stage that treatment should be most effective.

References

1. Chedid A, Mendenhall CL, Gartside P, *et al:* Prognostic factors in alcoholic liver disease. *Am J Gastroenterol* 86:210–216, 1991.
2. Lieber CS, Leo MA: Alcohol and the liver, in CS Lieber (ed): *Medical and Nutritional Complications of Alcoholism: Mechanisms and Management.* New York, Plenum Press, 1992, pp 185–240.
3. Lieber CS: Alcohol and the liver: 1994 Update. *Gastroenterology* 106:1085–1105, 1994.
4. Lieber CS: Medical disorders of alcoholism. *N Engl J Med* 333:1058–1065, 1995.
5. Lieber CS: Hepatic and other medical disorders of alcoholism: From pathogenesis to treatment. *J Stud Alcohol* 59:9–25, 1998.
6. Faller J, Fox IH: Evidence for increased urate production by activation of adenine nucleotide turnover. *N Engl J Med* 307:1598–1602, 1982.
7. Teschke R, Wiese B: Sex-dependency of hepatic alcohol metabolizing enzymes. *J Endocrinol Invest* 5:243–250, 1982.
8. Maly PI, Sasse D: Intra-acinar profiles of alcohol dehydrogenase and aldehyde dehydrogenase activities in human liver. *Gastroenterology* 101:1716–1723, 1991.
9. Zorzano A, Herrera E: *In vivo* ethanol elimination in man, monkey and rat: A lack of relationship between the ethanol metabolism and the hepatic activities of alcohol and aldehyde dehydrogenases. *Life Sci* 46:223–230, 1990.
10. Hernandez-Muñoz R, Caballeria J, Baraona E, *et al:* Human gastric alcohol dehydrogenase: Its inhibition by H_2-receptor antagonists, and its effect on the bioavailability of ethanol. *Alcoholism: Clin Exp Res* 14:949–950, 1990.
11. Baraona E, Yokoyama A, Ishii H, *et al:* Lack of alcohol dehydrogenase isoenzyme activities in the stomach of Japanese subjects. *Life Sci* 49:1929–1934, 1991.
12. Moreno A, Parés X: Purification and characterization of a new alcohol dehydrogenase from human stomach. *J Biochem* 266:1128–1133, 1991.
13. Satre MA, Zgombic-Knight M, Duester G: The complete structure of human class IV alcohol dehydrogenase (retinol dehydrogenase) determined from the ADH 7 gene. *J Biol Chem* 269:15605–15612, 1994.
14. Yokoyama H, Baraona E, Lieber CS: Molecular cloning of human class IV alcohol dehydrogenase. *Biochem Biophys Res Commun* 203:219–224, 1994.

15. Yokoyama H, Baraona E, Lieber CS: Molecular cloning and chromosomal localization of ADH7 gene encoding human class IV ADH. *Genomics* 31:243–245, 1996.
16. Haber PS, Gentry T, Mak KM, *et al:* Metabolism of alcohol by human gastric cells: Relation to first-pass metabolism. *Gastroenterology* 111:863–870, 1996.
17. Frezza M, Di Padova C, Pozzato G, *et al:* High blood alcohol levels in women. The role of decreased gastric alcohol dehydrogenase activity and first-pass metabolism. *N Engl J Med* 322:95–99, 1990.
18. DiPadova C, Worner TM, Julkunen RJK, *et al:* Effects of fasting and chronic alcohol consumption on the first pass metabolism of ethanol. *Gastroenterology* 92:1169–1173, 1987.
19. Roine RP, Gentry RT, Hernández-Muñoz R, *et al:* Aspirin increases blood alcohol concentrations in human after ingestion of ethanol. *JAMA* 264:2406–2408, 1990.
20. Caballeria J, Baraona E, Rodamilans M, *et al:* Effects of cimetidine on gastric alcohol dehydrogenase activity and blood ethanol levels. *Gastroenterology* 96:388–392, 1989.
21. Di Padova C, Roine R, Frezza M, *et al:* Effects of ranitidine on blood alcohol levels after ethanol ingestion: Comparison with other H_2-receptor antagonists. *JAMA* 267:83–86, 1992.
22. Caballeria J, Baraona E, Deulofeu R, *et al:* Effects of H_2-receptor antagonists on gastric alcohol dehydrogenase activity. *Dig Dis Sci* 36:1673–1679, 1991.
23. Palmer RH, Frank WO, Nambi P, *et al:* Effects of various concomitant medications on gastric alcohol dehydrogenase and first pass metabolism of ethanol. *Am J Gastroenterol* 86:1749–1755, 1991.
24. Seitz HK, Simanowski UA, Egerer G, *et al:* Human gastric alcohol dehydrogenase: *In vitro* characteristics and effect of cimetidine. *Digestion* 51:80–85, 1992.
25. Mirmiran-Yazdy SA, Haber PS, Korsten MA, *et al:* Metabolism of ethanol in rat gastric cells and in inhibition by cimetidine. *Gastroenterology* 108:737–742, 1995.
26. Hernández-Muñoz R, Caballeria J, Baraona E, *et al:* Human gastric alcohol dehydrogenase: Its inhibition by H_2-receptor antagonists, and its effect on the bioavailability of ethanol. *Alcohol Clin Exp Res* 14:946–950, 1990.
27. Fraser AG, Hudson M, Sawyerr AM, *et al:* Short report: The effect of ranitidine on postprandial absorption of a low dose of alcohol. *Aliment Pharmacol Ther* 6:267–271, 1992.
28. Gupta AM, Baraona E, Lieber CS: Significant increase of blood alcohol by cimetidine after repetitive drinking of small alcohol doses. *Alcohol Clin Exp Res* 19:1083–1087, 1995.
29. Seitz HK, Veith S, Czygan P, *et al: In vivo* interactions between H_2-receptor antagonists and ethanol metabolism in man and in rats. *Hepatology* 4:1231–1234, 1984.
30. Guram M, Howden CW, Holt S: Further evidence for an interaction between alcohol and certain H_2-receptor antagonists. *Alcohol Clin Exp Res* 15:1084–1085, 1991.
31. Sharma R, Gentry RT, Lim RT, *et al:* First pass metabolism of alcohol: Absence of diurnal variation and its inhibition by cimetidine after an evening meal. *Dig Dis Sci* 40:2091–2097, 1995.
32. Feely J, Wood AJ: Effect of cimetidine on the elimination and actions of ethanol. *JAMA* 247:2819–2821, 1982.
33. Raufman JP, Notar-Francesco V, Raffaniello RD, *et al:* Histamine$_2$-receptor antagonists do not alter serum ethanol levels in fed, nonalcoholic men. *Ann Intern Med* 118:488–494, 1993.
34. Roine RP, Gentry RT, Lim Jr RT, *et al:* Effect of concentration of ingested ethanol on blood alcohol levels. *Alcohol Clin Exp Res* 15:734–738, 1991.
35. Seitz HK, Egerer G, Simanowski UA, *et al:* Human gastric alcohol dehydrogenase activity: Effect of age, gender and alcoholism. *Gut* 34:1433–1437, 1993.
36. *Nutrition and Your Health: Dietary Guidelines for Americans.* Washington, DC, US Department of Agriculture, US Department of Health and Human Services, Home and Garden Bulletin No. 232, 3rd ed, 1990.
37. Wald A, Van Thiel DH, Hoechstetter L: Effect of pregnancy on gastrointestinal transit. *Dig Dis Sci* 27:1015–1018, 1982.
38. Arora S, Baraona E, Lieber CS: Ranitidine increases blood alcohol levels in social drinkers. *Gastroenterology* 112:1214, 1997.

39. Feinman L, Korsten MA, Lieber CS: Alcohol and the digestive tract, in Lieber CS (ed): *Medical and Nutritional Complications of Alcoholism: Mechanisms and Management*, New York, Plenum Press, 1992, pp 307–340.
40. Pateron D, Fabre M, Ink O, *et al:* Influence de l'alcool et de la cirrhose sur la présence de *Helicobacter pylori* dans la muqueuse gastrique. *Gastroenterol Clin Biol* 14:555–568, 1990.
41. Salmela KS, Salaspuro M, Gentry RT, *et al: Helicobacter* infection and gastric ethanol metabolism. *Alcohol Clin Exp Res* 18:1294–1299, 1994.
42. Roine RP, Salmela KS, Salaspuro M: Alcohol metabolism in *Helicobacter pylori*-infected stomach. *Ann Med* 27:583–588, 1995.
43. Uppal R, Lateef SK, Korsten MA, *et al:* Chronic alcoholic gastritis: Roles of alcohol and *Helicobacter pylori. Arch Intern Med* 151:760–764, 1991.
44. Lieber CS, DeCarli LM: Ethanol oxidation by hepatic microsomes: Adaptive increase after ethanol feeding. *Science* 162:917–918, 1968.
45. Lieber CS, DeCarli LM: Hepatic microsomal ethanol oxidizing system: *In vitro* characteristics and adaptive properties *in vivo. J Biol Chem* 245:2505–2512, 1970.
46. Tsutsumi M, Lasker JM, Shimizu M, *et al:* The intralobular distribution of ethanol-inducible P450IIE1 in rat and human liver. *Hepatology* 10:437–446, 1989.
47. Takahashi T, Lasker JM, Rosman AS, *et al:* Induction of P4502E1 in human liver by ethanol is due to a corresponding increase in encoding mRNA. *Hepatology* 17:236–245, 1993.
48. Tsyrlov IB, Salmela KS, Kessova IG, *et al:* Effect of combined ethanol and 3-methylcholanthrene treatment on hepatic microsomal P4502E1 and P4501A2 in rats. *Alcohol Clin Exp Res* 10:A37, 1996.
49. Shimizu M, Lasker JM, Tsutsumi M, *et al:* Immunohistochemical localization of ethanol-inducible P450IIE1 in the rat alimentary tract. *Gastroenterology* 99:1044–1053, 1990.
50. Koivisto T, Mishin VM, Mak KM, *et al:* Induction of cytochrome P-4502E1 by ethanol in rat Kupffer cells. *Alcohol Clin Exp Res* 20:207–212, 1996.
51. Lieber CS: Interactions of alcohol noncardiovascular medications, in Wassef M, Zakhari S (eds.): *Alcohol and the Cardiovascular System,* NIAAA Research Monograph No. 31, NIH-NIAAA Publication No. 96–4133, Washington, DC, US Government Printing Office, Superintendent of Documents, 1996, pp 679–712.
52. Hetu C, Joly J-G: Differences in the duration of the enhancement of liver mixed function oxidase activities in ethanol-fed rats after withdrawal. *Biochem Pharmacol* 34:1211–1216, 1985.
53. Borowsky SA, Lieber CS: Interaction of methadone and ethanol metabolism. *J Pharmacol Exp Ther* 207:123–129, 1978.
54. Hetu C, Dumont A, Joly JG: Effect of chronic ethanol administration on bromobenzene liver toxicity in the rat. *Tox Appl Pharm* 67:166–167, 1983.
55. Siegers CP, Heidbuchel K, Younes M: Influence of alcohol, dithiocarb and (+)-catechin on the hepatotoxicity and metabolism of vinylidene chloride in rats. *J Appl Toxicol* 3:90–95, 1983.
56. Tsutsumi R, Leo MA, Kim C, *et al:* Interaction of ethanol with enflurane metabolism and toxicity: Role of P450IIE1. *Alcohol Clin Exp Res* 14:174–179, 1990.
57. Kharasch ED, Thummel KE: Identification of cytochrome P4502E1 as the predominant enzyme catalyzing human liver microsomal defluorination of sevoflurane, isoflurane, and methoxyflurane. *Anesthesiology* 79:795–897, 1993.
58. Takagi T, Ishii H, Takahashi H, *et al:* Potentiation of halothane hepatotoxicity by chronic ethanol administration in rat: An animal model of halothane hepatitis. *Pharmacol Biochem Behav* 18:(Suppl 1) 461–465, 1983.
59. Beskid M, Bialck J, Dzieniszewski J, *et al:* Effect of combined phenylbutazone and ethanol administration on rat liver. *Exp Pathol* 18:487–491, 1980.
60. Raucy JL, Lasker JM, Lieber CS, *et al:* Acetaminophen activation by human liver cytochromes P450IIE1 and P4501A2. *Arch Biochem Biophys* 271:283–273, 1989.
61. Black M: Acetaminophen hepatotoxicity. *Ann Rev Med* 35:577–593, 1984.
62. Seef LB, Cuccherini BA, Zimmerman HJ, *et al:* Acetaminophen hepatotoxicity in alcoholics. (Clinical review). *Ann Intern Med* 104:399–404, 1986.

63. Sato C, Matsuda Y, Lieber CS: Increased hepatotoxicity of acetaminophen after chronic ethanol consumption in the rat. *Gastroenterology* 80:140–148, 1981.
64. Whitecomb DC, Block GD: Association of acetaminophen hepatotoxicity with fasting and ethanol use. *JAMA* 272:1845–1850, 1994.
65. Hirano T, Kaplowitz N, Tsukamoto H, *et al:* Hepatic mitochondrial glutathione depletion and progression of experimental alcoholic liver disease in rats. *Hepatology* 6:1423–1427, 1992.
66. Leo MA, Rosman A, Lieber CS: Differential depletion of carotenoids and tocopherol in liver diseases. *Hepatology* 17:977–986, 1993.
67. Dicker E, Cederbaum AI: Increased oxygen radical-dependent inactivation of metabolic enzymes by liver microsomes after chronic ethanol consumption. *FASEB J* 2:2901–2906, 1988.
68. Lieber CS, Casini A, DeCarli LM, *et al: S*-adenosyl-L-methionine attenuates alcohol-induced liver injury in the baboon. *Hepatology* 11:165–172, 1990.
69. Lieber CS, Garro A, Leo MA, *et al:* Alcohol and cancer. *Hepatology* 6:1005–1019, 1986.
70. Leo MA, Lieber CS: Hepatic vitamin A depletion in alcoholic liver injury. *N Engl J Med* 307:597–601, 1982.
71. Sato M, Lieber CS: Hepatic vitamin A depletion after chronic ethanol consumption in baboons and rats. *J Nutr* 111:2015–2023, 1981.
72. Leo MA, Kim CI, Lieber CS: NAD^+-dependent retinol dehydrogenase in liver microsomes. *Arch Biochem Biophys* 259:241–249, 1987.
73. Leo MA, Lieber CS: New pathway for retinol metabolism in liver microsomes. *J Biochem* 260:5228–5231, 1985.
74. Leo MA, Lieber CS: Hypervitaminosis A: A liver lover's lament. *Hepatology* 8:412–417, 1988.
75. Leo MA, Arai M, Sato M, *et al:* Hepatotoxicity of vitamin A and ethanol in the rat. *Gastroenterology* 82:194–205, 1982.
76. Leo MA, Lieber CS: Hepatic fibrosis after long-term administration of ethanol and moderate vitamin A supplementation in the rat. *Hepatology* 2:1–11, 1983.
77. Keilin D, Hartree EF: Properties of catalase: Catalysis of coupled oxidation of alcohols. *Biochem J* 39:293–301, 1945.
78. Sies H, Chance B: The steady state level of catalase compound I in isolated hemoglobin-free perfused rat liver. *FEBS Lett* 11:172–176, 1970.
79. Oshino N, Chance B, Sies H, *et al:* The role of H_2O_2 generation in perfused rat liver and the reaction of catalase compound I and hydrogen donors. *Arch Biochem Biophys* 154:117–131, 1973.
80. Handler JA, Thurman RG: Fatty acid-dependent ethanol metabolism. *Biochem Biophys Res Commun* 133:44–51, 1985.
81. Williamson JR, Scholz R, Browning ET, *et al:* Metabolic effects of ethanol in perfused rat liver. *J Biol Chem* 25:5044–5054, 1969.
82. Handler JA, Thurman RG: Redox interactions between catalase and alcohol dehydrogenase pathways of ethanol metabolism in the perfused rat liver. *J Biol Chem* 265:1510–1515, 1990.
83. Inatomi N, Kato S, Ito D, *et al:* Role of peroxisomal fatty acid beta-oxidation in ethanol metabolism. *Biochem Biophys Res Commun* 163:418–423, 1989.
84. Takagi T, Alderman J, Geller J, *et al:* Assessment of the role of non-ADH ethanol oxidation *in vivo* and in hepatocytes from deermice. *Biochem Pharmacol* 35:3601–3606, 1986.
85. Kato S, Alderman J, Lieber CS: Respective roles of the microsomal ethanol oxidizing system (MEOS) and catalase in ethanol metabolism by deermice lacking alcohol dehydrogenase. *Arch Biochem Biophys* 254:586–591, 1987.
86. Kato S, Alderman J, Lieber CS: Ethanol metabolism in alcohol dehydrogenase deficient deermice is mediated by the microsomal ethanol oxidizing system, not by catalase. *Alcohol Alcohol Suppl* 1:231–234, 1987.
87. Thurman RG, Brentzel HJ: The role of alcohol dehydrogenase in microsomal ethanol oxidation and the adaptive increase in ethanol metabolism due to chronic treatment with ethanol. *Alcohol Clin Exp Res* 1:33–38, 1977.

88. Teschke R, Matsuzaki S, Ohnishi K, *et al:* Microsomal ethanol oxidizing system (MEOS): Current status of its characterization and its role. *Alcohol Clin Exp Res* 1:7–15, 1977.
89. Kaikaus RM, Chan WK, Lysenko N, *et al:* Induction of liver fatty acid binding protein (L-FABP) and peroxisomal fatty acid ω-oxidation by peroxisome proliferators (PP) is dependent on cytochrome p-450 activity. *Hepatology* 12:A248, 1990.
90. Hasumura Y, Teschke R, Lieber CS: Acetaldehyde oxidation by hepatic mitochondria: Its decrease after chronic ethanol consumption. *Science* 189:727–729, 1975.
91. Korsten MA, Matsuzaki S, Feinman L, *et al:* High blood acetaldehyde levels after ethanol administration: Differences between alcoholic and non-alcoholic subjects. *N Engl J Med* 292:386–389, 1975.
92. Lieber CS, Baraona E, Hernandez-Munoz R, *et al:* Impaired oxygen utilization: A new mechanism for the hepatotoxicity of ethanol in sub-human primates. *J Clin Invest* 83:1682–1690, 1989.
93. Pikkarainen PH, Gordon ER, Lebsack ME, *et al:* Determination of plasma free acetaldehyde levels during the oxidation of ethanol: Effects of chronic ethanol feeding. *Biochem Pharmacol* 30:799–802, 1981.
94. Espina N, Lima V, Lieber CS, *et al: In vitro* and *in vivo* inhibitory effect of ethanol and acetaldehyde on O^6methylguanine transferase. *Carcinogenesis* 9:761–766, 1988.
95. Arai M, Leo MA, Nakano M, *et al:* Biochemical and morphological alterations of baboon hepatic mitochondria after chronic ethanol consumption. *Hepatology* 4:165–174, 1984.
96. Baraona E, Leo MA, Borowsky SA, *et al:* Pathogenesis of alcohol-induced accumulation of protein in the liver. *J Clin Invest* 60:546–554, 1977.
97. Wondergem R, Davis J: Ethanol increases hepatocyte water volume. *Alcohol Clin Exp Res* 18:1230–1236, 1994.
98. Israel Y, Hurwitz E, Niëmelä O, *et al:* Monoclonal and polyclonal antibodies against acetaldehyde-containing epitopes in acetaldehyde–protein adducts. *Proc Natl Acad Sci USA* 83:7923–7927, 1986.
99. Hoerner M, Behrens UJ, Worner T, *et al:* Humoral immune response to acetaldehyde adducts in alcoholic patients. *Res Commun Chem Pathol Pharmacol* 54:3–12, 1986.
100. Hoerner M, Behrens UJ, Worner TM, *et al:* The role of alcoholism and liver disease in the appearance of serum antibodies against acetaldehyde adducts. *Hepatology* 8:569–574, 1988.
101. Niemela O, Klajner F, Orrego H, *et al:* Antibodies against acetaldehyde-modified protein epitopes in human alcoholics. *Hepatology* 7:1210–1214, 1987.
102. Müller A, Sies H: Inhibition of ethanol- and aldehyde-induced release of ethane from isolated perfused rat liver by pargyline and disulfiram. *Pharmacol Biochem Behav* 18:429–432, 1983.
103. Shaw S, Rubin KP, Lieber CS: Depressed hepatic glutathione and increased diene conjugates in alcoholic liver disease: Evidence of lipid peroxidation. *Dig Dis Sci* 28:585–589, 1983.
104. Speisky H, MacDonald A, Giles G, *et al:* Increased loss and decreased synthesis of hepatic glutathione after acute ethanol administration. *Biochem J* 225:565–572, 1985.
105. Shaw S, Lieber CS: Increased hepatic production of alpha-amino-*n*-butyric acid after chronic alcohol consumption in rats and baboons. *Gastroenterology* 78:108–113, 1980.
106. Barclay LR: The cooperative antioxidant role of glutathione with a lipid-soluble and a water-soluble antioxidant during peroxidation of liposomes initiated in the aqueous phase and in the lipid phase. *J Biol Chem* 263:16138–16142, 1988.
107. Shaw S, Jayatilleke E, Ross WA, *et al:* Ethanol induced lipid peroxidation: Potentiation by long-term alcohol feeding and attenuation by methionine. *J Lab Clin Med* 98:417–425, 1981.
108. Zhang H, Loney LA, Potter BJ: Effect of chronic alcohol feeding on hepatic iron status and ferritin uptake by rat hepatocytes. *Alcohol Clin Exp Res* 17:394–400, 1993.
109. Valenzuela A, Fernandez V, Videla LA: Hepatic and biliary levels of glutathione and lipid peroxides following iron overload in the rat: Effect of simultaneous ethanol administration. *Toxicol Appl Pharmacol* 70:87–95, 1983.
110. Tsukamoto H: Oxidative stress, antioxidants, and alcoholic liver fibrogenesis. *Alcohol* 10: 465–467, 1993.

111. Rankin JG: The natural history and management of the patient with alcoholic liver disease, in Fisher MM, Rankin JG (eds): *Alcohol and the Liver*. New York, Plenum Press, 1977, pp 365–381.
112. Morgan MY, Sherlock S: Sex-related differences among 100 patients with alcoholic liver disease. *Br Med J* 1:939–941, 1977.
113. Pequignot G, Tuyns AJ, Berta JL: Ascitic cirrhosis in relation to alcohol consumption. *Int J Epidemiol* 7:113–120, 1978.
114. Parrish KM, Dufour MC, Stinson FS, *et al:* Average daily alcohol consumption during adult life among decedents with and without cirrhosis: The 1986 National Mortality Followback Survey. *J Stud Alcohol* 54:450–456, 1993.
115. Fukunage T, Sillanaukee P, Eriksson CJP: Occurrence of blood acetaldehyde in women during ethanol intoxication: Preliminary findings. *Alcohol Clin Exp Res* 17:1198–1200, 1993.
116. Kato R, Yamazoe Y: Sex-specific cytochrome P450 as a cause of sex- and species-related differences in drug toxicity. *Toxicol Lett* 64/65:661–667, 1992.
117. Ma XL, Baraona E, Lieber CS: Alcohol consumption enhances fatty acid ω-oxidation, with a greater increase in male than in female rats. *Hepatology* 18:1247–1253, 1993.
118. Pignon J-P, Bailey NC, Baraona E, *et al:* Fatty acid-binding protein: A major contributor to the ethanol-induced increase in liver cytosolic proteins in the rat. *Hepatology* 7:865–871, 1987.
119. Shevchuk O, Baraona E, Ma X-L, *et al:* Gender differences in the response of hepatic fatty acids and cytosolic fatty acid-binding capacity to alcohol consumption in rats. *Proc Soc Exp Biol Med* 198:584–590, 1991.
120. Gomberg ESL: Women and alcohol: Use and abuse. *J Nerv Ment Dis* 181:211–219, 1993.
121. Potter JF, James OFW: Clinical features and prognosis of alcoholic liver disease in respect of advancing age. *Gerontology* 33:380–387, 1987.
122. Linnoila M, Erwin CW, Ramm D, *et al:* Effects of age and alcohol on psychomotor performance of men. *J Stud Alcohol* 41:488–541, 1980.
123. Lumeng L, Crabb DW: Genetic aspects and risk factors in alcoholism and alcoholic liver disease. *Gastroenterology* 107:572–578, 1994.
124. Kendler KS, Heath AC, Neale MC, *et al:* A population-based twin study of alcoholism in women. *JAMA* 268:1877–1882, 1992.
125. Blum K, Noble EP, Sheridan PJ, *et al:* Ailelic association of human dopamine D2 receptor gene in alcoholism. *JAMA* 263:2055–2060, 1990.
126. Higuchi S, Muramatsu T, Murayama M, *et al:* Association of structural polymorphism of the dopamine D2 receptor gene and alcoholism. *Biochem Biophys Res Commun* 204:1199–1205, 1994.
127. Bolos AM, Dean M, Lucas-Derse S, *et al:* Population and pedigree studies reveal a lack of association between the dopamine D2 receptor gene and alcoholism. *JAMA* 264:356–360, 1990.
128. Gejman PV, Ram A, Gelernter J, *et al:* No structural mutation in the dopamine D_2 receptor gene in alcoholism or schizophrenia. Analysis using denaturing gradient gel electrophoresis. *JAMA* 271:204–208, 1994.
129. Day CP, Bashir R, James O, *et al:* Investigation of the role of polymorphisms at the alcohol and aldehyde dehydrogenase loci in genetic predisposition to alcohol-related end-organ damage. *Hepatology* 14:798–801, 1991.
130. Poupon RE, Napalas B, Coutelle C, *et al:* Polymorphism of the alcohol dehydrogenase, alcohol and aldehyde dehydrogenase activities: Implications in alcoholic cirrhosis in white patients. *Hepatology* 15:1017–1022, 1992.
131. Weiner FR, Eskreis D, Compton KV, *et al:* Haplotype analysis of type I collagen gene and its association with alcoholic cirrhosis in man. *Mol Aspects Med* 10:159–168, 1988.
132. Bashir R, Day CP, James OFW, *et al:* No evidence for involvement of type I collagen structural genes in "genetic predisposition" to alcoholic cirrhosis. *J Hepatol* 16:316–319, 1992.
133. Hrubec Z, Omenn GS: Evidence of genetic predisposition to alcoholic cirrhosis and psychosis: Twin concordances for alcoholism and its biological end points by zygosity among male veterans. *Alcohol Clin Exp Res* 5:207–215, 1981.

134. Savolainen VT, Pajarinen J, Perola M, *et al:* Glutathione-*S*-transferase GST M1 null genotype and the risk of alcoholic liver disease. *Alcohol Clin Exp Res* 20:1340–1345, 1996.
135. Lieber CS, DeCarli LM: Hepatotoxicity of ethanol. *J Hepatol* 12:394–401, 1991.
136. Lane BP, Lieber CS: Ultrastructural alterations in human hepatocytes following ingestion of ethanol with adequate diets. *Am J Pathol* 49:593–603, 1966.
137. Lieber CS, DeCarli LM: An experimental model of alcohol feeding and liver injury in the baboon. *J Med Primatol* 3:153–163, 1974.
138. Lieber CS, DeCarli LM, Rubin E: Sequential production of fatty liver, hepatitis and cirrhosis in sub-human primates fed ethanol with adequate diets. *Proc Natl Acad Sci USA* 72:437–441, 1975.
139. Lieber CS: Perspectives: Do alcohol calories count? *Am J Clin Nutr* 54:976–982, 1991.
140. Worner TM, Lieber CS: Perivenular fibrosis as precursor lesion of cirrhosis. *JAMA* 254:627–630, 1985.
141. Hasumura Y, Minato Y, Nishimura M, *et al:* Hepatic fibrosis in alcoholics: Morphologic characteristics, clinical diagnosis, and natural course. *Pathobiol Hepatic Fibrosis* 7:23–24, 1985.
142. Popper H, Lieber CS: Histogenesis of alcoholic fibrosis and cirrhosis in the baboon. *Am J Pathol* 98:695–716, 1980.
143. Lieber CS, DeCarli LM, Mak KM, *et al:* Attenuation of alcohol-induced hepatic fibrosis by polyunsaturated lecithin. *Hepatology* 12:1390–1398, 1990.
144. Lieber CS, Robins SJ, Li J, *et al:* Phosphatidylcholine protects against fibrosis and cirrhosis in the baboon. *Gastroenterology* 106:152–159, 1994.
145. Lieber CS, Robins SJ, Leo MA: Hepatic phosphatidylethanolamine methyltransferase activity is decreased by ethanol and increased by phosphatidylcholine. *Alcohol Clin Exp Res* 18:592–595, 1994.
146. Mak KI, Lieber CS: Lipocytes and transitional cells in alcoholic liver disease: A morphometric study. *Hepatology* 8:1027–1033, 1988.
147. Friedman SL: The cellular basis of hepatic fibrosis. *N Engl J Med* 328:1828–1835, 1993.
148. Moshage H, Casini A, Lieber CS: Acetaldehyde stimulates collagen production in cultured rat liver fat-storing cells but not in hepatocytes. *Hepatology* 12:511–518, 1990.
149. Casini A, Cunningham M, Rojkind M, *et al:* Acetaldehyde increases procollagen type I and fibronectin gene transcription in cultured rat fat-storing cells through a protein synthesis-dependent mechanism. *Hepatology* 13:758–765, 1991.
150. Yamada S, Mak KM, Lieber CS: Chronic ethanol consumption alters rat liver plasma membranes and potentiates release of alkaline phosphatase. *Gastroenterology* 88:1799–1806, 1985.
151. Arai M, Leo MA, Nakano M, *et al:* Biochemical and morphological alterations of baboon hepatic mitochondria after chronic ethanol consumption. *Hepatology* 4:165–174, 1984.
152. Arai M, Gordon ER, Lieber CS: Decreased cytochrome oxidase activity in hepatic mitochondria after chronic ethanol consumption and the possible role of decreased cytochrome aa3 content and changes in phospholipids. *Biochim Biophys Acta* 797:320–327, 1984.
153. Navder KP, Baraona E, Lieber CS: Polyenylphosphatidylcholine attenuates alcohol-induced fatty liver and hyperlipemia in rats. *J Nutr* 21:1057–1062, 1997.
154. Li J-J, Kim C-I, Leo MA, *et al:* Polyunsaturated lecithin prevents acetaldehyde-mediated hepatic collagen accumulation by stimulating collagenase activity in cultured lipocytes. *Hepatology* 15:373–381, 1992.
155. Li J-J, Rosman AS, Leo MA, *et al:* Tissue inhibitor of metalloproteinase is increased in the serum of precirrhotic and cirrhotic alcoholic patients and can serve as a marker of fibrosis. *Hepatology* 19:1418–1423, 1994.
156. McClain C, Hill D, Schmidt J, *et al:* Cytokines and alcoholic liver disease. *Semin Liver Dis* 13:170–182, 1993.
157. Paronetto F: Immunologic reactions in alcoholic liver disease. *Semin Liver Dis* 13:183–195, 1993.
158. Rosman AS, Paronetto F, Galvin K, *et al:* Hepatitis C virus antibody in alcoholic patients: Association with the presence of portal and/or lobular hepatitis. *Arch Intern Med* 153:965–969, 1993.

159. Leo MA, Kim CI, Lowe N, *et al:* Interaction of ethanol with β-carotene: Delayed blood clearance and enhanced hepatotoxicity. *Hepatology* 15:883–891, 1992.
160. Krinsky NI, Deneke SM: Interaction of oxygen and oxy-radicals with carotenoids. *J Natl Cancer Inst* 69:205–210, 1982.
161. Krinsky NI: Antioxidant functions of carotenoids. *Free Radic Biol Med* 7:617–635, 1989.
162. Burton GW, Ingold KU: β-carotene: An unusual type of lipid antioxidant. *Science* 224:569–573, 1984.
163. Halevy O, Sklan D: Inhibition of arachidonic acid oxidation by beta-carotene, retinol and alpha-tocopherol. *Biochim Biophys Acta* 918:304–307, 1987.
164. Lomnitski L, Bar-Natan R, Sklan D, *et al:* The interaction between β-carotene and lipoxygenase in plant and animal systems. *Biochim Biophys Acta* 1167:331–338, 1993.
165. Mobarhan S, Bowen P, Andersen B, *et al:* Effects of β-carotene repletion of β-carotene absorption, lipid peroxidation, and neutrophil superoxide formation in young men. *Nutr Cancer* 14:195–206, 1990.
166. Alam SQ, Alam BS: Lipid peroxide, α-tocopherol and retinoid levels in plasma and liver of rats fed diets containing β-carotene and 13-*cis*-retinoic acid. *J Nutr* 113:2608–2614, 1983.
167. Jenkins MY, Sheikh MN, Mitchell GV, *et al:* Dietary carotenoids influenced biochemical but not morphological changes in adult male rats fed a choline-deficient diet. *Nutr Cancer* 19:55–65, 1993.
168. Kunert KJ, Tappel AL: The effect of vitamin C on *in vitro* lipid peroxidation in guinea pigs as measured by pentane and thane production. *Lipids* 18:271–274, 1983.
169. Palozza P, Krinsky NI: The inhibition of radical-initiated peroxidation of microsomal lipids by both α-tocopherol and β-carotene. *Free Radic Biol Med* 11:407–414, 1991.
170. Kim-Jun H: Inhibitory effects of α- and β-carotene on croton oil-induced or enzymatic lipid peroxidation and hydroperoxide production in mouse skin epidermis. *Int J Biochem* 25:911–915, 1993.
171. Ahmed S, Leo MA, Lieber CS: Interactions between alcohol and beta-carotene in patients with alcoholic liver disease. *Am J Clin Nutr* 60:430–436, 1994.
172. Forman MR, Beecher GR, Lanza E, *et al:* Effect of alcohol consumption on plasma carotenoid concentrations in premenopausal women: A controlled dietary study. *Am J Clin Nutr* 62:131–135, 1995.
173. Alpha-Tocopherol, β-Carotene and Cancer Prevention Study Group: The effect of vitamin E and beta carotene on the incidence of lung cancer and other cancers in male smokers. *N Engl J Med* 330:1029–1035, 1994.
174. Albanes D, Heinonen OP, Taylor PR, *et al:* α-tocopherol and β-carotene supplements and lung cancer incidence in the Alpha-Tocopherol, Beta-Carotene Cancer Prevention Study: Effects of base-line characteristics and study compliance *J Natl Cancer Inst* 88:1560–1571, 1996.
175. Finkelstein JD, Martin JJ: Methionine metabolism in mammals. Adaptation to methionine excess. *J Biol Chem* 261:1582–1587, 1986.
176. Horowitz JH, Rypins EB, Henderson JM, *et al:* Evidence for impairment of transsulfuration pathway in cirrhosis. *Gastroenterology* 81:668–675, 1981.
177. Duce AM, Ortiz P, Cabrero C, *et al:* *S*-adenosyl-L-methionine synthetase and phospholipid methyltransferase are inhibited in human cirrhosis. *Hepatology* 8:65–68, 1988.
178. Lieber CS: Prevention and therapy with *S*-adenosyl-L-methionine and polyenylphosphatidylcholine, in Arroyo V, Bosch J, Rodes J (eds): *Treatments in Hepatology.* Barcelona, Spain, Masson, 1995, pp 299–311.
179. Bjørneboe GEA, Bjørneboe A, Hagen BF, *et al:* Reduced hepatic tocopherol content after long-term administration of ethanol to rats. *Biochem Biophys Acta* 918:236–241, 1987.
180. Kawase T, Kato S, Lieber CS: Lipid peroxidation and antioxidant defense systems in rat liver after chronic ethanol feeding. *Hepatology* 10:815–821, 1989.
181. von Herbay A, de Groot H, Hegi U, *et al:* Low vitamin E content in plasma of patients with alcoholic liver disease, hemochromatosis and Wilson's disease. *J Hepatol* 20:41–46, 1994.
182. Pia de la Maza M, Petermann M, Bunout D, *et al:* Effects of long-term vitamin E supplementation in alcoholic cirrhotics. *J Am Coll Nutr* 14:192–196, 1995.

183. Seitz HK, Poschl G: Antioxidant drugs and colchicine in the treatment of alcoholic liver disease, in Arroyo V, Bosch J, Rodes J (eds): *Treatments in Hepatology.* Barcelona, Spain, Masson, 1995, pp 271–276.
184. Lieber CS, Leo MA, Aleynik SI, *et al:* Polyenylphosphatidylcholine (PPC) decreases oxidant stress and protects against alcohol-induced liver injury in the baboon. *Hepatology* 22:A225A 1995.
185. Aleynik SI, Leo MA, Ma X, *et al:* Polyenylphosphatidylcholine prevents carbon tetrachloride induced lipid peroxidation while it attenuates liver injury and fibrosis. *J Hepatology* 26:554–561, 1997.
186. Takeshige U, Leo MA, Aleynik M, *et al:* Dilinoleoylphosphatidylcholine protects against lipid peroxidation and cell injury produced by arachidonate in hepatoma cells. *Hepatology* 24:A240 1996.
187. Halliwell B, Gutteridge JMC: *Free Radicals in Biology and Medicine,* 2nd ed. Oxford, England, Clarendon Press, 1989.
188. Parfitt VJ, Desomeaux K, Bolton CH, *et al:* Effects of high monounsaturated and polyunsaturated fat diets on plasma lipoproteins and lipid peroxidation in type 2 diabetes mellitus. *Diabet Med* 11:85–91, 1994.
189. Sosenko IRS, Innis SM, Frank L: Polyunsaturated fatty acids and protection of newborn rats from oxygen toxicity. *J Pediatr* 112:630–637, 1988.
190. Sosenko IRS, Innis SM, Frank L: Menhaden fish oil, *n*-3 polyunsaturated fatty acids and protection of newborn rats from oxygen toxicity. *Pediatr Res* 25:399–404, 1989.
191. Sosenko IRS, Innis SM, Frank L: Intralipid increases lung polyunsaturated fatty acids and protects newborn rats from oxygen toxicity. *Pediatr Res* 30:413–417, 1991.
192. Dennery PA, Kramer CM, Alpert SE: Effect of fatty acid profiles on the susceptibility of cultured rabbit tracheal epithelial cells to hyperoxic injury. *Am J Respir Cell Mol Biol* 3:137–144, 1990.
193. Spitz DR, Kinter MT, Kehrer JP, *et al:* The effect of monounsaturated and polyunsaturated fatty acids on oxygen toxicity in cultured cells. *Pediatr Res* 32:366–372, 1992.
194. Lieber CS, Leo MA, Aleynik SI, *et al:* Polyenylphosphatidylcholine decreases alcohol-induced oxidative stress in the baboon. *Alcohol Clin Exp Res* 21:375–379, 1997.
195. Ha YL, Storkson J, Pariza MW: Inhibition of benzo(*a*)pyrene-induced mouse forestomach neoplasia by conjugated dienoic derivatives of linoleic acid. *Cancer Res* 50:1097–1101, 1990.
196. Ip C, Carter CA, Ip MM: Requirement of essential fatty acid for mammary tumorigenesis in the rat. *Cancer Res* 45:1997–2001, 1985.
197. Helman RA, Temko MH, Nye SW, *et al:* Alcoholic hepatitis: Natural history and evaluation of prednisolone therapy. *Ann Intern Med* 74:311–321, 1971.
198. Lesesne HR, Bozymski EM, Fallon JH: Liver physiology and disease: Treatment of alcoholic hepatitis with encephalopathy—comparison of prednisolone with caloric supplements. *Gastroenterology* 74:169–173, 1978.
199. Maddrey WC, Boitnott JK, Bedine MS, *et al:* Corticosteroid therapy of alcoholic hepatitis. *Gastroenterology* 75:193–199, 1978.
200. Carithers RL Jr, Herlong FH, Diehl AM, *et al:* Methylprednisone therapy in patients with severe alcoholic hepatitis. A randomized multicentre trial. *Ann Intern Med* 110:685–690, 1989.
201. Ramond MJ, Paynard T, Rueff B: A randomized trial of prednisolone in patients with severe alcoholic hepatitis. *N Engl J Med* 326:507–512, 1992.
202. Mathurin P, Duchatelle V, Ramond MJ, *et al:* Survival and prognostic factors in patients with severe alcoholic hepatitis treated with prednisolone. *Gastroenterology* 110:1847–1853, 1996.
203. Mendenhall CL, Moritz TE, Roselle GA, *et al:* A study of oral nutritional support with oxandrolone in malnourished patients with alcoholic hepatitis: Results of a Department of Veterans Affairs Cooperative Study. *Hepatology* 17:564–576, 1993.
204. Lieber CS, Leo MA, Mak KM, *et al:* Choline fails to prevent liver fibrosis in ethanol-fed baboons but causes toxicity. *Hepatology* 5:561–572, 1985.
205. Sundler R, Akesson B: Regulation of phospholipid biosynthesis in isolated rat hepatocytes. *J Biol Chem* 250:3359–3367, 1975.

206. Fox JM: Polyene phosphatidylcholine: Pharmacokinetics after oral administration—a review, in Avogaro P, Macini M, Ricci G, Paoletti R (eds): *Phospholipids and atherosclerosis.* New York, Raven Press, 1983, pp 65–80.
207. Zierenberg O, Grundy SM: Intestinal absorption of polyenylphosphatidylcholine in man. *J Lipid Res* 23:1136–1142, 1982.
208. Parthasarathy S, Subbaiah PV, Ganguly J: The mechanism of intestinal absorption of phosphatidylcholine in rats. *Biochem J* 140:503–508, 1974.
209. Rodgers JB, O'Brien RJ, Balint JA: The absorption and subsequent utilization of lecithin by the rat jejunum. *Am J Dig Dis* 20:208–211, 1975.
210. Lekim D, Betzing H: The incorporation of essential phospholipids into the organs of intact and galactosamine intoxicated rats. *Drug Res* 24:1217–1221, 1974.
211. Arnesjö B, Nilsson Å, Barrowman J, *et al:* Intestinal digestion and absorption of cholesterol and lecithin in the human: Intubation studies with a fat-soluble reference substance. *Scand J Gastroenterol* 4:653–656, 1969.
212. Nilsson BE: Conditions contributing to fracture of the femoral neck. *Acta Chir Scand* 136:338–384, 1970.
213. Patton GM, Clark SB, Fasulo JM, *et al:* Utilization of individual lecithins in intestinal lipoprotein formation in the rat. *J Clin Invest* 73:231–240, 1984.
214. Holz J, Wagner H: Uber den Einbau von intraduodenal appliziertem $^{14}C/^{32}$-P-Polyenephosphatidylcholin in die Leber von Ratten und seine Ausscheidung durch die Galle. *Z Naturforsch* 26:1151–1158, 1971.
215. Lekim D, Betzing H, Stoffel W: Incorporation of complete phospholipid molecules in cellular membranes of rat liver after uptake from blood serum. *Hoppe-Seyler's Z Physiol Chem* 353S:929–946, 1972.
216. Lekim D, Graf E: Tierexperimentelle Studien zur Pharmakokinetik der "essentiellen" Phospholipids (EPL). *Arzneimittelforschung* 26:1772–1782, 1976.
217. Ma X, Svegliati-Baroni G, Poniachik J, *et al:* Collagen synthesis by liver stellate cells is released from its normal feedback regulation by acetaldehyde-induced modification of carbon-terminal propeptide of procollagen. *Alcohol Clin Exp Res* 21:1204–1211, 1997.
218. Ma X, Zhao J, Lieber CS: Polyenylphosphatidylcholine attenuates non-alcoholic hepatitis fibrosis and accelerates its regression. *J Hepatol* 24:604–613, 1996.
219. Ehrlich HP, Ross R, Bornstein P: Effects of antimicrotubular agents on the secretion of collagen. *J Cell Biol* 62:390–405, 1974.
220. Kershenobich D, Uribe M, Suarez GI, *et al:* Treatment of cirrhosis with colchicine. A double-blind randomized trial. *Gastroenterology* 77:532–536, 1979.
221. Kershenobich D, Vargas F, Garcia-Tsao G, *et al:* Colchicine in the treatment of cirrhosis of the liver. *N Engl J Med* 318:1709–1713, 1988.
222. Boyer LJ, Ransohoff FD: Is colchicine effective therapy for cirrhosis? *N Engl J Med* 318:1751–1752, 1988.
223. Plevris JN, Hayes PC, Bouchier IAD: Ursodeoxycholic acid in the treatment of alcoholic liver disease. *Eur J Gastroenterol Hepatol* 3:653–656, 1991.
224. Ferenci P, Dragosics B, Dittrich H, *et al:* Randomized controlled trial of silymarin treatment in patients with cirrhosis of the liver. *J Hepatol* 9:105–113, 1989.
225. Trinchet JC, Coste T, Levy VG, *et al:* Treatment of alcoholic hepatitis with silymarin: A double-blind comparative study in 116 patients. *Gastroenterol Clin Biol* 13:120–124, 1989.
226. Keiding S, Badsberg JH, Becker U, *et al:* The prognosis of patients with alcoholic liver disease. An international randomized, placebo-controlled trial on the effect of malotilate on survival. *J Hepatol* 20:454–460, 1994.
227. Nanji AA, Khettry U, Sadradeh SMH, *et al:* Severity of liver injury in experimental alcoholic liver disease: Correlation with plasma endotoxin, prostaglandin E_2, leukotriene B_4, and thromboxane B_2. *Am J Pathol* 142:367–373, 1993.
228. Shibayama Y, Asaka S, Nakata K: Endotoxin hepatotoxicity augmented by ethanol. *Exp Mol Pathol* 55:196–301, 1991.

229. Khoruts A, Stahnke L, McClain CJ, *et al:* Circulating tumor necrosis factor, interleukin-1 and interleukin-6 concentrations in chronic alcoholic patients. *Hepatology* 13:267–276, 1991.
230. Sheron N, Bird G, Goka J, *et al:* Elevated plasma interleukin-6 and increased severity and mortality in alcoholic hepatitis. *Clin Exp Immunol* 84:449–453, 1991.
231. Czaja MJ, Xu J, Alt E: Prevention of carbon tetrachloride-induced rat liver injury by soluble tumor necrosis factor receptor. *Gastroenterology* 108:1849–1954, 1995.
232. Mahler KM, Torrance DS, Smith CA, *et al:* Soluble tumor necrosis factor (TNF) receptors are effective therapeutic agents in lethal endotoxemia and function simultaneously as both TNF carriers and TNF antagonists. *J Immunol* 151:1548–1561, 1993.
233. Fisher CJ, Agosti JM, Opal SME, *et al:* Treatment of septic shock with the tumor necrosis factor receptor: Fc Fusion protein. *N Engl J Med* 334:1697–1702, 1996.
234. Brenner A, Alcorn J: Therapy for hepatic fibrosis. *Semin Liver Dis* 10:75–83, 1990.
235. Mezey E: Treatment of alcoholic liver disease. *Semin Liver Dis* 13:210–216, 1993.
236. Kumar S, Stauber RE, Gavaler JS, *et al:* Orthotopic liver transplantation for alcoholic liver disease. *Hepatology* 11:159–164, 1990.
237. Rosman AS, Lieber CS: Biochemical markers of alcohol consumption. *Alcohol Health Res World* 14:210–218, 1990.
238. Litten R, Allen J: *Measuring Alcohol Consumption; Psychosocial and Biochemical Methods.* Totowa, NJ, Humana, 1992.
239. Stibler H, Borg S, Joustra M: Microanion exchange chromatography of carbohydrate-deficient transferrin in serum in relation to alcohol consumption (Swedish Patent 8400587-5). *Alcohol Clin Exp Res* 10:535–544, 1986.
240. Behrens, UJ, Worner TM, Braly LF, *et al:* Carbohydrate-deficient transferrin (CDT), a marker for chronic alcohol consumption in different ethnic populations. *Alcohol Clin Exp Res* 12:427–432, 1988.
241. Sörensen TIA, Orholm M, Bentsen KD, *et al:* Prospective evaluation of alcohol abuse and alcoholic liver injury in man as predictors of development of cirrhosis. *Lancet* 2:241–244, 1984.
242. Nakano M, Worner T, Lieber CS: Perivenular fibrosis in alcoholic liver injury: Ultrastructure of histologic progression. *Gastroenterology* 83:777–785, 1982.
243. Worner TM, Lieber CS: Perivenular fibrosis as precursor lesion of cirrhosis. *JAMA* 254:627–630, 1985.
244. Mak KM, Leo MA, Lieber CS: Alcoholic liver injury in baboons: Transformation of lipocytes to transitional cells. *Gastroenterology* 87:188–200, 1984.
245. Lieber CS: Pathogenesis and treatment of liver fibrosis: 1997 update. *Dig Dis* 15:42–66, 1997.

2

Alcohol and the Pancreas

Steven Schenker and Ruth Montalvo

Abstract. Alcoholic pancreatitis may be one of the most serious adverse consequences of alcohol abuse. Its diagnosis, as it has for many years, depends primarily on clinical acumen in interpreting properly the symptoms and signs of abdominal distress, buttressed by elevated pancreatic enzymes (amylase and lipase). More recently, the use of computerized tomography (CT) in selected situations has been both of confirmatory and prognostic value. Severity of abnormality by CT correlates reasonably well with a variety of clinical–laboratory clusters (APACHE system, Ranson's criteria, etc.) and aids in therapy.

The pathogenesis of alcoholic pancreatitis is not fully defined. The ultimate picture is one of tissue autolysis by activated proteolytic enzymes. The triggers for such activation, however, are still not known. They are represented by three main theories: (1) large duct obstruction and/or increased permeability relative to pancreatic secretion, (2) small duct obstruction due to proteinaceous precipitates, and (3) a direct toxic–metabolic effect of ethanol on pancreatic acinar cells. While not mutually exclusive, we favor the last hypothesis as being most consistent with the effects of ethanol on other organ systems. The direct effects of ethanol and/or its metabolites may be mediated, at least in part, via oxidative stress or the generation of fatty acid ethyl esters. Autolysis (regardless of proximate mechanism(s)) leads to inflammation likely mediated via release of various cytokines. It also should be appreciated that "acute" pancreatitis (the topic of this chapter) likely represents an acute process within a chronic pancreatic exposure and injury from alcoholic abuse. The key question of why pancreatitis develops in only a small number of alcohol abusers is not resolved.

Therapy depends on the severity of alcoholic pancreatitis, which is defined by clinical–laboratory and often CT criteria. Mild pancreatitis usually resolves acutely with alcohol abstention and supportive therapy. Severe pancreatitis has a significant morbidity and mortality, mainly related to the degree of pancreatic necrosis and infection. It requires meticulous combined medical–surgical care.

Steven Schenker and Ruth Montalvo • Department of Medicine, Division of Gastroenterology and Nutrition, The University of Texas Health Science Center at San Antonio, San Antonio, Texas 78284-7878.

Recent Developments in Alcoholism, Volume 14: The Consequences of Alcoholism, edited by Galanter. Plenum Press, New York, 1998.

1. Introduction

Alcohol abuse is the most common cause of pancreatic injury in the United States. The exact incidence of pancreatic damage in patients abusing alcohol varies with the populations and countries studied,[1,2] the definition and assessment of what constitutes increased alcohol consumption, and the methods (terminology) used for the diagnosis of pancreatitis.[1] For example, *clinical* evidence of pancreatitis is reported in about 5% of alcohol abusers in the United States,[2,3] but at autopsy changes consistent with chronic pancreatitis have been reported in up to 75% of the patients, even in the absence of symptoms of pancreatitis during life.[4–8] This is many times greater than in nondrinkers. There are also data that asymptomatic alcoholics often exhibit abnormal pancreatic secretory response after secretin–pancreozymin stimulation[4] and an abnormal pancreatogram on endoscopic retrograde cholangiopancreatography (ERCP).[9] Thus, symptomatic pancreatitis may only be the tip of the iceberg in terms of pancreatic injury due to alcohol abuse. A similar phenomenon is seen with alcoholic liver damage and myocardial injury due to alcohol.[10,11] These observations have implications for the pathogenesis of alcohol-induced pancreatic damage, an area of considerable ongoing debate and uncertainty.[1,2,12,13]

Despite a low prevalence of clinically relevant disease, alcoholic pancreatitis with its multiple recurrences is a major cause of chronic patient suffering and disability, and in a minority of individuals with pancreatic necrosis and/or infection, death may ensue.[14] However, because of its relatively inaccessible location and lack of suitable animal models until fairly recently, progress in understanding the pathogenesis, developing new diagnostic and prognostic tools for the disease, and developing appropriate treatment has lagged. In the last decade, however, this has changed considerably with the development of new imaging techniques (sonography, computed tomography),[15–17] various animal models of pancreatitis[18] (mostly acute to be sure), methodology that assesses various aspects of intrapancreatic enzyme production[19] and of inflammation (i.e., cytokines),[20–23] and the availability of antibiotics that penetrate well into tissues.[24–26] This brief review chapter will consider sequentially the pathogenesis, the diagnosis, the prognostic aspects, and the therapeutic aspects of alcoholic pancreatitis, in light of these new developments. Our emphasis will be on the acute disease, as discussion of the complications of chronic pancreatic disease (pancreatic pseudocysts, biliary obstruction, pancreatic ascites, etc.) deserve an extensive assessment on their own. It should be appreciated, however, that episodes of alcohol-induced acute clinical pancreatitis very likely represent individual episodes in the course of protracted alcohol abuse and more chronic (pathological) pancreatic injury.[27–30]

2. Pathogenesis

2.1. *General Concepts*

A number of general points are worthy of mention before specific mechanisms of pancreatitis are discussed:

1. It has been known since at least 1896[31] that the ultimate key mechanism of pancreatitis (of all types, not just alcoholic) depends on autodigestion of the tissue by the pancreas's own proteolytic enzymes. It is the manner in which these proenzymes are activated that has not been fully established.

2. Although trypsin is usually considered a key player in this autolytic process, recent studies with isolated rat pancreatic acinar cells[32] show clearly that other enzymes (elastase and, to a lesser extent, chymotrypsin, phospholipase A_2, and lipase) have a much greater potential to damage the pancreas than trypsin (Fig. 1). Elastase damaged pancreatic cells in nanomolar concentrations, chymotrypsin and lipase in micromolar amounts, and for trypsin even millimolar concentrations were not noxious. Clearly, the presence of substrate also contributed to enzyme activity as shown for lipase.[32] It appears that trypsin activation may serve as a "trigger" for the cascade of the other autolytic enzymes. If confirmed *in vivo,* this may mean that future therapeutic agents should be also directed at these enzymes, in addition to trypsin.

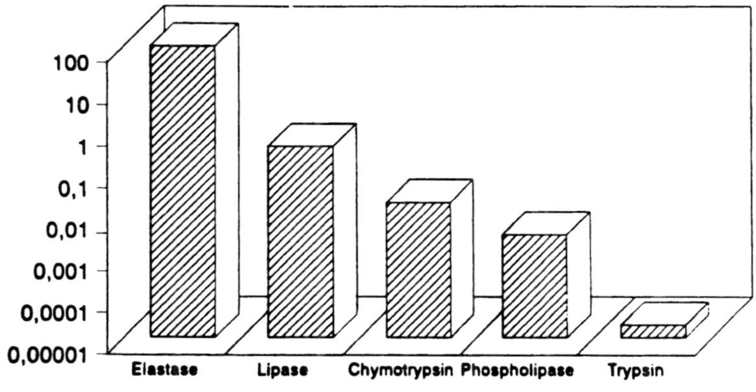

Figure 1. Comparison of noxious potential of different pancreatic enzymes, studied on a molar basis. Comparison was done with that enzyme concentration that caused 20% cell damage after 90 min of incubation. Trypsin, even at the highest concentration of 2 mmole/liter, was not able to cause 20% cell damage. For illustrative reasons, 2 mmole/liter concentration was used for calculation, although the value shown overestimates the noxious potential of trypsin. The difference between the noxious potential of elastase versus trypsin is probably greater than six orders of magnitude. (From Niederau *et al.*,[32] with permission.)

3. Whatever the proximate (initiating) mechanism for alcoholic pancreatitis, it has to explain the acute exacerbations of illness so characteristic of this clinical process.

4. Many of the present concepts about human alcoholic pancreatitis derive, in part, from animal models of pancreatitis. This is because, unlike in the liver wherein serial liver biopsies are feasible, longitudinal examination of pancreatic tissue, as pancreatitis evolves, is not possible in humans. Aside from the difficulties of extrapolating from smaller animals to man, most experimental models of pancreatitis are not based on ethanol use–abuse. They consist of low choline-ethionine or cerulein (cholecystokinelike agent) feeding or retrograde administration of bile salts into the pancreatic duct.[18] These techniques produce a much more extensive pancreatic injury than has been reported for experimental alcohol administration.[2] Acute alcohol administration to rats enhances pancreatic triglyceride synthesis at the expense of phospholipids but causes no serious tissue injury.[2] Chronic alcohol administration in various animals does result in pancreatic fat deposition, accumulation of some fatty acid ethyl esters (nonoxidative products of ethanol metabolism),[33,34] evidence of mitochondrial alteration, autophagic vacuoles, and ultimately some patchy atrophy of acini, ductular dilation, and fibrosis but no necrosis or inflammation (reviewed in ref. 2). Such longer-term studies often suffer from inadequate control for decreased dietary intake with alcohol consumption, although this actually may be similar to the human disease state. In any event, pathologically, the animal model of alcoholic pancreatitis does not mimic the human condition, hence caution is needed in mechanistic data extrapolation. As to physiological studies on pancreatic secretion, the data in animals and man are complex and depend on prior secretory state and acute versus chronic or oral versus intravenous alcohol administration. In most instances, however, animal and human data tend to correspond in that acute ethanol is hypersecretory and chronic alcohol tends to enhance the response of the pancreas to secretin and over a shorter time (3 months) to cholecystokinin, as well (reviewed in ref. 2). Overall, in our view, a faithful model of human alcoholic pancreatitis has not yet been produced in lower experimental animals, and to our knowledge, no significant pancreatic injury exists in baboons fed alcohol over a long time.[35]

5. Although pancreatic fibrosis is seen in many chronic alcohol abusers at autopsy, the large majority of them are asymptomatic prior to death. It is thus essential to determine what factors can induce clinically overt pancreatitis (superimposed on mild chronic injury) in these patients.

The subject has been elegantly discussed in a recent review[13] and editorial.[36] One conclusion of these reports is that the process takes time. The duration of alcohol abuse in the United States averages 9 years, in South Africa 5–15 years, and in Japan, about 18 years before the disease is clinically evident.[7,36] Beyond this, there are few, if any, predictors. Thus, amount (beyond the level of abuse) and type of alcoholic beverage did not correlate with the development of pancreatitis.[13] Drinking pattern (binge vs. steady use) did not clearly emerge as a precipitant and smoking also did not seem to exert a particularly negative effect. Should decreased pancreatic blood flow contribute to alcoholic pancreatitis, smoking could aggravate this process. However, evidence that alcohol impairs pancreatic blood flow early on in the development of pancreatitis is not compelling (reviewed in ref. 13).

Diet has been discussed as a possible component of pancreatitis. Diet is often deficient in alcoholics.[37] Pancreatic secretion is altered in malnourished alcoholics,[38] accompanied by morphological changes in the organ.[39] However, dietary assessment in alcoholics with pancreatitis has not shown evidence of reduced nutrition.[40] On the other hand, the possibility was also raised that a high fat diet may contribute to the pancreatitis.[41–43] This could relate mechanistically to the production of hyperlipidemia and/or the provision of substrate (unsaturated fat) for production of free radicals (oxidative stress).[44] Well-controlled studies, however, did not document a contribution of high fat intake to alcoholic pancreatitis.[40,45] Hypertriglyceridemia of high grade is known to produce pancreatitis (likely by a vascular mechanism) in the absence of alcohol, and alcohol intake, as well as alcoholic pancreatitis, may potentiate a preexisting lipid disorder (reviewed in ref. 13); however, there is no good evidence that plasma triglyceride levels were consistently higher in alcoholics with than without pancreatitis.[13,46]

Genetic factors could also play a significant role in the proclivity for pancreatitis. A number of HLA antigens have been cited as potential markers,[13] but the studies were not internally consistent for any given antigen and were usually not controlled for alcoholism alone. There is some preliminary evidence that the alcohol dehydrogenase *ADH31* gene encoding the high-activity *ADHG1* isozyme may be statistically more frequent in patients with alcoholic pancreatitis (reviewed in ref. 13). This, however, was not confirmed in another persuasive recent report that showed a significantly higher frequency of the *ADH2*2/ADH2*2* genotype in alcoholics with pancreatitis as compared to other apropriate controls.[47] More confirmatory genetic studies are needed to resolve this controversy. In a very small Chinese study, patients with alcoholic pancreatitis did not manifest changes in the cytochrome P4502E1 genetic markers as compared to other groups,[48] and this was recently confirmed in a larger Japanese population.[47] In summary, the reason why only a small number of patients who abuse alcohol develop overt, clinically apparent "acute" pancreatitis is not certain. This is similar to alcoholic liver disease, which is seen in severe form in only about 20% of alcohol abusers, although fatty liver is very common. In the past it was believed that alcoholic cirrhosis and pancreatitis rarely coexisted, implying a predisposition to one or another organ damage. However, postmortem studies suggest a high prevalence of both lesions in the same person.[49,50]

2.2. *Specific Initiating Mechanisms*

In the absence of longitudinal studies in individual patients and without availability of a good animal model of alcoholic pancreatitis, as discussed above, it is understandable that the specific initiating process that leads to eventual pancreatic autodigestion with alcohol abuse has not been established. There are three main concepts of such initiation and they will be discussed sequentially.

2.2.1. Large Duct Hypothesis. This mechanism implies some type of pancreatic juice flow disturbance and/or duodenal content reflux in the larger pancreatic ducts. Historically, the concept likely derives from observations with biliary calculi and the demonstration that retrograde injection of bile salts into the pancreatic ducts can induce greater pancreatic damage in animals given ethanol than in controls.[51] The implications of this hypothesis are that alcohol can impair normal flow of pancreatic juice (or permit duodenal reflux) either by an effect on the sphincter of Oddi and/or directly on the pancreatic duct pressure and permeability. However, the effects of alcohol on the sphincter of Oddi are not clear,[52,53] and the pancreatic–duodenal gradient usually does not favor reflux.[54] Nevertheless, pancreatography often shows distorted pancreatic ducts in chronic alcoholic pancreatitis.[55] Probably of more relevance, pancreatic ducts are normally impermeable to molecules larger than 3,000 Da, but ethanol has been shown to render the ductal epithelium permeable to molecules as high as 20,000 Da.[56,57] This might allow pancreatic enzymes to enter pancreatic interstitial tissue space, and if activated, to proceed to tissue digestion. Such an activation could theoretically occur if enhanced permeability is accompanied by increased pressure and interstitial colocalization of hydrolytic processes and the proenzymes. Because the process would require both penetration of the ductal barrier and enzyme activation, this concept (although viable) is probably the least popular at present. In fact, such a study was carried out in experimental animals, and increased lysosomal activity was seen in biliary pancreatitis models, but no clear correlation with pancreatitis was observed.[58]

2.2.2. Small Duct–Proteinaceous Precipitate Hypothesis. This widely discussed concept, popularized by Sarles,[59,60] stipulates that ethanol abuse results in the precipitation of proteinaceous material in small pancreatic ducts with resulting obstruction of pancreatitic ductules, increase in pancreatic pressure, and release of activated pancreatic enzymes into the extracellular space. The precipitated protein, often complexed to calcium, may be deposited in the small ducts because of ethanol-induced altered homeostasis that normally solubilizes these complexes. A key component of such postulated altered homeostasis is a decrease in pancreatic stone protein (lithostatin), a 14,000-Da phosphoglucoprotein with a high content of acidic amino acids.[61]

There is significant evidence of such a process in morphological and biochemical studies of experimental animals and patients, although dissenting data have also been published (reviewed in refs. 1, 12, and 59). Two major questions are whether the protein precipitates are the cause of or a result of pancreatitis, and how can such a process explain the acute clinical exacerbations of pancreatitis.[1] This concept, however, is consistent with the prolonged alcohol intake needed to establish the process and with the chronicity of the disease and could account for the development of severe acute disease in only a small number of such patients, possibly under genetic control of protein secretion. Further comparative longitudinal studies of pancreatic protein in the pancreatic juice of alcoholics without and in the early and later stages of alcohol-induced pancreatitis may differentiate causal from casual biochemical events.

2.2.3. Toxic–Metabolic Hypothesis. This concept implies that alcohol and/or its primary metabolite, acetaldehyde, may have a direct toxic effect on pancreatic acinar cells. This is generally felt to be because of altered lipid metabolism with increased cell membrane (largely composed of lipids) permeability,[1] accompanied by increased secretion of pancreatic enzymes,[19] and possibly an increase of lysosomal fragility due to exposure to fatty acid ethyl esters.[34] It is postulated that these events may all combine to induce disruption of pancreatic acini *in situ*.

It is usually felt that ethanol per se may be toxic to the pancreas as *in vitro* exposure of pancreas demonstrated ethanol-induced alterations of lipid metabolism.[62] However, using an isolated perfused canine pancreas preparation, it was shown that infusion of 250 mg/hr of acetaldehyde (accompanied by ischemia, and in the presence of xanthine oxidase) induced more pancreatic edema, hemorrhage, and hyperamylasemia as compared to ischemia and ethanol controls.[63] This toxic effect of acetaldehyde may have been mediated via free radical release, as it was inhibited by free radical scavengers and allopurinol as a xanthine oxidase inhibitor.[63] Moreover, fatty acid ethyl esters (nonoxidative ethanol metabolites) added to the rat pancreatic lysosomes increased their fragility as measured by the release of lysosomal enzyme markers.[34] Thus, the precise cause of ethanol-induced pancreatic damage—parent drug and/or its metabolites—is still uncertain. There is a general impression that it is the interaction of ethanol-induced increased enzyme synthesis shown in the pancreas experimentally *in vivo*[19] and their release from more fragile (acidified) lysosomal–zymogen storage sites that promotes enzyme hydrolysis and subsequent pancreatic necrosis.[1] Such a composite colocalizational effect also has been postulated in other forms of pancreatitis,[18] perhaps with pH-dependent autoactivation of trypsinogen as a trigger for other proenzymes.[18,64] Unfortunately, raising the pH of pancreatic acinar cells by administration of chloroquine did not prevent experimental pancreatitis,[65] hence the issue of pH and enzyme activation needs further study. Other effects of alcohol could be on disruption of the actin tight junctions between acinar and pancreatic duct cells as shown with cerulein-induced pancreatitis in rats.[66]

Other intracellular mechanisms may also occur with exposure to ethanol. With increased pancreatic edema, changes in microcirculation may ensue. Microvascular injury could also be influenced by severe hyperlipidemia. Alcohol cytotoxicity also has been ascribed to oxidative stress with membrane lipid oxidation.[44] This has been extensively documented in various forms of experimental pancreatitis,[67] and indeed various antioxidants and free radical scavengers have been shown to be of some benefit in these studies, but usually only if given prior to the injury.[68]* Documentation of such benefit has been difficult in alcoholic pancreatitis in patients, although at least one study demonstrated markers of oxidative stress in acute human pancreatitis[70] and possible benefit from antioxidant therapy in terms of pain control and prevention of relapse.[71] Carefully controlled studies are needed to confirm these very preliminary impressions. The possible role of nitric oxide and other mediators on pancreatic blood flow and on the oxidative injury is also controversial[44,72,73] and in need of further study.

It should be emphasized that autolysis leads to inflammation and that there is experimental evidence that cytokines released by the injured tissue may participate in and propagate the injury.[74] Thus, release of tumor necrosis factor (TNF),[23] interleukin-6,[20] and localization of transforming growth factor B_1[22] are seen in experimental and human chronic pancreatitis, respectively, and attest to the importance of these secondary mediators. Amelioration of experimental pancreatitis by anti-TNF antibody[23] and interleukin-10[21] corroborates this, and may eventually have clinical implications. There is evidence that cerulein (as a cause of experimental pancreatitis) stimulates the pancreatic production of platelet-activating factor (PAF), which, in turn, mediates apoptosis and neutrophil chemotaxis. Neutrophils, in turn, may convert apoptolic cells into necrotic ones.[75] The toxic–metabolic concept of initial injury has been reinforced lately by sequential pathological–clinical observations over time in patients with this disease.[29,30]

2.3. *Conclusions*

It is evident from the above comments that the initiating mechanism(s) for eventual pancreatic autodigestion from alcohol abuse have not been established. The toxic–metabolic concept for us is the most persuasive, as it would agree with present understanding (direct cytotoxic effect) of the pathogenesis of alcohol-induced liver, heart, and fetal damage. Thus, it would be a unitary and parsimonious view. The more specific production of free radicals via oxidative stress and membrane lipid alteration also seems to rest on reasonable data. This, of course, does not imply that the other mechanisms could not contribute and indeed in some individuals may be primary noxious influ-

* Formation of an α-hydroxyethyl radical adduct from ^{13}C-ethanol in pancreatic secretions from rats exposed to intragastric ethanol was very recently documented. However, pancreatic enzymes were not increased and only very minor histological changes were seen after 4 weeks of alcohol.[69]

ences. Alcohol abuse has so many adverse physiological–biochemical effects that it would surprise us if the mechanism of pancreatic injury were very simple. A tentative, schematic overview of the pathogenesis of alcoholic pancreatitis is shown in Fig. 2. The issue of individual sensitivity (or conversely of resistance) of the pancreas to alcohol abuse should consider the possibility of genetic factors. This could be similar to the genetically determined proclivity for hereditary pancreatitis that has been linked to chromosome 7q35,[76] and through identification of the gene itself appears to point to a decrease in normal trypsin degradation through a mutation in cationic trypsinogen.[77] The concentration of such inhibitors (i.e., antioxidants) or initiators could define the propensity for tissue injury. Other intrinsic protective mechanisms in the normal pancreas are the segregated locations and secretory pathways of the digestive enzymes and lysosomal hydrolases (i.e., cathepsin-β) as triggers for proenzymic activation.[78] It is their proclivity for disruption that may determine the onset of pancreatitis. In our view, a good animal model and longitudinal studies in patients are needed to better understand the mechanism(s) of this disease.

This discussion of the mechanisms of alcohol-induced pancreatitis has benefited from a number of elegant reviews,[1,2,12,44] which served as source material.

3. Diagnosis

The diagnosis of acute pancreatitis (or the acute process in the setting of chronic disease) has depended traditionally on classical clinical symptoms

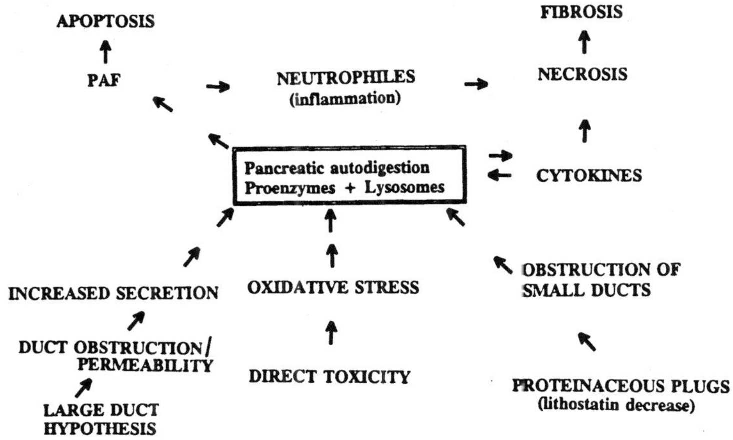

Figure 2. Tentative scheme of causation of alcoholic pancreatitis. Direct toxic alcohol pathway is favored by us. **PAF**, platelet activating factor.

and signs, elevation of pancreatic enzymes (amylase/lipase) in blood, and exclusion of other causes of abdominal distress. The symptoms of pancreatic disease characteristically consist of midepigastric pain with radiation to the back and with relief on flexing the spine.[79,80] This may be accompanied by nausea and vomiting, as well as by fever. The abdomen is tender, with decreased or absent bowel sounds, but usually is not as rigid as with other intra-abdominal disorders. Elevation of pancreatic enzymes in blood is a key aspect of the diagnosis, especially if they are more than fivefold the upper limit of normal.[81] It should be appreciated, however, that (1) not all cases of pancreatitis exhibit a high amylase or lipase, (2) these enzymes may be elevated due to other disorders (i.e., perforated/ischemic small bowel), and (3) increased amylase (not macroamylase) may be present in blood over a long period of time without the presence of any disease state.[82] Short of surgery or autopsy, tissue diagnosis is not available. Fortunately, a new diagnostic approach has appeared more recently in the form of imaging with sonography or with computerized tomography (CT), which has greater sensitivity.[17,81,83] This provides corroboration of the presence of pancreatitis (especially with severe disease), gives prognostic information as to the extent of disease, and helps to exclude other causes of abdominal pain. In mild disease, imaging may not be sensitive enough to detect the pancreatitis. However, in case of doubt as to the diagnosis, or with apparently severe and/or progressive disease, imaging is indicated. For example, the presence of severe disease clinically and/or by laboratory tests and a normal CT scan of the pancreas should lead to a reevaluation of the diagnosis of pancreatitis. Diagnosis of specific aspects of pancreatitis (i.e., necrosis and infection) is considered below.

Once the diagnosis of pancreatitis is made, it is essential to determine that alcohol abuse is the cause of the pancreatitis. Diagnosis of alcohol abuse depends on a good history, with collateral confirmation, and is helped by the use of various serum markers such as sialic acid deficient transferrin, gamma-glutamyl peptidase, and increased red blood cell mean corpuscular volume. Thus, other causes of the disease (i.e., biliary calculi, drugs, hyperlipidemia, etc.) need to be excluded. Treatment for these other disorders may be different than for alcoholic pancreatitis.

4. Prognosis

For many years, the terminology of pancreatitis was confusing in that it mixed pathology and clinical aspects, as well as using unclear descriptions (i.e., phlegmon). An international symposium in 1992 developed a classification system that permitted a clear stratification of severity, including the diagnosis of pancreatic necrosis by dynamic CT.[84] Assessment of severity is a key to prognosis and management of this disorder.[14,85] In about 80% of patients, the pancreas is inflamed but exhibits no necrosis—so-called interstitial pancreatitis. The mortality is less than 2% and supportive therapy is adequate.[14] In the remainder of patients, necrosis is documented by areas of nonperfusion on CT. The necrosis is believed to be the result of lipolysis of peripancreatic fat and disruption of pancreatic microcirculation and acini by enzymatic digestion. The necrosis may be sterile (mortality of 10%) or infected (mortality of about 30%).[14]

Identification of necrosis and severe pancreatitis depend on the use of clinical, laboratory, and CT criteria according to established guidelines, tested over time.[14,85] Such classification is not only of prognostic value, but is also an important guide to management (i.e., transfer and monitoring in intensive care, serial CTs, diagnostic aspiration and drainage, or surgical tissue removal). The terminology of acute pancreatitis is shown in Table I, and the factors that generally define a severe case are cited in Table II.[14] More detailed assessment of severity of pancreatitis can be carried out using purely clinical criteria (Table III),[86] a combination of mainly laboratory tests (Table IV),[87] simplified prognostic criteria (SPC) (Table V),[88] or the acute physiology and chronic health evaluation (APACHE) systems.[89] Clinical assessment alone (Table III) was helpful in defining mild cases, but was not valuable in identifying severe ones. Using Ranson's early prognostic criteria (Table IV), a score of < three positive signs carries no mortality, three to five signs a mortality of 10–20%, and more than six signs (likely necrotizing disease) a mortality of more than 50%.[14] Figure 3 shows the relationship of these prognostic signs versus complications and mortality.[85] The limitations of this system are the large number of signs, the requirement for a 48-hr observation period, and some lack of precision in the intermediate 2- to 5-sign group. The SPC system (Table V) showed no mortality with no SPC present to an 84% complication and 32% mortality in patients with two or more SPC (see Figs. 4 and 5).[85,88] The APACHE system correlated well with prognosis.[85] Although each system has its advocates and detractors, in general, they have similar predictive potential for severity of disease and prognosis.[85] Even such simple markers such as serum urea and blood glucose may serve as predictors of severe disease.[90]

Another very valuable approach to assessing the severity of acute pancre-

Table I. Terminology of Acute Pancreatitis[a]

Acute interstitial pancreatitis
Necrotizing pancreatitis
Sterile necrosis
Infected necrosis
Pancreatic fluid collection
Sterile
Infected
Pancreatic pseudocyst
Sterile
Pancreatic abscess

[a]From Banks,[14] with permission.

Table II. Severe Acute Pancreatitis[a]

Organ failure[b] and/or
Local complications
Necrosis
Abscess
Pseudocyst

[a]From Banks,[14] with permission.
[b]Shock: systolic BP < 90 mm Hg; pulmonary insufficiency: $Pao_2 \leq 60$ mm Hg; renal failure: creatinine > 2 mg/dl; GI bleeding: > 500 ml/24 hr.

atitis (and influencing the management of the patient) depends on the use of the dynamic CT.[91] The object in this setting is to define the presence and extent of pancreatic necrosis. A CT is clearly not indicated if the diagnosis is evident and the course (see above) suggests a mild pancreatitis. Moreover, the use of intravenous contrast in performing a dynamic CT has been reported to enhance acute experimental pancreatic necrosis in the rat.[92] Whereas it is uncertain if this has any relevance to humans, it is usually unnecessary to perform a dynamic CT on patients during the first few (3) days of acute pancreatitis, as infection is unlikely to occur so early, and, thus, the need for diagnostic aspiration usually is also not needed then.[14] If it is felt to be necessary, a CT without contrast will provide a reasonable grading of pancreatic disease severity and the likelihood of future infection.[14,91] Some, however, proceed with a dynamic CT early on in severe cases of pancreatitis. Clearly, renal disease and allergy are other contraindications for the use of contrast material. Individualization is essential. The value of a dynamic (contrast) CT is that it helps to distinguish necrotizing from interstitial severe pancreatitis, with areas of nonenhancement in the former. Grading of severity of acute pancreatitis is readily accomplished by the CT index (Table VI).[91] There is good evidence that the severity index on CT correlates well with severity of clinical disease and degree of pancreatic necrosis.[91] The accuracy of the CT for

Table III. Bank's Clinical Criteria[a]

Cardiac	Shock, tachycardia > 130, arrhythmia, EKG changes
Pulmonary	Dyspnea, rales, $Po_2 < 60$ mm Hg, adult respiratory distress syndrome
Renal	Urine output < 50 ml/hr, rising blood urea nitrogen and/or creatinine
Metabolic	Low or falling calcium, pH; albumin decrease
Hematological	Falling hematocrit, disseminated intravascular coagulation (low platelets, split products)
Neurological	Irritability, confusion, localizing signs
Hemorrhagic	On signs or peritoneal tap
Tense distension	Severe ileus, fluid + +
Interpretation	≥ 1 = severe (potentially lethal) disease

[a]From Bank *et al.*,[86] with permission.

Table IV. Ranson's Criteria of Severity[a]

At admission	
	Age > 55 yr
	WBC > 16,000/mm^3
	Glucose > 200 mg/dl
	LDH > 350 IU/liter
	AST > 250 U/liter
During initial 48 hr	
	Hct decrease of > 10
	BUN increase of > 5 mg/dl
	CA^{2+} < 8mg/dl
	Pao_2 < 60 mm Hg
	Base deficit > 4 mEq/liter
	Fluid sequestration > 6 liter

[a]From Ranson and Pasternack,[87] with permission.

pancreatic necrosis increases with the extent of necrosis, and it has a false-negative rate of only 21% with more than 50% necrosis.[83] The risk of infection also rises with the degree of necrosis.[91] There is still debate, however, as to how much the CT index adds to information obtained from the combined clinical and laboratory assessment (see above).[94] In conclusion, we believe that the dynamic CT should be used selectively in severe acute pancreatitis. In chronic pancreatitis, the indications for the CT will be different (pseudocyst, extrapancreatic necrosis/inflammation, follow-up).

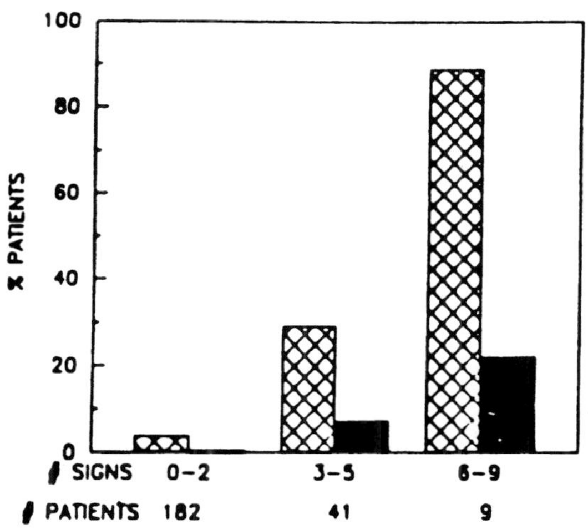

Figure 3. Relationship between Ranson's early prognostic signs and complications (⊠) and mortality (■) in acute pancreatitis. (From Ranson and Pasternack,[87] with permission.)

Table V. Simplified Prognostic Criteria[a]

During initial 48 hr	
Cardiac	BP < 90 mm Hg and/or tachycardia > 130/min
Pulmonary	Po_2 < 60 mm Hg
Renal	Urinary output < 50 ml/hr
Metabolic	Calcium < 8 mg/dl; and/or albumin < 3.2 g/dl

[a]From Agarwal and Pitchumoni,[88] with permission.

Various other laboratory markers have also been used to assess the severity of acute pancreatitis. These are the C-reactive protein (CRP) (an acute phase reactant),[20] interleukin-6,[20] antiendotoxin core antibody,[95] and pancreatitis-associated protein.[96–98] CRP is elevated in a large majority of patients with pancreatic damage, tends to remain high somewhat longer than serum amylase, and does rise more in necrotizing than edematous pancreatitis[98] (Fig. 6). Similarly, more elevated CRP was reported in severe pancreatitis by others.[95] In one group of 20 patients with severe acute pancreatitis, the sensitivity of the CRP was 85% and specificity 88%.[98] In a series of 24 patients with acute pancreatitis, interleukin-6 (another acute-phase protein response) had a sensitivity of 90% and a specificity of 79%.[20] It correlated well with CRP in the same patients (n = 0.73), but peaked earlier. In another report, however, a poor correlation was seen.[95] Again, the values of interleukin-6 were higher in the more severe cases.[95]

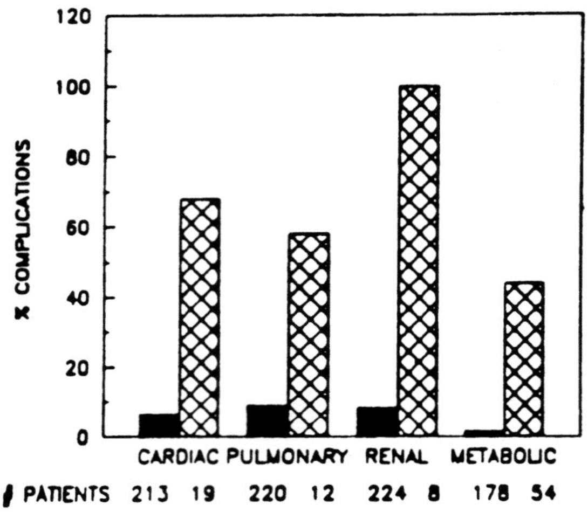

Figure 4. Relationship between individual simplified prognostic criteria (SPC) and complications in acute pancreatitis. ■, Criteria absent; ⊠, criteria present. (From Agarwal and Pitchumoni,[85] with permission.)

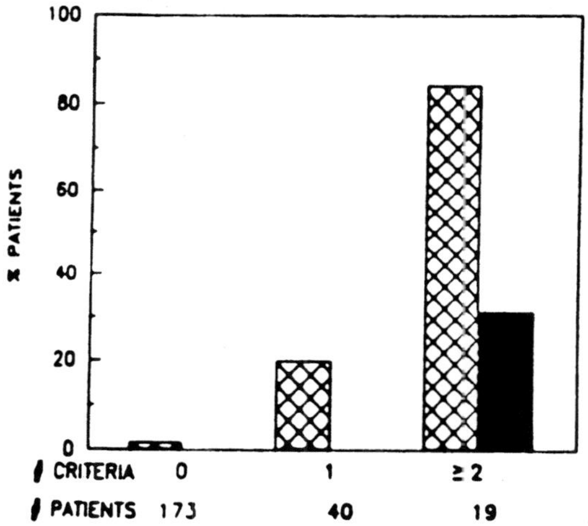

Figure 5. Relationship between number of simplified prognostic criteria (SPC) and complications (☒) and mortality (■) in acute pancreatitis. (From Agarwal and Pitchumoni,[85] with permission.)

The basis for measuring serum antiendotoxin antibody is the presence of endotoxemia in pancreatitis. The antibody presumably binds to the endotoxin and a fall in antibody may relate to more severe disease. Indeed, in 23 patients with severe pancreatitis by clinical assessment, the IgG antibody fell more compared to that in 10 mild cases.[95] This rather indirect approach to assessing severity of pancreatitis needs to be verified in a larger patient sample and should be compared with other prognostic modalities.

Table VI. CT Severity Index in Acute Pancreatitis[a,b]

	Points
Grade of acute pancreatitis	
A, normal pancreas	0
B, pancreatic enlargement alone	1
C, inflammation confined to the pancreas and peripancreatic fat	2
D, One peripancreatic fluid collection	3
E, two or more fluid collections	4
Degree of pancreatic necrosis	
No necrosis	0
Necrosis of one third of pancreas	2
Necrosis of one half of pancreas	4
Necrosis of more than one half of pancreas	6

[a]CT severity index, grade points, and degree of necrosis points.
[b]Modified from Balthazar *et al.*[91]

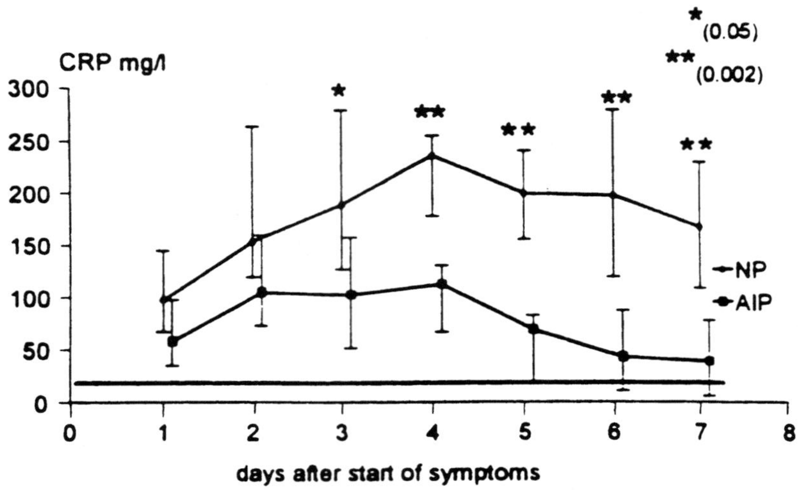

Figure 6. Medians and quartiles of C-reactive protein in patients with acute pancreatitis in relation to the beginning of the disease. NP, necrotizing pancreatitis; AIP, edematous pancreatitis. (From Schmid *et al.*,[98] with permission.)

An initial retrospective study of pancreatitis-associated protein (PAP) suggested that the serum assay may be helpful in diagnosing severe pancreatitis and its follow-up will correlate with the disease course.[96] This protein, which is released from the diseased pancreatic cytosol, has been identified as procarboxy peptidase B.[99] In other studies it was shown that the PAP concentration paralleled the extent of pancreatic necrosis by dynamic CT (Fig. 7),although there was a substantial overlap in PAP values.[98] More importantly,

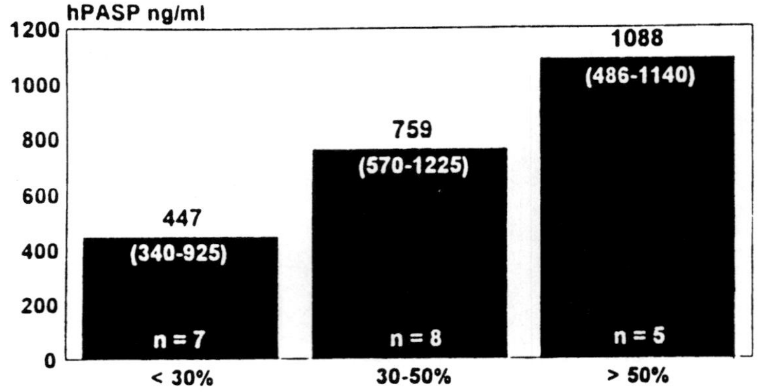

Figure 7. Correlation of peak values of pancreatic protein (hPASP) with the extent of pancreatic necrosis revealed by contrast-enhanced CT scanning. (From Schmid *et al.*,[98] with permission.)

assay for PAP did not improve on the sensitivity or specificity of CRP.[98] In another recent study wherein PAP was measured on admission as a diagnostic–prognostic tool,[97] the sensitivity and specificity of this test to detect acute pancreatitis or severe acute pancreatitis were not very impressive.[97] Regrettably, we are not aware of studies that compare all of these assays with the clinical–laboratory assessments in the same patients. As will be evident from the therapy section, the severity of acute pancreatitis is a critical factor in its therapy.

5. Therapy

The current therapeutic approach for acute pancreatitis involves the provision of supportive care, the elimination of causal agents (i.e., alcohol), and the treatment of complications. Approximately 80% of patients with acute pancreatitis will follow an uncomplicated course, and for these patients a supportive regimen is sufficient to ensure recovery from the acute phase of the illness (Table VII). A supportive regimen will include total fasting, appropriate parenteral analgesia, and correction of hemodynamic abnormalities by aggressive replacement of deficits in volume and electrolytes.[100,101] Whereas mild pancreatitis can usually be managed safely on an open floor, severe pancreatitis (patients with increased Ranson's signs and/or increased APACHE II points on presentation, or signs of organ failure) invariably requires treatment in an intensive care unit. As indicated in more detail earlier, if the diagnosis is uncertain, if there is evidence of organ failure, or if the clinician considers it of great importance to know whether the patient has necrotizing pancreatitis, a CT scan of the abdomen should be obtained. Other additional forms of therapy are more controversial and are discussed below. These general comments apply to alcoholic pancreatitis. Other causes, i.e., biliary tract, may require other therapeutic approaches.

For many years, nasogastric suction was part of the standard treatment for acute pancreatitis. However, several controlled clinical trials have demonstrated that nasogastric suction delays resumption of bowel activity, prolongs the duration of pain, and increases analgesic requirements when compared

Table VII. Supportive Management of Acute Alcoholic Pancreatitis

• Total fasting/pancreatic rest
• Analgesia
• Volume and electrolytes replacement
• Nasogastric suction[a]
• Nutritional support for moderate to severe cases

[a]See text for indications.

with fasting alone.[102–106] Nasogastric suction should then be reserved for patients who present with intestinal ileus, nausea, or vomiting, or if the patient has a depressed mental status and is at risk for aspiration.

Histamine$_2$ (H_2)-receptor antagonists were also introduced into the treatment of acute pancreatitis because they were thought to reduce the delivery of acid into the duodenum, thus decreasing pancreatic secretions. However, they have failed to demonstrate any beneficial effect in a number of clinical trials.[103,104,106–108] At present, H_2-antagonists cannot be recommended for treatment of acute pancreatitis, although they may decrease stress ulceration of the stomach.

The role of peritoneal lavage in the treatment of severe acute pancreatitis has been a controversial one. Two prospective, randomized, placebo-controlled trials concluded that the outcome of severe pancreatitis was not greatly influenced by peritoneal lavage of 3–4 days duration.[109,110] On the other hand, Ranson and Berman[111] showed that long-term peritoneal lavage (7 days) significantly reduced both the frequency and mortality rate of pancreatic sepsis in severe pancreatitis as compared to a lavage of 2 days. Further clinical studies will be helpful before deciding whether or not peritoneal lavage should be recommended for the treatment of severe acute pancreatitis, but at present it appears that only a week or more of such treatment could be beneficial.

A number of pancreatic enzymes have been suggested as factors for tissue autolysis in acute pancreatitis. In particular, the relationship between proteases and antiproteases has been examined extensively, based on the suspicion that an imbalance between them is a central factor in the pathogenesis of acute pancreatitis. This subject has been elegantly reviewed recently by Schmid, Uhl, and Buchler.[112] Aprotinin was the first antiprotease drug to be entered into clinical trials. Animal studies showed a positive effect of aprotinin on survival, but human studies have been disappointing.[113] Its lack of efficacy, given its molecular weight, was related to an inability to enter the acinus to exert its effect. Subsequent trials have been conducted with a lower-molecular-weight agent, gabexate mesilate. Although the first studies with this drug were promising, a prospective randomized multicenter study showed no statistical differences between placebo and gabexate mesilate, either in mortality or in complications associated with severe acute pancreatitis.[114] It seems that protease inhibitors are only beneficial when given prophylactically, or very early in the initial phase of pancreatic damage (< 12 hr), as shown in experimental pancreatitis.

Whereas, in interstitial pancreatitis, the prognosis is excellent (< 1% infection, < 1% mortality), in necrotizing pancreatitis, the prognosis is far more severe. In the presence of necrotizing pancreatitis, if there is evidence of clinical deterioration/toxicity, such as fever and leukocytosis, and/or systemic complications, such as shock or progressive respiratory failure, the distinction between sterile necrosis and infected necrosis needs to be made. This can be achieved accurately by a CT-guided percutaneous aspiration of fluid from the necrotic areas. If infected necrosis is confirmed, surgical debridement should be performed; otherwise, the process carries a mortality of at least 30%.[14] If the guided percutaneous aspiration is negative, treatment choices are either continuation of medical therapy or debridement of the sterile necrosis.

The clinical management of sterile necrosis is still a matter of debate. In 1995, Rau *et al.*[115] published a retrospective study comparing the clinical course and outcome of patients with sterile necrotizing pancreatitis treated surgically or nonsurgically. They concluded that most patients with limited and sterile necrosis responded to intensive care treatment and that indication for surgery should be based on persistent or advancing organ complications despite therapy.[115]

It is important to note that there are forms of pancreatic infection in addition to infected necrosis. Pancreatic pseudocysts may become secondary infections, or purulent material may collect in the pancreas approximately 6 weeks after the onset of acute pancreatitis. These two forms of pancreatic abscess can usually be drained successfully by percutaneous or surgical techniques, and in general the mortality is lower than in infected necrosis.[14] Pancreatic infection is the most important cause of fatal outcome in acute pancreatitis. Bacterial contamination of pancreatic necrosis has been shown in 40–70% of patients with necrotizing pancreatitis.[116] Not surprisingly, the therapeutic role of antibiotics in acute pancreatitis has been much discussed. Clinical trials in the 1980s discovered the prophylactic use of antibiotics.[117,118] Moreover, in recent years, new knowledge has accumulated about infected necrosis and about pancreatic penetration by a number of antibiotics.[119,120] Most recent clinical trials are leaning toward antibiotic prophylaxis for necrotizing pancreatitis.[25,121] In a recent randomized, placebo-controlled study, Mithofer *et al.*[116] investigated the effect of two broad-spectrum antibiotics with known high pancreatic bioavailability—imipenem and ciprofloxacin—on experimental acute necrotizing pancreatitis. The antibiotics significantly reduced the number of infected pancreatic specimens and survival was also significantly improved.[116] More clinical studies are needed to apply these experimental results to human pancreatitis before one can confidently recommend the widespread use of such prophylactic antibiotics. Their use in severe pancreatitis, however, seems reasonable.

What about nutrition in acute pancreatitis? Most patients with mild uncomplicated pancreatitis do not benefit from nutritional support.[122] However, in patients with moderate to severe disease, with a course of more than a few days, nutrition seems to be important and generally used. The decision of whether to use parenteral or enteral nutritional support remains controversial.[123,124] Enteral nutrition is much less expensive, maintains gastrointestinal integrity, and preserves the gut mucosal barrier. This may facilitate prevention of systemic sepsis and multisystem organ failure. Ragins *et al.*[125] studied the effect of gastric, duodenal, and jejunal administration of elemental diet in dogs. Jejunal feedings resulted in no significant increase in volume or protein or bicarbonate content of pancreatic secretions. The question remains, however, whether enteral feedings can truly maintain the pancreas "at rest." The data on this subject are still controversial, although jejunal nutrition is increasingly used.[123]

Total parenteral nutrition (TPN) has been shown more consistently to maintain pancreatic rest as compared to jejunal elemental feedings.[124] Disadvantages of TPN are the expense and the possibility of catheter sepsis, although the incidence may be as low as 2.2% if the catheter is managed appropriately.[126] Others cite a higher rate of infection.[127] In general, TPN is likely the preferable route during severe, acute episodes of pancreatic inflammation. However, jejunal feedings should be initiated as soon as the acute inflammation episode begins to resolve.[123–125] Enteral regimens, however, should be avoided in patients with respiratory complications.

Ideally, the patient should be maintained in a positive nitrogen balance. Modified amino acid solutions providing 0.5 to 0.8 g/kg per day of branched-chain amino acids have been shown to improve nitrogen balance. Carbohydrate has been shown to be a safe and effective source of nonprotein calories. Available data indicate that intravenous lipid infusions are safe and effective forms of caloric support in patients with nonhyperlipidemic acute pancreatitis. Provision of 4–8% of total daily caloric needs as linolic and linolenic acid is adequate to prevent essential fatty acid deficiency.[124,128]

In conclusion, it would seem to us that only better understanding of the early pathogenesis of acute pancreatitis secondary to alcohol abuse will lead to more specific early therapy, most likely with inhibitors of pancreatic enzymes.

References

1. Korsten MA, Wilson JS: Alcohol and the pancreas: Clinical aspects and mechanisms of injury. *Alcohol Health Res World* 17:292–298, 1993.
2. Korsten MA, Pirola RC, Lieber CS: Alcohol and the pancreas, in Lieber SC (ed): *Medical and Nutritional Complications of Alcoholism.* New York, Plenum Medical, 1992, pp 341–358.
3. Singh M, Simsek H: Ethanol and the pancreas: Current status. *Gastroenterology* 98:1051–1062, 1990.
4. Clark E: Pancreatitis in acute and chronic alcoholism. *Am J Dig Dis* 9:428–431, 1942.
5. Pitchumoni CS, Glasser M, Saran RM, *et al:* Pancreatic fibrosis in chronic alcoholics and nonalcoholics without clinical pancreatitis. *Am J Gastroenterol* 79:383–388, 1984.
6. Stigendal L, Olsson R: Alcohol consumption pattern and serum lipids in alcoholic cirrhosis and pancreatitis. A comparative study. *Scand J Gastroenterol* 19:582–587, 1984.
7. Suda K, Akai J, Nakamura T: Pancreatic fibrosis in patients with alcoholic dependence syndrome. *Arch Pathol Lab Med* 117:1013–1016, 1993.
8. Goebell H, Bode C, Bastian R, *et al:* Clinical asymptomatic functional disorders of the exocrine pancreas in chronic alcoholics. *Dtsch Med Wochenschr* 95:808–814, 1970.
9. Elsborg L, Bruusgard A, Strandgaard L, *et al:* Endoscopic retrograde pancreatography and the exocrine pancreatic function in chronic alcoholism. *Scand J Gastroenterol* 16:941–944, 1981.
10. Lelbach WK: Epidemiology of alcoholic liver disease, in Popper J, Schaffner F (eds): *Progress in Liver Disease,* vol 5. New York, Grune & Stratton, 1976, pp 494–515.
11. Rubin E, Doria J: Alcoholic cardiomyopathy. *Alcohol Health Res World* 14:277–284, 1996.
12. Malagelada J-R: The pathophysiology of alcoholic pancreatitis. *Pancreas* 1:270–278, 1986.

13. Haber P, Wilson J, Apte M, *et al:* Individual susceptibility to alcoholic pancreatitis: Still an enigma. *J Lab Clin Med* 125:305–312, 1995.
14. Banks PA: Acute pancreatitis: Medical and surgical management. *Am J Gastroenterol* 89:S78–S85, 1994.
15. DiMagno EP: Laboratory assessment of pancreatic impairment, in Haubrich WS, Schaffner F, Berk JE (eds): *Bockus Gastroenterology,* ed 5. Philadelphia, WB Saunders, 1995.
16. Thoeori RF, Blankenberg F: Pancreatic imaging computed tomography and magnetic resonance imaging. *Radiol Clin North Am* 31:1085–1113, 1993.
17. Lucarotti ME, Virjee J, Alderson D: Patient selection and timing of dynamic computed tomography in acute pancreatitis. *Br J Surg* 80:1393–1395, 1993.
18. Bettinger JR, Grendell JH: Intracellular events in the pathogenesis of acute pancreatitis. *Pancreas* 6:S2–S6, 1991.
19. Apte MV, Wilson JS, McCaughan GW, *et al:* Ethanol-induced alterations in messenger RNA levels correlate with glandular content of pancreatic enzymes. *J Lab Clin Med* 125:634–640, 1995.
20. Heath DI, Cruickshank A, Gudgeon M, *et al:* Role of interleukin-6 in mediating the acute phase protein response and potential as an early means of severity assessment in acute pancreatitis. *Gut* 34:41–45, 1993.
21. Van Laethem J-L, Marchant A, Delvaux A, *et al:* Interleukin 10 prevents necrosis in murine experimental acute pancreatitis. *Gastroenterology* 108:1917–1922, 1995.
22. Van Laethem J-L, Deviere J, Resibois A, *et al:* Localization of transforming growth factor β1 and its latent binding protein in human chronic pancreatitis. *Gastroenterology* 108:1873–1881, 1995.
23. Grewal HP, Mohey el Din A, Gaber L, *et al:* Amelioration of the physiologic and biochemical changes of acute pancreatitis using an anti-TNF-α polyclonal antibody. *Am J Surg* 167:214–218, 1994.
24. Buchler M, Malfertheiner P, Fries H, *et al:* Human pancreatic tissue concentration of bactericidal antibodies. *Gastroenterology* 103:1902–1908, 1992.
25. Pederzoli P, Bassi C, Vesentini, *et al:* A randomized multicenter clinical trial of antibiotic prophylaxis of septic complications in acute necrotizing pancreatitis with imipenem. *Surg Gynecol Obstet* 176:480–483, 1993.
26. Bassi C, Pederzoli P, Vesentini S, *et al:* Behavior of antibiotics during human necrotizing pancreatitis. *Antimicrob Agents Chemother* 38:830–836, 1994.
27. Ammann RW, Muellhaupt B: Progression of alcoholic acute to chronic pancreatitis. *Gut* 35:552–556, 1994.
28. Kloppel G, Maillet B: Pathology of acute and chronic pancreatitis. *Pancreas* 8:659–670, 1993.
29. Longnecker DS: Role of the necrosis–fibrosis sequence in the pathogenesis of alcoholic chronic pancreatitis. *Gastroenterology* 111:258–259, 1996.
30. Ammann RW, Hertz PV, Kloppel G: Course of alcoholic chronic pancreatitis: A prospective clinicomorphological long term study. *Gastroenterology* 111:224–231, 1996.
31. Chiari H: Uber die Selbstverdavung des Menschlichen Pancreas. *Z Heilk* 17:69–96, 1896.
32. Niederau C, Fronhoff K, Klonowski H, *et al:* Active pancreatic digestive enzymes show striking differences in their potential to damage isolated rat pancreatic acinar cells. *J Lab Clin Med* 125:265–275, 1995.
33. Laposata EA, Lange LG: Presence of nonoxidative ethanol metabolism in human organs commonly damaged by ethanol abuse. *Science* 231:497–499, 1986.
34. Haber PS, Wilson JC, Apte MV, *et al:* Fatty acid ethyl esters increase rat pancreatic lysosomal fragility. *J Lab Clin Med* 121:759–764, 1993.
35. Lieber CS, De Carli LM, Rubin E: Sequential production of fatty liver, hepatitis and cirrhosis in subhuman primates fed ethanol with adequate diets. *Proc Natl Acad Sci USA* 72:437–441, 1974.
36. Meier PB: Who gets and what causes pancreatitis? *J Lab Clin Med* 125:298–300, 1995.
37. Schenker S, Halff GA: Nutritional therapy in alcoholic liver disease. *Semin Liver Dis* 13:196–209, 1993.

38. Mezey E, Jow E, Slavin RE, *et al:* Pancreatic function and intestinal absorption in chronic alcoholism. *Gastroenterology* 59:657–664, 1970.
39. Pitchumeni CS: Pancreas in primary malnutrition disorders. *Am J Clin Nutr* 9:389–403, 1973.
40. Wilson JS, Bernstein L, Mcdonald C, *et al:* Diet and drinking habits in relation to the development of alcoholic pancreatitis. *Gut* 26:882–887, 1985.
41. Raino OJ: Antecedent long term ethanol consumption in combination with different diets alters the severity of experimental acute pancreatitis in rats. *Gut* 28:64–69, 1987.
42. Tuskamoto H, Towner SJ, Yu GSM, *et al:* Potentiation of ethanol-induced pancreatic injury by dietary fat. *Am J Pathol* 131:246–257, 1988.
43. Pitchumoni CS, Sonnenschein M, Candido FM, *et al:* Nutrition in the pathogenesis of alcoholic pancreatitis. *Am J Clin Nutr* 33:631–636, 1980.
44. Sweiry JH, Mann GE: Role of oxidative stress in the pathogenesis of acute pancreatitis. *Scand J Gastroenterol* 31(Suppl 219):10–15, 1996.
45. Johnson CD, Hoshing S: National statistics for diet, alcohol consumption and chronic pancreatitis in England and Wales, 1960–1988. *Gut* 32:1401–1405, 1991.
46. Haber PS, Wilson JS, Apte MV, *et al:* Lipid intolerance does not account for susceptibility to alcoholic and gallstone pancreatitis. *Gastroenterology* 106:742–748, 1994.
47. Matsumoto M, Takahashi H, Maruyama K, *et al:* Genotypes of alcohol-metabolizing enzymes and the risk for alcoholic chronic pancreatitis in Japanese alcoholics. *Alcohol Clin Exp Res* 20:289A–292A, 1996.
48. Chao Y-C, Young T-H, Chang W-K, *et al:* An investigation of whether polymorphisms of cytochrome P4502E1 are genetic markers of susceptibility to alcoholic end-stage organ damage in a Chinese population. *Hepatology* 22:1409–1414, 1995.
49. Seligson V, Cho JW, Shre T, *et al:* Clinical course and autopsy findings in acute and chronic pancreatitis. *Acta Chir Scand* 148:269–274, 1987.
50. Angelini G, Mergio F, Degani G, *et al:* Association of chronic alcoholic liver disease and pancreatic disease: A prospective study. *Am J Gastroenterol* 80:998–1003, 1985.
51. Jalovaara P, Apapa M: Alcohol and acute pancreatitis. An experimental study in the rat. *Scand J Gastroenterol* 13:703–709, 1978.
52. Goff JS: The effect of ethanol on the pancreatic duct sphincter of Oddi. *Am J Gastroenterol* 88:656–660, 1993.
53. Guelrud M, Mendoza S, Rossiter G, *et al:* Effect of local instillation of alcohol on the sphincter of Oddi motor activity: Combined ERCP and manometric study. *Gastrointest Endosc* 37:428–432, 1991.
54. Geenen JE, Hogan WJ, Dodds WJ, *et al:* Intraluminal pressure recording from the human sphincter of Oddi. *Gastroenterology* 78:317–324, 1980.
55. Nagata A, Homma T, Tamai K, *et al:* A study of chronic pancreatitis by serial endoscopic pancreatography. *Gastroenterology* 81:884–891, 1981.
56. Reber HA, Roberts C, Way LW: The pancreatic duct mucosal barrier. *Am J Surg* 137:128–134, 1979.
57. Wedgwood KR, Adler G, Kern H, *et al:* Effects of oral agents on pancreatic duct permeability: A model of acute alcoholic pancreatitis. *Dig Dis Sci* 31:1081–1088, 1986.
58. Luther R, Niederau C, Niederau M, *et al:* Influence of ductal pressure and infusates on activity and subcellular distribution of lysosomal enzymes in the rat pancreas. *Gastroenterology* 109:573–581, 1995.
59. Sarles H: Chronic calcifying pancreatitis—chronic alcoholic pancreatitis. *Gastroenterology* 66:604–616, 1974.
60. Sarles H, Figarella C, Tisurina O, *et al:* Chronic calcifying pancreatitis (CCP). Mechanism of formation of the lesions. New data and critical study, in Fitzgerald PJ, Morrison AB (eds): *The Pancreas,* International Academy of Pathology Monograph. Baltimore, Williams & Wilkins, 1980, pp 48–66.
61. Grendell JH, Cello JP: Chronic pancreatitis, in Sleisenger MH, Fordtran JS (eds): *Gastrointestinal Disease, Pathophysiology, Diagnosis, Management,* ed 5. Philadelphia, WB Saunders, 1993, pp 1654–1681.

62. Calderon-Attas P, Furnelle J, Christophe J: *In vitro* effects of ethanol and ethanol metabolism in the rat pancreas. *Biochem Biophys Acta* 620:387–399, 1980.
63. Nordback IH, MacGowan S, Potter JJ, *et al:* The role of acetaldehyde in the pathogenesis of acute alcoholic pancreatitis. *Ann Surg* 214:671–678, 1991.
64. Patel AG, Toyama MT, Alvarez C, *et al:* Pancreatic interstitial pH in human and feline chronic pancreatitis. *Gastroenterology* 109:1639–1645, 1995.
65. Lerch MM, Saluga AK, Dawra R, *et al:* The effect of chloroquine administration on two experimental models of acute pancreatitis. *Gastroenterology* 104:1768–1779, 1993.
66. Fallon MB, Gorelick FS, Anderson JM, *et al:* Effect of cerulein hyperstimulation on the paracellular barrier of rat exocrine pancreas. *Gastroenterology* 108:1863–1872, 1995.
67. Schoenberg MH, Buchler M, Beger HG: The role of oxygen radicals in experimental acute pancreatitis. *Free Radic Biol Med* 12:515–522, 1992.
68. Niederau C, Niederau M, Borchard F, *et al:* Effects of antioxidants and free radical scavengers in three different models of acute pancreatitis. *Pancreas* 7:486–496, 1992.
69. Iimuro Y, Bradford BU, Gao W, *et al:* Detection of α-hydroxyethyl free radical adducts in the pancreas after chronic exposure to alcohol in the rat. *Mol Pharmacol* 50:656–661, 1996.
70. Braganza JM, Rinderknecht H: Free radicals and acute pancreatitis. *Gastroenterology* 94:1111–1112, 1988.
71. Uden S, Main C, Hunt LP, *et al:* Placebo-controlled double-blind trial of antioxidant supplements in patients with recurrent pancreatitis. *Clin Sci* 77(Suppl 21):26–27, 1989.
72. Dabrowski A, Gabryelewicz A: Nitric oxide contributes to multiorgan oxidative stress in acute experimental pancreatitis. *Scand J Gastroenterol* 29:943–948, 1994.
73. Molero Z, Guarner F, Salas A, *et al:* Nitric oxide modulates pancreatic basal secretion and response to cerulein in the rat: Effects in acute pancreatitis. *Gastroenterology* 108:1855–1862, 1995.
74. Kusske AM, Rongione AJ, Reber HA: Cytokines and acute pancreatitis. *Gastroenterology* 110:639–642, 1996.
75. Sandoval D, Gukovskaya A, Reavey P, *et al:* The role of neutrophils and platelet-activating factor in mediating experimental pancreatitis. *Gastroenterology* 111:1081–1091, 1996.
76. Whitcomb DC, Preston RA, Aston CE, *et al:* A gene for hereditary pancreatitis maps to chromosome 7q35. *Gastroenterology* 110:1975–1980, 1996.
77. Walsh JH: Tripping up trypsin: Supermutant causes hereditary pancreatitis. *Gastroenterology* 112:3–4, 1997.
78. Banks PA: Modern concepts in pancreatitis. *Mt Sinai J Med* 60:170–174, 1993.
79. Chauffard MA: Le cancer du corps du pancreas. *Bull Acad Med* 60:242–255, 1908.
80. Schenker S, Balint J, Schiff L: Differential diagnosis of jaundice: Report of a prospective study of 61 proved cases. *Am J Dig Dis* 7:449–463, 1960.
81. Soergel KH: Acute pancreatitis, in Sleissenger MH, Fordtran JS (eds): *Gastroeintestinal Disease, Pathophysiology, Diagnosis, Management,* ed 5. Philadelphia, WB Saunders, 1993, pp 1628–1653.
82. Gullo L: Chronic nonpathological hyperamylasemia of pancreatic origin. *Gastroenterology* 110:1905–1906, 1996.
83. Balthazar EJ, Freeny PC, vanSonnenberg E: Imaging and intervention in acute pancreatitis. *Radiology* 193:297–306, 1994.
84. Bradley EL III: A clinically based classification system for acute pancreatitis. *Arch Surg* 128:586–590, 1993.
85. Agarwal N, Pitchumoni CS: Assessment of severity in acute pancreatitis. *Am J Gastroenterol* 86:1385–1391, 1991.
86. Bank S, Wise L, Gersten M: Risk factors in acute pancreatitis. *Am J Gastroenterol* 78:637–640, 1983.
87. Ranson JHC, Pasternack BS: Statistical methods for quantifying the severity of clinical acute pancreatitis. *J Surg Res* 22:79–91, 1977.
88. Agarwal N, Pitchumoni CS: Simplified prognostic criteria in acute pancreatitis. *Pancreas* 1:69–73, 1986.

89. Knaus WA, Draper EA, Wagner DP, Zimmerman JE: APACHE II, A severity of disease classification system. *Crit Care Med* 13:818–829, 1985.
90. Fan S, Lai ECS, Mok FPT, *et al:* Prediction of the severity of acute pancreatitis. *Am J Surg* 166:262–268, 1993.
91. Balthazar EJ, Robinson DL, Megibow AJ, *et al:* Acute pancreatitis: Value of CT in establishing prognosis. *Radiology* 174:331–336, 1990.
92. Foitzik T, Bass DG, Schmidt J, *et al:* Intravenous contrast medium accentuates the severity of acute necrotizing pancreatitis in the rat. *Gastroenterology* 106:207–214, 1994.
93. Vesentini S, Bassi C, Talamini G, *et al:* Prospective comparison of C-reactive protein, Ranson score and contrast-enhanced computed tomography in the prediction of septic complications of acute pancreatitis. *Br J Surg* 80:755–757, 1993.
94. London NSM, Neoptolemus JP, Lovelle J, *et al:* Contrast-enhanced abdominal computed tomography scanning and prediction of severity of acute pancreatitis: A prospective study. *Br J Surg* 76:268–272, 1989.
95. Windsor JA, Fearon KCH, Ross JA, *et al:* Role of serum endotoxin and antiendotoxin core antibody levels in predicting the development of multiple organ failure in acute pancreatitis. *Br J Surg* 80:1042–1046, 1993.
96. Iovanna JL, Keim V, Nordback I, *et al:* Serum levels of pancreatitis-associated protein as indicators of the course of acute pancreatitis. *Gastroenterology* 106:728–734, 1994.
97. Kemppainen E, Sand J, Puolakkainen P, *et al:* Pancreatitis-associated protein as an early marker of acute pancreatitis. *Gut* 39:675–678, 1996.
98. Schmid SW, Uhl W, Steinle A, *et al:* Human pancreas-specific protein. *Int J Pancreatol* 19:165–170, 1996.
99. Yamamoto K, Pousette A, Phoebe CH, *et al:* Isolation of a e-DNA encoding a human serum marker for acute pancratitis. *J Biol Chem* 267:2575–2581, 1992.
100. Skaife P, Kingsnorth AN: Acute pancreatitis: Assessment and management. *Postgrad Med J* 72:277–283, 1996.
101. Loser Chr, Folsch UR: A concept of treatment in acute pancreatitis—results of controlled trials, and future developments. *Hepatogastroenterology* 40:569–573, 1993.
102. Fuller RK, Loveland J, Frankel MH: An evaluation of the efficacy of nasogastric suction treatment in alcoholic pancreatitis. *Am J Gastroenterol* 75:349–353, 1981.
103. Navarro S, Ros E, Aused R, *et al:* Comparison of fasting, nasogastric suction and cimetidine in the treatment of acute pancreatitis. *Digestion* 30:224–230, 1984.
104. Loiudice TA, Lang J, Mehta H, *et al:* Treatment of acute alcoholic pancreatitis: The roles of cimetidine and nasogastric suction. *Am J Gastroenterol* 79:553–558, 1984.
105. Sarr MG, Sanfey H, Cameron JL: Prospective, randomized trial of nasogastric suction in patients with acute pancreatitis. *Surgery* 100:500–504, 1986.
106. Goff JS, Feinberg LE, Brugge WR: A randomized trial comparing cimetidine to nasogastric suction in acute pancreatitis. *Dig Dis Sci* 27:1085–1088, 1982.
107. Broe PJ, Zinner MJ, Cameron JL: A clinical trial of cimetidine in acute pancreatitis. *Surg Gynecol Obstet* 154:13–16, 1982.
108. Niederau C, Schulz H-U: Current conservative treatment of acute pancreatitis: Evidence from animal and human studies. *Hepatogastroenterology* 40:538–549, 1993.
109. Mayer D, McMahon MJ, Corfield AP, *et al:* Controlled clinical trial of peritoneal lavage for the treatment of severe acute pancreatitis. *N Engl J Med* 312:399–404, 1985.
110. Ihse I, Evander A, Holmberg JT, *et al:* Influence of peritoneal lavage on objective prognostic signs in acute pancreatitis. *Ann Surg* 204:122–127, 1986.
111. Ranson JHC, Berman RS: Long peritoneal lavage decreases pancreatic sepsis in acute pancreatitis. *Ann Surg* 211:708–718, 1990.
112. Schmid S, Uhl W, Buchler MW: Protease–antiprotease interactions and the rationale for therapeutic protease inhibitors. *Scand J Gastroenterol* 31(Suppl 219):47–50, 1996.
113. Steinberg WM, Schlesselmar SE: Treatment of acute pancreatitis: Comparison of animal and human studies. *Gastroenterology* 93:1420–1427, 1987.

114. Buchler M, Malfertheiner P, Uhl W, *et al:* Gabexate mesilate in human acute pancreatitis. *Gastroenterology* 104:1165–1170, 1993.
115. Rau B, Pralle U, Uhl W, *et al:* Management of sterile necrosis in instances of severe acute pancreatitis. *J Am Coll Surg* 191:279–288, 1995.
116. Mithofer K, Fernandez-Del Castillo C, Ferraro MJ, *et al:* Antibiotic treatment improves survival in experimental acute necrotizing pancreatitis. *Gastroenterology* 110:232–240, 1996.
117. Byrne JJ, Treadwell TL: Treatment of pancreatitis—When do antibiotics have a role. *Postgrad Med* 85:333–339, 1989.
118. Bradley EL: Antibiotics in acute pancreatitis—Current status and future directions. *Am J Surg* 158:472–477, 1989.
119. Buchler M, Malfertheiner P, Friess H, *et al:* Human pancreatic tissue concentration of bactericidal antibiotics. *Gastroenterology* 103:1902–1908, 1992.
120. Isenmann R, Friess H, Schlegel P, *et al:* Penetration of ciprofloxacin into the human pancreas. *Infection* 22:343–346, 1994.
121. Sainio V, Kemppainen E, Puolakkainen P, *et al:* Early antibiotic treatment in acute necrotising pancreatitis. *Lancet* 346(8976):663–667, 1995.
122. Sax HC, Warner BW, Talamini MA, *et al:* Early total parenteral nutrition in acute pancreatitis: Lack of beneficial effects. *Am J Surg* 153:117–124, 1987.
123. Pisters PWT, Ranson JHC: Nutritional support for acute pancreatitis. *Surgery* 175:275–284, 1992.
124. Havala T, Shronts E, Cerra F: Nutritional support in acute pancreatitis. *Gastroenterol Clin North Am* 18:525–542, 1989.
125. Ragins H, Levenson SM, Signer R, *et al:* Intrajejunal administration of an elemental diet at neutral pH avoids pancreatic stimulation. *Am J Surg* 126:606–614, 1973.
126. Copeland EM, McFadyen BJ, McGowan C, *et al:* The use of hyperalimentation in patients with potential sepsis. *Surg Gynecol Obstet* 138:377–380, 1974.
127. Grant JP, Jarnes S, Grabouski V, *et al:* Total parenteral nutrition in pancreatic disease. *Ann Surg* 200:627–631, 1984.
128. Edelman K, Valenzuela JE: Effect of intravenous lipid on human pancreatic secretion. *Gastroenterology* 85:1063–1066, 1983.

3

Alcohol and Cancer

Helmut K. Seitz, Gudrun Pöschl, and Ulrich A. Simanowski

Abstract. A great number of epidemiological data have identified chronic alcohol consumption as a significant risk factor for upper alimentary tract cancer, including cancer of the oropharynx, larynx, and the esophagus, and for the liver. In contrast to those organs, the risk by which alcohol consumption increases cancer in the large intestine and in the breast is much smaller. However, although the risk is lower, carcinogenesis can be enhanced with relatively low daily doses of ethanol. Considering the high prevalence of these tumors, even a small increase in cancer risk is of great importance, especially in those individuals who exhibit a higher risk for other reasons. The epidemiological data on alcohol and other organ cancers are controversial and there is at present not enough evidence for a significant association.

Although the exact mechanisms by which chronic alcohol ingestion stimulates carcinogenesis are not known, experimental studies in animals support the concept that ethanol is not a carcinogen, but under certain experimental conditions is a cocarcinogen and/or (especially in the liver) a tumor promoter. The metabolism of ethanol leads to the generation of acetaldehyde and free radicals. These highly reactive compounds bind rapidly to cell constituents and possibly to DNA. Acetaldehyde decreases DNA repair mechanisms and the methylation of cytosine in DNA. It also traps glutathione, an important peptide in detoxification. Furthermore, it leads to chromosomal aberrations and seems to be associated with tissue damage and secondary compensatory hyperregeneration. More recently, the finding of considerable production of acetaldehyde by gastrointestinal bacteria was reported. Other mechanims by which alcohol stimulates carcinogenesis include the induction of cytochrome P4502E1, associated with an enhanced activation of various procarcinogens present in alcoholic beverages, in association with tobacco smoke and in diets, a change in the metabolism and distribution of carcinogens, alterations in cell cycle behavior such as cell cycle duration leading to hyperregeneration, nutritional deficiencies such as methyl, vitamin A, folate, pyrridoxalphosphate, zinc and selenium deficiency, and alterations of the immune system, eventually resulting in an increased susceptibility to certain viral infections such as hepatitis B virus and hepatitis C virus. In addition, local mechanisms in the upper

Helmut K. Seitz, Gudrun Pöschl, and Ulrich A. Simanowski • Laboratory of Alcohol Research, Liver Disease and Nutrition, and Department of Medicine, Salem Medical Center, D-69121 Heidelberg, Germany.

Recent Developments in Alcoholism, Volume 14: The Consequences of Alcoholism, edited by Galanter. Plenum Press, New York, 1998.

gastrointestinal tract and in the rectum may be of particular importance. Such mechanisms lead to tissue injury such as cirrhosis of the liver, a major prerequisite for hepatocellular carcinoma. Thus, all these mechanisms, functioning in concert, actively modulate carcinogenesis, leading to its stimulation.

1. Introduction

The concept that chronic alcohol consumption enhances cancer risk in certain organs is not new. Almost a century ago, French pathologists discovered the association between heavy chronic alcohol consumption and the development of esophageal cancer.[1] This early observation was followed by a great number of epidemiological studies, which showed a striking positive correlation between chronic alcohol ingestion and the occurrence of cancer in the oropharynx, larynx, and esophagus. Alcohol intake also favors the development of liver cancer in the cirrhotic liver. In addition, during the last decade countless numbers of case–control and prospective studies have identified the large intestine, especially the rectum and the female breast, as additional target organs, in which alcohol even at lower doses stimulates cancer growth. In 1978, the first workshop on Alcohol and Cancer was held at the National Institutes of Health (NIH), and at this time the mechanisms by which alcohol affects carcinogenesis were completely unclear. Meanwhile, intensive research has focused on such mechanisms and has elucidated some cocarcinogenic and promoter effects of ethanol. This chapter will summarize the epidemiology on alcohol and cancer. However, major emphasis will be placed on the possible mechanisms by which chronic alcohol consumption stimulates carcinogenesis.

2. Epidemiology

Interpretation of the epidemiological data on alcohol and cancer may be difficult, especially when the ethanol effect is borderline. Factors that may influence these results are the types of beverages offered by different manufacturers in various geographic regions. Conclusions drawn from sales data may be problematic, as in the case of Luxembourg where many people from surrounding countries buy alcohol because of the lower prices.

2.1. *Upper Alimentary Tract Cancer*

In France, Lamu[1] reported at the beginning of this century on absinthe drinkers having an increased risk of developing esophageal cancer. Meanwhile, a great number of epidemiological studies have demonstrated a significant correlation between alcoholism and the development of oropharyngeal, laryngeal, and esophageal cancer.[2] It was demonstrated that heavy drinkers of highly concentrated alcoholic beverages have a 10- to 12-fold increased risk to develop tumors in the mouth, pharynx, and larynx, while this risk was significantly lower when beer and wine were consumed.[3] In addition, alcohol abuse is often associated with heavy smoking. These factors have a synergistic effect on carcinogenesis in the upper alimentary tract. In a carefully designed French study, Tuyns[4] was able to demonstrate that alcohol consumption of more than 80 g/day (approximately 1 bottle of wine) increases the relative risk (RR) of esophageal cancer by a factor of 18, while smoking alone of more than 20 cigarettes has an increased RR by a factor of 5. Both together stimulate the risk synergistically by a factor of 44.[4] It was calculated that 76% of all cancers could be prevented by avoiding smoking and alcohol consumption.[2] More recently, an epidemiological study by Maier and co-workers[5] showed that 90% of all patients with head and neck cancer consumed alcohol regularly in amounts almost double the amount in a control group. They found a significant dose–response relationship. If the RR for a person with a daily alcohol consumption of 25 g was assumed to be 1, the controlled RR increases steadily with increasing alcohol dosage and reaches a value of 32.4 when 100 g/day of alcohol were consumed. These RR values are comparable with those reported by others. Tuyns and co-workers[6] found an RR of 12.5 for hypopharynx carcinoma, 10.6 for epipharynx carcinoma, 2.0 for supraglottic larynx carcinoma, and 3.4 for glottic and subglottic larynx carcinoma when 121 g alcohol was consumed daily. Furthermore, Bruguere and co-workers[7] found a significantly higher RR for oral cancer, which was 13.5, when 100–159 g alcohol were consumed daily. They found an RR of 15.2 for oropharynx carcinoma and 28.6 for hypopharynx carcinoma. It is noteworthy that even with those high daily alcohol dosages, the alcohol-associated cancer risk is not saturable. If alcohol is consumed excessively with more than 160 g/day, there is a further increase in cancer risk (oral cancer RR = 70; oropharyngal cancer RR = 70; hypopharyngal cancer RR = 143). Chronic alcohol consumption and smoking have an independent risk on cancer development in the head and neck area. Tuyns *et al.*[6] emphasized that 68% of the risk of those tumors are solely due to alcohol. As expected, smoking has a higher risk compared to alcohol abuse for the oral cavity and the pharynx, while this relation is reversed for the esophagus.

2.2. *Liver Cancer*

Cirrhosis of the liver is the major prerequisite for the development of hepatocellular cancer (HCC). Since infection with hepatitis B (HBV) and C virus (HCV) also leads to cirrhosis of the liver followed by an increased occurrence of HCC, and since alcoholics are often infected by those viruses, the exact risk of alcohol as compared to HBV and HCV etiology in the development of HCC is still not exactly defined. Almost all prospective and retrospective case–control studies in Western countries indicate that the incidence of HCC among alcoholics is above the expected level.[8] However, variable prevalences of HCC in alcoholic cirrhosis have been reported. With some exceptions, generally lower incidence rates have been reported in Western countries (<15%), which have showed some increased trends within the last two decades, while in Japan the prevalence of HCC in alcoholic cirrhosis increased at the rate of 1.0% per year during 1976 to 1985, reaching a 25% incidence rate.[9] The higher prevalence in Asia may be linked to the increased concomitant viral infection. The observed increase of the incidence of HCC worldwide may be related partially to the prolongation of survival time for patients with alcoholic cirrhosis because of improved treatment.

Although the effect of abstinence on the development of HCC was variable in various studies, it has been reported that after cessation of drinking the risk to develop HCC increased; therefore, it was speculated that this may be due to changes in cell regeneration after alcohol withdrawal which will be discussed below. However, abstinence improves hepatocellular damage due to alcohol and prolongs survival time significantly, which by itself increases the chance to develop HCC.

2.3. Colorectal Cancer

In 1974, Breslow and Enstrom[10] were the first to consider the possibility of an association between beer consumption and the occurrence of rectal cancer. To date, 7 correlational studies, 34 case–control studies, and 17 prospective cohort studies have been performed to elucidate the role of alcohol in the development of colorectal cancer.[11] An association was found in 5 of the 7 correlational studies and in half of the 34 case–control studies. In the majority of the case–control studies (10 out of 12) using community controls, such a correlation was detected, suggesting that the absence of an association when hospital controls were used is due to a high prevalence of alcohol consumption–alcohol-related diseases in hospital controls. Eleven of the 17 cohort studies also demonstrate a positive association with alcohol. A positive trend with respect to dose–response was found in five of the ten case–control studies and in all prospective cohort studies in which this factor has been taken into consideration.

Six studies have investigated the effect of chronic alcohol consumption on the occurrence of adenomatous polyps of the large bowel.[11] In five of these, such a correlation was observed. In addition, an RR increase of hyperplastic polyps of the distal colon and rectum was also observed by increasing amounts of alcohol.[12] When more than 30 g alcohol per day were consumed, the RR for men was 1.8 and for women 2.5.

Finally, alcohol may influence the adenoma–carcinoma sequence at different early steps, as very recently reported by Boutron *et al.*[13] In conclusion, epidemiological data are still somewhat controversial, but it seems that chronic ethanol ingestion even at low daily intake (10–40 g), especially consumed as beer, results in a 1.5- to 3.5-fold risk of rectal and to a lesser extent of colonic cancer in both sexes, but predominantly in males. Most recently these data have been reviewed in detail by a panel of European experts at a World Health Organization (WHO) Consensus Conference on Nutrition and Colorectal Cancer in Stuttgart, Germany, and it was stated that more than 20 g alcohol per day increase the risk of colorectal cancer.

2.4. *Breast Cancer*

During the last decade a great number of epidemiological studies have identified alcohol as one of several risk factors for breast cancer, usually but not always showing a 1.2- to 2.0-fold RR, as reported in 1994 in a large meta-analysis of the data available at this time.[14] Strong evidence was found supporting a dose–response relation in both case–control and follow-up epidemiological data. The RR of breast cancer at an alcohol intake of 24 g of absolute alcohol per day relative to nondrinkers was found to be 1.4 in the case–control and 1.7 in the prospective studies. In a recent review article on breast cancer, various risk factors for breast cancer were compared and it was interesting to note that the RR for breast cancer was about 2 when three drinks or more per day were consumed as compared to an RR of 3 associated with the exposure to radiation due to the atomic bomb explosion in Hiroshima.[15] At the 8th Congress of the International Society for Biomedical Research on Alcoholism (ISBRA), a symposium was held on the interaction between alcohol and other risk factors for breast cancer and it was concluded that there is enough epidemiological evidence that supports a modest association between alcohol ingestion and breast cancer risk.[16] An international panel of experts at a recent WHO Consensus Conference on Nutrition and Cancer in Stuttgart, Germany, came to a similar conclusion.

2.5. *Other Organs*

Epidemiological research also has found other organs in which chronic alcohol consumption increases cancer risk, including stomach, pancreas, lungs, bladder, prostate, and skin (melanoma). However, these data are controversial and to date there is not enough evidence to link chronic alcohol consumption as a risk factor to those cancer sites.

3. Animal Experiments

The results of animal experiments on alcohol and cancer depend on the experimental design, the type of carcinogen used, and the route, time, duration, and dosage of carcinogen and alcohol administration. One of the most important factors seems to be the means of alcohol application. If alcohol is added to the drinking water, ethanol intake may be extremely low, but nutritional deficiencies may occur that can influence carcinogenesis. The administration of ethanol as a liquid diet, first introduced by Lieber and DeCarli in 1970, guarantees an adequate ethanol intake and considers nutritional factors.

Table I summarizes the effect of chronic ethanol consumption on chemically induced upper digestive tract carcinogenesis. It shows that local application of alcohol on the oral and esophageal mucosa increases the occurrence of tumors probably due to an irritational effect of alcohol.[17–21] When ethanol was given systemically, in most of the studies,[22–30] with some exceptions,[26,27,29,31,32] a stimulatory effect on carcinogenesis was noted. Surprisingly, both an enhancement of tumor initiation[24] and promotion[29] has been reported.

Table II summarizes the effect of chronic alcohol consumption on colorectal cancer. In two of the eight studies ethanol was given in the drinking water,[33,34] and the results of these experiments therefore have to be questioned. When the two procarcinogens dimethylhydrazine (DMH) and azoxymethane (AOM) were used to induce colorectal tumors, different results were reported depending on the experimental conditions.[35–38] In these studies it is important to note that both compounds need metabolic activation by cytochrome P450-dependent microsomal enzymes to become carcinogenic. The results of these studies depend on the ethanol dose used and on the timing of ethanol administration. The conclusions derived from those experiments are as follows:

1. The modulation of experimental colonic tumorigenesis by chronic dietary beer and ethanol consumption is because of alcohol rather than to other beverage constituents.
2. The tumorigenesis in the right and left colorectum is affected differently by alcohol and may depend on the levels of alcohol consumption. Thus, high alcohol intake (18–33% of total calories) inhibits carcinogenesis in the right colon and has no effect on the left colon, while lower ethanol consumption (9–12% of total calories) enhances tumor development in the left colon without effect on the right colon.
3. Ethanol affects carcinogenesis during the preinduction and/or induction phase, including carcinogen metabolism, but not in the postinduction phase (promotion).
4. An interaction between ethanol and procarcinogen metabolism does occur and this may influence tumor incidences.

It must be emphasized that in one experiment with DMH, ethanol ingestion only enhanced tumor development in the rectum, but not in the remaining large intestine.[35] In this study, ethanol was given during acclimatization and initiation, but at the time of procarcinogen application ethanol was not present in the body. In a similar study by McGarrity and co-workers,[36] these results could not be confirmed. In addition, in two other animal experiments, the primary carcinogen acetoxymethylmethylnitrosamine (AMMN) was used to induce rectal tumors.[39,40] This carcinogen does not need metabolic activa-

Table I. Influence of Ethanol on Chemically Induced Upper Digestive Tract Carcinogenesis

Species	Carcinogen	Ethanol application	Target organ	Ethanol effect	Reference
Local effect on skin and mucosa[a]					
Mouse	BP, oral	As a solvent	Esophagus	Stimulation	17
Hamster	DMBA, local	As a solvent	Oral Mucosa	Stimulation	18
Hamster	DMBA, local	As a solvent	Oral mucosa	Stimulation	19
Mouse	DMBA, local	As a solvent	Skin	Stimulation	20
Hamster	DMBA, local	Before ethanol diet	Oral mucosa	Stimulation	21
Digestive Tract					
Rat	DENA, i.g.	30% i.g., with carcinogen	Esophagus	Stimulation	22
Rat	NMBA,i.g.	4% DW, continuously, Zn-deficiency	Esophagus	Stimulation	23
Rat	MPNA, s.c.	25% DW, continuously	Esophagus	No effect	31
Rat	NNP, in diet	50% intrapharyngeal and 10% DW	Esophagus	No effect	32
Rat	NMBA	5% LD, before and with carcinogen	Esophagus	Inhibition	29
Rat	NMBA	5% LD, after carcinogen	Esophagus	Stimulation	29
Rat	DMNA, p.o.	10% DW with carcinogen	Esophagus	Stimulation	24
Mouse	NMBA, i.g.	6% LD, after carcinogen	Esophagus	Stimulation	25
Hamster	NPYR, i.p.	5% LD, before and with carcinogen	Nasal cavity	Stimulation	26
Rat	NNN, p.o.	6% LD, before and with carcinogen	Nasal cavity	Stimulation	27
Rat	NNN, s.c.	6% LD, before and with carcinogen	Nasal cavity	No effect	27
Hamster	NNN, i.p.	5% LD, before and with carcinogen	Trachea	No effect	26
Mouse	DENA, p.o.	10% DW with carcinogen	Forestomach	Stimulation	28
Rat	MNNG, p.o.	20% i.p., after carcinogen	Stomach	Stimulation	30

[a]BP, Benzo-α-pyrene; DMBA, dimethylbenzanthracene; DENA, diethylnitrosamine; MPNA, methylphenylnitrosamine; NNP, *N*-Nitrosopiperidine; NPYR, *N*-nitrosopyrrolidine, NNN, *N*-Nitrosonornicotin; DMNA, dimethylnitrosoamine; NMBA, nitrosomethylbenzylamine; LD, liquid diet; DW, drinking water; i.g., introgastrically; i.p., intraperitoneally; p.o., orally; s.c., subcutaneously.

tion to exert its carcinogenic effect. It is applied locally to the rectal mucosa of rats and the animals were endoscoped regularly. Since chronic ethanol administration either as liquid diet or intragastrically accelerates the appearance of rectal tumors induced by AMMN, it seems most likely that alcohol enhances carcinogenesis, at least in part, by local mechanisms in the rectal mucosa and not only by increasing the activation of procarcinogens.

Most animal experiments with respect to hepatocarcinogenesis have been performed with nitrosamines as inducing agents. Almost all these studies showed an inhibition of carcinogenesis with alcohol, but on the other hand an enhancement in the incidence of extrahepatic tumors such as those in the nasal cavity, trachea, and esophagus.[22,26,27,41–43] Only if additional manipulations were added, such as the administration of a methyl-deficient[44] or low-carbohydrate[45] diet or partial hepatectomy,[46] was hepatic carcinogenesis stimulated by alcohol. A striking enhancement of hepatic carcinogenesis was also observed

Table II. Effect of Ethanol on Chemically Induced Colorectal Carcinogenesis in Rats

Carcinogen	Ethanol administration	Ethanol effect	Reference
DMH, s.c.	6% l.d. (36% total calories) preinduction	Increased rectal but not colonic tumors	35
DMH, s.c.	5% DW, induction	No effect	33
DMH, s.c.	5% DW, preinduction/induction	No effect	34
DMH, s.c.	6% LD (36% total calories), preinduction	No effect	36
AMMN, i.r.	6% LD (36% total calories), preinduction/induction	Increased rectal tumors	39
AOM, s.c.	LD (11%, 22%, 33% total calories), preinduction/induction, postinduction	Inhibition of tumor development in the left but less than in the right colon. Higher ethanol intake has a stronger inhibitory effect. No effect when ethanol is given in the postinduction phase	37
AOM, s.c.	LD (9%, 18% total calories ethanol), (12%, 23% total calories beer), preinduction/ induction	High ethanol inhibits tumors in the right, but not in the left colon, while low ethanol enhances tumors in the left colon, but not in the right colon. No effect of beer	38
AMMN, i.r.	i.g. (4.8g/kg body weight per day), preinduction/induction	Increased rectal tumors Carcinogenesis was further stimulated when cyanamide, an acetaldehyde dehydrogenase inhibitor, was administered additionally	40

DMH, 1,2-dimethylhydrazine; AMMN, azetoxymethyl-methylnitrosamine; AOM, azoxymethane; s.c., subcutaneously; i.r., intrarectally; i.g., intragastrically; LD, liquid diet; DW, drinking water.

when alcohol and the procarcinogen were given strictly alternatively to avoid an interaction between alcohol and carcinogen metabolism.[47,48]

Animal experiments with respect to breast cancer are limited. There is no consistent evidence that alcohol enhances the formation of either spontaneous or of dimethylbenzanthracene (DMBA)-induced mammary tumors when ethanol is consumed continuously at both stages of tumor development.[16] When ethanol consumption is limited to only the initiation or promotion stage, there is evidence that ethanol may be a weak cocarcinogen and/or promoter in the methylnitrosourea (MNO) and DMBA-induced mammary tumor models.[49,50] However, there is no consistent dose–response relationship between alcohol intake and carcinogenesis. Ethanol also seems to augment mammary tumor progression.[51]

4. General Mechanisms by Which Alcohol Modulates Carcinogenesis

Experiments in which alcohol was given chronically to rodents have shown that alcohol per se is not a carcinogen, since animals with a chronic lifelong exposure to alcohol do not develop more cancer than controls.[52] Since ethanol modulates chemically induced carcinogenesis, it has to be defined as a tumor promoter and/or cocarcinogen. Multiple mechanisms increase alcohol-associated cancer development. (Fig. 1) including the consequences of alcohol metabolism, cytochrome P4502E1 (CYP2E1) induction, modulation of cell regeneration, and nutritional deficiencies, which may be important for a variety of tissues but differ quantitatively and qualitatively locally. Since these factors may be involved in alcohol-associated cocarcinogenesis in general, they are discussed in this section. In addition, more specific local-acting pathogenic mechanisms in carcinogenesis linked to chronic alcohol consumption are discussed later.

4.1. Sources of Carcinogen Intake

Alcoholics who smoke have an increased carcinogen intake with two sources of carcinogens. First, certain alcoholic beverages, such as certain types of whisky, vermouth, sherry, beer, and wine, may contain carcinogenic substances including polycyclic hydrocarbons, nitrosamines, and asbestos fibers.[53] Second, an increased carcinogen load through smoking, since tobacco smoke contains a great number of various carcinogens including polycyclic hydrocarbons and nitrosamines. In addition, dietary carcinogens have also been considered. An epidemiological study on aflatoxin exposure demonstrated that the daily consumption of 24 g of ethanol or more increases the risk of developing HCC induced by 4 μg of dietary aflatoxin B1 (AFB1) by a factor of 35.[54] Finally, simultanous exposure to vinylchloride (VC) at the workplace and to alcohol enhances the occurrence of HCC in humans.[55]

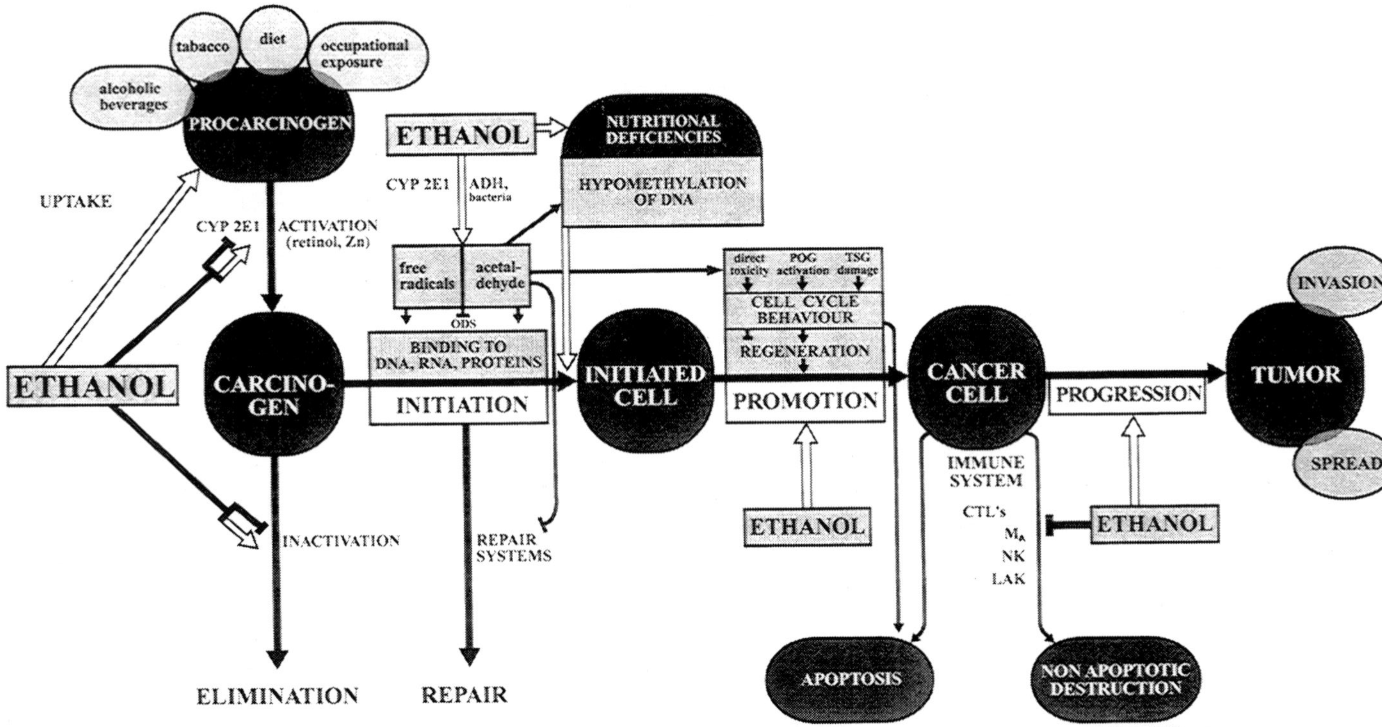

Figure 1. Effect of ethanol on carcinogenesis. Ethanol affects procarcinogen activation and possibly carcinogen inactivation. It also leads to an increased uptake of carcinogens into the cells. Ethanol is metabolized by CYP2E2 and ADH to free radicals and AA, both of which can bind to cell macromolecules including DNA, especially since detoxification systems are depressed by ethanol. Alcohol also leads to nutritional deficiencies, some of which (including vitamin A, E, and zinc deficiency) stimulate carcinogenesis. Methyl and folate deficiency together with the action of AA result in hypomethylation of DNA; in addition, AA inhibits the nuclear repair system. Direct toxicity (alcohol/AA) modulates cell cycle behavior, resulting in regenerativity changes. Alcohol also acts as a promoter, particularly in the liver, leads to an inhibition of the immune system, and may stimulate cancer progression (for more details see text). Abbreviations: AA, acetaldehyde; CYP2E1, cytochrome P4502E1; ADH, alcohol dehydrogenase; ODS, oxidative defense system; POG, proto-oncogen; TSG, tumor suppressor gene; CTL, cytotoxic thymus-dependent lymphocytes; Ma, activated macrophages; NK, natural killer cells; LAK, lymphokine-activated killer cells.

4.2. *Ethanol Metabolism and Its Link to Carcinogenesis*

As already discussed in Chapter 1 (this volume), ethanol is predominantly metabolized in the liver by alcohol dehydrogenase (ADH) and CYP2E1. Although quantitatively much lower, ethanol metabolism also occurs in a variety of other tissues and in gastrointestinal bacteria. Acetaldehyde (AA), the extremely toxic first intermediate of alcohol metabolism, binds rapidly to cellular proteins and possibly to DNA,[56] which results in morphological and functional impairment of the cell. In addition, AA adducts represent neoantigens leading to the production of specific antibodies.[57–60] AA has well-known mutagenic and carcinogenic effects that include inflammation and metaplasia of tracheal epithelium, induction of laryngeal carcinoma in animals, inhibition of DNA repair, delayed cell cycle progression, stimulation of apoptosis, and enhanced cell injury associated with hyperregeneration. According to the International Agency for Research on Cancer, there is sufficient evidence to identify AA as a carcinogen in animals.[61]

4.2.1. Generation of Acetaldehyde via ADH and by Gastrointestinal Bacteria. ADH is not only present in the liver, but also in the gastrointestinal mucosa. In contrast to the liver, gastrointestinal mucosa contains not only class I ADH, but also class IV ADH (σ-ADH). Its highest activity exists in the epithelium of the esophagus and the oropharynx. Although its Km is high, because of the high ethanol concentration in the upper alimentary tract, the enzyme is completely saturated after ethanol intake. σ-ADH also metabolizes longer alcohols such as butanol or propanol to their corresponding aldehydes, which have been shown to affect mucosal integrity. σ-ADH also detoxifies the dietary carcinogen nitrobenzaldehyde; it is of considerable interest that a large percentage of Japanese lack this enzyme, since nitrobenzaldehyde occurs in food and gastric cancer is the most common cancer in Japan.[62] Thus, the production of AA via σ-ADH is especially high in the upper alimentary tract. AA is further metabolized by various AA-dehydrogenases (ALDH). Recently, a deficiency of ALDH2 was found in alcoholics who are susceptible to esophageal cancer.[63]

Class I and class IV ADH also occur in the colorectal mucosa, and it seems at least from one study that its activity is higher in the rectum than in the remaining colon, which could lead to higher AA concentration in the rectal mucosa.[64] Most recently, a change in ADH pattern during colorectal carcinogenesis has been observed demonstrating an increased expression of σ-ADH in adenomatous polyps as compared to the adjacent normal mucosa.[65]

AA can also be produced from ethanol by gastrointestinal bacteria, including *Helicobacter pylori*[66] and those present in the oropharynx and in the feces.[67–69] AA production by oropharyngeal bacteria may be especially important in heavy alcoholics with poor dental status and bacterial overgrowth. More recent data have shown that AA is also produced by colorectal bacteria.[40,69] This production is extremely high, leading to mucosal AA concentrations that are per gram of tissue much higher than those observed in the liver.[40] Since AA concentrations measured in the colorectal mucosa correlated significantly with tissue regenerativity, it was speculated that AA results in mucosal injury, leading to secondary compensatory hyperregeneration.[60]

4.2.2. Induction of Cytochrome P4502E1 (CYP2E1) and Production of Free Radicals. It is important to note that chronic alcohol consumption leads to an induction of microsomal CYP2E1, which is capable of metabolizing ethanol to AA. This cytochrome is also involved in the metabolism of various xenobiotics, including procarcinogens.[70] More recently it has been shown in the liver that the concentration of CYP2E1 can be correlated with the generation of hydroxyethyl radicals, and thus with lipidperoxidation.[71] These biochemical observations are associated with changes in liver morphology. The induction of CYP2E1 resulted in an enhanced hepatocellular injury, and inhibition of CYP2E1 was associated with an improvement of the liver lesions. It was concluded that this is mainly because of stimulation and inhibition of free radical formation.

Besides the hydroxyethyl radical, other types of free oxygen radicals and also radicals of unsaturated fatty acids do occur during intermediary metabolism. Other sources for radical generation are the mitochondrial electron transport system of the respiratory chain, leading to superoxide radicals, the NADH-dependent cytochrome *c* reductase, the aldehyde and xanthine oxidase, and the NADPH oxidase in neutrophils.[72] Free radicals initiate predominantly lipid peroxidation, but they also react rapidly with cell constituents, including DNA, and may lead to cancer initiation. Oxygen radicals can indeed lead to copper-dependent formation of etheno-DNA adducts in the liver.[73] Under normal conditions such toxic free radicals are detoxified by several defense mechanisms, including the action of glutathione, α-tocopherol, superoxide dismutase, catalase, and glutathione peroxidase. Since chronic alcohol consumption leads to a decrease of all these factors,[74] an adequate detoxification of free radicals does not occur in the chronic alcoholic.

The role of free radicals in upper alimentary tract cancer has been demonstrated most recently in an animal study. Eskelson and co-workers[25] reported that chronic alcohol consumption increases the carcinogenesis induced by *N*-nitrosomethylbenzylamine (NMBA) in the esophagus, which was associated with an increased free radical production and which was inhibited by administration of the scavenger α-tocopherol.

4.2.3. Enhanced CYP2E1-Mediated Procarcinogen Activation. The induction of CYP2E1 also increases the conversion of various xenobiotics including procarcinogens to potentially toxic metabolites including dimethylnitrosamine (DMN), AFB1, VC, and possibly nitrosopyrrolodine (NPY) and DMH.[70] The induction of CYP2E1 not only takes place in the liver, but also in the gastrointestinal tract. Increased CYP2E1 concentrations after chronic ethanol ingestion up to threefold have been reported in the oropharynx[75] and in the mucosa of the small[76] and large intestine[77] of rodents and more recently in the oral mucosa of man.[78] Enhanced activation of many structurally diverse carcinogens by microsomes from various tissues including those from liver, lungs, intestine and esophagus[70,79–82] has been observed after inductive pretreatment with ethanol. The carcinogens used in these studies have included compounds and mixtures found in tobacco smoke and diets such as amino acid pyrolizates, polycyclic hydrocarbons, and nitrosamines. Induction of CYP2E1 in the esophagus may be particularly relevant to carcinogenesis at this site because of the low concentrations of other detoxifying enzyme systems in this tissue.[79] The lack of such enzyme systems may further enhance DNA alkylations and carcinogenesis.

At the same time, ethanol is capable of inhibiting the metabolism of these compounds when present in sufficiently high concentrations. Whether the microsomal metabolism of procarcinogens is enhanced or inhibited depends on the presence or absence of ethanol in the organism. In some instances the inductive effect exhibits tissue, substrate, gender, and species specifities.[70]

The interaction of ethanol and nitrosamine metabolism has been investigated intensively.[43] It has been shown that chronic alcohol consumption induces low Km–DMN–demethylase activity,[80] leading to an increased activation of the carcinogen both in rats[80] and in man.[83] On the other hand, ethanol is an effective competitive inhibitor of DMN–demethylase activity.[84–86] This capacity to act as both an inducer and inhibitor may explain the conflicting results of ethanol influence on DMN-mediated carcinogenicity in the liver when the route of exposure and the presence or absence of ethanol at the time of exposure are taken into account. In most of the studies published, the coadministration of ethanol with nitrosamines has resulted in a large increase of tumors in extrahepatic target organs.[43] The results are very similar to those observed when the CYP2E1 inhibitor disulfiram was administered. The tumors that occurred were cancer of the nasal cavity and trachea in hamsters; olfactory mucosal, lung, kidney, and forestomach tumors in mice; and esophageal and nasal cavity tumors in rats. It has been a consistent, reproducible, and general finding.

When DMN is given orally, it undergoes a first-pass metabolism in the liver, up to a dose of 30 μg/kg bodyweight.[86] At higher doses the hepatic enzymes are saturated and the methylation of other organs such as the kidney or the esophagus occurs. When ethanol is given to rats at low levels, it inhibits the first-pass metabolism of DMN by competing with the hepatic microsomal enzymes. As a result, more nitrosamine can bypass the liver and extrahepatic organs are exposed to higher concentrations of the procarcinogen. When given to rats in relatively low amounts equivalent to a person drinking 0.5 liters of beer, ethanol prevents the clearance of DMN and can produce a fivefold increase in the methylation of kidney DNA. Measurements of DNA metabolism in liver slices and esophageal epithelium suggest that the changes in alkylation of esophageal DNA can be the result of a selective inhibition of DMN metabolism in the liver.[86] This goes along with the fact that no increased methylation of hepatic DNA was detected when radioactively labeled DMN was given to ethanol-fed and control rats. However, labeling of the esophageal DNA was enhanced after alcohol.[87] Furthermore, ethanol administration also increased DMN-derived *O*6-methylguanine (*O*6-MG) in gastrointestinal mucosal DNA of monkeys.[88] Following the administration of the esophageal carcinogen NMBA, the formation of *O*6-methyldeoxyguanosine in the esophagus was increased threefold by 20% ethanol. Various alcoholic beverages such as brandy, scotch whyskey, white wine, or beer had the same effect. However, red burgundy and calvados exhibited the most striking increase in DNA alkylation.[89]

These biochemical data on the interaction between ethanol and nitrosamine metabolism in the liver and extrahepatic tissue at least in part may explain why alcohol does not stimulate the nitrosamine-induced hepatocarcinogenesis, but does stimulate the development of extrahepatic tumors. This may possibly be related to the fact that the hepatic inactivating enzyme activities are also increased after prolonged ingestion of ethanol or more likely that the presence of ethanol in the liver during procarcinogen application inhibited hepatic activation of nitrosamines.

Some experiments with DMN as a tumor-inducing agent underline the importance of the induction of CYP2E1 and the promoting effect of ethanol in the liver. Most recently, Tsutsumi *et al.*[48] reported on the occurrence of preneoplastic hepatic changes in the liver of rats that were treated with low amounts of DMN and alcohol chronically. These changes were neither observed in the alcohol- nor in the carcinogen-treated group alone. It was emphazised that to avoid interaction between ethanol and DMN metabolism both compounds were administered in the diets alternatively. A similar enhancement of DMN-induced hepatocarcinogenesis by ethanol when given during promotion was reported by Driver and McLean.[47] Other experiments show that hepatic carcinogenesis is enhanced by chronic alcohol administration when carcinogenesis was further modulated by other stimulators, namely by the administration of a methyl-deficient[44] or a low carbohydrate[45] diet or by partial hepatectomy to stimulate hepatic regeneration.[46]

Nitrosamine metabolism is also influenced by dietary factors such as zinc and vitamin A.[53] Zinc deficiency leads to a strikingly enhanced rate of NMBA metabolism in mucosal microsomes from the esophagus.[90] Zinc seems to inhibit the CYP2E1-dependent activation of the nitrosamine. Alcohol consumption also results in a severe depression of hepatic vitamin A levels. Since ethanol, DMN, and retinol share the same CYP2E1 species, chronic ethanol consumption results not only in an enhanced retinol metabolism, leading to decreasing hepatic vitamin A levels, but also in an increased activation of DMN, which if further enhanced by diminishing competitive inhibition of DMN activation due to low vitamin A.[91]

An enhanced metabolism of AOM by CYP2E1 may be an important

mechanism of the cocarcinogenic effect of ethanol on the rectum.[92] It has been shown that ethanol inhibits the hepatic microsomal activation of AOM, while the activation of the procarcinogen was strikingly enhanced following chronic ethanol consumption when ethanol was withdrawn. The conversion of AOM to methyl-azoxy-methanol (MAM) is catalyzed by a microsomal cytochrome P450-dependent *N*-hydroxylase in the liver and in the colon. Pretreatment of animals with microsomal enzyme inducers such as phenobarbital, chrysene, or ethanol leads to an increased metabolism of AOM to carbon monoxide, probably through an induction of the microsomal enzyme. On the other hand, agents that inhibit DMH metabolism also inhibit DMH-induced colorectal carcinogenesis *in vivo*.[2] It therefore seems possible that the effect of ethanol observed in the animal experiment with DMH and AOM can be attributed, at least in part, to the alcohol-related changes in the metabolism of the procarcinogen. In the light of these facts, it is understandable why high ethanol intake results in an inhibition of colorectal carcinogenesis, whereas low alcohol intake does not.[37,38] The presence of ethanol during tumor initiation also inhibits tumor development, while its absence at a stage of enzyme induction enhances the carcinogenic process.

Other compounds relevant in carcinogenesis and metabolized by CYP2E1 are AFB1 and VC. With respect to AFB1-induced hepatocarcinogenesis, controversial results have been obtained. While one study reported an enhancement of AFB1-induced carcinogenesis by ethanol,[93] which is in agreement with the reported increased activation of AFB1,[94] another study reported no effect.[95] It was suggested that the metabolism of AFB1 to aflatoxin M1 is favored, while the metabolism to aflatoxin Q1 is depressed by alcohol administration.

Metabolism of VC is also mediated by CYP2E1 and it is inhibited by ethanol. The animals who received alcohol and VC had a doubling in incidence of angiosarcoma in the liver compared to VC alone.[96] This is consistent with liver blood vessel endothelium representing an intraorgan downstream target receiving increased doses of the carcinogen as a result of inhibition of metabolism in the hepatocyte. On the other hand, in humans it has been shown that large quantities of ethanol in addition to exposure to VC led to the development of both angiosarcoma and HCC, possibly as a result of an increased activation of VC to its toxic metabolite at the workplace where no alcohol was present in the blood.[55]

In summary, chronic ethanol consumption increases the capacity of microsomes to activate many classes of chemical carcinogens in different tissues. This effect is gender and species dependent. The significance of this effect of ethanol vis-à-vis actual cancer risk will be influenced by other factors operating *in vivo* including the carcinogen detoxifying capacity of various tissues, the route of carcinogen exposure, and, in the alcohol abuser in particular, the presence or absence of ethanol in the circulation at the time of carcinogen exposure.

4.3. *Alcohol Effects on DNA*

As pointed out in Section 4.2, AA inhibits DNA methylation[97] and may directly bind to DNA.[56] It has been reported that it induces sister chromatide exchanges (SCE) in tissue cultures.[98] Also, an elevation of chromosomal aberrations in lymphocytes of alcoholics has been found.[99] The potential significance of these observations with respect to tumor promotion is related to the hypothesis that compounds with SCE activity may act as promoters. By increasing the frequency of SCEs, such compounds could theoretically enhance recessive mutations being converted from heterozygous to a homozygous state, and thereby lead to tumor development. More recently, it has been reported that AA induces *c-fos* and *c-jun* proto-oncogen expression in fat storing cells associated with enhanced fibrogenesis.[100]

Besides an increased activation of DMN, an enhanced *O*6-MG DNA adduct formation is additionally caused by an inhibition of the capacity of cells to repair carcinogen-induced DNA damage.[58] Indeed, it was reported that DMN-induced hepatic DNA alkylation persisted for longer periods in ethanol-fed animals than in controls. This effect appeared to be specific for *O*6-MG repair. The enzyme responsible for the repair of *O*6-MG adducts is *O*6-MG transferase, which transfers methyl- or ethylgroups from the *O*6 position of guanine to a cysteine residue located in the enzyme, which in turn inactivates the transferase. Chronic ethanol consumption was found to reduce this enzyme activity significantly.[58] Since alkylation at the *O*6 position of guanine is associated with both mutagenesis and carcinogenesis, the apparently decreased *O*6-MG transferase activity in alcohol fed rats could be an important mechanism in alcohol-associated cancer risk.

More recently, by using microgel electrophoresis, DNA damage has been detected in rectal biopsies from chronic alcoholics (HK Seitz, personal communication).

4.4. *The Effect of Alcohol on Cell Regeneration and Its Link to Carcinogenesis*

Cell proliferation is an important measure and characteristic of tissues. In general there are two different entities of changes in mucosal cell regeneration. One is related to tissue damage and indicates reparative growth and the other is concerned with the acute and chronic progressive changes during cancer development. Abnormal cellular regeneration is a hallmark of neoplasia. Actively proliferating cells are more susceptible to initiators of carcinogenesis and genetic alterations. A substantial body of literature indicates that in the colon a sequence of events after crypt cell production and during migration and differentiation is disordered in carcinogenesis.[101]

Morphometric analysis in rats who were fed with alcohol over 6 months has shown an enlargement of the size of the nuclei of the basal cells of the oral mucosa from the floor of the mouth and from the edge and the base of the tongue.[102] The size of the basal cell layer in these rats was also increased and the stratification of the cells was altered. The percentage of cells in the S-phase of the cell cycle was significantly higher in ethanol-fed rats as compared to controls. Mean epithelium thickness of the mucosa from the floor of the mouth was significantly reduced after chronic alcohol ingestion. This indicates an atrophy of the mucosa and it is remarkable that this finding was most pronounced for a location within the oral cavity that is believed to have the most intensive contact with alcoholic beverages. A reduction of epithelial thickness increases the vulnerability of the epithelium to chemical and physical noxae.

Acute[103] and chronic ethanol consumption[104,105] also enhances cell replication in the rat esophagus. Eight weeks of feeding an ethanol-containing liquid diet doubled the labeling index in the esophagus. The thickness of the epithelium was increased, but no overt changes in morphology were detected. Simanowski *et al.*[105] found a significant increase of cell proliferation in the middle part of the esophagus of male F-344 rats. This enhancement of cell proliferation was particularly obvious in young and middle-aged animals. Age alone did not significantly effect cell regeneration.[105] When the effect of ethanol was investigated in Wistar rats with and without sialoadenectomy using proliferative cellular nuclear antigen (PCNA) immunohistology, proliferative index values were significantly increased in the intact alcohol-consuming animals, whereas this effect of alcohol was completely abolished after sialoadenectomy. No detectable mucosal damage was observed by light microscopy.

In an attempt to mimic more closely the situation as it occurs in humans, alcoholic solutions were administered to rats using an intubation tube long enough to prevent the solution from passing into the lungs, but as short as possible to allow maximum flow through the esophagus. One day after treatment, the animals were given bromodesoxyuridine and it was found that the intubation of 64% ethanol had no detectable effect on basal cell replication; however, when 2-methylbutanol was dissolved in ethanol, the mixture produced a dramatic increase in replication.[106] This effect could well explain the dependence of risk on the type of beverage consumed.

A similar hyperregeneration was observed in the rectum after alcohol consumption.[36,60107] This was associated with a marked extension of the proliferative compartment and with a reduced life span of functional epithelium cells. In addition, aging further increased this ethanol-associated proliferation. Furthermore, using PCNA labeling technique, cell regeneration was also found to be increased in rectal biopsies from chronic alcoholics as compared to age- and sex-matched controls.[108] Mucosal hyperregeneration observed after chronic ethanol ingestion is paralleled by a significant increase in rectal mucosal ornithin decarboxylase (ODC) activity, a marker for high risk with respect to colorectal cancer.[40]

4.5. Alcohol-Associated Nutritional Deficiencies and Carcinogenesis

The ethanol-induced malnutrition is of clinical significance. Various deficiencies of vitamins and trace elements that occur in chronic alcoholics lead to certain diseases, including alcohol-associated cancer.[74] The principal mechanisms involved are described in the following sections.

4.5.1. A Decrease of the Oxidative Defense System. (See also Section 4.2.2.) The increased oxidative stress observed during ethanol metabolism leads to an increased requirement for glutathione and α-tocopherol. In addition, glutathione is trapped by AA and its regeneration is restricted by a limited availability of cysteine and methionine. Catabolism of methionine is stimulated to generate cysteine and replenish glutathione, but this is compensated by an attempt to conserve methionine through a futile cycle of enhanced choline oxidation. As a result, a striking wastage of methyl groups occurs.[109] It has been shown that glutathione inhibits oral carcinogenesis.[110]

Ethanol also produces an increased breakdown of other lipid-soluble vitamins such as hepatic α-tocopherol,[111] possibly secondary to a marked increase in the formation of α-tocopherol–quinone, a metabolite of α-tocopherol by free radical reaction. This may lead additionally to an increased hepatic lipid peroxidation seen in alcoholics.

4.5.2. Methyl Deficiency including an Alteration of Methyl Transfer. Chronic alcoholism increases the requirement for methyl groups[109] and dietary methyl deficiency enhances hepatic carcinogenesis.[94] Methionine obtained from the diet and synthesized by several reactions is the sole precursor of *S*-adenosylmethionine (SAM), the primary methyl donor in the body. Disruption in methionine metabolism and methylation reaction may be involved in the cancer process. SAM is involved in the methylation of a small percentage of cytosine bases of the DNA. Findings suggest that enzymatic DNA methylation is an important component of gene control and may serve as a silencing mechanism for gene function. Some carcinogens interfere with enzymatic DNA methylation, and thus may allow oncogene activation. DNA hypomethylation has been observed in many cancer cells and tumors. Chronic ethanol consumption decreases dietary intake of methionine and its conversion to SAM.[112,113]

Folate deficiency, which is common in the alcoholic, may additionally contribute to an inhibition of transmethylation, since it is an important factor in one-carbon transport.[114] Decreased folate levels after alcohol intake are caused by, among others, a decreased ability to retain folate in the liver or to an increased breakdown of folate.[74] Most recently it has been demonstrated that vitamin B6 deficiency, which also occurs following chronic ethanol ingestion, also leads to a decrease of SAM.[115]

Another factor for DNA hypomethylation is the AA-mediated inhibition of methyltransferase activity.[97]

4.5.3. Vitamin A Deficiency. Vitamin A regulates among others epithelial cell function via metabolism to retinoic acid, and pleiotrophic regulator of gene expression. Vitamin A decreases in the liver after chronic ethanol consumption, predominantly due to an enhanced metabolism via CYP2E1.[72,91] It interferes with the metabolism of ethanol via ADH and with that of nitrosamines via CYP2E1. Extrahepatic tissue exhibits an increased vitamin A level after chronic alcohol consumption due to increased mobilization of vitamin A from the liver to peripheral tissues.[72,91,116] This seems of special importance with respect to age since cellular vitamin A binding protein decreases with age, which may lead to an increased toxicity of vitamin A in those tissues.[116] It has been reported that even β-carotene has an increased toxicity when alcohol is consumed.[117] Epidemiological studies have shown that the supplementation of β-carotene in smokers does not prevent lung cancer. In contrast, those who received β-carotene had an increased occurrence of lung cancer, and this has been attributed to the concomitant consumption of alcohol.[118] It has been reported experimentally that chronic alcohol consumption leads to the generation of toxic intermediates of vitamin A and β-carotene due to their increased metabolism via CYP2E1.[72,91,117]

4.5.4. Zinc and Selenium Deficiency. A deficiency of zinc and selenium may also contribute to cancer development.[119] Besides the effect of zinc on nitrosamine activation by CYP2E1,[90] it is important to note that zinc deficiency also leads to disturbances in vitamin A metabolism, since zinc is an important factor in the conversion of retinol to retinal, as well as in the synthesis and secretion of retinol-binding protein in the liver. Many other enzyme systems are impaired by zinc deficiency in alcoholic subjects. One classical example is the altered activity of zinc–copper superoxide dismutase, which plays an important role in the protection of oxidative tissue damage. Because of the altered zinc status with altered superoxide dismutase activity, the hepatocytes become more vulnerable to oxidative stress.[74]

Zinc deficiency also reduces glutathione transferase, an enzyme important in the detoxification of carcinogens *in vivo*, and increases cell proliferation in the esophageal mucosa.[119]

Selenium deficiency leads to a decreased activity of the selenium-containing enzyme glutathione peroxidase, which guarantees an adequate availability of glutathione.[74]

5. Specific Pathogenesis of Alcohol-Associated Organ Cancer

5.1. *Upper Alimentary Tract Cancer*

The effect of alcohol on upper alimentary tract carcinogenesis includes a local production of AA from ethanol either via mucosal σ-ADH or via bacterial metabolism and the production of free radicals through CYP2E1 induction.

Both AA and free radicals may damage mucosal cells, which may lead to tumor initiation and could also play a role in tumor promotion by the stimulation of secondary compensatory cell hyperregeneration. In addition, the induction of CYP2E1 may lead to an increased activation of procarcinogens, which are mainly inhaled by tobacco smoking. When alcohol is present, nitrosamine metabolism is inhibited in the liver and the exposure of extrahepatic organs to these carcinogens, as shown in animal experiments, is enhanced. Vitamin deficiencies such as those of riboflavin and zinc may be of additional importance. However, no significant difference in vitamins A and E concentrations could be detected in oral biopsies from alcoholics with oropharyngeal cancer and controls.[120]

Ethanol may facilitate the uptake of environmental carcinogens especially from tobacco smoke, through cell membranes that are damaged and changed in their molecular composition by the direct effect of alcohol. Furthermore, it is postulated that alcohol acts as a solvent that enhances the penetration of carcinogenic compounds into the mucosa.[53] Therefore, both factors may have relevance to the upper gastrointestinal tract, particularly, since chronic alcohol abuse leads to atrophy and lipomatic metamorphosis of the parenchyma of the parotic and submandibulary gland and this morphological alteration results in functional impairment including reduction of saliva flow and increased viscosity of saliva.[121] Thus, the mucosa surface will be insufficiently rinsed. Therefore, higher concentrations of locally effective carcinogens in addition to a prolongation of the contact time of those substances with the mucosa can be observed.

Other local mechanisms include the direct toxic effect of highly concentrated alcoholic beverages on the squamous epithelium, the impaired motility of the esophagus due to alcohol, and the enhanced gastroesophageal reflux, which lead to esophagitis and Barrett's metaplasia.

5.2. *Liver Cancer*

The exact role of alcohol itself, of the alcohol-induced cirrhosis of the liver, or of the concomitant HBV or HCV infection, or of a combination of all three has not been determined. In addition, many other variables including geographic exposure to carcinogens, ethnicity, and diet, all influence the results in studies correlating chronic alcohol ingestion with hepatocarcinogenesis. A major prerequisite for HCC in the alcoholic is the presence of cirrhosis of the liver. Mechanisms by which chronic alcohol consumption leads to liver cirrhosis are discussed in detail elsewhere in this book. In addition, HBV and HCV infection of patients with alcoholic cirrhosis is high. Studies from Japan show that HCV infections are more closely related to HCC in heavy drinkers than is HBV infection.[8,9,122] Nevertheless, the incidence of HCC was significantly higher among chronic HBV carriers who were drinkers than among HBV carriers who were abstinent.[8,9] Among drinkers, HCC developed at a younger age.[123] It was concluded that hepatic cell injury caused by alcohol may enhance the development of HCC caused by HBV.

It also has been shown that HCV infection is more important for the pathogenesis of HCC and that a high prevalence of HCV antibodies have been detected in alcoholic liver disease, especially in cirrhosis and HCC.[124–126] It seems that alcohol abuse enhances the development of HCC related to hepatitis virus infection through the interaction with the replication and oncogenicity of HCV and through the promoter action superimposed on HBV oncogenicity. Results from Japan have identified chronic alcohol consumption as a promoter in viral-associated hepatic carcinogenesis.[8,9]

In addition to cirrhosis of the liver and concomitant viral infection, alcohol per se may influence hepatic carcinogenesis. The mechanism by which alcohol acts includes possibly an increased activation of procarcinogen through microsomal CYP2E1, an inhibition of the nuclear DNA repair system by small amounts of AA, nutritional deficiencies such as methyl and vitamin A deficiency, the promoting action of ethanol, and changes in cell proliferation. Some of these factors have been discussed already in detail. Some controversy exists as to whether alcohol is a promoter in hepatocarcinogenesis. Recent studies have found that numbers and areas of enzyme-altered foci were significantly increased in chronically alcohol-treated rats. These changes were similar to those in the phenobarbital-treated animals. In alcohol- and phenobarbital-treated groups, the numbers of visible nodules were also significantly increased. The visible nodules showed preneoplastic histological changes. These results indicated that ethanol may act as a promoting agent in hepatocarcinogenesis.[9,48]

It is interesting that Mallory body (MB) formation is significantly high in HCC and the incidence of HCC is significantly elevated in cirrhosis with MBs than in those without.[127] Therefore it was hypothesized that MBs may be a phenotypical expression of carcinogenesis of hepatocytes, especially since gammaglutamyltranspeptase activity was observed in those hepatocytes with MB from the early stage of development of HCC.[128] Another histological abnormality is the occurrence of oval cells in the liver after long-term alcohol exposure, resulting in an alteration of the cellular composition of the liver similar to that observed after the administration of a choline-deficient, ethionine-supplemented diet, which is known to stimulate hepatocarcinogenesis.[129]

Finally, it was observed that alcohol inhibits hepatocellular regeneration. The fact that in some studies HCC was observed after the cessation of alcohol led to the theory that the inhibition of regeneration was omitted and that therefore the increased cell regenerativity contributed to the carcinogenesis. However, chronic alcohol consumption leads to hepatocellular injury accompanied by cell death and fibrogenesis, a process that is associated with an increased renewal. Such hyperregenerativity during the development of hepatic cirrhosis may indeed be a pathogenetic factor. Rats with hepatic hyperregenerativity after partial hepatectomy developed more liver tumors after nitrosamine application and alcohol.[46]

The significance of ethanol-mediated changes in immune function including depression of B and T lymphocytes, macrophages, neutrophils, and natural killer cells associated with increased cytokine concentrations in hepatocarcinogenesis needs to be further determined.[130]

5.3. Colorectal Cancer

Although the enhanced activation of procarcinogens due to chronic ethanol consumption could be important in ethanol-associated colorectal cocarcinogenesis, local mechanisms may predominate. As already pointed out, chronic ethanol consumption leads to hyperproliferation and expansion of the proliferative compartment of the rectal crypt toward the intestinal lumen in the rat model and also in humans.[40,60,107,108] ODC activity was found to be significantly enhanced after chronic alcohol consumption.[44] It was also shown that the hyperregenerative effect of chronic ethanol consumption on the rectal mucosa was further increased in old age, which by itself is a risk factor in colorectal cancer.[60] Mucosal AA concentrations correlated significantly with cell regeneration. Thus, it was suspected that AA injures the rectal mucosa. The rectal hyperproliferation observed after alcohol ingestion may be of a secondary compensatory nature, since light microscopy of rectal mucosa from alcoholics reveals superficial cell damage, which returns to normal following alcohol abstinence for 2 weeks[131] and since the life span of functional epithelial cells in the rectal crypt is reduced.[107]

Significantly high concentrations of AA were found in the distal colon after alcohol application. These AA concentrations were significantly elevated compared to the proximal colon and to the liver when calculated per gram of tissue.[40] Data on the effect of ethanol on AMMN-induced rectal cancer further support the concept that AA is involved in the ethanol-associated rectal carcinogenesis. Animals who received ethanol and cyanamide, a potent AA-dehydrogenase inhibitor, exhibited an earlier occurrence of rectal tumors compared to animals who received ethanol alone.[40] In these experiments, AA concentrations were significantly elevated in the serum and in the colonic mucosa following the application of cyanamide. All these experiments underline the role of AA in ethanol rectal cocarcinogenicity.

Since the ethanol concentration in the rectal lumen is similar to that in the blood, it seems unclear how AA is generated and why more AA associated with increased cell regeneration is found in the rectum compared to other large intestinal segments. Increased ADH activity was found in the mucosa derived from the distal colon when compared to the proximal large intestine, which may favor AA accumulation through ethanol oxidation.[35] Meanwhile, the presence of increased mucosal ADH activity in the rectum has also been found in humans.[64] However, it seems impossible that the rectal ADH with its low activity is capable of producing the striking accumulation of AA seen in the rectum. It is therefore more likely that bacterial production of AA, especially in the distal colon (where the highest bacteria count occurs), may be responsible for the AA formation.[40] Indeed, Jokelainen *et al.*[69] reported increasing AA production when human colonic content was incubated with increasing ethanol concentrations starting already at 2.75 mM ethanol. The question whether different types of alcoholic beverages such as beer and wine may affect fecal bacteria quantitatively and qualitatively, affecting AA generation, still remains.

In addition, folate deficiency may also enhance colorectal carcinogenesis.[132] The mechanisms have already been discussed.

5.4. *Breast Cancer*

Factors other than those already discussed for gastrointestinal and liver cancer may be involved in alcohol-associated mammary carcinogenesis. Since many breast cancers are estrogen-dependent, the observation of increased serum sex hormone levels in women with breast cancer and elevated estrogen and androgen serum concentrations after alcohol ingestion may have pathogenic importance.[16] Only limited information exists on the effect of chronic ethanol consumption on estrogen-receptor-positive and -negative breast cancer as well as for women who reported ever using estrogen replacement therapy. Another possibility by which alcohol may affect mammary carcinogenesis may be by increasing cell proliferation of the mammary gland. In cell cultures, ethanol selectively stimulated cell proliferation of estrogen-receptor-positive, but not estrogen-receptor-negative human breast cancer cells.[133] Also, a positive association of ethanol intake with circulating prolactin levels has been reported in animals.[19] The evidence of an effect of ethanol on carcinogen metabolism in mammary tissue is rather small. Finally, an increased mammary tumor metastasis has been observed following alcohol administration, which may be linked to an impairment of natural killer cell activity, suggesting that impaired immune function leads to increased tumor progression.[51]

Note Added in Proof. An important finding regarding alcohol and cancer has recently been reported. Chronic ethanol administration to rats resulted in a striking reduction in retinoic acid and in a concomitant enhanced expression of the protooncogenes *c-fos* and *c-jun* (AP-1) in the liver of these animals. The low retinoic acid concentrations are probably due to the fact that retinol metabolism via ADH is inhibited by ethanol.[134]

References

1. Lamu L: Etude de statistique clinique de 131 cas de cancer de l'oesophage et du cardia. *Arch Mal Appar Dig Mal Nutr* 4:451–456, 1910.
2. Seitz HK, Pöschl G: Alcohol and cancer: Pathogenetic mechanisms. *Addict Biol* 2:19–33, 1996.

3. Wynder EL, Mabushi K: Etiological and environmental factors in esophageal cancer. *JAMA* 226:1546–1548, 1973.
4. Tuyns A: Alcohol and cancer. *Alcohol Health Res World* 2:20–31, 1978.
5. Maier H, Dietz A, Zielinski D, Jünemann KH, *et al:* Risikofaktoren bei Patienten mit Plattenepithelkarzinomen der Mundhöhle, des Oropharynx, des Hypopharynx und des Larynx. *Deutsche Medizinische Wochenschrift* 115:843–850, 1990.
6. Tuyns AJ, Esteve J, Raymond L, *et al:* Cancer of the larynx/hypopharynx, tobacco and alcohol: IARC International case–control study in Turin and Varese (Italy), Zaragoza and Navarra (Spain), Geneva (Switzerland), and Calvados (France). *Int J Cancer* 41:483–492, 1988.
7. Bruguere J, Guenel P, Leclerc A, *et al:* Differential effects of tobacco and alcohol in cancer of the larynx, pharynx and mouth. *Cancer* 57:391–397, 1986.
8. Ohnishi K: Alcohol and hepatocellular carcinoma, in Watson RR (ed): *Alcohol and Cancer.* Boca Raton, FL, CRC Press, 1992, pp 179–202.
9. Takada A, Takase S, Tsutsumi M: Alcohol and hepatic carcinogenesis, in Yirmiya R, Taylor AN (eds): *Alcohol, Immunity and Cancer.* Boca Raton, FL, CRC Press, 1993, pp 187–210.
10. Breslow NE, Enstrom JE: Geographic correlations between mortality rates and alcohol, tobacco consumption in the United States. *J Natl Cancer Inst* 53:631–639, 1974.
11. Kune GA, Vitetta L: Alcohol consumption and the etiology of colorectal cancer: A review of the scientific evidence from 1957 to 1991. *Nutr Cancer* 18:97–111, 1992.
12. Kearney J, Giavamnucci E, Rimm EB, *et al:* Diet, alcohol and smoking and the occurrence of hyperplastic polyps of the colon and rectum. *Cancer Causes Contr* 6:45–56, 1995.
13. Boutron MC, Faivre J, Dop MC, *et al:* Tobacco, alcohol and colorectal tumors: A multistep process. *Am J Epidemiol* 141:1038–1046, 1995.
14. Longnecker N: Alcohol beverage consumption in relation to risk of breast cancer: Meta-analysis and review. *Cancer Causes Contr* 5:73–82, 1994.
15. Harris JR, Lippman ME, Veronesi U, *et al:* Breast cancer. *N Engl J Med* 327:319–328, 1992.
16. Singletary KW, Meadows GG: Alcohol and breast cancer: Interaction between alcohol and other risk factors. *Alcohol Clin Exp Res* 20(Suppl):57A–61A, 1996.
17. Horie A, Kohchi S, Karatsune M: Carcinogenesis in the esophagus II. Experimental production of esophageal cancer by administration of ethanolic solution of carcinogens. *Gann* 56:429–441, 1965.
18. Henefer EP: Ethanol 30% and hamster pouch carcinogenesis. *J Dent Res* 45:838–844, 1966.
19. Elzay RR: Local effect of alcohol in combination with DMBA on hamster cheek pouch. *J Dent Res* 45:1788–1795, 1966.
20. Stenback F: The tumorigenic effect of alcohol. *Acta Pathol Microbiol Scand* 77:325–326, 1969.
21. Nachiappan V, Mufti SI, Eskelson CD: Ethanol-mediated promotion of oral carcinogenesis in hamsters: Association with lipid peroxidation. *Nutr Cancer* 20:293–302, 1993.
22. Gibel VW: Experimentelle Untersuchungen zur Synkarzinogenese beim Ösophaguskarzinom. *Arch Geschwulstforsch* 30:181–189, 1967.
23. Gabrial GN, Schrager TF, Newberne PM: Zinc deficiency, alcohol and retinoid: Association with esophageal cancer in rats. *J Natl Cancer Inst* 68:785–789, 1982.
24. Aze Y, Toyoda K, Furukawa F, *et al:* Enhancing effect of ethanol on esophageal tumor development in rats by initiation of diethylnitrosamine. *Carcinogenesis* 14:37–40, 1993.
25. Eskelson CD, Odeleye OE, Watson RR, *et al:* Modulation of cancer growth by vitamin E and alcohol. *Alcohol Alcohol* 28:117–126, 1993.
26. McCoy GD, Hecht SS, Katayama, *et al:* Differential effects of chronic ethanol consumption on the carcionogenicity of *N*-nitrosopyrrolidine and *N*-nitrosonornicotine in male Syrian hamsters. *Cancer Res* 41:2849–2854, 1981.
27. Castonguay A, Rivenson A, Trushin N, *et al:* Effect of chronic ethanol consumption on the metabolism and carcinogenicity of *N*-nitrosonornicotine in F344 rats. *Cancer Res* 44:2285–2290, 1984.
28. Anderson LM, Carter JP, Driver CL, *et al:* Enhancement of tumorigenesis by *N*-nitrosodiethylamine, *N*-nitrosopyrrolidine and N^6(methylnitroso)-adenosine by ethanol. *Cancer Lett* 68:61–66, 1993.

29. Mufti SI, Becker G, Sipes IG: Effect of chronic dietary ethanol consumption on the initiation and promotion of chemically induced esophageal carcinogenesis in experimental rats. *Carcinogenesis* 10:303–309, 1989.
30. Ishii H, Tatsuta M, Baba M, *et al:* Promotion by ethanol of gastric carcinogenesis induced by *N*-methyl-*N*-nitro-*N*-nitroso-guanidine in Wistar rats. *Br J Cancer* 59:719–721, 1989.
31. Schmähl D: Investigations of esophageal carcinogenicity by methylphenyl nitrosamine and ethyl-alcohol in the rat. *Cancer Lett* 1:215–218, 1976.
32. Konishi N, Kitahori Y, Shimoyama T, *et al:* Effects of sodium chloride and alcohol on experimental esophageal carcinogenesis induced by *N*-nitrospiperidine in rats. *Gann* 77:446–451, 1986.
33. Howarth AE, Phil E: High fat diet promotes and causes distal shift of experimental rat colonic cancer—beer and alcohol do not. *Nutr Cancer* 6:229–235, 1985.
34. Nelson RL, Samelson SL: Neither dietary ethanol nor beer augments experimental colon carcinogenesis in rats. *Dis Col Rectum* 28:460–462, 1985.
35. Seitz HK, Czygan P, Waldherr R, *et al:* Enhancement of 1,2-dimethylhydrazine induced rectal carcinogenesis following chronic ethanol consumption in the rat. *Gastroenterology* 86:886–891, 1984.
36. McGarrity TJ, Via EA, Colony PC: Changes in tissue sialic acid content and staining in dimethylhydrazine(DMH)-induced colorectal cancer: Effects of ethanol (abstract). *Gastroenterology* 90:1543, 1986.
37. Hamilton SR, Sohn OS, Fiala ES: Effects of timing and quantity of chronic dietary ethanol consumption on azoxymethane induced colonic carcinogenesis and azoxymethane metabolism in Fischer 344 rats. *Cancer Res* 47:4305–4311, 1987.
38. Hamilton SR, Hyland J, McAvinchey D, *et al:* Effects of chronic dietary beer and ethanol consumption on experimental colonic carcinogenesis by azoxymethane in rats. *Cancer Res* 47:1551–1559, 1987.
39. Garzon FT, Simanowski UA, Berger MR, *et al:* Acetoxymethyl-methylnitrosamine(AMMN)-induced colorectal carcinogenesis is stimulated by chronic alcohol consumption. *Alcohol Alcohol* Suppl 1:501–502, 1987.
40. Seitz HK, Simanowski UA, Garzon FZ, *et al:* Possible role of acetaldehyde in ethanol related rectal carcinogenesis in the rat. *Gastroenterology* 98:1–8, 1990.
41. Anderson LM: Increased numbers of *N*-nitrosodimethylamine-initiated lung tumors in mice by chronic coadministration of ethanol. *Carcinogenesis* 9:1717–1721, 1988.
42. Griciute L, Castegnaro M, Bereziat JC: Influence of ethyl alcohol on carcinogenesis with *N*-nitrosodimethylamine. *Cancer Lett* 13:345–352, 1981.
43. Anderson LM: Modulation of nitrosamine metabolism by ethanol: Implications of cancer risk, in Watson RR (ed): *Alcohol and Cancer.* Boca Raton, FL, CRC Press, 1992, pp 17–54.
44. Porta EA, Markell N, Dorado RD: Chronic alcoholism enhances hepatocarcinogenesis of dimethylnitrosamine in rats fed a marginally methyl-deficient diet. *Hepatology* 5:1120–1125, 1985.
45. Yonekura I, Matsumoto Y, Miura K, *et al:* Ethanol ingestion combined with lowered carbohydrate intake enhances the initiation of diethylnitrosamine liver carcinogenesis in rats. *Nutr Cancer* 17:171–178, 1992.
46. Takada A, Nei J, Takase S, *et al:* Effect of ethanol on experimental carcinogenesis. *Hepatology* 6:65–72, 1986.
47. Driver HE, McLean AEM: Dose–response relationship for initiation of rat liver tumors by dimethylnitrosamine and promotion by phenobarbital and alcohol. *Food Chem Toxicol* 24:241–245, 1986.
48. Tsutsumi M, Matsuda Y, Takada A: Role of cytochrome P4502E1 in the development of hepatocellular carcinoma by the chemical carcinogen *N*-nitrosomethylamine. *Hepatology* 18:1483–1489, 1993.
49. Singletary K, Nelshoppen J, Wallig N: Enhancement by chronic ethanol intake of *N*-methylnitrosourea-induced rat mammary tumorigenesis. *Carcinogenesis* 15:959–964, 1995.
50. Singletary K, McNary M, Odoms A, *et al:* Ethanol consumption and DMBA induced carcinogenesis in rats. *Nutr Cancer* 16:13–21, 1991.

51. Yimaya R, Ben-Eliyahu S, Gale R, *et al:* Ethanol increases tumor progression in rats: Possible involvement of natural killer cells. *Brain Behav Immun* 6:74–86, 1992.
52. Ketcham AS, Wexler H, Mantel N: Affects of alcohol in mouse neoplasia. *Cancer Res* 23:667–670, 1963.
53. Seitz HK, Simanowski UA: Alcohol and carcinogenesis. *Annu Rev Nutr* 8:99–119, 1988.
54. Bulatao-Jayme J, Almero EM, Castro CA, *et al:* A case–control dietary study of primary liver cancer risk from aflatoxin exposure. *Int J Epidemiol* 11:112–119, 1982.
55. Tamburro CH, Lee HM: Primary hepatic cancer in alcoholics. *Clin Gastroenterol* 10:457–477, 1981.
56. Fang JL, Vaca CE: Development of a ^{32}P-postlabelling method for the analysis of adducts arising through the reaction of acetaldehyde with 2′-deoxyguanosine-3′-monophosphate and DNA. *Carcinogenesis* 16:2177–2185, 1995.
57. Appelman LM, Wouterson RA, Feron VJ: Toxicity of acetaldehyde in rats. Acute and subacute studies. *Toxicology* 23:293–307, 1982.
58. Garro AJ, Espina N, Farinati F, *et al:* The effect of chronic ethanol consumption on carcinogen metabolism and on O6-methylguanine transferase-mediated repair of alkylated DNA. *Alcohol Clin Exp Res* 10:73S–77S, 1986.
59. Zimmerman Bt, Crawford GD, Dahl R, *et al:* Mechanism of acetaldehyde-mediated growth inhibition: Delayed cell cycle progression and induction of apoptosis. *Alcohol Clin Exp Res* 19:434–440, 1987.
60. Simanowski UA, Suter P, Russell RM, *et al:* Enhancement of ethanol induced rectal mucosal hyperregeneration with the age in F344 rats. *Gut* 35:1102–1106, 1994.
61. International Agency for Research on Cancer: Working Group on the Evaluation of the Carcinogenic Risk of Chemicals to Humans. Acetaldehyde. *IARC Monogr* 36:101–132, 1985.
62. Baraona E, Yokoyama A, Ishii H, *et al: Lack of alcohol dehydrogenase isoenzyme activities in the stomach of Japanese subjects. Life Sci* 49:1929–1934, 1991.
63. Jokoyama A, Muramatsu T, Higuchi S, *et al:* Esophageal cancer and aldehyde dehydrogenase-2 genotype in Japanese. *Alcohol Clin Exp Res* (Suppl)20:66A 1996.
64. Seitz HK, Egerer G, Oneta C, *et al:* Alcohol dehydrogenase in the human colon and rectum. *Digestion* 57:105–108, 1996.
65. Egerer G, Schulitz R, Gebhardt A, *et al:* Change of alcohol dehydrogenase phenotypes during colorectal carcinogenesis in men (abstract). *Gastroenterology* 112:A260, 1997.
66. Salmela KS, Roine RP, Höök-Nikanne J, *et al:* Acetaldehyde and ethanol production by *Helicobacter pylori. Scand J Gastroenterol* 29:309–312, 1994.
67. Pikkarainen PH, Baraona E, Jauhonen P, *et al:* Contribution of oropharynx microflora and of lung microsomes to acetaldehyde in exspired air after alcohol ingestion. *J Lab Clin Med* 97:617–621, 1979.
68. Homann N, Jousimies-Somo H, Jokelainen K, *et al:* High acetaldehyde levels in saliva after ethanol consumption: Methological aspects and pathogenetic implications. *Carcinogenesis* 18:1739–1743, 1997.
69. Jokelainen K, Roine RP, Väänänen H, *et al: In vitro* acetaldehyde formation by human colonic bacteria. *Gut* 35:1271–1274, 1994.
70. Seitz HK, Osswald BR: Effect of ethanol on procarcinogen activation, in Watson RR (ed): *Alcohol and Cancer.* Boca Raton, FL, CRC Press, 1992, pp 55–72.
71. Albano E, Clot P: Free radicals and ethanol toxicity, in Preedy VR, Watson RR (eds): *Alcohol and the Gastrointestinal Tract.* Boca Raton, FL, CRC Press, 1996, pp 57–68.
72. Lieber CS: Alcohol and the liver: 1994 update. *Gastroenterology* 106:1085–1105, 1994.
73. Nair J, Sone H, Nagao M, *et al:* Copper dependent formation of miscoding etheno-DNA adducts in the liver of Long Evans Cinnamon (LEC) rats developping hereditary hepatitis and hepatocellular carcinoma. *Cancer Res* 56:1267–1271, 1996.
74. Seitz HK, Suter PM: Ethanol toxicity and nutritional status in Kotsonis FM, McKey M, Hjelle J (eds): *Nutritional Toxicology.* New York, Raven Press, 1994, pp 95–116.
75. Shimizu M, Lasker JM, Tsutsumi M, *et al:* Immunohistochemical localization of ethanol inducible cytochrome P4502E1 in the rat alimentary tract. *Gastroenterology* 93:1044–1050, 1990.

76. Seitz HK, Korsten M, Lieber CS: Effect of chronic ethanol ingestion on intestinal metabolism and mutagenicity of benzo-alpha-pyrine. *Biochem Biophys Res Commun* 85:1061–1066, 1978.
77. Hakkak R, Korourian S, Ronis MJ, *et al:* The effects of diet and ethanol on the expression and localisation of cytochromes P450 2E1 and P450 2C7 in the colon of male rats. *J Chem Pharmacol* 51:61–69, 1996.
78. Baumgarten G, Waldherr R, Stickel F, *et al:* Enhanced expression of cytochrome P450 2E1 in the oropharyngeal mucosa in alcoholics with cancer (abstract). Annual Meeting International Society of Biomedical Researchers, Alcoholism, Washington DC, June 22–27, 1996.
79. Farinati F, Lieber CS, Garro AJ: Effects of chronic ethanol consumption on carcinogen activating and detoxifying systems in rat upper alimentary tract tissue. *Alcohol Clin Exp Res* 13:357–360, 1989.
80. Garro AJ, Seitz HK, Lieber CS: Enhancement of dimethylnitrosamine metabolism and activation to a mutagen following chronic ethanol consumption in the rat. *Cancer Res* 41:120–124, 1981.
81. Farinati F, Zhou Z, Bella HC, *et al:* Effect of chronic ethanol consumption on activation of nitrosopyrolidine to a mutagen by rat upper alimentary tract, lung and hepatic tissue. *Drug Metab Dispos Biol Fate Chem* 13:210–216, 1985.
82. Seitz HK, Garro AJ, Lieber CS: Enhanced pulmonary and intestinal activation of procarcinogens and mutagens after chronic ethanol consumption. *Eur J Clin Invest* 11:33–38, 1981.
83. Amelizad S, Appel KE, Schoepke M, *et al:* Enhanced dimethylase and dinitrosation of *N*-nitrosodimethylamine by human liver microsomes from alcoholics. *Cancer Lett* 46:43–48, 1989.
84. Peng R, Yong-Tu J, Yang CS: Induction and competitive inhibition of a high affinity microsomal nitrosodimethylamine dimethylase by ethanol. *Carcinogenesis* 3:1457–1461, 1982.
85. Hauber G, Frommberger R, Remmer G, *et al:* Metabolism of low concentrations of *N*-nitrosodimethylamine in isolated liver cells of guinea pig. *Cancer Res* 44:1343–1348, 1984.
86. Swann PF, Koe AM, Mace R: Ethanol and dimethylnitrosamine metabolism and disposition in the rat. Possible relevance in the influence of ethanol on human cancer incidence. *Carcinogenesis* 5:1337–1343, 1984.
87. Kouros M, Mönch W, Reifer FJ: The influence of various factors on the methylation of DNA by the esophageal carcinogen *N*-nitrosomethylbenzylamine:1. The importance of alcohol. *Carcinogenesis* 4:1081–1084, 1983.
88. Anderson LM, Souliotis VL, Chhabra SK, *et al:* *N*-nitrosodimethylamine-derived O6-methylguanine in DNA of monkey gastrointestinal and urogenital organs and enhancement by ethanol. *Int J Cancer* 66:130–134, 1996.
89. Yamada Y, Weller RO, Kleihues P, *et al:* Effects of ethanol and various alcoholic beverages on the formation of O^6-methyldeoxyguanosine from concurrently administered *N*-nitrosomethylbenzylamine in rats: A dose–response study. *Carcinogenesis* 13:1171–1175, 1992.
90. Barch DH, Kuemmerle SC, Holenberg PF, *et al:* Esophageal microsomal metabolism of *N*-nitrosomethylbenzylamine in the zinc deficient rat. *Cancer Res* 44:5629–5633, 1984.
91. Lieber CS, Garro AJ, Leo MA, *et al:* Alcohol and cancer. *Hepatology* 6:1005–1019, 1986.
92. Sohn OS, Fiala ES, Puz C, *et al:* Enhancement of rat liver microsomal metabolism of azoxymethane to methylazoxymethanol by chronic ethanol administration: Similarity to the microsomal metabolism of *N*-nitrosomethylamine. *Cancer Res* 47:3123–3129, 1987.
93. Tanaka T, Nishikara A, Iwata H: Enhanced effect of ethanol of aflatoxin B1 induced hepatocarcinogenesis in male ACI/N rats. *Jpn J Cancer Res* 80:526–530, 1989.
94. Seitz HK, Simanowski UA, Hörner M, *et al:* Alcohol and liver carcinoma, in Bannasch P, Keppler D, Weber G (eds): *Liver Cell Carcinoma.* Dordrecht, Kluwe Academic Publishers, 1989, pp 227–242.
95. Mendenhall CL, Chedid LA: Peliosis hepatis. Its relationship to chronic alcoholism, aflatoxin B1 and carcinogenesis in male Holtzman rats. *Dig Dis Sci* 25:587–594, 1980.
96. Radike MJ, Stemmer KL, Brown PB, *et al:* Effect of ethanol and vinylchloride on the induction of liver tumors. *Environ Health Perspect* 21:153–155, 1977.
97. Garro AJ, McBeth DL, Lima V, *et al:* Ethanol consumption inhibits fetal DNA methylation in mice: Implications for the fetal alcohol syndrome. *Alcohol Clin Exp Res* 15:395–398, 1991.

98. Obe G, Ristow H: Acetaldehyde but not alcohol induces cystochromatide exchanges in Chinese hamster cells *in vitro*. *Mut Res* 56:211–213, 1977.
99. Obe G, Ristow H: Mutagenic, carcinogenic and teratogenic effects of alcohol. *Mutat Res* 65:229–259, 1979.
100. Casini A, Galli G, Salcano R, *et al:* Acetaldehyde induces C-*phos* and C-*jun* protooncogenes in fat storing cell cultures through protein kinase C activation. *Alcohol Alcohol* 29:303–314, 1994.
101. Seitz HK, Simanowski UA: Cell turnover in the gastrointestinal tract and the effect of ethanol, in Preedy VR, Watson RR (eds): *Alcohol and the Gastrointestinal Tract*. Boca Raton, FL, CRC Press, 1996, pp 273–288.
102. Maier H, Weidauer H, Zöller J, *et al:* Effect of chronic alcohol consumption on the morphology of the oral mucosa. *Alcohol Clin Exp Res* 18:387–391, 1994.
103. Haentjens P, DeBacker A, Willems G: Effect of an apple brandy from Normandy and of ethanol on epithelial cell proliferation in the esophagus of rats. *Digestion* 37:184–192, 1987.
104. Mak KM, Leo MA, Lieber CS: Effect of ethanol and vitamin A deficiency on epithelial cell proliferation and structure in the rat esophagus. *Gastroenterology* 93:362–370, 1987.
105. Simanowski UA, Suter P, Stickel F, *et al:* Esophageal epithelial hyperregeneration following chronic ethanol consumption: effect of age and salivary gland function. *J Natl Cancer Inst* 85:2030–2033, 1993.
106. Craddock VM: Etiology of esophageal cancer: Some operative factors. *Eur J Cancer Press* 1:89–92, 1992.
107. Simanowski UA, Seitz HK, Baier B, *et al:* Chronic ethanol consumption selectively stimulates rectal cell proliferation in the rat. *Gut* 27:278–282, 1986.
108. Homann N, Seitz HK, Schuhmann H, *et al:* Immunhistochemical studies on cell regeneration, differentiation and regulatory genes in the rectal mucosa of alcoholics (abstract). *Alcohol Alcohol* 30:520, 1995.
109. Trimble KC, Molloy AM, Scott JM, *et al:* The effect of ethanol on one-carbon metabolism: Increased methionine catabolism and lipotrope methyl group wastage. *Hepatology* 18:984–989, 1993.
110. Trickler D, Shklar G, Schwartz J: Inhibition of oral carcinogenesis by glutathione. *Nutr Cancer* 20:139–144, 1993.
111. Meydani M, Seitz HK, Blumberg J, *et al:* Effect of chronic alcohol feeding on hepatic and extrahepatic distribution of vitamin E in rats. *Alcohol Clin Exp Res* 15:771–774, 1991.
112. Lieber CS, Casini A, DeCarli LM, *et al:* *S*-adenosyl-L-methionine attenuates alcohol induced liver injury in the baboon. *Hepatology* 11:165–172, 1990.
113. Halsted CH, Villanuewa J, Chandler CJ, *et al:* Ethanol feeding of micropigs alters methionine metabolism and increases hepatocellular apoptosis and proliferation. *Hepatology* 23:497–505, 1996.
114. Glynn SA, Albanez D: Folate and cancer: A review of literature. *Nutr Cancer* 22:101–119, 1994.
115. Stickel F, Kim Y, Selhub J, *et al:* Chronic ethanol intake increases plasma homocysteine in rats: Association with diminished pyridoxal 5′-phosphate status. *Ger J Gastroenterol* 35:802, 1997.
116. Mobarhan S, Seitz HK, Russell RM, *et al:* Age related effects of chronic ethanol intake and vitamin A status in rats. *J Nutr* 121:510–517, 1991.
117. Leo MA, Kim C, Lowe N, *et al:* Interaction of ethanol with β-carotene: Delayed blood clearance and enhanced hepatotoxicity. *Hepatology* 15:883–891, 1992.
118. Albanes D, Heinonen OP, Taylor PR, *et al:* α-tocopherol and β-carotene supplements and lung cancer incidence in the α-tocopherol, β-carotene cancer prevention study: Effects of baseline characteristics and study compliance. *J Natl Cancer Inst* 88:1560–1570, 1996.
119. Cho CH: Zinc: Absorption and role in gastrointestinal metabolism and disorders. *Dig Dis* 9:49–60, 1991.
120. Leo MA, Seitz HK, Maier H, *et al:* Carotinoid, retinoid and vitamin E status of the oropharyngeal mucosa in the alcoholic. *Alcohol Alcohol* 30:163–170, 1995.

121. Maier H, Born IA, Veith S, *et al:* The effect of chronic ethanol consumption on salivary gland morphology and function in the rat. *Alcohol Clin Exp Res* 10:425–427, 1986.
122. Tsutsumi M, Ishizaki M, Takada A: Relative risk for the development of hepatocellular carcinoma in alcoholic patients with cirrhosis: A multiple logistic-regression coefficient analysis. *Alcohol Clin Exp Res* 20:758–762, 1996.
123. Ohnishi K, Iida S, Iwama S, *et al:* The effect of chronic habitual alcohol intake on the development of liver cirrhosis and hepatocellular carcinoma: Relation to hepatitis B surface antigen carriers. *Cancer* 49:672–677, 1982.
124. Oshita M, Hayashi N, Kashara A, *et al:* Increased serum hepatitis C virus RNA levels among alcoholic patients with chronic hepatitis C. *Hepatology* 20:1115–1120, 1994.
125. Zignego AL, Foschi M, Laffi G, *et al:* Inapparent hepatitis B virus infection and hepatitis C virus replication in alcoholic subjects with and without liver disease. *Hepatology* 19:577–582, 1994.
126. Fong TL, Kanel GC, Conrad A, *et al:* Clinical significance of concomitant hepatitis C infection in patients with alcoholic liver disease. *Hepatology* 19:554–557, 1993.
127. Nakanuma Y, Ohta G: Is Mallory body formation a preneoplastic change? A study of 181 cases of liver bearing hepatocellular carcinoma and 82 cases of cirrhosis. *Cancer* 55:2400–2405, 1985.
128. Tazawa J, Irie T, French SW: Mallory body formation runs parallel to gammaglutamyl transferase induction in hepatocytes of griseofulvin fed mice. *Hepatology* 3:989–996, 1983.
129. Smith PG, Tee LB, Yeoh GC: Appearance of oval cells in the liver of rats after long-term exposure of ethanol. *Hepatology* 23:145–154, 1996.
130. Roselle G, Mendenhall Cl, Grossman CJ: Effects of alcohol on immunity and cancer, in Yirmiya R, Taylor AN (eds): Alcohol, Immunity and Cancer. Boca Raton, FL, CRC Press, 1993, pp. 3–22.
131. Brozinski S, Fami K, Grosberg JJ: Alcohol ingestion-induced changes in the human rectal mucosa: Light and electronmicroscopic studies. *Dis Colon Rectum* 21:329–335, 1979.
132. Giovannucci E, Rimm EB, Ascherio A, *et al:* Alcohol, low-methionine-low folate diets and risk of colon cancer in men. *J Natl Cancer Inst* 87:265–273, 1995.
133. Singletary K, Yan W: Ethanol and proliferation of human breast cancer cells. *FASEB J* 10:712–716, 1996.
134. Wang XD, Liu C, Chung J, *et al:* Chronic alcohol intake reduces plasma retinoic acid concentration but not retinoic acid receptor gene expression in rats. *FASEB J* 2040:A351, 1998.

4

Alcohol and Lipids

Enrique Baraona and Charles S. Lieber

Abstract. Alcoholic fatty liver and hyperlipemia result from the interaction of ethanol and its oxidation products with hepatic lipid metabolism. An early target of ethanol toxicity is mitochondrial fatty acid oxidation. Acetaldehyde and reactive oxygen species have been incriminated in the pathogenesis of the mitochondrial injury. Microsomal changes offset deleterious accumulation of fatty acids, leading to enhanced formation of triacylglycerols, which are partly secreted into the plasma and partly accumulate in the liver. However, this compensatory mechanism fades with progression of the liver injury, whereas the production of toxic metabolites increases, exacerbating the lesions and promoting fibrogenesis. The early presence of these changes confers to the fatty liver a worse prognosis than previously thought. Alcoholic hyperlipemia results primarily from increased hepatic secretion of very-low-density lipoprotein and secondarily from impairment in the removal of triacylglycerol-rich lipoproteins from the plasma. Hyperlipemia tends to disappear because of enhanced lipolytic activity and aggravation of the liver injury. With moderate alcohol consumption, the increase in high-density lipoprotein becomes the predominant feature. Its mechanism is multifactorial (increased hepatic secretion and increased extrahepatic formation as well as decreased removal) and explains part of the enhanced cholesterol transport from tissues to bile. These changes contribute to, but do not fully account for, the effects on atherosclerosis and/or coronary heart disease attributed to moderate drinking.

1. Introduction

The alcohol-induced changes of liver and serum lipids are a reflection of the interaction of the metabolism of ethanol and that of lipids in the liver, and

Enrique Baraona • Department of Medicine, Mount Sinai School of Medicine, New York, New York; and Bronx VA Medical Center, Bronx, New York 10468. **Charles S. Lieber** • Departments of Medicine and Pathology, Mount Sinai School of Medicine, New York, New York; and Alcohol Dependence Treatment Program and Section of Liver Disease and Nutrition, Bronx VA Medical Center, Bronx, New York 10468.

Recent Developments in Alcoholism, Volume 14: The Consequences of Alcoholism, edited by Galanter. Plenum Press, New York, 1998.

to a lesser extent of the direct effects of ethanol and its oxidation products. After prolonged alcohol abuse, the associated malnutrition and the development of liver injury also contribute to these effects.

2. Interaction of the Metabolism of Ethanol with Lipids

2.1. *Effects of Excessive Hepatic NADH Generation*

Except for minimal amounts produced endogenously, ethanol is essentially foreign to the body and its oxidation proceeds to the full capacity of available enzymatic systems, without efficient mechanisms for feedback regulation. Alcohol dehydrogenase (ADH), an enzyme involved in the metabolism of several endogenous substrates, becomes the predominant pathway for ethanol oxidation to acetaldehyde. The bulk of this activity resides in the liver.[1] Ethanol oxidation through this pathway results in the transfer of hydrogen to NAD. During this process, the redox potential of the liver shifts to a more reduced level, reflected in an increased NADH to NAD ratio. This excess NADH produces changes in the flux of other substrates and alters the ratio of those metabolites that are dependent for reduction or oxidation on the NADH–NAD couple.

In the absence of ethanol, the reducing equivalents utilized in the respiratory chain are provided mainly by the oxidation of fatty acids. During the oxidation of ethanol, the activity of the citric acid cycle is depressed,[2,3] partly because of a slowing of the reactions of the cycle that require NAD. The mitochondria then use the hydrogen equivalents originating from ethanol rather than from oxidation (through the citric acid cycle) of two carbon fragments derived from fatty acids. Thus, fatty acids that normally serve as the main energy source of the liver are supplanted by ethanol. The increased NADH to NAD ratio is also associated with a rise in the concentration of α-glycerophosphate,[4] the initial acyl receptor for glycerolipid synthesis.

After chronic ethanol consumption, the acute inhibitory effect of ethanol on fatty acid oxidation fades,[5] in keeping with the attenuation of the redox change.[6] This is most likely due to the development of microsomal pathways for ethanol oxidation that utilize rather than produce reducing equivalents. Methylene blue, which attenuated the redox changes produced by ethanol, did not prevent the development of alcoholic fatty liver in rats,[7] indicating the participation of other mechanisms after chronic alcohol consumption. Conversely, the low oxygen tension prevailing in perivenular zones of the liver enhances the redox shift produced by ethanol oxidation,[8,9] and this factor increases with the progression of liver injury as a result of further decreases in oxygen tension due to progressive reduction of hepatic blood flow.[10,11] Thus, the ethanol-induced shift of the redox potential is maximal in the perivenular area where the most severe injury occurs.

2.2. *Effects of the Interaction of Ethanol with Hepatic Microsomes*

Chronic ethanol feeding results in proliferation of the smooth endoplasmic reticulum. This change is linked to the fact that ethanol oxidation is also catalyzed by a specific microsomal cytochrome (P4502E1) and that this alternate pathway increases in activity after prolonged consumption.[12] In addition, chronic alcohol consumption accelerates the rate of triacylglycerol synthesis by stimulating the activities of the microsomal enzymes involved: the *sn*-glycerol-3-phosphate acyltransferase,[13] the phosphatidate phosphohydrolase,[14–16] and the acyl-CoA:1,2 diacylglycerol acyltransferase.[15] Increases in the activity of the latter two enzymes have also been observed after short-term ethanol administration.[17–19] The phosphatidate phosphohydrolase fulfills almost all criteria of a rate-limiting enzyme, and its activity changes, in most situations, in parallel to the rate of triacylglycerol synthesis.[20] The diacylglycerol acyltransferase, which branches the pathway toward the synthesis of triacylglycerols, is also a plausible site of regulation for the ethanol effect, since there is a much greater increase in triacylglycerols than in phospholipids.[21] The mechanism for these increases has not been fully elucidated.[22] There is, however, consensus that the availability of fatty acids is a major determinant of the synthesis and secretion of triacylglycerols.[23] Ethanol-fed rats show no changes in the activity of enzymes for *de novo* fatty acid synthesis,[24] but the availability of fatty acids is markedly enhanced by the impairments of mitochondrial β-oxidation (see Section 2.3). The hepatic fatty acid-binding protein (L-FABPc), which normally transports fatty acids in the cytosol, binds to microsomes and exerts a direct stimulatory effect on triacylglycerol-synthesizing enzymes, including the diacylglycerol acyltransferase.[25,26]

Liver biopsies from recently drinking alcoholics show a marked increase in triacylglycerol, with a smaller increase in cholesteryl ester and no significant changes in phospholipid concentrations.[27] Cholesteryl esters accumulate in the rat liver, as a result of both enhanced cholesterogenesis and decreased bile excretion.[28] The 3-hydroxy-3-methylglutaryl-coenzyme A (HMG-CoA) reductase activity was found to be increased in rats fed alcohol-containing diets,[29,30] but not in rats given alcohol in drinking water, in which the principal alteration was a decrease in 7α-hydroxylase activity,[31] a key enzyme for the synthesis of bile acids. The microsomal acyl coenzyme A–cholesterol acyltransferase (CAT) activity increased in male rats fed alcohol-containing diets[29] but not in females.[32]

Chronic alcohol administration also increased the cytochrome P450 4A1-catalyzed ω-hydroxylation of fatty acids in the microsomes.[33] This led to a rise in the hepatic concentration of dicarboxylic acids, products of oxidation of ω-hydroxy fatty acids by class III ADH. These increases were greater in male than in female rats. Consistent with the possibility of similar alterations in human subjects, dicarboxylic aciduria was found in male but not female alcoholics.[34] Also, the ratio of adipic–sebacic acid (an index of peroxisomal β-oxidation) increased in male but not in female alcoholics. These pathways normally play a minor quantitative role in fatty acid oxidation, but their contribution increases markedly under conditions in which mitochondrial β-oxidation decreases, such as alcohol consumption. This may explain how a typical peroxisomal proliferator, such as clofibrate, attenuated the ethanol-induced fatty liver.[35] Dicarboxylic acids (products of ω-oxidation) can activate the nuclear receptor for peroxisomal proliferators. The activated receptor then binds to response elements in the promoters of genes, such as those for peroxisomal fatty acyl-CoA oxidase, cytochrome P4504A1, and L-FABPc, stimulating their transcription.[36] This may represent an important homeostatic mechanism to maintain low concentrations of potentially deleterious fatty acids when their major site of oxidation in the mitochondria is impaired (Fig. 1). In keeping with this interpretation, L-FABPc was markedly increased in male rats fed alcohol-containing diets[37] and much less in females.[32] This was associated with more fatty acid accumulation and less esterification in the females than in the males. Accumulation of fatty acids to deleterious levels may contribute to the greater vulnerability of women than men to develop alcoholic liver injury.[38]

Total liver phospholipids increase after chronic ethanol consumption, probably reflecting the increased mass of microsomal membranes.[39] This results in a small increase in hepatic concentration in rats,[21] but not in primates.[15] In ethanol-fed rats, the activities of two enzymes specifically involved in phospholipid synthesis [choline phosphotransferase and phosphoethanolamine methyl transferase (PEMT)] were found to be increased.[40] However, after more prolonged administration of larger ethanol doses to baboons, PEMT activity was found to be decreased.[41] In the liver, a major control mechanism for the synthesis of phosphatidylcholine (the most abundant phospholipid in membranes) is the supply of methionine that determines the concentration of *S*-adenosylmethionine necessary for the methylation of phosphatidylethanolamine to phosphatidylcholine, a reaction-catalyzed by PEMT.

After alcohol consumption, the fatty acid composition of liver triacylglycerols[42,43] and phosphatidylcholine[44] closely resembles that of the diet. In addition, ethanol consumption increases linoleate and decreases arachidonate, which has been attributed to an inhibitory effect of ethanol on Δ5, Δ6, and Δ9 acyl CoA desaturase activities,[45–48] particularly the Δ5 and Δ6 ones.

Some of the microsomal changes seem to offset a possibly deleterious accumulation of fatty acids. However, compensatory mechanisms such as the increase in triacylglycerol-synthesizing enzymes[15] and in fatty acid-binding protein[49] fade during the progression of the liver injury, leading to further accumulation of fatty acids in the liver of patients with cirrhosis.[50] Other changes appear to reflect microsomal injury and are possibly linked to the fact that enhanced oxidation of ethanol via the microsomal pathway increases the production of potentially toxic metabolites, such as acetaldehyde, hydroxyethyl, and other radicals. Initiation of free radical events usually occurs by excessive formation of reactive oxygen species, such as the superoxide anion radical (O_2^-), which is converted by a superoxide dismutase into hydrogen peroxide (H_2O_2), removed in turn by glutathione peroxidase and catalase. They are produced, in part, from "leakage" of electrons in the mitochondrial electron transport chain and the microsomal cytochrome P4502E1 system. In small concentrations, they may play physiological roles. However, toxicity may result from excessive generation, impaired removal, or enhanced conversion by metals such as free iron (normally sequestered in macromolecules, such as ferritin) into hydroxyl radicals (HO^-), the principal initiator of peroxidative damage of lipids, proteins, and DNA. Acetaldehyde[51–54]

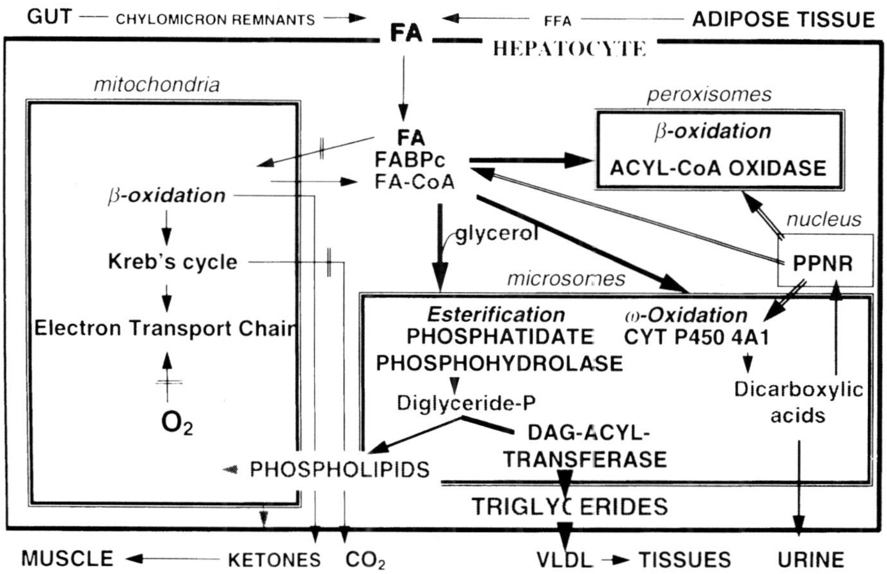

Figure 1. Schematic representation of the fatty acid (FA) changes, which are either enhanced (→) or inhibited (⇸) by alcohol consumption. The supply of fatty acids from gut, adipose tissue, and liver synthesis is increased under some conditions, but the main alteration resides in the mitochondria, where the uptake and oxidation of FA is markedly impaired. The FA, bound to a fatty acid-binding protein of the cytosol (FABPc), undergo esterification in the microsomes where the activity of key triacylglycerol-synthesizing enzymes increases, leading to the formation of triacylglycerols that are partly secreted as VLDL or accumulate in the liver (fatty liver). The increased availability of FA also stimulates alternate pathways for their oxidation (microsomal ω-oxidation and peroxisomal β-oxidation). The capacity of these pathways is believed to increase as a result of the activation by dicarboxylic acids (products of ω-oxidation) of the peroxisomal proliferator nuclear receptor (PPNR), which increases transcription of FABPc, acyl-CoA oxidase, and cytochrome P4504A1 (key components of these pathways) by binding to response element in the promoter region of the corresponding genes.

and hydroxyethyl radicals,[55] as well as aldehyde intermediates of lipoperoxidation,[56] form adducts that may alter the function of biologically important proteins.

2.3. *Effects of Acetaldehyde and Other Reactive Products of Ethanol on Mitochondrial Lipid Metabolism*

After chronic alcohol consumption, the acute inhibition of fatty acid oxidation by ethanol metabolism is followed by structural[57] and functional alterations of this organelle, which persist after the disappearance of ethanol from the body. Mitochondria from ethanol-fed rats display decreased capacity to oxidize two-carbon fragments of fatty acids[58,59] with no changes in β-oxidation,[60] which determines that an important fraction of the accumulated acetyl-CoA is diverted to the formation of ketones.[61] Also, the transport of fatty acids into the mitochondria has been found to be limited by the decreased activity of palmitoyltransferase I and increased sensitivity of this enzyme to the inhibition by malonyl-CoA.[62] Mitochondria are sensitive targets for ethanol toxicity, and impairments can be detected with relatively modest ethanol consumption.[63,64] With higher levels of alcohol consumption, in alcohol-fed baboons, Arai and co-workers[65] found marked alterations in the phospholipid composition of the mitochondrial membranes (characterized by decreases in phosphatidylcholine and cardiolipin), which were associated with a marked decrease in cytochrome oxidase activity. Reconstitution of this enzyme with synthetic phospholipids restored its activity. Phosphatidylcholine and cardiolipin were more efficient reactivators than phosphatidylethanolamine. A possible mechanism for the decrease in phosphatidylcholine is the reduction of PEMT activity.[41]

Acetaldehyde is one of the agents incriminated in the pathogenesis of the mitochondrial alterations. The concentration of this reactive metabolite is maintained very low, because acetaldehyde is readily oxidized to acetate in the mitochondria via aldehyde dehydrogenase, with further reduction of NAD to NADH. However, if its production is increased, acetaldehyde by itself can depress the oxidative capacity of liver mitochondria, including its own oxidation.[66] This creates a vicious circle, which results in a progressive increase in the concentration of this metabolite and further deterioration of this organelle upon chronic alcohol consumption. The inhibition of fatty acid oxidation by acetaldehyde was particularly prominent when mitochondria were isolated from animals fed alcohol chronically.[59] In baboons fed alcohol-containing diets for several years, acute ethanol administration markedly increased the output of acetaldehyde in hepatic venous blood.[67] This was associated with defective utilization of oxygen, striking accumulation of reducing equivalents in the mitochondria, and leakage of enzymes from the mitochondrial matrix into the hepatic vein.[67] The decreased activity of palmitoyltransferase I was also reproduced by incubation of hepatocytes with acetaldehyde.[62] Part of the acetate, a product of acetaldehyde oxidation, ends up incorporated into lipids, but most of it is secreted into the plasma.[68]

Mitochondria are also a rich source of reactive oxygen radicals, mainly as superoxide anions produced in the electron transport chain. The oxidation of reduced glutathione (GSH) is the main mechanism to maintain low levels of these radicals. Chronic ethanol administration impairs the uptake of cytosolic GSH by hepatic mitochondria, which increases their susceptibility to oxidative injury, aggravating the deficits in oxidation of other substrates.[69,70] Acetaldehyde binding to cysteine and/or glutathione may contribute to the decrease in GSH.[71] In addition, alcohol feeding increases the activity of NADH–cytochrome reductase of the outer mitochondrial membranes, which, in the presence of iron, generates hydroxyl radicals[72] that in turn can initiate a cascade of autocatalytic lipoperoxidation reactions and damage of cell membranes.

2.4. *Nonmetabolic Effects of Ethanol*

Some changes may be produced by the incorporation of ethanol per se into membrane lipids. It has been shown that clinically relevant concentrations of ethanol (20–80 mM) increase the fluidity of the plasma membranes of erythrocytes and synaptosomes *in vitro*.[73] After chronic alcohol consumption, however, those membranes become more resistant to the *in vitro* fluidizing effect of ethanol.[74] At variance with other membranes, hepatic plasma membranes show increased fluidity (assessed by fluorescence anisotropy) after chronic ethanol feeding.[75–77] These alterations may be due in part to changes in composition that could be related to metabolic effects of ethanol.

Lipids also accumulate in tissues that do not oxidize significant amounts of ethanol, such as the heart,[78,79] lungs,[80] or pancreas.[81] Ethanol forms esters with fatty acids, and these ethyl esters have been identified in total body lipid extracts,[82] heart,[83] pancreas, brain, adipose tissue, and other organs[84] commonly damaged by ethanol abuse. This reaction is catalyzed by a specific fatty acyl ethyl ester synthase,[85] in addition to nonspecific esterases. The presence of fatty acid ethyl esters in human serum recently has been documented after alcohol ingestion,[86] with concentrations up to 42 μM.[87] The esters are bound to lipoproteins and albumin. Low-density lipoprotein (LDL) reconstituted with fatty acid ethyl esters inhibited protein synthesis and proliferation of human hepatoblastoma cells, although at concentrations much higher (400–800 μM) than those found in LDL of intoxicated subjects (3 μM).[88] Moreover, fatty acid ethyl esters can act as uncouplers of oxidative phosphorylation in heart mitochondria[89] and can destabilize rat pancreatic lysosomes.[90] Since cells actively hydrolyze the esters to ethanol and fatty acids,[91] the question has been raised whether the toxicity is due to the esters or to the fatty acids.[92]

Another potentially deleterious compound is phosphatidylethanol, which has been found in brain, liver, and other tissues after alcohol consumption.[93] It results from the reaction between ethanol and phosphatidic acid, an important intermediate in phospholipid synthesis and signal transduction.

3. Alcoholic Fatty Liver

The accumulation of lipids in the hepatocyte (steatosis) is one of the earliest and most striking manifestations of alcoholic liver injury. In addition to fat accumulation, the early manifestations include alterations of protein metabolism, subcellular organelles, and mesenchymal cells, which are probably the major determinants of the progression of the lesions. Fatty liver is associated with a worse prognosis than previously thought. In a large prospective study,[94] the development of cirrhosis over 10 to 13 years increased in proportion to the degree of steatosis found in the first biopsy.

The concept that malnutrition is primarily responsible for the development of alcoholic fatty liver was challenged by its experimental reproduction through administering ethanol while maintaining adequate nutrition by incorporation of ethanol into nutritionally adequate liquid diets that were given as the only source of food and fluids.[21] The administration of ethanol to volunteers (either as a supplement to a normal or enriched diet, or as substitution for other calories) produced up to a 25-fold rise in hepatic triacylglycerol concentrations.[95–97]

3.1. Pathogenesis

Excessive accumulation of fat in the liver may result from an increased supply of lipids to the liver (from either the intestine, the adipose tissue, or the liver itself) or from decreased disposition of liver lipids (by oxidation, by release into plasma lipoproteins, or by biliary excretion of cholesterol and phospholipids). The predominance of one mechanism over the others depends, to a large extent, on the experimental conditions. After administration of a single large dose of alcohol, the resulting fatty liver is associated with enhanced mobilization of fatty acids from adipose tissue with increased serum concentrations of free fatty acid (FFA).[98] These effects are mediated in part by the release of catecholamines during alcoholic intoxication.[99] A number of factors that prevent the release or the action of catecholamines on FFA mobilization also prevent to a great extent the development of fatty liver after an acute ethanol dose.[100,101]

In rats given 36% of their energy requirement as ethanol, hepatic lipid accumulation reached a maximum in about 4 weeks.[21,102] The steatosis was exaggerated by increasing the amount of dietary fat, but it was not fully prevented when dietary fat was reduced to supply only the essential fatty acids.[103] No differences were noted when the fat contained mainly saturated (coconut oil) or unsaturated (linseed oil) fatty acids,[42] but steatosis was markedly decreased when the dietary triacylglycerols contained medium-chain fatty acids.[3] Despite continuous consumption of ethanol for the life span of this species, there was no further progression of the liver lesions.[103] Attempts to increase ethanol intake decreased food consumption and promoted undernutrition. In baboons, up to 50% of the energy requirement could be given as ethanol without impairing nutrition.[104] This not only resulted in a more severe fatty liver but also produced most of the spectrum of alcoholic liver disease, including cirrhosis. The principal mechanisms of the fatty liver under these conditions is the inhibition of fatty acid oxidation in the mitochondria and the enhanced activity of triacylglycerol-synthesizing enzymes in the microsomes. Ethanol increases the output of triacylglycerol-carrying lipoproteins from the liver both in man[105] and experimental animals,[15,106,107] which may play some compensatory role in diminishing hepatic fat accumulation. However, this mechanism is relatively inefficient, probably because ethanol consumption also impairs the secretion of plasma proteins.[108] This impairment is due, at least in part, to acetaldehyde-mediated disruption of liver microtubules,[108–112] the integrity of which is required for normal secretion. This secretion defect aggravates but probably does not initiate the fatty liver. At the blood ethanol concentrations reached in these animals, the levels of plasma FFA actually decrease in men[113] and in rats,[114] as well as the turnover of FFA,[115] an effect found to be mediated by acetate[116] and acetaldehyde.[114]

More recently, a rat model based on continuous intragastric infusion of ethanol[117] has prompted considerable interest, because, in a relatively short time, it results in the development not only of fatty liver but also of perivenular necroinflammatory lesions.[118] An increase in dietary fat[119] (from 5 to 35% of calories), especially that containing polyunsaturated fatty acids.[120] resulted in the appearance of perivenular fibrosis and thin fibrous septa. By contrast, beef fat (tallow) was found to prevent all manifestations of alcoholic liver injury in the rats force-fed ethanol.[121] This was consistent with some epidemiological studies indicating a positive correlation between the development of cirrhosis with the consumption of polyunsaturated fatty acids and a negative one with the consumption of saturated fatty acid and cholesterol.[122,123] The feeding of ω3 fatty acids of fish oil (menhaden oil) produced the most severe liver lesions.[124,125] However, the saturated "protective" oil in the latter study[125] contained as much linoleate as the one previously reported to be hepatotoxic. Furthermore, this report[125] contrasts with previous findings that administration of menhaden oil to rats pair-fed ethanol-containing and control diets resulted in a trend for a decrease in fatty liver and the hyperlipemia.[126] An important difference between the intragastric infusion model and the spontaneous consumption of ethanol-containing diets is the production of marked fluctuation of blood alcohol levels (from less than 10 mg/dl to greater than 450 mg/dl),[117] which could produce multiple episodes of hypoxia (during the periods of intense intoxication) and reperfusion injury.

Ethanol feeding increases the susceptibility of rats to develop hypoxic injury with centrolobular necrosis and inflammation.[127,128] Rats[129] or baboons[10,130] chronically consuming ethanol by the oral route showed no evidence of shortage in oxygen supply, whereas rats force-fed ethanol intragastrically did.[131] The decrease in hepatic ATP in these animals[132,133] was associated with decreased arterial PO_2 and corrected by oxygen administration. By contrast, the decrease in ATP found in rats fed ethanol orally[134] was attributed to the mitochondrial alterations rather than to shortage in oxygen supply. The combination of consumption of unsaturated fatty acids with hypoxia appears to be optimal for the production of intense lipoperoxidation and secondary alterations, but one wonders to what extent these rather extreme conditions can be extrapolated to the majority of alcoholics.

3.2. *Role of Lipoperoxidation*

Manifestations of lipoperoxidation have been a feature in all models of alcoholic liver injury, including human alcoholics.[71,135] It was first demonstrated by the increased production of malondialdehyde after a large acute dose of ethanol[136,137] and subsequently confirmed in various models of chronic ethanol administration either in the drinking fluid[138,139] or in liquid diets.[140] In the rats fed alcohol-containing diets, an increase in conjugated dienes was found only after acute ethanol administration, whereas these changes were more intense in baboons fed ethanol-containing diets for several years and persisted after alcohol withdrawal.[140] In the latter model, there was also an increase in 4-hydroxynonenal and F_2-isoprostane.[141] The lipoperoxidative changes were associated with a decrease in GSH and were partially attenuated by administration of its precursor, methionine. The fatty liver produced by an acute large dose of alcohol was prevented by the administration of α-tocopherol and *N-N′*-diphenyl-*p*-phenylenediamine (DPPD),[137] another antioxidant, whereas they had no effect on the fatty liver of rats chronically consuming alcohol by the oral route.[142] The manifestations of lipoperoxidation (such as the production of conjugated dienes or 8-isoprostane) were markedly exaggerated in rats force-fed intragastrically the combination of ethanol and unsaturated fatty acids and correlated with the severity of the lesions.[143,144] The liver injury in these rats was also associated with increased levels of endotoxin in the blood, elevations of thromboxane B_2 and leukotriene B_4, and decreased levels of prostaglandins E_2 and I_2,[145,146] which may contribute to further aggravation of the lesions.

Lipoperoxidation thus appears to be an important factor in the progression of the lesions. Acetaldehyde, another incriminated factor, also promotes lipid peroxidation when added to the perfused liver.[147] In addition, both acetaldehyde[148,149] and lipoperoxidation products[150] promotes the synthesis of collagen. Recently, an agent (polyenylphosphatidylcholine, or PPC), which prevented the appearance of fibrosis and cirrhosis in ethanol-fed baboons[151] and opposed the rise in 4-hydroxynonenal and F_2-isoprostanes,[141] also attenuated the fatty liver in ethanol-fed rats,[152] an effect that was not reproduced by equivalent amounts of choline or linoleic acid. The prevention was associated with restoration of the ethanol-induced decrease of mitochondrial cytochrome oxidase activity and of the oxidation of fatty acids and other substrates.[153] These effects may be related to the high bioavailability of dilinoleoylphosphatidylcholine (the main component of PPC) and to its effective incorporation *in toto* in cell membranes.

4. Alcoholic Hyperlipemia

Different clinical entities are recognized within the common denomination of "alcoholic hyperlipemia." They include episodic hypertriglyceridemia after bouts of excessive drinking, chronic forms of hyperlipemia affected by the concomitant consumption of alcohol and isolated elevations of high-density lipoprotein (HDL) cholesterol in moderate drinkers, as well as the striking lipoprotein abnormalities observed in severe forms of alcoholic liver disease. Since they share many pathogenetic features, they will be discussed as a single entity. The main mechanisms for the lipoprotein changes are summarized in Fig. 2.

4.1. Chylomicrons and Very-Low-Density Lipoproteins

The plasma triacylglycerols are the major determinants of the serum lactescence or turbidity found after bouts of excessive drinking. They increase in all lipoprotein fractions, but proportionally more in those lipoproteins that are normally rich in triacylglycerols: very-low-density lipoprotein (VLDL) and chylomicrons or chylomicronlike particles. Thus, alcoholic hyperlipemia is usually classified as type IV or type V. However, the phenotypic pattern changes rapidly after alcohol withdrawal, from type V to type IV and to type II, because of the rapid clearance of chylomicrons, followed by that of VLDL and the slower clearance of cholesterol and phospholipids that predominate in LDL and HDL.[154] As a consequence, the frequency and intensity of the hypertrigliceridemia in alcoholics is likely to be minimized by the measurement in fasting samples.

The incidence of hypertriglyceridemia varies with the population studied. Among hyperlipemic patients, alcohol constitutes the second major cause, following diabetes.[155] In epidemiological studies, plasma triacylglycerol levels correlate with alcohol consumption.[156] However, significant increases in plasma triacylglycerols are rather rarely encountered in patents hospitalized for alcoholism or its complications. Only 27–28% of hospitalized alcoholics had fasting triacylglycerol levels over normal limits (2 mM) and 17% over 3 mM, with phenotypes IV, II, or V, in that order of frequency.[157] This hypertriglyceridemia is frequently seen in patients with fatty liver but rarely among cirrhotics.[158,159] In severe liver diseases, striking alterations of

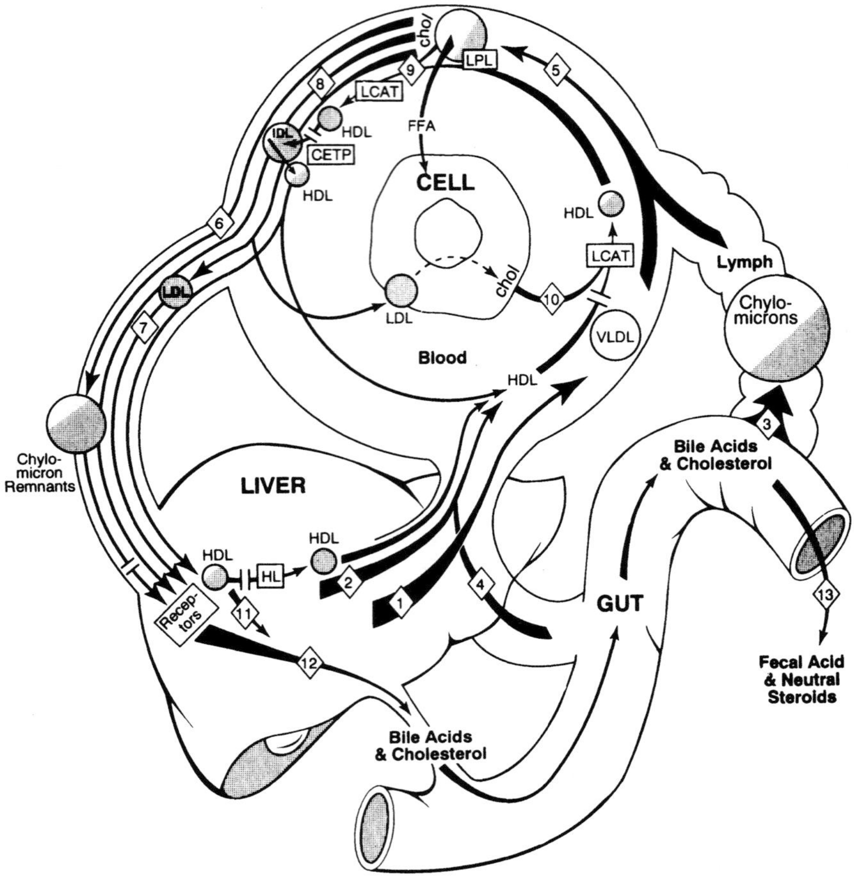

Figure 2. Schematic representation of the lipoprotein metabolic steps reported to be enhanced (—◇→) or inhibited (⫩) by alcohol consumption. Alcohol consumption stimulates the hepatic production of VLDL (1) and HDL (2) and the intestinal production of chylomicrons (3) and probably HDL (4). The triglyceride-rich lipoproteins (VLDL and chylomicrons) undergo hydrolysis of the triglycerides to fatty acids by lipoprotein lipase (LPL), the activity of which increases after chronic alcohol consumption (5), leading to attenuation of the hypertriglyceridemia. In addition to fatty acids, this reaction generates cholesteryl ester-rich chylomicron remnants (6), LDL (7), and intermediate density lipoproteins (IDL) (or VLDL remnants) (8), and increases the supply of free cholesterol and apoAI to HDL from the excess membranes of partially hydrolyzed triglycerides-rich particles (9). The four sources of free cholesterol for HDL, namely hepatic and intestinal nascent HDL (2 and 4), and membranes of both cells (10) and triglyceride-rich particles (9) are increased by chronic alcohol consumption. The free cholesterol is esterified by action of the lecithin cholesterol acyltransferase (LCAT), transported in the core of the HDL particles and transferred to products of VLDL degradation by the action of the cholesteryl ester transfer protein (CETP). LDL becomes a major source of cholesterol for the tissues, including the liver. Excess cholesterol is removed by the liver via receptor-mediat-

serum lipoprotein occur, regardless of the etiologic agent. Such alterations are found in patients with alcoholic hepatitis or advanced cirrhosis. Electrophoretically, there is a marked decrease or disappearance of both pre-β and α-lipoproteins, with the appearance of a broad β-band[159] and, chemically, by a decreased cholesteryl ester–free cholesterol ratio. These changes are associated with decreases in lecithin cholesterol acyltransferase (LCAT) activity[160,161] and in apoAI (the major activator of LCAT), the catabolism of which was found to be increased in patients with severe alcoholic hepatitis.[162] HDL deficient in cholesteryl esters and apoAI but markedly enriched in apoE appear in the plasma as stacked discoidal particles similar to nascent HDL with corresponding decreases in VLDL and LDL apoE.[161,163] The diminished transfer of apoE from HDL to triacylglycerol-rich lipoproteins may result in decreased hepatic removal of the remnants of these particles and hypertriglyceridemia with a type III phenotype.

4.1.1. Effects of Ethanol Administration and Associated Conditions. Acute administration of a single ethanol dose, which results in blood concentration over 100 mg/dl and mild intoxication, increases triacylglycerols in the plasma of normal volunteers,[164–166] whereas the administration of smaller doses does not.[167] One fourth of the subjects drinking 1 g ethanol per kg of body weight in the evening showed a type IV hyperlipemia in the fasting serum samples obtained the next morning.[168]

Chronic ethanol administration exaggerates the effects of ethanol on plasma triacylglycerols. Either as a supplement to a normal diet[95,169,170] or as substitution for other foods,[153] ethanol produced a fourfold increase in plasma triacylglycerols and less increases in cholesterol and phospholipids. Daily administration of 75 g ethanol for 2 weeks slightly increased serum triglycerides (mainly as VLDL) and apoB.[171] Smaller doses of ethanol given to normal subjects in substitution for other calories did not produce significant hypertriglyceridemia.[172]

Dietary fat markedly enhances the lipemic response to acute ethanol administration.[173–175] The increase includes both VLDL and chylomicrons.[176] Preprandial drinking of a moderate dose of alcohol for 1 week significantly increased fasting triacylglycerol levels in the plasma.[177] Alcohol consumption

←

ed uptake of LDL, IDL, and chylomicron remnants or via direct uptake of HDL free cholesterol (11) and excreted in the bile as such or converted to bile acids (12). Fecal excretion of acid and neutral steroids (intestinal products of bile acids and cholesterol) are increased by alcohol consumption (13). Usually after higher consumption of alcohol and more advanced liver injury, some activities are decreased, such as those of CETP (leading to further accumulation of HDL cholesteryl esters), hepatic removal of remnants (producing accumulation of these particles), HL (contributing to the increase in HDL), and LCAT (responsible for the accumulation of discoidal HDL and other alterations in severe forms of liver disease). Chol, free cholesterol; □, triglycerides; ▩, cholesterol esters.

for 2 weeks exaggerated the postprandial response to a diet containing alcohol, but not to a diet without alcohol.[175] However, in patients with alcoholic fatty liver, administration of a high-fat meal, even in the absence of ethanol, produced a striking increase in serum triacylglycerols.[178,179] Alcoholics who were not hyperlipemic in the fasting state became hyperlipemic in the postprandial state. The enhanced lipemic response to dietary lipids tends to disappear with the progression of the liver damage from fatty liver to cirrhosis. Contrasting with the potentiating effect of usual fat mixtures. ω3 fatty-acid rich fish oil lowers the ethanol-induced increases in blood lipids.[126]

The lipemic response of human volunteers to chronic ethanol administration is usually transient: After reaching maximal levels in several days or weeks, serum lipids decrease and even normalize despite continuation of the ethanol intake.[95,160,180] Conversely, some individuals exhibit enhanced susceptibility to the lipemic effects of ethanol. This condition is generally suspected by the lack of response to the usual treatment for hyperlipemia and the improvement after abstinence from alcohol.[181,182] Alcohol consumption may even unmask subclinical defects in lipid metabolism, especially those associated with reduced activity of lipoprotein lipase[153,154] or overproduction of VLDL.[168,183–185] Obese subjects are more susceptible to the hyperlipemic effects of alcohol.[186] In pregnant women who do not abstain from alcohol, the physiological hyperlipemia of late gestation is exaggerated,[187] possibly due to increased VLDL production and decreased lipase activities. Moreover, a large percentage of patients with marked and sustained alcoholic hyperlipemia have relatives with hyperlipemia.[188] Thus, the participation of an underlying defect in lipid metabolism should be suspected in any alcoholic with severe hyperlipemia. Conversely, the lack of response to the usual treatment for hyperlipemia should lead to a search for alcoholism.

4.1.2. Pathogenesis of the Hypertriglyceridemia. The striking enhancement of alcoholic hypertriglyceridemia by dietary fat suggests that the lipids accumulated in the plasma may originate in the intestine (mechanism 3 in Fig. 2). In the absence of malnutrition, alcohol can increase both fat absorption[189] and the production of both triacylglycerol[190,191] and cholesterol[192] by the intestine. In pair-fed rats, acute ethanol administration to the controls increased the mesenteric lymph flow and the output of both dietary[193] and nondietary[194] lipids. But even the largest increase in dietary lymph lipids was insufficient to produce significant hyperlipemia in rats fed the same diet. By contrast, when postprandial hyperlipemia was markedly enhanced by chronic ethanol administration, there was no increase in lymph lipid output.[107,193] In fact, a decrease was observed after ethanol administration to rats fed a low-fat diet.[195] The *in vitro* inhibitory effects of ethanol on the absorption of fatty acids and other nutrients were prevented by feeding rats saturated fatty acids.[196] The dissociation between the effects of ethanol on serum lipids and the changes in lymph lipid output indicates that the postprandial hyperlipemia is not merely due to changes in intestinal absorption or production of lipids.

Mesenteric lymph diversion prevented the development of alcoholic hyperlipemia; however, hyperlipemia reappeared in the ethanol-fed rats (but not in the pair-fed controls) when equal loads of lymph lipids were infused intravenously to the lymph-diverted rats.[107] Moreover, the administration of orotic acid, an agent that inhibits hepatic but not intestinal release of triacylglycerols, abolished ethanol-induced hyperlipemia in rats.[197] Thus, the supply of lipids via the mesenteric lymph seems to play more a permissive than causal role for the development of alcoholic hyperlipemia.

An alternate possibility is that the chylomicrons could be poorly hydrolyzed by lipoprotein lipase (LPL) or their remnant slowly removed by the liver after alcohol consumption (mechanisms 5 and 6 in Fig. 2). Most of the early studies focused on the total postheparin LPL activity and found no change after acute[198] or chronic[199] ethanol administration. More recently, a large dose of ethanol has been found to produce a slight decrease in LPL activity and some delay in the clearance of serum triacylglycerols[180,200,201] The decreased clearance was greater when ethanol was given with saturated than with polyunsaturated fat and was associated with a concomitant reduction in the appearance of plasma FFA of dietary origin, a finding consistent with decreased LPL activity.[202] Crouse and Grundy[186] also found decreased clearance of chylomicron triglycerides, but without changes in LPL or the hepatic triglyceride lipase (HL).

The possibility that alcohol consumption could interfere with the removal of cholesteryl ester-enriched remnants by the liver was supported by the finding that, after the injection of chylomicrons doubly labeled in the triacylglycerol and cholesteryl ester moieties to alcohol-fed rats, the clearance of chylomicron–cholesteryl esters was impaired to a greater extent than that of chylomicron triacylglycerol.[203,204] In the rat, Lakshman and co-workers[205] provided direct evidence that hepatocytes isolated from alcohol-fed animals have a decreased uptake of remnants. An incomplete feedback inhibition of HMG-CoA reductase activity by chylomicron remnants from alcohol-fed rats was also reported.[204] In alcohol-fed baboons with hyperlipemia, Savolainen and co-workers[206] found a decrease in the fractional removal of chylomicron triglycerides, namely in the percent of such particles taken up by the liver. However, the total hepatic removal of both chylomicron and VLDL triglycerides were markedly increased in the alcohol-fed animals, suggesting that the primary mechanism for the hyperlipemia was excessive production rather than decreased removal. Furthermore, after alcohol administration for 4 weeks to human volunteers, the delayed clearance of chylomicron triacylglycerols was marked in those patients who developed the greatest increase in the hepatic synthesis of VLDL triacylglycerols.[186] The defect in chylomicron removal could be due, at least in part, to saturation of either LPL or the hepatic uptake by the excessive supply of products of both endogenous and dietary origin sharing similar mechanisms of removal from the blood.

Chronic alcohol administration to rats significantly increased the incorporation of intravenously injected [^{14}C]lysine into VLDL.[106] This effect persisted after complete diversion of the mesenteric lymph,[107] incriminating the liver as the major source for the increased lipoprotein production (mechanism 1 in Fig. 2). The increased production of plasma triacylglycerol in alcohol-fed rats was also demonstrated after blocking triacylglycerol removal from plasma with Triton WR-1339.[106]

Direct evidence of an increase in hepatic VLDL and other lipoprotein production was obtained by hepatic vein catherization. In three normal volunteers undergoing catheterization, ethanol infusion to produce low blood concentrations (3–5 mM) increased hepatic secretion of tryacylglycerols.[105] In nonhuman primates, Savolainen and co-workers[206] have shown by catherization studies that the livers of alcohol-fed baboons at early stages of liver injury secrete more VLDL triacylglycerols than the livers of the pair-fed controls; the main part of the increased hepatic output of VLDL was due to an enhanced production of abnormally large VLDL particles with flotation characteristics similar to those of chylomicrons ($S_f > 400$). These particles were found in the hepatic venous but not in the portal blood, indicating that their production occurs in the liver rather than the intestine. This may account for the observation of chylomicronlike particles in the fasting blood of some alcoholics.[154] The contribution of the enhanced hepatic production of VLDL to the serum lipid changes observed in recently drinking alcoholics without liver disease was supported by documentation of an increase in the total turnover and synthetic rates of VLDL triacylglycerols, even in the absence of high levels of VLDL.[207] Similarly, the synthetic rate of apoB was also found to be increased after chronic alcohol administration[208] and even in alcoholics with type V hyperlipemia[209] in whom postheparin LPL activity was decreased.[210] This reflects the predominant role of increased lipoprotein production, at least at early stages of alcoholic liver disease.

Several factors contribute to the disappearance of the hypertriglyceridemia in the course of prolonged alcohol consumption. One is the progressive impairment of liver functions. Progression of alcoholic liver injury from fatty liver to fibrosis in baboons fed an alcohol-containing diet for several years resulted in decreased hepatic induction of triacylglycerol-synthesizing activities and disappearance of the hypertriglyceridemia.[15] This is consistent with previous results in alcoholics showing decreased incorporation of fatty acids into plasma triacylglycerols of hepatic origin with progression of the liver injury.[211]

Protein[212] as well as choline[213] deficiencies in rats impair lipoprotein secretion and aggravate fat accumulation in the liver. It is possible that associated protein malnutrition may also contribute to the lack of hyperlipemia in some alcoholics.

In contrast to the acute effects of ethanol, chronic consumption has been found to increase the activity of extrahepatic LPL in the majority of alcoholics[214,215] but not in moderate drinkers.[216] Mordasini and co-workers[217] documented that the rise in plasma triacylglycerol (mainly VLDL) is associated with an initial decrease in LPL activity, whereas the return of triacylglycerol to normal levels (despite continuous ethanol intake) is associated with increased LPL activity. Also, according to a kinetic study,[207] the increase in the total turnover and synthetic rates were associated with a 23% increase in the fractional catabolic rate of VLDL triacylglycerols. This may account for the transient nature of hypertriglyceridemia during alcohol administration,[95,170] the modest degree of hypertriglyceridemia found in the majority of alcoholics, and the paradoxical increase in VLDL and LDL due to normalization of the lipoprotein lipase activity during the initial period of abstinence.[214]

4.2. HDL

In patients with marked hypertriglyceridemia, plasma cholesterol and phospholipids are also increased.[95] They are components of all lipoprotein fractions, but most of it is transported in LDL and HDL. In hospitalized alcoholics, total plasma cholesterol was not significantly increased.[157] However, in 86% of recently drinking alcoholics, a prominent α-lipoprotein band was found in electrophoresis,[218] which reflects an increase in HDL cholesterol.[219,220] These changes are more persistent than those in triacylglycerols and also occur at lower levels of alcohol consumption, constituting the principal serum lipid change in moderate drinkers. Acute ethanol administration produced hypertriglyceridemia without significant changes in plasma cholesterol.[221] Conversely, administration of smaller doses of ethanol to normal subjects did not produce significant hypertriglyceridemia, but HDL cholesterol was increased.[165,170,222,223] Since only a few other factors (chronic administration of some drugs and vigorous physical exercise) can increase HDL cholesterol, this has been proposed as a useful biological marker of alcoholism.[224,225]

Because of the inverse relationship between high HDL levels and the development of atherosclerosis, the rise in HDL associated with alcohol consumption has been the subject of extensive clinical studies[156,226–228] that confirmed this association. With higher alcohol consumption (in alcoholics), no correlation was found between the level of consumption and the rise in HDL cholesterol.[220,229] The increase in HDL cholesterol occurs in women (who normally have higher HDL cholesterol) as well as in men,[225] teenagers,[230] and both older and younger men,[231] inactive or active.[216,223,232] Obesity attenuated the effects of moderate alcohol consumption on HDL.[233] In teenagers, it has been estimated that for every ounce of alcohol consumed, the increase in HDL cholesterol is higher in females than in males.[230] A similar gender difference was observed by Weidner and co-workers[234]: a very low level of alcohol consumption (1 drink per day or less) was positively associated with the levels of HDL cholesterol in women but not in men, possibly due to the higher alcohol bioavailability in the female gender.[235]

HDL particles are heterogenous in size, hydrated density, and apoprotein composition. The alcohol-induced increase in HDL involves the light (HDL_2) and the heavy (HDL_3) subfractions. In individuals with a relatively high intake of alcohol, the increase affected primarily the HDL_2.[233,234] By contrast, moderate doses of ethanol (about 12–51 g of absolute ethanol/day) raised levels of HDL_3 but not those of HDL_2,[236–239] whereas in another study there was a transient increase in both HDL_2 and HDL_3.[240] In pregnant women who do not abstain from alcohol, the increase in VLDL was associated with a decrease in LDL and HDL_2 and an increase in HDL_3,[187] possibly due to increased VLDL production and decreased lipase activities.

The rise in HDL includes the apolipoproteins AI and AII.[216,222,241–243] Several investigators have found a more pronounced effect of alcohol on apoAII than on apoAI.[238,244,245] HDL has been fractionated, by affinity chromatography, into two main populations: one containing only apoAI (Lp AI) and another containing both AI and AII (Lp AI, AII). In a large group of subjects, Lp AI,AII rose as the alcohol consumption increased from less than 30 g to almost 120 g/day, whereas Lp AI decreased.[246]

Alcoholics with advanced liver disease failed to show the increase in HDL cholesterol shortly after their last drink, nor did they show a significant change after abstinence.[219] Contrasting with the increases in HDL and apolipoproteins AI and AII found at early stages of liver disease, subnormal values were found in cirrhotics and these were associated with decreased ratios of cholesteryl esters–cholesterol, HDL_2–HDL_3, and apoAI–apoAII.[244,247] LDL, with a similar alteration of the cholesterol esterification ratio, also increased with the severity of liver injury, whereas no significant changes were noted in VLDL, apoB, or triacylglycerol levels.[244] The decrease in apoAI was found to have an independent and discriminative value for the diagnosis of fibrosis.[243]

4.2.1. Pathogenesis of the Changes in HDL. The mechanism for the ethanol-induced increase in HDL appears to be multiple.

4.2.1a. Increased Hepatic Production of HDL. In addition to VLDL, the liver normally secretes HDL, containing apoAI, apoAII, apoC, and apoE, whereas apoAI and apoAIV are also major constituents of intestinally produced HDL (mechanisms 2 and 4 in Fig. 2). In alcoholics, as well as after chronic administration of phenobarbital, a correlation between the plasma levels of HDL and hepatic microsomal activities has been reported.[248,249] In rats fed ethanol-containing diets, a good correlation has been found between the increase in HMG-CoA reductase activity and the increase in plasma HDL cholesterol,[30] suggesting a contribution of increased hepatic synthesis to the rise in HDL cholesterol. In squirrel monkeys fed alcohol-containing diets, Cluette and coworkers[250] found increased incorporation of mevalonate into free cholesterol of HDL, particularly that of the HDL_3 subclass. Malmendier and Delcroix[208] have performed kinetic studies of HDL apoAI in healthy volunteers before and after a 4-week period of alcohol intake and found the synthetic rate of this apolipoprotein to be increased, providing evidence in favor of increased HDL production. A role of the liver in this increased HDL production was supported by the recent finding of increased levels of apoAI mRNA in liver biopsies of alcoholics with steatosis.[251] The mechanism of such induction is unknown. Furthermore, primary cultures of hepatocytes from ethanol-fed rats secreted more apoAI, apoE, and apoAIV than those of controls.[252] Moreover, in two human hepatoma cell lines without alcohol dehydrogenase, in which ethanol oxidation depends on the microsomal ethanol oxidizing system, incubation with ethanol increased the production of apoAI and apoB, with accumulation of VLDL and LDL in the media.[253] The apoAI secreted by ethanol-stimulated hepatocytes can promote the efflux cholesterol from human fibroblasts.[254]

4.2.1b. Increased Extrahepatic Production of HDL. During lipolysis, surface components (cholesterol, phospholipids, apoproteins) of VLDL and chylomicrons may be an important source of the increased mass of HDL in alcoholics (mechanism 9 in Fig. 2). Many, but not all, investigators have found that LPL activity increases with chronic alcohol consumption, and some claim this to be the principal mechanism for the HDL increase after moderate drinking.[255]

The role of the hepatic triglyceride lipase (HL) on the ethanol-induced alterations of HDL is much less clear. Acute ethanol administration decreased HL activity[180,200,221,240] or retarded the response to heparin.[256] The microsomal production of HL and its secretion into the media were decreased in primary hepatocyte cultures from ethanol-fed rats.[257] In alcoholics with mild liver injury, this hepatic activity was found to be unchanged[214] or increased,[215] but it may decrease in more severe forms of liver impairment, such as in alcoholic hepatitis.[258,259]

4.2.1c. Decreased Removal of HDL from Plasma. In addition to the enhanced hepatic and extrahepatic production of HDL, alcohol consumption can affect plasma levels of HDL cholesterol by interfering with the reverse transport of cholesterol toward the liver for excretion into the bile (mechanisms 10–13 in Fig. 2). In humans and other primates, only part of the HDL cholesterol may be taken up by the liver as such; probably most returns to the liver as LDL cholesterol, after transfer of cholesterol esters from HDL to the VLDL–LDL pathway by the action of a cholesterol ester transfer protein (CETP). In alcohol-fed baboons, the increase in HDL affects mainly the esterified cholesterol. The latter was found to be associated with decreased turnover due to delayed transfer of esterified cholesterol from HDL to LDL.[260] In alcohol-fed squirrel monkeys, a delayed transfer of cholesteryl esters from LDL to HDL has also been documented.[261] In alcoholics, CETP has been found to be significantly decreased.[262–264] The decrease was not due to the presence of the CETP inhibitor described in human plasma; but HDL and LDL isolated from alcoholics further decreased the transfer activity, suggesting that changes in the donor and receptor lipoproteins can also contribute to the decreased transfer activity of the alcoholics. The decrease in CETP activity correlated with the low LDL cholesterol–HDL cholesterol ratio observed in these patients. LDL was found to be particularly depleted in cholesteryl esters and enriched in triacylglycerols.[264] The effects on CETP activity have been less consistent in moderate drinkers, in whom no changes[233,255,265] or even an increase[266] have been reported.

By contrast, the smaller increase in HDL free cholesterol of ethanol-fed baboons was associated with increased turnover in the plasma, increased splanchnic uptake, and increased fecal excretion of plasma cholesterol, mainly as neutral steroid.[260] These observations are consistent with kinetic data indicating that the HDL free cholesterol is a better precursor of bile cholesterol and bile salts than HDL esterified cholesterol.[267–268] Cholesterol extraction exceeded the release in the splanchnic vascular bed, suggesting that the excess of cholesterol excreted in the feces originated in extrasplanchnic tissues.[260] Similar increases in fecal steroid excretion after ethanol have been found in squirrel monkeys,[269] pigs,[270] and rats.[271] In patients with alcoholic hyperlipemia, the increased excretion of fecal steroids involved mainly the acid rather than the neutral steroids.[272] In addition, alterations in the catabolism of HDL apoproteins have also been reported. In alcohol-fed squirrel monkeys, a decreased fractional catabolic rate of HDL apoAI was found,[273] whereas increased catabolism was reported in patients with alcoholic hepatitis.[162]

4.3. LDL

Contrasting with the strong positive correlation between alcohol consumption and plasma HDL cholesterol, in epidemiological studies there was a weaker but significant negative correlation with LDL cholesterol.[156,227] LDL cholesterol has been found to be reduced in alcoholics.[215] The decrease of LDL observed in alcoholics is associated with a particularly striking decrease in apoB, resulting in high cholesterol–apoB ratios and an increase in the light LDL subfractions.[274] Over the range of moderate alcohol consumption, however, the changes in LDL levels are either very small[227] or nonsignificant.[186,240] The administration of 24–50% of energy as alcohol to animals produces significant increases in at least some of the LDL components.[107,206,261,275] In ethanol-fed squirrel monkeys, as in alcoholics,[274] the increase has been found in the light LDL subfractions (LDL_{1a} and LDL_{1b}), whereas the more dense LDL_2 (probably more atherogenic) did not change.[276] Also, a possible role of associated undernutrition at high alcohol consumption has not been excluded. In any event, the increases in LDL (when present) were much smaller than the changes in VLDL or HDL.

4.3.1. Pathogenesis of the Changes in LDL. The decrease in LDL and apoB observed in alcoholics has been puzzling, since one would expect that the increase in VLDL production and enhanced lypolysis would result in increased levels of LDL. The decreased transfer of cholesterol esters from HDL can explain low LDL cholesterol levels, but does not explain the larger decrease in apoB. This suggests that alcoholics may have accelerated clearance of LDL apoB or decreased conversion of VLDL to LDL apoB. In both men[277] and rats,[278] the formation of LDL–acetaldehyde adducts *in vitro* increased the catabolism of this lipoprotein. The *in vivo* presence of such adducts has been documented in actively drinking alcoholics.[279] They were particularly abundant in VLDL, less in LDL, and nondetectable in HDL, suggesting that the acetaldehyde-induced modification of apoB occurs in the liver prior to the secretion of VLDL. Acetaldehyde adducts were much more abundant in apoB-containing lipoproteins than in nonlipoprotein proteins of the plasma. This is probably due to the presence of lysine clusters in apoB, since a common acetaldehyde reaction is ethylation of the epsilon amino group of this amino acid.

In addition, ethylation by acetaldehyde, as well as other modifications of apoB lysine, has been shown to render this protein immunogenic.[51] Autoantibodies against apoB-containing lipoproteins of the IgG isotype also have been found recently in alcoholics and to a much lesser extent even in nonalcoholics who consume alcohol occasionally.[279] These antibodies reacted more strongly with lipoproteins isolated from alcoholics than from nonalcoholics. It is conceivable that the humoral immune response to acetaldehyde-induced neoantigens may increase the clearance of VLDL, decrease the conversion of VLDL to LDL, and/or increase the catabolism of LDL. This is consistent with the increase in fractional catabolic rates of LDL apoB after alcohol administration for 8 weeks to human subjects.[208] However, in alcoholics, Kervinen and co-workers[280] found no changes in LDL apoB catabolism between the first and the eighth day after withdrawal. In alcohol-fed squirrel monkeys, in which LDL levels were significantly increased, Hojnacki and co-workers[273] found a decreased fractional catabolic rate.

5. Alcohol and Atherosclerosis

The long-standing discussions on whether moderate alcohol consumption protects against the development of atherosclerosis and coronary heart disease (CHD) has culminated in numerous recent epidemiological studies that confirm this association. Many of the objections to earlier studies (younger age of alcoholics, lower socioeconomic status,[281] differences in dietary habits,[282] inclusion of ex-drinkers in the control group,[283] and the likelihood of alcoholics to die from the first heart attack before hospitalization[283]) have been taken into account in the more recent studies.[285–288] It is still possible that the teetotalers, used as controls, may differ from moderate drinkers in ways other than alcohol intake that may also affect coronary complications. However, the fact that this association has been reproduced experimentally in rabbits[289] or primates[275] suggests that the protection is not merely due to selection of the controls.

The protective action pertains to a population comprising moderate rather than heavy drinkers.[290–293] An overall decrease in mortality was associated with an alcohol consumption of two drinks per day or less, whereas higher alcohol consumption was associated with a rise in mortality for cancer and stroke,[292,294,295] resulting in a U- or J-shaped survival curve. Moreover, it is generally agreed that such high alcohol intakes are not associated with protection against CHD.[295–297] Women and younger persons appear to be more susceptible to the increased mortality risk of heavy drinking.[287]

Some observations suggest that the pattern of alcohol intake might also be important: while significantly lower levels of coronary occlusion were observed in moderate drinkers who drank relatively constant amounts, drinkers with variable drinking patterns had higher occlusion scores regardless of amount consumed.[298] However, others found significant protection in occasional drinkers.[295,299]

The type of drink has been an issue raised by the low incidence of CHD disease in France despite a high intake of saturated fat and cholesterol levels. This "French paradox" has been attributed to the higher alcohol consumption, particularly in the form of red wines.[300] However, several large prospective studies do not find a consistently preferential benefit of a particular type of alcoholic beverage.[285,293,301,302]

The mechanism of this protective effect of moderate alcohol consumption remains unknown. From epidemiological studies, it has been estimated that approximately half of the protection by alcohol could be linked to the rise in HDL.[286,303] Consistent with this possibility, genetically induced increases of apoAI and HDL in transgenic mice inhibit atherogenesis.[304] The implicit assumption has been that the ethanol-induced increase in HDL reflects an enhancement of the reverse cholesterol transport from vessels to the liver for excretion into the bile. Transhepatic measurements in alcohol-fed baboons[260] partially support this hypothesis: The hepatic extraction of cholesterol exceeded the release of cholesterol from the liver, suggesting increased mobilization of extrahepatic cholesterol. Moreover, this was associated with increased cholesterol excretion in the feces, as also shown in other species,[269–271] including man.[272] However, as discussed before, the alcohol-induced increase in HDL cholesterol did not reflect exclusively the enhancement of reverse transport of cholesterol. Moreover, these results pertain to a relatively high alcohol consumption. Studies in hyperlipemic mice confirm inhibitory effects of alcohol on the development of fatty-streak atherosclerotic lesions in a dose-dependent manner, but this was unrelated to the levels of HDL cholesterol, which decreased in a dose-dependent manner.[305] Similarly, in mice with genetically knockout LDL receptor, alcohol feeding retarded the development of atherosclerosis, but the protective effect was not entirely attributable to the rise in HDL apoAI.[306]

The HDL subfractions more frequently increased by moderate alcohol consumption (HDL_3 and Lp AI,AII) were less consistently associated with prevention of CHD than HDL_2 or LpAI.[246,307–309] However, more recently, the levels of all subfractions have been shown to be independent predictors of myocardial infarction.[288,310–312]

Much less attention has been paid to the effects of alcohol consumption on LDL, the main atherogenic lipoprotein, probably because of the modest or no change in plasma concentration with moderate alcohol consumption. As discussed above, there are decreases in apoB and LDL cholesterol in alcoholics, despite the increase in VLDL production. Either no changes or decreases in the fractional catabolic rate of LDL have been reported,[276,280] but a more important determinant for the development of atherosclerosis seems to be the uptake of modified LDL by vascular monocytes, leading to the formation of foam cells.[313] This has been well documented in the case of oxidized LDL, but the atherogenic potential of the acetaldehyde-modified LDL[279] is unknown. Oxidized LDL (an atherogenetic product of lipoperoxidation) was found to be increased in alcoholics.[314] This could contribute to the U- or J-shaped relation between alcohol consumption and CHD. Flavonoids present in red wines protected against LDL oxidation *in vitro*,[315,316] whereas conflicting results have been obtained *in vivo*.[316–318]

Another proatherogenic and possibly prothrombotic lipoprotein, Lp(a), was found to be markedly decreased in heavy alcohol consumers,[319] particularly in wine drinkers.[320] Alcohol by itself has a lowering effect on this lipoprotein.[321,322] Lp(a) recovers after abstinence in parallel to α1-antitrypsin, haptoglobin, and the decrease in carbohydrate-deficient transferrin, suggesting that these effects are due to inhibition of protein sialylation by ethanol.[323]

Mechanisms other than lipoproteins might also explain the protective effect of alcohol on cardiovascular disease. Among current drinkers, patients with either nonfatal myocardium infarction or coronary death were found to have significantly lower alcohol consumption in the preceding 24-hr period than similar unaffected drinkers questioned at random,[324] suggesting that alcohol could have acute protective effects on coronary heart disease. Inhibition of platelet aggregation and increased fibrinolytic activity have been suggested as alternative explanations. Moderate alcohol consumption has been shown to prolong the bleeding time and to decrease platelet aggregation in response to collagen and ADP,[325] an effect that was more intense with red than white wine.[300] Ethanol produces vasodilation and may decrease platelet aggregation by production of acetaldehyde, which is a potent stimulus of vascular production of prostacyclin,[326] a vasodilator and platelet antiaggregator. In addition, HDL has been shown to stimulate the synthesis of prostacyclin (PGI_2),[327] an effect that was enhanced by chronic alcohol consumption.[328] In addition to its effects on prostacyclin, HDL has been reported to decrease thromboxane formation by platelets.[329] Also, ethanol inhibits platelet thromboxane production both *in vitro*[330] and *in vivo*.[331,332] With heavy alcohol consumption, the effects on platelet aggregation appears to be different. An increased reactivity of the platelets to aggregant agents has also been found in severe alcoholics.[333,334] Such changes might explain in part the opposite effects of moderate and large doses of alcohol on cardiovascular disease. After alcohol withdrawal, the ratio of the vasodilator prostanoids (prostaglandin E and prostacyclin) to the vasoconstrictor prostanoid (thromboxane A_2) was found to be lower than in normal subjects.[335]

A positive association has been found between moderate alcohol consumption and plasma fibrinolytic activity, especially that of tissue-type plasminogen activator (tPA) in the plasma,[336–338] whereas heavy drinking increases both tPA and the type I inhibitor of this activator.[339] Thus, it is possible that the prevention of coronary heart disease by moderate alcohol consumption may be related only in part or not at all to the alcohol-induced alterations of serum lipoproteins. Along with these possibilities are the puzzling observations that the apparent protection was found in people who have only one drink per week[295] or even one per month.[299]

References

1. Kitson KE, Weiner H: Symposium. Ethanol and acetaldehyde metabolism: Past, present and future. *Alcohol Clin Exp Res* 20:82A–92A, 1996.
2. Forsander OA, Mäenpää PH, Salaspuro MP: Influence of ethanol on the lactate/pyruvate and β-hydroxybutyrate/acetoacetate ratios in rat liver experiments. *Acta Chem Scand* 19: 1770–1771, 1965.
3. Lieber CS, Lefèvre A, Spritz N, *et al:* Difference in hepatic metabolism of long- and medium-chain fatty acids: The role of fatty acid chain length in the production of the alcoholic fatty liver. *J Clin Invest* 46:1451–1460, 1967.
4. Nikkilä EA, Ojala K: Role of hepatic L-α-glycerolphosphate and triglyceride synthesis in production of fatty liver by ethanol. *Proc Soc Exp Biol Med* 113:814–817, 1963.
5. Salaspuro MP, Shaw S, Jayatilleke E, *et al:* Attenuation of the ethanol induced hepatic redox changes after chronic alcohol consumption in baboons: Metabolic consequences *in vivo* and *in vitro*. *Hepatology* 1:33–38, 1981.
6. Domschke S, Domschke W, Lieber CS: Hepatic redox state: Attenuation of the acute effects of ethanol induced by chronic alcohol consumption. *Life Sci* 15:1327–1334, 1974.
7. Ryle PR, Chakraborty J, Thomson AD: The effect of methylene blue on the hepatocellular redox state and liver lipid content during chronic ethanol feeding in the rat. *Biochem J* 232:877–882, 1985.
8. Quistorff B, Chance B, Takeda H: Two- and three-dimensional redox heterogeneity. Effects of anoxia and alcohol on lobular redox pattern, in Dutton LP, Leigh LS, Scarpa A (eds): *Frontiers of Biological Energetics: Electrons to Tissues*. New York, Academic Press, 1978, pp 1487–1497.
9. Jauhonen VP, Baraona E, Lieber CS, Hassinen IE: Dependence of ethanol-induced redox shift on hepatic oxygen tensions prevailing *in vivo*. *Alcohol* 2:163–167, 1985.
10. Jauhonen P, Baraona E, Miyakawa H, Lieber CS: Mechanism for the selective hepatotoxicity of ethanol. *Alcohol Clin Exp Res* 6:350–357, 1982.
11. Baraona E, Jauhonen P, Miyakawa H, Lieber CS: Zonal redox changes as a cause of selective perivenular hepatotoxicity of alcohol. *Pharmacol Biochem Behav* 96:306–315, 1983.
12. Lieber CS, DeCarli LM: Hepatic microsomal ethanol oxidizing system: *In vitro* characteristics and adaptive properties *in vivo*. *J Biol Chem* 245:2505–2512, 1970.
13. Joly JG, Feinman L, Ishii H, Lieber CS: Effect of chronic ethanol feeding on hepatic microsomal glycerophosphate acyltransferase activity. *J Lipid Res* 14:337–343, 1973.
14. Lamb RG, Wood CK, Fallon HJ: The effect of acute and chronic ethanol intake on hepatic glycerolipid biosynthesis in the hamster. *J Clin Invest* 63:14–20, 1979.
15. Savolainen MJ, Baraona E, Pikkarainen P, *et al:* Hepatic triacylglycerol synthesizing activity during progression of alcoholic liver injury in the baboon. *J Lipid Res* 25:813–820, 1984.
16. Day CP, James OFW, Brown ASM, *et al:* The activity of the metabolic form of hepatic phosphatidate phosphohydrolase correlates with the severity of alcoholic fatty liver in human beings. *Hepatology* 18:832–838, 1993.
17. Savolainen MJ: Stimulation of hepatic phosphatidate phosphohydrolase activity by a single dose of ethanol. *Biochem Biophys Res Commun* 75:511–518, 1977.
18. Pritchard PH, Bowley M, Burditt SD, *et al:* The effects of acute ethanol feeding and of chronic benfluorex administration on the activities of some enzymes of glycerolipid synthesis in rat liver and adipose tissue. *Biochem J* 166:639–642, 1977.
19. Simpson KJ, Venkatesan S, Martin A, *et al:* Effect of alcohol on the activity and subcellular

distribution of phosphatidate phosphohydrolase in rat liver. *Biochim Biophys Acta* 1201:411–414, 1994.

20. Fallon HJ, Lamb RG, Jamdar SC: Phosphatidate phosphohydrolase and the regulation of glycerolipid biosynthesis. *Biochem Soc Trans* 5:37–40, 1977.
21. Lieber CS, Jones DP, DeCarli LM: Effects of prolonged ethanol intake: Production of fatty liver despite adequate diets. *J Clin Invest* 44:1009–1021, 1965.
22. Day CP, Yeaman SJ: The biochemistry of alcohol-induced fatty liver. *Biochim Biophys Acta* 1215:33–48, 1994.
23. Ide T, Ontko JA: Increased secretion of very low density lipoprotein triglyceride following inhibition of long chain fatty acid oxidation in isolated rat liver. *J Biol Chem* 256:10247–10255, 1981.
24. Tijburg LBM, Maquedano A, Bijleveld C, *et al:* Effects of ethanol feeding on hepatic lipid synthesis. *Arch Biochem Biophys* 267:568–579, 1988.
25. O'Doherty PJA, Kuksis A: Stimulation of triacylglycerol synthesis by Z protein in rat liver and intestinal mucosa. *FEBS Lett* 60:256–258, 1975.
26. Gossett RE, Frolov AA, Roths JB, *et al:* Acyl-CoA binding proteins: Multiplicity and function. *Lipids* 31:895–918, 1996.
27. Cairns SR, Peters TJ: Biochemical analysis of hepatic lipid in alcoholic and diabetic and control subjects: *Clin Sci* 65:645–652, 1983.
28. Lefèvre AF, DeCarli LM, Lieber CS: Effect of ethanol on cholesterol and bile acid metabolism. *J Lipid Res* 13:48–55, 1972.
29. Field FJ, Boydstun JS, LaBrecque DR: Effect of chronic ethanol ingestion on hepatic and intestinal acyl coenzyme A: Cholesterol acyltransferase and 3-hydroxy-3-methylglutaryl coenzyme A reductase in the rat. *Hepatology* 5:133–138, 1985.
30. Maruyama S, Murawaki Y, Hirayama C: Effects of chronic ethanol administration on hepatic cholesterol and bile acid synthesis in relation to serum high density lipoprotein cholesterol in rats. *Res Commun Chem Pathol Pharmacol* 53:3–21, 1986.
31. Lakshman MR, Veech RL: Short-term and long-term effects of ethanol administration *in vivo* on rat liver HMG-CoA reductase and cholesterol 7α-hydroxylase activities. *J Lipid Res* 18:325–330, 1977.
32. Shevchuk O, Baraona E, Ma X-L, Lieber CS: Gender differences in the response of hepatic fatty acids and cytosolic fatty acid-binding capacity to alcohol consumption in rats. *Proc Soc Exp Biol Med* 198:584–590, 1991.
33. Ma X, Baraona E, Lieber CS: Alcohol consumption enhances fatty acid ω-oxidation, with a greater increase in males than in female rats. *Hepatology* 18:1247–1253, 1993.
34. Ma X, Baraona E, Goozner N, Lieber CS: Increased vulnerability of women to alcoholic liver injury as indicated by the lack of dicarboxylic aciduria after alcohol consumption. *Alcohol Clin Exp Res* 19 (Suppl):97A 1995.
35. Spritz N, Lieber CS: Decrease of ethanol-induced fatty liver by ethyl α-*p*-chlorophenoxyisobutyrate. *Proc Soc Exp Biol Med* 121:147–149, 1966.
36. Kaikaus RM, Chan WK, Ortiz de Montellana PR, Bass NM: Mechanisms of regulation of liver fatty acid-binding protein. *Mol Cell Biochem* 123:93–100, 1993.
37. Pignon JP, Bailey NC, Baraona E, Lieber CS: Fatty acid binding protein: A major contributor to the ethanol-induced increase in liver cytosolic proteins in the rat. *Hepatology* 7:865–871, 1987.
38. Lieber CS: Women and alcohol: Gender differences in metabolism and susceptibility, in Wilsnack RW, Wilsnack SC (eds): *Gender and Alcohol.* Piscataway, NJ, Rutgers Center of Alcohol Studies, 1997, pp 77–89.
39. Ishii H, Joly J-G, Lieber CS: Effect of ethanol on the amount and enzyme activities of hepatic rough and smooth microsomal membranes. *Biochim Biophys Acta* 291:411–420, 1973.
40. Uthus EO, Skurdal DN, Cornatzer WE: Effect of ethanol ingestion on choline phosphotransferase and phosphatidyl ethanolamine methyltransferase activities in liver microsomes. *Lipids* 11:641–644, 1976.
41. Lieber CS, Robins SJ, Leo MA: Hepatic phosphatidylethanolamine methyltransferase is

decreased by ethanol and increased by phosphatidylcholine *Alcohol Clin Exp Res* 18:592–595, 1994.
42. Lieber CS, Spritz N, DeCarli LM: Role of dietary, adipose and endogenously synthesized fatty acids in the pathogensis of the alcoholic fatty liver. *J Clin Invest* 45:51–62, 1966.
43. Lieber CS, Spritz N: Effect of prolonged ethanol intake in man: Role of dietary, adipose, and endogenously synthesized fatty acids in the pathogenesis of the alcoholic fatty liver. *J Clin Invest* 45:1400–1411, 1966.
44. Mendenhall CL, Bradford RH, Furman RH: Effect of ethanol on fatty acid composition of hepatic phosphatidylcholine and phosphatidylethanolamine and on microsomal fatty acyl-CoA: lysophosphatide transferase activities in rats fed corn oil or coconut oil. *Biochim Biophys Acta* 187:510–519, 1969.
45. Nervi AM, Peluffo RO, Brenner RR, Leikin AI: Effect of ethanol administration on fatty acid desaturation. *Lipids* 15:263–268, 1980.
46. Rao GA, Lew G, Larkin EC: Alcohol ingestion and levels of hepatic fatty acid synthetase and stearoyl-CoA desaturase activities in rats. *Lipids* 19:151–153, 1984.
47. Wang DL, Reitz RC: Ethanol ingestion and polyunsaturated fatty acids: effects on the acyl-CoA desaturases. *Alcohol Clin Exp Res* 7:220–226, 1983.
48. Nakamura MT, Tang AB, Villanueva J, *et al:* Reduced tissue arachidonic acid concentration with chronic ethanol feeding in miniature pigs. *Am J Clin Nutr* 56:467–474, 1992.
49. Kamisaka K, Maezawa H, Inagaki T, Okano K: A low molecular weight binding protein for organic anions (Z protein) from human hepatic cytosol: Purification and quantitation. *Hepatology* 1:221–227, 1981.
50. Mavrelis PG, Ammon HV, Gleysteen JJ, *et al:* Hepatic free fatty acids in alcoholic liver disease and morbid obesity. *Hepatology* 3:226–231, 1983.
51. Nomura F, Lieber CS: Binding of acetaldehyde to rat liver microsomes: Enhancement after chronic alcohol consumption. *Biochem Biophys Res Commun* 100:131–137, 1981.
52. Steinbrecher UP, Fisher MJL, Witztun JL, Curtiss LK: Immunogenicity of homologous low density lipoproteins after methylation, ethylation, acetylation, or carbamylation: Generation of antibodies specific for derivatized lysine. *J Lipid Res* 25:1109–1116, 1984.
53. Israel Y, Hurwitz E, Niëmelä O, Arnon R: Monoclonal and polyclonal antibodies against acetaldehyde-containing epitopes in acetaldehyde–protein adducts. *Proc Natl Acad Sci USA* 83:7923–7927, 1986.
54. Behrens UH, Hoerner M, Lasker JM, Lieber CS: Formation of acetaldehyde adducts with ethanol-inducible P450IIE1 *in vivo. Biochem Biophys Res Commun* 154:584–590, 1988.
55. Moncada C, Torres G, Varghese E, *et al:* Ethanol-derived immunoreactive species formed by free radical mechanisms. *Mol Pharmacol* 46:786–791, 1994.
56. Niëmelä O, Parkkila S, Ylä-Herttuala S, *et al:* Covalent protein adducts in the liver as a result of ethanol metabolism and lipid peroxidation. *Lab Invest* 70:537–546, 1994.
57. Lane BP, Lieber CS: Ultrastructural alterations in human hepatocytes following ingestion of ethanol with adequate diets. *Am J Pathol* 49:593–603, 1966.
58. Rubin E, Beattie DS, Toth A, Lieber CS: Structural and functional effects of ethanol on hepatic mitochondria. *Fed Proc* 31:131–140, 1972.
59. Matsuzaki S, Lieber CS: Increased susceptibility of hepatic mitochondria to the toxicity of acetaldehyde after chronic ethanol consumption. *Biochem Biophys Res Commun* 75:1059–1065, 1977.
60. Cederbaum AI, Lieber CS, Beattie DS, Rubin E: Effect of chronic ethanol ingestion on fatty acid oxidation by hepatic mitochondria. *J Biol Chem* 250:5122–5129, 1975.
61. Lefèvre A, Adler H, Lieber CS: Effects of ethanol on ketone metabolism. *J Clin Invest* 49:1775–1782, 1970.
62. Guzmán M, Geelen MJH: Effects of ethanol feeding on the activity and regulation of hepatic carnitine palmitoyltransferase. *Arch Biochem Biophys* 267:580–588, 1988.
63. Zentella de Piña M, Villalobos-Molina R, Saavedra-Molina A, *et al:* Effects of moderate chronic ethanol consumption on rat liver mitochondrial fractions. *Alcohol* 6:3–7, 1989.

64. Quintanilla ME, Tampier L: Ethanol intake: Effect on liver and brain mitochondrial function and acetaldehyde oxidation. *Alcohol* 9:375–380, 1992.
65. Arai M, Gordon ER, Lieber CS: Decreased cytochrome oxidase activity in hepatic mitochondria after chronic ethanol consumption and the possible role of decreased cytochrome aa_3 content and changes in phospholipids. *Biochim Biophys Acta* 797:320–327, 1984.
66. Hasumura Y, Teschke R, Lieber CS: Characteristics of acetaldehyde oxidation in rat liver mitochondria. *J Biol Chem* 251:4908–4913, 1976.
67. Lieber CS, Baraona E, Hernández-Muñoz R, *et al:* Impaired oxygen utilization. A new mechanism for the hepatotoxicity of ethanol in sub-human primates. *J Clin Invest* 83:1682–1690, 1989.
68. Lundquist E, Tygstrup N, Winkler K, *et al:* Ethanol metabolism and production of free acetate in the human liver. *J Clin Invest* 41:955–961, 1962.
69. Fernández-Checa J, García-Ruiz C, Ookhtens M, Kaplowitz N: Impaired uptake of glutathione by hepatic mitochondria from chronic ethanol-fed rats. Tracer kinetic studies *in vitro* and *in vivo* and susceptibility to oxidant stress. *J Clin Invest* 87:397–405, 1991.
70. García-Ruiz C, Colell A, Morales A, *et al:* Role of oxidative stress generated from the mitochondrial electron transport chain and mitochondrial glutathione status in loss of mitochondrial function and activation of transcription factor nuclear factor-*k*B: Studies with isolated mitochondria and rat hepatocytes. *Mol Pharmacol* 48:825–834, 1995.
71. Shaw S, Rubin KP, Lieber CS: Depressed hepatic glutathione and increased diene conjugates in alcoholic liver disease. Evidence of lipid peroxidation. *Dig Dis Sci* 28:585–589, 1983.
72. Kukielka E, Dicker E, Cederbaum AI: Increased production of reactive oxygen species by rat liver mitochondria after chronic ethanol treatment. *Arch Biochem Biophys* 309:377–386, 1994.
73. Chin JH, Goldstein DB: Effects of low concentration of ethanol on the fluidity of spin-labeled erythrocyte and brain membranes. *Mol Pharmacol* 13:435–441, 1977.
74. Chin JH, Parson LM, Goldstein DR: Increased cholesterol content of erythrocyte and brain membranes in ethanol-tolerant mice. *Biochem Biophys Acta* 513:358–363, 1978.
75. Polokoff MA, Simon TJ, Harris RA, *et al:* Chronic ethanol increases liver plasma membrane fluidity. *Biochemistry* 24:3114–3120, 1985.
76. Yamada S, Lieber CS: Decrease in microviscosity and cholesterol content of rat liver plasma membranes after chronic ethanol feeding. *J Clin Invest* 74:2285–2289, 1984.
77. Kim CI, Leo MA, Lowe N, Lieber CS: Effects of vitamin A and ethanol on liver plasma membrane fluidity. *Hepatology* 8:735–741, 1988.
78. Kikuchi T, Kako KJ: Metabolic effects of ethanol on the rabbit heart. *Circulation Res* 26:625–634, 1970.
79. Vasdev SC, Subrahmanyam D, Chakravarti RN, Wahi PL: Effect of chronic ethanol feeding on the major lipids of red blood cells, liver and heart of Rhesus monkey. *Biochim Biophys Acta* 369:323-330, 1974.
80. Liau DF, Hashim SA, Pierson RN, Ryan SF: Alcohol-induced lipid change in the lung. *J Lipid Res* 22:680–686, 1981.
81. Wilson JS, Colley PW, Sasula L, *et al:* Alcohol causes a fatty pancreas. A rat model of ethanol-induced pancreatic steatosis. *Alcohol Clin Exp Res* 6:117–121, 1982.
82. Goodman DS, Deykin D: Fatty acid ethyl ester formation during ethanol metabolism *in vivo*. *Proc Soc Exp Biol Med* 113:65–67, 1963.
83. Lange LG, Bergmann SR, Sobel BE: Identification of fatty acid ethyl esters as products of rabbit myocardial ethanol metabolism. *J Biol Chem* 256:12968–12973, 1981.
84. Laposata EA, Lange LG: Presence of nonoxidative ethanol metabolism in human organs commonly damaged by ethanol abuse. *Science* 231:497–499, 1986.
85. Mogelson S, Lange LG: Nonoxidative ethanol metabolism in rabbit myocardium: Purification to homogeneity of fatty acyl ethyl ester synthase. *Biochemistry* 23:4075–4071, 1984.
86. Doyle KM, Cluette-Brown JE, Dube DM, *et al:* Fatty acid ethyl esters in the blood as markers for ethanol intake. *JAMA* 276:1152–1156, 1994.
87. Laposata M, Szczepiorkowski ZM, Brown, JE: Fatty acid ethyl esters: Non-oxidative metabolites of ethanol. *Prostaglandins Leukot Essent Fatty Acids* 52:87–91, 1995.

88. Szczepiorkowski ZM, Dickersin GR, Laposata M: Fatty acid ethyl esters decrease human hepatoblastoma cell proliferation and protein synthesis. *Gastroenterology* 108:515–522, 1995.
89. Lange LG, Sobel BE: Mitochondrial dysfunction induced by fatty acid ethyl esters, myocardial metabolites of ethanol. *J Clin Invest* 72:724–731, 1983.
90. Haber PS, Wilson JS, Apte MV, Pirola RC: Fatty acid ethyl esters increase rat pancreatic lysosomal fragility. *J Lab Clin Med* 121:759–764, 1993.
91. Laposata EA, Harrison EH, Hedberg EB: Synthesis and degradation of fatty acid ethyl esters by culture hepatoma cells exposed to ethanol. *J Biol Chem* 265:9688–9693, 1990.
92. Spector AA: Fatty acid ethyl esters: insight of intoxication? *Gastroenterology* 108:605–607, 1995.
93. Alling C, Gustavsson L, Änggård E: An abnormal phospholipid in rat organs after ethanol treatment. *FEBS Lett* 152:24–28, 1983.
94. Sørensen TIA, Orholm M, Bentsen KD, *et al:* Prospective evaluation of alcohol abuse and alcoholic liver injury in men as predictors of development of cirrhosis. *Lancet* 2:241–244, 1984.
95. Lieber CS, Jones DP, Mendelson J, DeCarli LM: Fatty liver, hyperlipemia and hyperuricemia produced by prolonged alcohol consumption, despite adequate dietary intake. *Trans Assoc Am Physicians* 76:289–300, 1963.
96. Lieber CS, Rubin E: Alcoholic fatty liver in man on a high protein and low fat diet. *Am J Med* 44:200–207, 1968.
97. Rubin E, Lieber CS: Alcohol induced hepatic injury in non-alcoholic volunteers. *N Engl J Med* 278:869–876, 1968.
98. Brodie BB, Butler WM, Horning MG, *et al:* Alcohol-induced triglyceride deposition in liver through derangement of fat transport. *Am J Clin Nutr* 9:432–435, 1961.
99. Mallov S: Effect of ethanol intoxication on plasma free fatty acids in the rat. *J Stud Alcohol* 22:250–253, 1961.
100. Rebouças G, Isselbacher KJ: Studies on the pathogenesis of the ethanol-induced fatty liver. I. Synthesis and oxidation of fatty acids by the liver. *J Clin Invest* 40:1355–1362, 1961.
101. Kalant H, Khanna JM, Seymour F, Loth J: Acute alcoholic fatty liver. Metabolism or stress. *Biochem Pharmacol* 24:431–434, 1975.
102. DeCarli LM, Lieber CS: Fatty liver in the rat after prolonged intake of ethanol with a nutritionally adequate new liquid diet. *J Nutr* 91:331–336, 1967.
103. Lieber CS, DeCarli LM: Quantitative relationship between amount of dietary fat and severity of alcoholic fatty liver. *Am J Nutr* 23:474–478, 1970.
104. Lieber CS, DeCarli LM: An experimental model of alcohol feeding and liver injury in the baboon. *J Med Primatol* 3:153–163, 1974.
105. Wolfe BM, Havel JR, Marliss EB, *et al:* Effect of a 3-day fast and of ethanol on splanchnic metabolism of FFA, amino acids, and carbohydrates in healthy young men. *J Clin Invest* 57:329–340, 1976.
106. Baraona E, Lieber CS: Effects of chronic ethanol feeding on serum lipoprotein metabolism in the rat. *J Clin Invest* 49:769–778, 1970.
107. Baraona E, Pirola R, Lieber CS: The pathogenesis of postprandial hyperlipemia in rats fed ethanol-containing diets. *J Clin Invest* 52:296–303, 1973.
108. Baraona E, Leo MA, Borowsky SA, Lieber CS: Pathogenesis of alcohol-induced accumulation of protein in the liver. *J Clin Invest* 60:546–554, 1977.
109. Matsuda Y, Baraona E, Salaspuro M, Lieber CS: Effects of ethanol on liver microtubules and Golgi apparatus. Possible role in altered hepatic secretion of plasma protein. *Lab Invest* 41:455–463, 1979.
110. Baraona E, Matsuda Y, Pikkarainen P, Lieber CS: Effects of ethanol on hepatic protein secretion and microtubules. Possible mediation by acetaldehyde. *Curr Alcohol* 8:421–434, 1981.
111. Jennett RB, Sorrell MF, Saffari-Fard A, *et al:* Preferential covalent binding of acetaldehyde to the *a*-chain of purified rat liver tubulin. *Hepatology* 9:57–62, 1989.
112. Smith SL, Jennett RB, Sorrell MF, Tuma DJ: Acetaldehyde substoichiometrically inhibits bovine neurotubulin polymerization. *J Clin Invest* 84:337–341, 1989.

113. Lieber CS, Leevy CM, Stein SW, *et al:* Effect of ethanol on plasma free fatty acids in man. *J Lab Clin Med* 59:826–832, 1962.
114. Jauhonen VP, Hassinen IE: Metabolic and hormonal changes during intravenous infusion of ethanol, acetaldehyde and acetate in normal and adrenalectomized rats. *Arch Biochem Biophys* 191:358–366, 1978.
115. Jones DP, Perman ES, Lieber CS: Free fatty acid turnover and triglyceride metabolism after ethanol ingestion in man. *J Lab Clin Med* 66:804–813, 1965.
116. Crouse JR, Gerson CS, DeCarli LM, Lieber CS: Role of acetate in the reduction of plasma free fatty acids produced by ethanol in man. *J Lipid Res* 2:509–512, 1968.
117. Tsukamoto H, French SW, Reidelberger RD, Largman C: Cyclical pattern of blood alcohol levels during continuous intragastric ethanol infusion in rats. *Alcohol Clin Exp Res* 9:31–37, 1985.
118. Tsukamoto H, French SW, Benson N, *et al:* Severe and progressive steatosis and focal necrosis in rat liver induced by continuous intragastric infusion of ethanol and low fat diet. *Hepatology* 5:224–232, 1985.
119. French SW, Miyamoto K, Tsukamoto H: Ethanol-induced hepatic fibrosis in the rat: Role of the amount of dietary fat. *Alcohol Clin Exp Res* 10(Suppl):13S–19S, 1886.
120. Nanji AA, French SW: Dietary linoleic acid is required for development of experimentally induced alcoholic liver injury. *Life Sci* 44:223–227, 1989.
121. Nanji AA, Mendenhall CL, French SW: Beef fat prevents alcoholic liver disease in the rat. *Alcohol Clin Exp Res* 13:15–19, 1989.
122. Nanji AA, French SW: Relationship between pork consumption and cirrhosis. *Lancet* 1:681–683, 1985.
123. Nanji AA, French SW: Dietary factors and alcoholic cirrhosis. *Alcohol Clin Exp Dis* 10:271–273, 1986.
124. French SW: Nutrition in the pathogenesis of alcoholic liver disease. *Alcohol Alcohol* 28:97–100, 1992.
125. Nanji AA, Sadrzadeh SMH, Yang EK, *et al:* Dietary saturated fatty acids: A novel treatment for alcoholic liver disease. *Gastroenterology* 109:547–554, 1995.
126. Lakshman MR, Chirtel SJ, Chambers LL: Roles of ω3 fatty acids and chronic ethanol in the regulation of plasma and liver lipids and plasma apoproteins A_1 and E in rats. *J Nutr* 118:1299–1303, 1988.
127. Israel Y, Kalant H, Orrego, *et al:* Experimental alcohol induced hepatic necrosis: Suppression by propylthiouracil. *Proc Natl Acad Sci USA* 72:1137–1141, 1975.
128. French SW, Benson NC, Sun PS: Centrilobular necrosis induced by hypoxia in chronic ethanol-fed rats. *Hepatology* 4:912–917, 1984.
129. Bredfelt JE, Riley EM, Groszman RJ: Compensatory mechanisms in response to an elevated hepatic oxygen consumption in chronically ethanol-fed rats. *Am J Physiol* 248: G507–G511, 1985.
130. Shaw S, Heller EA, Friedman HS, *et al:* Increased hepatic oxygenation following ethanol administration in the baboon. *Proc Soc Exp Biol Med* 156:509–513, 1977.
131. Tsukamoto H, Xi XP: Incomplete compensation of enhanced hepatic oxygen consumption in rats with alcoholic centrilobular liver necrosis. *Hepatology* 9:302–306, 1989.
132. Miyamoto K, French SW: Hepatic adenine nucleotide metabolism measured *in vivo* in rats fed ethanol and a high fat-low protein diet. *Hepatology* 8:53–60, 1988.
133. Takahashi H, Geoffrion Y, Butler KW, French SW: *In vivo* hepatic energy metabolism during progression of alcoholic liver disease: A noninvasive ^{31}P nuclear magnetic resonance study in rats. *Hepatology* 11:65–73, 1990.
134. Helzberg JH, Brown MS, Smith DJ, *et al:* Metabolic state of the rat liver with ethanol: Comparison of *in vivo* ^{31}phosphorus nuclear magnetic resonance spectroscopy with freeze clamp assessment. *Hepatology* 7:83–88, 1987.
135. Suematsu T, Matsumura T, Sato N, *et al:* Lipid peroxidation in alcoholic liver disease in humans. *Alcohol Clin Exp Res* 5:427–430, 1981.
136. DiLuzio NR: Prevention of the acute ethanol-induced fatty liver by the simultaneous administration of antioxidants. *Life Sci* 3:113–118, 1964.

137. Comporti M, Hartman A, DiLuzio NR: Effect of *in vivo* and *in vitro* ethanol administration on liver lipid peroxidation. *Lab Invest* 16:616–624, 1967.
138. MacDonald CM: The effects of ethanol on hepatic lipid peroxidation and on the activities of glutathione reductase and peroxidase. *FEBS Lett* 25:227–230, 1973.
139. Reitz RC: A possible mechanism for the peroxidation of lipids due to chronic ethanol ingestion. *Biochim Biophys Acta* 380:145–154, 1975.
140. Shaw S, Jayatilleke E, Ross WA, Lieber CS: Ethanol-induced lipid peroxidation: Potentiation by long-term alcohol feeding and attenuation by methionine. *J Lab Clin Med* 98:417–424, 1981.
141. Lieber CS, Leo MA, Aleynik SI, *et al:* Polyenylphosphatidylcholine decreases alcohol-induced oxidative stress in the baboon. *Alcohol Clin Exp Res* 21:375–379, 1997.
142. Lieber CS, DeCarli LM: Study of agents for the prevention of the fatty liver produced by prolonged alcohol intake. *Gastroenterology* 50:316–322, 1966.
143. Nanji AA, Zhao S, Lamb RG, *et al:* Changes in microsomal phospholipases and arachidonic acid in experimental alcoholic liver injury: Relationship to cytochrome P450 2E1 induction and conjugated diene formation. *Alcohol Clin Exp Res* 17:598–603, 1993.
144. Nanji AA, Khwaja S, Tahan SR, Sadrzadeh SMH: Plasma levels of a novel noncyclooxygenase-derived prostanoid (8-isoprostane) correlate with severity of liver injury in experimental alcoholic liver disease. *J Pharmacol Exp Ther* 269:1280–1285, 1994.
145. Nanji AA, Khettry U, Sadrzadeh SMH, Yamanaka T: Severity of liver injury in experimental alcoholic liver disease. Correlation with plasma endotoxin, prostaglandin E2, leukotriene B4, and thromboxane B2. *Am J Pathol* 142:367–373, 1993.
146. Nanji AA, Khwaja S, Sadrzadeh SMH: Eicosanoid production in experimental alcoholic liver disease is related to vitamin E levels and lipid peroxidation. *Mol Cell Biochem* 140:85–89, 1994.
147. Müller A, Sies H: Role of alcohol dehydrogenase activity and of acetaldehyde in ethanol-induced ethane and pentane production by isolated perfused rat liver. *Biochem J* 206:153–156, 1982.
148. Savolainen E-R, Leo MA, Timpl R, Lieber CS: Acetaldehyde and lactate stimulate collagen synthesis in cultured baboon myofibroblasts. *Gastroenterology* 87:777–787, 1984.
149. Moshage H, Casini A, Lieber CS: Acetaldehyde selectively stimulates collagen production in cultured rat liver fat-storing cells but not in hepatocytes. *Hepatology* 12:511–518, 1990.
150. Lee KS, Buck M, Houglum K, Chojkier M: Activation of hepatic stellate cells by TGFα and collagen type I is mediated by oxidative stress through c-*myb* expression. *J Clin Invest* 96:2461–2468, 1995.
151. Lieber CS, Robins SJ, Li J, *et al:* Phosphatidylcholine protects against fibrosis and cirrhosis in the baboon. *Gastroenterology* 106:152–159, 1994.
152. Navder KP, Baraona E, Lieber CS: Polyenylphosphatidylcholine (PPC) attenuates alcohol-induced fatty liver and hyperlipemia in rats. *J Nutr* 127:1800–1806, 1997.
153. Navder KP, Baraona E, Lieber CS: Restoration of ethanol-induced mitochondrial dysfunction by polyenylphosphatidylcholine (PPC) in rats. *FASEB J* 11:A383, 1997.
154. Losowsky MS, Jones DP, Davidson CS, Lieber CS: Studies of alcoholic hyperlipemia and its mechanism. *Am J Med* 35:794–803, 1963.
155. Chait A, February AE, Mancini M, Lewis BL: Clinical and metabolic study of alcoholic hyperlipidemia. *Lancet* 2:62–64, 1972.
156. Castelli WP, Gordon T, Hjortland MC, *et al:* Alcohol and blood lipids. *Lancet* 2:153–155, 1977.
157. Böttiger LE, Carlson LA, Hultman EM, Romanus V: Serum lipids in alcoholics *Acta Med Scand* 199:357–361, 1976.
158. Marzo S, Ghirardi P, Sardini D, *et al:* Serum lipids and total fatty acids in chronic alcoholic liver disease at different states of cell damage. *Klin Wochen* 48:949–950, 1970.
159. Papadopolous NM, Charles MA: Serum lipoprotein patterns in liver disease. *Proc Soc Exp Biol Med* 134:797–799, 1970.
160. Day RC, Harry DS, Owen JS, *et al:* Lecithin-cholesterol acyltransferase and the lipoprotein abnormalities of parenchymal liver disease. *Clin Sci* 56:575–583, 1979.

161. Sabesin SM, Hawkins HL, Kuiken L, *et al:* Abnormal plasma lipoproteins and lecithin-cholesterol acyltransferase deficiency in alcoholic liver disease. *Gastroenterology* 72:510–518, 1977.
162. Nestel PJ, Tada N, Fidge NH: Increased catabolism of high density lipoprotein in alcoholic hepatitis. *Metabolism* 29:101–104, 1980.
163. Weidman SW, Ragland JB, Sabesin SM: Plasma lipoprotein composition in alcoholic hepatitis: Accumulation of apolipoprotein E-rich high density lipoprotein and preferential reappearance of "light"-HDL during partial recovery. *J Lipid Res* 23:556–569, 1982.
164. Jones DP, Losowsky MS, Davidson CS, Lieber CS: Effects of ethanol on plasma lipids in man. *J Lab Clin Med* 62:675–682, 1963.
165. Belfrage P, Berg B, Cronholm T, *et al:* Prolonged administration to ethanol to young, healthy volunteers: Effects on biochemical, morphological and neurophysiological parameters. *Acta Med Scand* [Suppl] 552:1–44, 1973.
166. Avogaro P, Cazzolato G: Changes in the composition and physico-chemical characteristics of serum lipoproteins during ethanol-induced lipemia in alcoholic subjects. *Metabolism* 24:1231–1242, 1975.
167. Friedman M, Rosenman RH, Byers SO: Effect of moderate ingestion of alcohol upon serum triglyceride responses of normo-hyperlipemic subjects. *Proc Soc Exp Biol Med* 120:696–698, 1965.
168. Taskinen M-R, Nikkilä EA: Nocturnal hypertriglyceridemia and hyperinsulinemia following moderate evening intake of alcohol. *Acta Med Scand* 202:173–177, 1997.
169. Schapiro RH, Scheig RL, Drummey GD, *et al:* Effect of prolonged ethanol ingestion on transport and metabolism of lipids in man. *N Engl J Med* 272:610–615, 1965.
170. Belfrage P, Berg B, Hägerstrand I, *et al:* Alterations of lipid metabolism in healthy volunteers during long-term ethanol intake. *Eur J Clin Invest* 7:127–131, 1977.
171. Contaldo F, D'Arrigo E, Carandente V, *et al:* Short-term effects of moderate alcohol consumption on lipid metabolism and energy balance in normal men. *Metabolism* 38:166–171, 1989.
172. Glueck CJ, Hogg E, Allen C, Gartside PS: Effects of alcohol ingestion on lipids and lipoproteins in normal men: Isocaloric metabolic studies. *Am J Clin Nutr* 33:2287–2293, 1980.
173. Talbot GD, Keating BM: Effects of preprandial whiskey on postalimentary lipemia. *Geriatrics* 17:802–808, 1962.
174. Barboriak JJ, Meade RC: Enhancement of alimentary lipemia by preprandial alcohol. *Am J Med Sci* 255:245–251, 1968.
175. Superko HR: Effects of acute and chronic alcohol consumption on postprandial lipemia in healthy normotriglyceridemic men. *Am J Cardiol* 69:701–704, 1992.
176. Wilson DE, Schreibman PH, Brewster AC, Arky RA: The enhancement of alimentary lipemia by ethanol in man. *J Lab Clin Med* 75:264–274, 1970.
177. Barboriak JJ, Hogan WJ: Preprandial drinking and plasma lipids in man. *Atherosclerosis* 4:323–325, 1976.
178. Borowsky SA, Perlow W, Baraona E, Lieber CS: Relationship of alcoholic hypertriglyceridemia to stage of liver disease and dietary lipid. *Dig Dis Sci* 25:22–27, 1980.
179. Avgerinos A, Chu P, Greenfield C, *et al:* Plasma lipid and lipoprotein response to fat feeding in alcoholic liver disease. *Hepatology* 3:349–355, 1983.
180. Schneider J, Panne E, Braun H, *et al:* Ethanol-induced hyperlipoproteinemia. Crucial role of preceding ethanol intake in the removal of chylomicrons. *J Lab Clin Med* 101:114–122, 1983.
181. Lewis B, Chait A, Simmons P: Lipid abnormalities in alcoholism and chronic renal failure. *Adv Exp Biol Med* 38:155–159, 1973.
182. Janus ED, Lewis B: Alcohol and abnormalities of lipid metabolism. *Clin Endocrinol Metab* 7:321–332, 1978.
183. Mendelson JH, Mello NK: Alcohol-induced hyperlipidemia and beta lipoproteins. *Science* 180:1372–1374, 1973.
184. Ginsberg H, Olefsky J, Farquhar JW, Reaven GM: Moderate ethanol ingestion and plasma triglyceride levels. *Ann Intern Med* 80:143–149, 1974.

185. Debry G, Mejean L, Max JP, *et al:* Effects of alcohol intake on several metabolic parameters in primary hyperlipoproteinemia. In Avogaro P, Sirtori CR, Tremoli F (eds): *Metabolic Effects of Alcohol.* Amsterdam, The Netherlands, Elsevier/North Holland Biomedical Press, 1979, pp 227–234.
186. Crouse JR, Grundy SM: Effects of alcohol on plasma lipoproteins and cholesterol and triglyceride metabolism in man. *J Lipid Res* 25:486–496, 1984.
187. Välimäki M, Halmesuaki E, Keso L, *et al:* Serum lipids and lipoproteins in alcoholic women during pregnancy. *Metabolism* 39:486–493, 1990.
188. DeGennes JL, Thomopoulus P, Truffert J, Labrouse de Tregomain B: Hyperlipémies dépendantes de l'alcool. *Nutr Metabol* 14:141–158, 1972.
189. Lindenbaum J, Lieber CS: Effects of chronic ethanol administration on intestinal absorption in man in the absence of nutritional deficiency. *Ann NY Acad Sci* 252:228–234, 1975.
190. Carter EA, Drummey GD, Isselbacher KJ: Ethanol stimulates triglyceride synthesis by the intestine. *Science* 174:1245–1247, 1971.
191. Baraona E, Pirola RC, Lieber CS: Acute and chronic effects of ethanol on intestinal lipid metabolism. *Biochim Biophys Acta* 388:19–28, 1975.
192. Middleton WRJ, Carter EA, Drummey GD, Isselbacher KJ: Effect of oral ethanol administration on intestinal cholesterogenesis in the rat. *Gastroenterology* 60:880–887, 1971.
193. Baraona E, Lieber CS: Intestinal lymph formation and fat absorption: Stimulation by acute ethanol administration and inhibition by chronic ethanol feeding. *Gastroenterology* 68:495–502, 1975.
194. Mistilis SP, Ockner RK: Effects of ethanol on endogenous lipids and lipoprotein metabolism in small intestine. *J Lab Clin Med* 80:34–46, 1972.
195. Hayashi H: Lipid metabolism in the intestinal tract and its modification by ethanol. In Preddy VR, Watson RR (eds): *Alcohol and the gastrointestinal tract.* Boca Raton, FL, CRC Press, 1996, pp 289–309.
196. Thomson ABR, Keelan M, Clandinin MT: Feeding rats diets enriched with saturated fatty acids prevent the inhibitory effects of acute and chronic ethanol exposure on the *in vitro* uptake of hexoses and lipids. *Biochim Biophys Acta* 1084:122–128, 1991.
197. Hernell O, Johnson O: Effects of ethanol on plasma triglycerides in male and female rats. *Lipids* 8:503–508, 1973.
198. Barboriak JJ: Effect of ethanol on lipoprotein lipase activity. *Life Sci* 5:237–241, 1966.
199. Kudzma DJ, Schonfeld G: Alcoholic hyperlipidemia: Induction by alcohol but not by carbohydrate. *J Lab Clin Med* 77:384–389, 1971.
200. Nikkilä EA, Taskinen M-R, Huttunen JK: Effect of acute ethanol load on postheparin plasma lipoprotein lipase and hepatic lipase activities and intravenous fat tolerance. *Horm Metab Res* 10:220–223, 1978.
201. Nilsson-Ehle P, Carlstrom S, Belfrage P: Effects of ethanol intake on lipoprotein lipase activity in adipose tissue of fasting subjects. *Lipids* 13:433–437, 1978.
202. Pownall HJ: Dietary ethanol is associated with reduced lipolysis of intestinally derived lipoproteins. *J Lipid Res* 35:2105–2113, 1994.
203. Redgrave TG, Martin G: Effects of chronic ethanol consumption on the catabolism of chylomicron triacylglycerol and cholesteryl ester in the rat. *Atherosclerosis* 28:69–80, 1977.
204. Lakshman MR, Ezekiel M: Relationship of alcoholic hyperlipidemia to the feedback regulation of hepatic cholesterol synthesis by chylomicron remnant. *Alcohol Clin Exp Res* 6:482–496, 1982.
205. Lakshman MR, Ezekiel M, Campbell BS, Muesing RA: Binding, uptake, and metabolism of chylomicron remnants by hepatocytes from control and chronic ethanol-fed rats. *Alcohol Clin Exp Res* 10:412–418, 1986.
206. Savolainen M, Baraona E, Leo MA, Lieber CS: Pathogenesis of the hypertriglyceridemia at early stages of alcoholic liver injury in the baboon. *J Lipid Res* 27:1073–1083, 1986.
207. Sane T, Nikkilä EA, Taskinen M-R, *et al:* Accelerated turnover of very low density lipoprotein triglycerides in chronic alcohol users. A possible mechanism for the up-regulation of high density lipoprotein by ethanol. *Atherosclerosis* 53:185–193, 1984.

208. Malmendier CL, Delcroix C: Effect of alcohol intake on high and low density lipoprotein metabolism in healthy volunteers. *Clin Chim Acta* 152:281–288, 1985.
209. Sigurdsson G, Nicoll A, Lewis B: The metabolism of low density lipoprotein in endogenous hypertriglyceridemia. *Eur J Clin Invest* 6:167–177, 1976.
210. Breier C, Lisch H-J, Drexel H, Braunsteiner H: Post-heparin lipolytic activities and alterations of the chemical composition of high density lipoproteins in alcohol-induced type V hyperlipidemia. *Atherosclerosis* 52:317–328, 1984.
211. Alexander RH, Friedberg SJ, Bogdonoff MD, Estes EH: Hepatic cirrhosis. Correlation of clinical severity and abnormality in triglyceride metabolism. *Metabolism* 12:197–206, 1963.
212. Seakins A, Waterlow JC: Effect of a low-protein diet on the incorporation of amino acids into rat serum lipoproteins. *Biochem J* 129:793–795, 1972.
213. Lombardi BP, Pani P, Schlunk FF: Choline-deficiency fatty liver: Impaired release of hepatic triglycerides. *J Lipid Res* 9:437–446, 1968.
214. Ekman R, Fex G, Johansson BG, *et al:* Changes in plasma high density lipoproteins and lipolytic enzymes after long-term, heavy consumption. *Scand J Clin Lab Invest* 41:709–715, 1981.
215. Taskinen M-R, Välimäki M, Nikkilä EA, *et al:* High density lipoprotein subfractions and postheparin plasma lipases in alcoholic men before and after ethanol withdrawal. *Metabolism* 31:1168–1174, 1982.
216. Hartung GH, Foreyt JP, Reeves RS, *et al:* Effect of alcohol dose on plasma lipoprotein subfractions and lipolytic enzyme activity in active and inactive men. *Metabolism* 39:81–86, 1990.
217. Mordasini R, Kaffarnik H, Schneider J, Riesen W: Alkohol und Plasmalipoproteine im akut und Langzeitversuch. *Schweiz Med Wochen* 112:1928–1931, 1982.
218. Johansson BC, Medhus A: Increase in plasma α-lipoproteins in chronic alcoholics after acute abuse. *Acta Med Scand* 195:273–277, 1974.
219. Devenyi P, Robinson GM, Roncari DAK: Alcohol and high-density lipoproteins. *Can Med Assoc J* 123:981–984, 1980.
220. LaPorte R, Valvo-Gerard L, Kuller L, *et al:* The relationship between alcohol consumption, liver enzymes and high-density lipoprotein cholesterol. *Circulation* 64(Suppl III):67–72, 1981.
221. Taskinen M-R, Välimäki M, Nikkilä EA, *et al:* Sequence of alcohol-induced initial changes in plasma lipoproteins. *Metabolism* 34:112–119, 1985.
222. Fraser GE, Anderson JT, Foster W, *et al:* The effect of alcohol on serum high density lipoprotein (HDL). *Atherosclerosis* 46:275–286, 1983.
223. Hartung GH, Foreyt JP, Mitchell RE, *et al:* Effect of alcohol intake on high-density lipoprotein cholesterol levels in runners and inactive men. *JAMA* 249:747–750, 1983.
224. Danielsson B, Ekman R, Fex G, *et al:* Changes in plasma high density lipoproteins in chronic male alcoholics during and after abuse. *Scand J Clin Lab Invest* 38:113–119, 1978.
225. Barboriak JJ, Jacobson GR, Cushman P, *et al:* Chronic alcohol abuse and high density lipoprotein cholesterol. *Alcoholism: Clin Exp Res* 4:346–349, 1980.
226. Ernst N, Fisher M, Smith W, *et al:* The association of plasma high-density lipoprotein cholesterol with dietary intake and alcohol consumption. The Lipid Research Clinics Prevalence Study. *Circulation* 62(Suppl IV):41–52, 1980.
227. Hulley SB, Gordon S: Alcohol and high-density lipoprotein cholesterol: Causal inference from diverse study designs. *Circulation* 64(Suppl 3):57–63, 1981.
228. Phillips NR, Havel RJ, Kane JP: Levels and interrelationships of serum and lipoprotein cholesterol and triglycerides. Association with adiposity and the consumption of ethanol, tobacco and beverages containing caffeine. *Arteriosclerosis* 1:13–24, 1981.
229. Bell H, Strømme JH, Steensland H, Bache-Wiig JE: Plasma HDL-cholesterol and estimated ethanol consumption in 104 patients with alcohol dependence syndrome. *Alcohol Alcohol* 20:35–40, 1985.
230. Glueck CJ, Heiss G, Morrison JA, *et al:* Alcohol intake, cigarette smoking and plasma lipids and lipoproteins in 12–19-year-old children. *Circulation* 64(Suppl III):48–56, 1981.
231. Barrett-Connor E, Sharez L: A community study of alcohol and other factors associated with

the distribution of high density lipoprotein cholesterol in older vs younger men. *Am J Epidemiol* 115:888–893, 1982.
232. Willet W, Hennekens CH, Siegel AJ, *et al:* Alcohol consumption and high density lipoprotein cholesterol in marathon runners. *N Engl J Med* 303:1159–1161, 1980.
233. Hagiage M, Marti C, Rigau D, *et al:* Effect of moderate alcohol intake on the lipoproteins of normotriglyceridemic obese subjects compared to normoponderal controls. *Metabolism* 41:856–861, 1992.
234. Weidner G, Connor SL, Chesney MA, *et al:* Sex differences in high density lipoprotein cholesterol among low-level alcohol consumers. *Circulation* 83:176–180, 1991.
235. Frezza M, DiPadova C, Pozzato G, *et al:* High blood alcohol levels in women: Role of decreased gastric alcohol dehydrogenase activity and first pass metabolism. *N Engl J Med* 322:95–99, 1990.
236. Haskell WL, Camargo C Jr, Williams PT, *et al:* The effect of cessation and resumption of moderate alcohol intake on serum high-density-lipoprotein subfractions. A controlled study. *N Engl J Med* 310:805–810, 1984.
237. Haffner SM, Applebaum-Bowden D, Wahl PW, *et al:* Epidemiological correlates of high density lipoprotein subfractions, apolipoproteins A-I, A-II, and D, and lecithin cholesterol acyltransferase. Effects of smoking, alcohol, and adiposity. *Arteriosclerosis* 5:169–177, 1985.
238. Williams PT, Kraus RM, Wood PD, *et al:* Associations of diet and alcohol intake with high-density lipoprotein subclasses. *Metabolism* 34:524–530, 1985.
239. Välimäki M, Taskinen M-R, Ylikahri R, *et al:* Comparison of the effects of two different doses of alcohol on serum lipoproteins, HDL-subfractions and apolipoproteins A-I and A-II: A controlled study. *Eur J Clin Invest* 18:472–480, 1988.
240. Goldberg CS, Tall AR, Krumholz S: Acute inhibition of hepatic lipase and increase in plasma lipoproteins after alcohol intake. *J Lipid Res* 25:714–720, 1984.
241. Malmendier CL, Mailier EL, Amerijckx JP, Fischer ML: Plasma levels of apolipoproteins A-I, A-II in alcoholism in relation to the degree of histological liver damage, and to liver function tests. *Hepatogastroenterology* 30:236–239, 1983.
242. Camargo CA, Williams PT, Vranizan KM, *et al:* The effect of moderate alcohol intake on serum apolipoproteins A-I and A-II. *JAMA* 253:2854–2857, 1985.
243. Poynard T, Abella A, Pignon JP, *et al:* Apolipoprotein A-I and alcoholic liver disease. *Hepatology* 6:1391–1395, 1986.
244. Duhamel G, Nalpas B, Goldstein S, *et al:* Plasma lipoprotein and apolipoprotein profile in alcoholic patients with and without liver disease: On the relative roles of alcohol and liver injury. *Hepatology* 4:577–585, 1984.
245. Puchois P, Fontan M, Gentilini J-L, *et al:* Serum apolipoprotein A-II, a biochemical indicator of alcohol abuse. *Clin Chim Acta* 185:185–189, 1984.
246. Puchois P, Ghalin N. Zylberberg G, *et al:* Effect of alcohol intake on human apolipoprotein A-I-containing lipoprotein subfractions. *Arch Intern Med* 150:1638–1641, 1990.
247. Sabesin SM, Weidman SW: Lipoprotein profiles in chronic alcoholics: Use of high-density lipoprotein subspecies levels to differentiate subpopulations. *Hepatology* 4:737–738, 1984.
248. Cushman P, Barboriak JJ, Liao A, Hoffman NE: Association between plasma high density lipoprotein cholesterol and antipyrine metabolism in alcoholics. *Life Sci* 30:1721–1724, 1982.
249. Luoma PV, Sotaniemi EA, Pelkonen RO, Enholm C: High-density lipoproteins and hepatic microsomal enzyme induction in alcohol consumers. *Res Commun Chem Pathol Pharmacol* 37:91–96, 1982.
250. Cluette JE, Mulligan JJ, Noring R, *et al:* Ethanol enhances *de novo* synthesis of high density lipoprotein cholesterol. *Proc Soc Exp Biol Med* 176:508–511, 1984.
251. Mathurin P, Vidaud D, Bedossa P, *et al:* Quantification of apolipoprotein A-I and B messenger RNA in heavy drinkers according to liver disease. *Hepatology* 23:44–51, 1996.
252. Lin RC, Lumeng L, Phelps VL: Serum high-density lipoprotein particles of alcohol-fed rats are deficient in apolipoprotein E. *Hepatology* 9:307–313, 1989.
253. Tam S-P: Effect of ethanol on lipoprotein secretion in two human hepatoma cell lines, HepG2 and Hep3B. *Alcohol Clin Exp Res* 16:1021–1028, 1992.

254. Amasuriya RN, Gupta AK, Civen M, *et al:* Ethanol stimulates apolipoprotein A-I secretion by human hepatocytes: Implications for a mechanism for atherosclerosis protection. *Metabolism* 41:827–832, 1992.
255. Nishiwaki M, Ishikawa T, Ito T, *et al:* Effects of alcohol in lipoprotein lipase, hepatic lipase, cholesteryl ester transfer protein, and lecithin:cholesterol acyltransferase in high-density lipoprotein cholesterol elevation. *Atherosclerosis* 111:99–109, 1994.
256. Mishra L, Le N-A, Brown V, Mezey E: Effect of acute intravenous alcohol on plasma lipoproteins in man. *Metabolism* 40:1128–1130, 1991.
257. Parkes JG, Auerbach W, Goldberg DM: Effect of alcohol in lipoprotein metabolism. II. Lipolytic activities and mixed function oxidases. *Enzyme* 43:47–55, 1990.
258. Muller P, Fellin R, Lambrecht J. *et al:* Hypertriglyceridaemia secondary to liver disease. *Eur J Clin Invest* 4:419–428, 1974.
259. Freeman M, Kuiken L, Ragland JB, Sabesin SM: Hepatic triglyceride lipase deficiency in liver disease. *Lipids* 12:443–445, 1977.
260. Karsenty C, Baraona E, Savolainen MJ, Lieber CS: Effects of chronic ethanol intake on mobilization and excretion of cholesterol in baboons. *J Clin Invest* 75:976–986, 1985.
261. Cluette-Brown J, Mulligan J, Igoe F, Hojnacki JL: Ethanol induced alterations in low and high density lipoproteins. *Proc Soc Exp Biol Med* 178:495–499, 1985.
262. Savolainen MJ, Hannuksela M, Sepuanen S, *et al:* Increased high-density lipoprotein cholesterol concentration in alcoholics is related to low cholesteryl ester transfer protein activity. *Eur J Clin Invest* 20:593–599, 1990.
263. Hannuksela M, Marcel YL, Kesäniemi YA, Savolainen MJ Reduction in the concentration and activity of plasma cholesteryl ester transfer protein by alcohol. *J Lipid Res* 33:737–744, 1992.
264. Hirano K-I, Yamashita S, Sakai N, *et al:* Low-density lipoproteins in hyperalphalipoproteinemic heavy alcohol drinkers have reduced affinity for the low density lipoprotein receptor. *Clin Biochem* 25:357–362, 1992.
265. Ridker PM, Vaughan DE, Stampfer MJ, *et al:* A cross-sectional study of endogenous tissue plasminogen activator, total cholesterol, HDL cholesterol and apolipoproteins A-I, A-II, and B100. *Arterioscler Thromb* 13:1587–1592, 1993.
266. van Tol A, Groener JEM, Scheek LM, *et al:* Induction of net mass lipid transfer reactions in plasma by wine consumption with dinner. *Eur J Clin Invest* 25:390–395, 1995.
267. Schwartz CC, Halloran LG, Vlahcevic ZR, *et al:* Preferential utilization of free cholesterol from high-density lipoproteins for biliary cholesterol secretion in man. *Science* 200:62–64, 1978.
268. Schwartz CC, Vlahcevic ZR, Berman M, *et al:* Central role of high density lipoprotein in plasma free cholesterol metabolism. *J Clin Invest* 70:105–116, 1982.
269. Cluette JE, Mulligan JJ, Noring R, *et al:* Effect of ethanol on lipoprotein synthesis and fecal sterol excretion. *Nutr Res* 5:45–56, 1985.
270. Topping DL, Weller RA, Nader CJ, *et al:* Adaptive effects of dietary ethanol in the pig: Changes in plasma high-density lipoproteins and fecal steroid excretion and mutagenicity. *Am J Clin Nutr* 36:245–250, 1982.
271. Cohen BI, Raicht RF: Sterol metabolism in the rat: Effect of alcohol on sterol metabolism in two strains of rats. *Alcohol Clin Exp Res* 5:225–229, 1981.
272. Nestel PJ, Simons LA, Homma Y: Effects of ethanol on bile acid and cholesterol metabolism. *Am J Clin Nutr* 29:1007–1015, 1976.
273. Hojnacki JL, Cluette-Brown JE, Dawson M, *et al:* Alcohol delays clearance of lipoproteins from the circulation. *Metabolism* 41:1151–1153, 1992.
274. Maruszewicz M, Mirkiewicz E, Wehr H: Abnormal low density lipoprotein composition in some chronic alcoholics: A possible mechanism. *Alcohol Alcohol* 25:533–538, 1990.
275. Rudel LL, Leathers CW, Bond MG, Bullock BC: Dietary ethanol-induced modifications in hyperlipoproteinemia and atherosclerosis in non-human primates (*Macaca nemestrina*). *Atherosclerosis* 1:144–155, 1981.
276. Hojnacki JL, Cluette-Brown JE, Dawson M, *et al:* Alcohol dose and low density lipoprotein heterogeneity in squirrel monkeys (*Saimiri sciureus*). *Atherosclerosis* 94:249–261, 1992.

277. Kesäniemi YA, Kervinen K, Miettinen TA: Acetaldehyde modification of low density lipoprotein accelerates its catabolism in man. *Eur J Clin Invest* 17:29–36, 1987.
278. Savolainen MJ, Baraona E, Lieber CS: Acetaldehyde binding increases the catabolism of rat serum low-density lipoproteins. *Life Sci* 40:841–846, 1987.
279. Wehr H, Rodo M, Lieber CS, Baraona E: Acetaldehyde adducts and autoantibodies against VLDL and LDL in alcoholics. *J Lipid Res* 34:1237–1244, 1993.
280. Kervinen K, Savolainen MJ, Kesäniemi YA: Multiple changes in apoprotein B containing lipoproteins after ethanol withdrawal in alcoholic men. *Ann Med* 23:407–413. 1991.
281. Cullen KJ, Knuiman MW, Ward NJ: Alcohol and mortality in Busselton, Western Australia. *Am J Epidemiol* 137:242–248, 1993.
282. Popham RE, Schmidt W, Israel Y: Variation in mortality from ischemic heart disease in relation to alcohol and milk consumption. *Med Hypotheses* 12:321–329, 1983.
283. Shaper AG, Wannamethee G, Walker M: Alcohol and mortality in British men: Explaining the U-shaped curve. *Lancet* 2:1267–1273, 1988.
284. Fraser GE, Upsdell M: Alcohol and other discriminants between cases of sudden death and myocardial infarction. *Am J Epidemiol* 114:462–476, 1981.
285. Rimm EB, Giovannucci EL, Willett WC, *et al:* Prospective study of alcohol consumption and risk of coronary heart disease in men. *Lancet* 338:464–468, 1991.
286. Suh I, Shaten J, Cutler JA, Kuller LH: Alcohol use and mortality from coronary heart disease: The role of high-density lipoprotein cholesterol. *Ann Intern Med* 116:881–887, 1992.
287. Klatsky AL, Armstrong MA, Friedman GD: Alcohol and mortality. *Ann Intern Med* 117:646–654, 1992.
288. Gaziano JM, Buring JE, Breslow JL, *et al:* Moderate alcohol intake, increased levels of high density lipoprotein and its subfractions, and decreased risk of myocardial infarction. *N Engl J Med* 329:1829–1834, 1993.
289. Eberhard TP: Effect of alcohol on cholesterol-induced atherosclerosis in rabbits. *Arch Pathol* 21:616–622, 1936.
290. Barboriak JJ, Anderson AJ, Rimm AA, Tristani FE: Alcohol and coronary arteries. *Alcohol Clin Exp Res* 3:29–32, 1979.
291. Hennekens CH, Rosner B, Cole DS: Daily alcohol consumption and fatal coronary heart disease. *Am J Epidemiol* 107:196–200, 1978.
292. Marmot MG, Rose G, Shipley MJ, Thomas BJ: Alcohol and mortality: A U-shaped curve. *Lancet* 1:580–583, 1981.
293. Yano K, Rhoads GG, Kagan A: Coffee, alcohol and risk of coronary heart disease among Japanese men living in Hawaii. *N Engl J Med* 297:405–409, 1977.
294. Blackwelder WC, Yano K, Rhoads GG, *et al:* Alcohol and mortality: The Honolulu heart study. *Am J Med* 68:164–169, 1980.
295. Boffeta P, Garfinkel L: Alcohol drinking and mortality among men enrolled in an American Cancer Society prospective study. *Epiodemiology* 1:342–348, 1990.
296. Castelli WP: Diet, smoking, and alcohol: Influence on coronary heart disease risk. *Am J Kidney Dis* 16:41–46, 1990.
297. Jackson R, Scragg R, Beaglehole R: Alcohol consumption and risk of coronary heart disease. *Br Met J* 303:211–216, 1991.
298. Gruchow HW, Hoffmann RG, Anderson AJ, Barboriak JJ: Effects of drinking patterns on the relationship between alcohol and coronary occlusion. *Atherosclerosis* 43:393–404, 1982.
299. Gronbaek M, Deis A, Sorensen TIA, *et al:* Mortality associated with moderate intake of wine, beers or spirits. *Br Med J* 310:1165–1169, 1995.
300. Renaud S, de Logeril M: Wine, alcohol, platelets, and the French paradox for coronary heart disease. *Lancet* 339:1523–1526, 1992.
301. Stampfer MJ, Colditz GA, Willett WC, *et al:* A prospective study of moderate alcohol consumption and the risk of coronary disease and stroke in women. *N Engl J Med* 319:267–273, 1988.
302. Parker DR, McPhillips JB, Derby CA, *et al:* High-density-lipoprotein cholesterol and types of alcoholic beverages consumed among men and women. *J Public Health* 86:1022–1027, 1996.

303. Langer RD, Criqui MH, Reed DM: Lipoproteins and blood pressure as biological pathways for effect of moderate alcohol consumption on coronary heart disease. *Circulation* 85:919–915, 1992.
304. Rubin EM, Krauss RM, Spangler EA, *et al:* Inhibition of early atherogenesis in transgenic mice by human apolipoprotein A-I. *Nature* 353:265–267, 1991.
305. Emerson EE, Manaves V, Singer T, Tabesh M: Chronic alcohol feeding inhibits atherogenesis in C57BL/6 hyperlipidemic mice. *Am J Pathol* 147:1749–1758, 1995.
306. Dai J, Miller BA, Lin RC: Alcohol feeding impedes early atherosclerosis in low-density lipoprotein receptor knockout mice: Factors in addition to high-density lipoprotein–apolipoprotein A1 are involved. *Alcohol Clin Exp Res* 21:11–18, 1997.
307. Miller NE, Hammett F, Saltissi S, *et al:* Relation of angiographically defined coronary artery disease to plasma lipoprotein subfractions and apolipoproteins. *Br Med J* 282:1741–1744, 1981.
308. Ballantyne FC, Clark RS, Simpson HS, and Ballantyne D: High density and low density lipoprotein subfractions in survivors of myocardial infarction and in control subjects. *Metabolism* 31:433–437, 1982.
309. Gofman JW, Young W, Tandy R: Ischemic heart disease, atherosclerosis, and longevity. *Circulation* 34:679–697, 1966.
310. Stampfer MJ, Sacks FM, Salvini S, *et al:* A prospective study of cholesterol, apolipoproteins, and the risk of myocardial infarction. *N Engl J Med* 325:373–381, 1991.
311. Buring JE, O'Connor GT, Goldhaver SZ, *et al:* Decreased HDL_2 and HDL_3 cholesterol, apo A-I and apo A-II, and increased risk of myocardial infarction. *Circulation* 85:22–29, 1992.
312. Sillanaukee P, Koivula T, Jokela H, *et al:* Relationship of alcohol consumption to changes in HDL-subfractions. *Eur J Clin Invest* 23:486–491, 1993.
313. Steinberg D, Pearson TA, Kuller LH: Alcohol and atherosclerosis. *Ann Intern Med* 114:967–976, 1991.
314. Lin RC, Dai J, Lumeng L, *et al:* Serum low density lipoprotein of alcoholic patients is chemically modified in vivo and induces apolipoprotein E synthesis by macrophages. *J Clin Invest* 95:1979–1986, 1995.
315. Frankel E, Kanner J, German J, *et al:* Inhibition of oxidation of human low-density lipoprotein by phenolic substances in red wines. *Lancet* 341:454–457, 1993.
316. Whitehead TP, Robinson D, Allaway S, *et al:* Effect of red wine ingestion on the antioxidant capacity of serum. *Clin Chem* 41:32–35, 1995.
317. Fuhrman B, Lavy A, Aviram M: Consumption of red wine with meals reduces the susceptibility of human plasma and low-density lipoproteins to lipid peroxidation. *Am J Clin Nutr* 61:549–554, 1995.
318. de Rijke JB, Demacker PNM, Assen NA, *et al:* Red wine consumption does not affect oxidizability of low-density lipoproteins in volunteers. *Am J Clin Nutr* 63:329–334, 1996.
319. Marth E, Cazzolato G, Bon B, *et al:* Serum concentrations of Lp(a) and other lipoprotein parameters in heavy alcohol consumers. *Ann Nutr Metab* 26:56–62, 1982.
320. Sharper PC, McGrath LT, McClean E, *et al:* Effect of red wine consumption on lipoprotein(a) and other risk factors for atherosclerosis. *Q J Med* 88:101–108, 1995.
321. Kervinen K, Savolainen MJ, Kesäniemi YA: A rapid increase in lipoprotein(a) levels after ethanol withdrawal in alcoholic men. *Life Sci* 48:2183–2188, 1991.
322. Välimäki M, Kahri J, Laitinen K, *et al:* High density lipoprotein subfractions, apolipoprotein A-I containing lipoproteins, lipoprotein(a), and cholesterol ester transfer protein activity in alcoholic women before and after alcohol withdrawal. *Eur J Clin Invest* 23:406–417, 1993.
323. Delarue J, Husson M, Schellenberg F, *et al:* Serum lipoprotein(a) in alcoholic men: Effect of withdrawal. *Alcohol* 13:309–314, 1996.
324. Jackson R, Scragg R, Beaglehole R: Does recent alcohol consumption reduce the risk of acute myocardial infarction and coronary death in regular drinkers? *Am J Epidemiol* 136:819–824, 1992.
325. Renaud SC, Beswick AD, Fehily AM, *et al:* Alcohol and platelet aggregation: The Caerphilly Prospective Heart Disease Study. *Am J Clin Nutr* 55:1012–1017, 1992.

326. Guivernau M, Baraona E, Lieber CS: Acute and chronic effects of ethanol and its metabolites on vascular production of prostacyclin in rats. *J Pharmacol Exp Ther* 240:59–64, 1987.
327. Fleisher LN, Tall AR, Witte LD, *et al:* Stimulation of arterial endothelial cell prostacyclin synthesis by high density lipoproteins. *J Biol Chem* 257:6653–6655, 1982.
328. Guivernau M, Baraona E, Soong J, Lieber CS: Enhanced stimulatory effect of HDL and other agonists on vascular prostacyclin production in rats fed alcohol-containing diets. *Biochem Pharmacol* 38:503–508, 1989.
329. Beitz J, Block H-U, Beitz A, *et al:* Endogenous lipoproteins modify the thromboxane formation capacity of platelets. *Atherosclerosis* 60:95–99, 19896.
330. Mikkhailidis DP, Jeremy JY, Barradas MA, *et al:* Effect of ethanol on vascular prostacyclin (prostaglandin I2) synthesis, platelet aggregation, and platelet thromboxane release. *Br Med J* 287:1495–1498, 1983.
331. Kangasaho M, Hillbom M, Kaste M, Vapaatalo H: Effects of ethanol intoxication and hangover on plasma levels of thromboxane B2 and 6-keto prostaglandin F1a and on thromboxane B2 formation by platelets in man. *Throm Haemost* 48:232–234, 1982.
332. Kontula K, Vilnikka L, Ylikorkala O, Ylikahri R: Effect of acute ethanol intake on thromboxane and prostacyclin in human. *Life Sci* 31:261–264, 1982.
333. Arai M, Okuno F, Nagata S, *et al:* Platelet dysfunction and alteration of prostaglandin metabolism after chronic alcohol consumption (Abstract). *Scand J Gastroenterol* 21:1091, 1986.
334. Hillborn M, Kangasaho M, Lowbeer C, *et al:* Effects of ethanol on platelet function. *Alcohol* 2:429–432, 1985.
335. Förstermann U, Feuerstein TJ: Decreased systemic formation of prostaglandin E and prostacyclin, and unchanged thromboxane formation, in alcoholics during withdrawal as estimated from metabolites in urine. *Clin Sci* 73:277–283, 1987.
336. Meade TW, Chakrabarti R, Haines AP, *et al:* Characteristics affecting fibrinolytic activity and plasma fibrinogen concentrations. *Br Med J* 1:153–156, 1979.
337. Hendriks HFJ, Veenstra J, Velthuis-te-Wierik EJM, *et al:* Effect of moderate alcohol does with the evening meal on fibrinolytic activity. *Br Med J* 308:1003–1006, 1994.
338. Ridker PM, Vaughan DE, Stampfer MJ, *et al:* Association of moderate alcohol consumption and plasma concentration of endogenous tissue-type plasminogen activator. *JAMA* 272:929–933, 1994.
339. Iso H, Folsom AR, Koike KA, *et al:* Antigens of tissue plasminogen activator and plasminogen activator inhibitor I: Correlates in nonsmoking Japanese and Caucasian men and women. *Thromb Haemost* 70:475–480, 1993.

5

Cardiovascular Effects of Alcohol

Howard S. Friedman

Abstract. The ingestion of one or two alcoholic drinks can affect heart rate, blood pressure, cardiac output, myocardial contractility, and regional blood flow. These actions generally are not clinically important. In the presence of cardiovascular disease, however, even such small quantities of alcohol might result in transient unfavorable hemodynamic changes. Moreover, alcohol abuse can produce cardiac arrhythmias, hypertension, cardiomyopathy, stroke, and even sudden death. In contrast, moderate alcohol use produces changes that have an overall favorable effect on atherosclerotic-related vascular diseases. Because cardiovascular disease due to atherosclerosis is the leading cause of death in Western society, this desirable effect of alcohol use outweighs its detrimental actions, resulting in favorable findings in population studies. Nevertheless, the body of evidence argues against encouraging alcohol use for its cardiovascular effects.

1. Introduction

Moderate use of alcohol (defined as no more than two unit drinks per day in men and no more than one unit drink per day in women) has come to be viewed as having some health benefit.[1] The change in public health recommendations regarding alcohol use reflects the frequently repeated observation in population studies that when used in moderation, alcohol use is associated with a reduction of deaths due to coronary heart disease; this effect is not offset by deaths related to alcohol use, thereby resulting in lower all-causes mortality rates.[2] Moreover, these findings correlate with the quantity of alcohol used[3] and relate to concurrent favorable changes in the blood lipid profile,[4] thereby providing both statistical and biological plausibility for the

Howard S. Friedman • Department of Medicine, Long Island College Hospital, Brooklyn, New York; and Department of Medicine, SUNY Health Sciences Center at Brooklyn, Brooklyn, New York 11201.

Recent Developments in Alcoholism, Volume 14: The Consequences of Alcoholism, edited by Galanter. Plenum Press, New York, 1998.

observations. Despite these favorable trends, there is equally persuasive evidence that even such small quantities of alcohol might have adverse effects in some individuals, and consumption of larger amounts can result in serious cardiovascular complications. The cardiovascular effects of alcohol have recently been reviewed in depth.[5] This chapter will update that overview of the subject.

2. Acute Myocardial Effects of Ethanol

Ethanol, even at concentrations as low as 50 mg/dl,[6] has consistently been shown to depress myocardial contractility.[6–8] Because ethanol and its metabolites also have adrenergic[9] and vasodilatory effect,[10] the direct myocardial depressant actions of alcohol may be obscured when cardiac "pump" function is assessed following ethanol administration. Cardiac output generally increases following alcohol ingestion in healthy subjects, reflecting the changes in heart rate and peripheral vascular resistance that ensue.[11,12] However, more sensitive indices of cardiac function, such as left ventricular ejection fraction, generally worsen.[9,13] Figure 1 illustrates this effect in anesthetized dogs.

Although the acute effects of alcohol on myocardial metabolism have been extensively studied, these investigations have not provided an explanation for the cardiac muscle depressant actions of alcohol. Recent investigations using isolated myocyte tissue culture and measurements of the cyclic fluctuations of cytosolic calcium (calcium transients), however, have demonstrated abnormalities of myocardial electromechanical coupling at concentra-

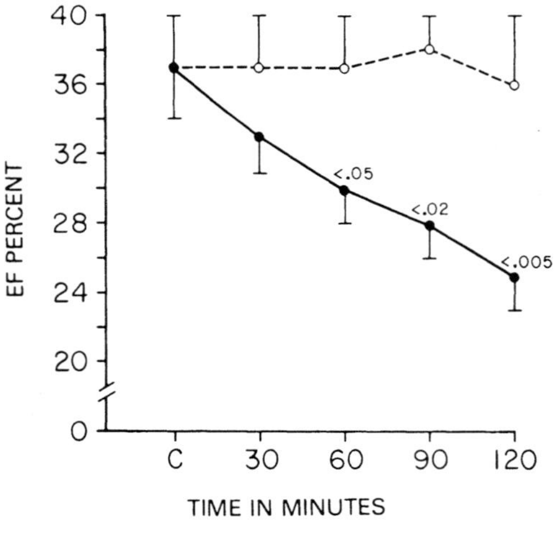

Figure 1. Effects of ethanol (●—●, $n = 8$) on cardiac function. During an infusion of ethanol in anesthetized dogs, which produced an average concentration of 118 mg/dl at 30 min and 294 mg/dl at 120 min, ejection fraction (EF) declined. Saline (control, ○—○, $n = 5$), did not produce such a change. (Reprinted with permission from Friedman *et al.*[63])

tions of ethanol relevant to human use, and therefore may provide important insights into ethanol's acute myocardial depressant effects.

The heart lacks alcohol dehydrogenase.[14] Even in pharmacological concentrations under conditions in which myocardial depressant effects are still evident, myocardial oxidation of ethanol has not been observed.[15] However, nonoxidative metabolism with formation of abnormal alcohol esters has recently been demonstrated.[16,17] In a series of reports, Lang and co-workers have demonstrated fatty acid ethyl esters in hearts obtained at autopsy,[16] and experimentally they have been generated from myocardial tissue.[18] These substances bind to myocardial mitochondria and can uncouple mitochondrial oxidative phosphorylation at concentrations found in human hearts.[19] Moreover, hydrolysis of these esters produces fatty acids that are also potent uncouplers of oxidative phosphorylation.[19] Ethanol has in fact been shown to depress acutely mitochondrial respiration.[20,21] However, despite these observations, even at pharmacological concentrations (>2 gm/dl) ethanol has not been found to alter myocardial intracellular pH or phosphocreatine and it only slightly reduces adenosine triphosphate concentration.[22] Thus, changes in myocardial energetics are not likely to explain the acute myocardial depressant effects of ethanol.

Ethanol has been shown to affect acutely the metabolism of free fatty acids,[23–25] the major fuel of the heart in the fasted state, and in some studies protein metabolism,[26–28] but not glucose metabolism.[15] For more than 30 years, ethanol's alterations of cardiac lipid metabolism have been known: free fatty acid myocardial extraction and oxidation are reduced and their incorporation into triglycerides increased.[23,24] This metabolic defect produced by alcohol, at least partially, can be reversed with carnitine, suggesting that the changes may be due to a defect in the transfer of fatty acyl coenzyme A (CoA) derivatives from the cytosol to the mitochondria for oxidation.[25] Because these changes are not reflected in a disturbance of myocardial energetics, they would not explain ethanol's acute myocardial depressant actions. The administration of ethanol has also been shown to depress the rate of myofibrillar (contractile) and sarcoplasmic (noncontractile) protein synthesis in rats, an effect that is markedly enhanced by the acetaldehyde inhibitor, cyanamide.[27] Under identical conditions, ethanol has been observed to inhibit ventricular mitochondrial protein synthesis (subsarcolemmal and interfibrillar).[28] These changes in myocardial protein synthesis, even if relevant to humans, would not explain ethanol's acute depression of myocardial contractility, albeit, if sustained, might contribute to the long-term detrimental effects of alcohol.

With the development of methods to study directly the physical and biochemical changes occurring during myocardial contraction, evidence for direct effects of ethanol on the contractile process has emerged. The propagation of a wave of electrical excitation provides the signal for cardiac contraction, evoking a complex cascade of events beginning with calcium entry into the myocote and the release of calcium from the sarcoplasmic reticulum (SR), measured as calcium transients; this makes calcium available to the contractile proteins, which leads to myocardial shortening and force development.

Ethanol has been shown to reduce the amplitude, duration, and rate of rise of the myocardial transmembrane action potential, an effect that is related directly to a reduction of contractile force, at moderate ethanol concentrations (<100 mg/dl) in human fetal tissue.[8] The propensity of ethanol to shorten the myocardial action potential is a property of alcohols in general, increasing with the length of their carbon chain, and consequently their lipophilic property.[29] Although alcohols have been demonstrated to reduce the calcium inward current,[30,31] ethanol does this only in pharmacological concentrations, and in fact increases calcium entry at low concentrations (<50 mg/dl) in frog isolated ventricular cells, an effect that is *not* adrenergically mediated.[31] Despite this apparent lack of effect on calcium entry, the total calcium made available, reflected by light-indicator measured calcium transients, is decreased by ethanol at relevant concentrations[32–34] (an effect that correlates with myocardial depression), is reversible with removal of ethanol, and is attenuated by beta-agonists and by increasing external calcium concentration.[33,34]

Although the effects of ethanol on the SR (uptake, binding, release, and content) would be pertinent to explaining the changes in calcium transients, the abnormalities observed have generally occurred at concentrations not relevant to human use.[34–36] Of interest, SR vesicles obtained from hearts of guinea pigs acutely treated with more relevant concentrations of ethanol (average peak concentration of 210 mg/dl) demonstrated reduced calcium uptake but no change in SR calcium-dependent ATPase.[37] This apparent enzymatic uncoupling of calcium uptake by the SR and other studies requiring pharmacological concentrations of ethanol to affect the calcium kinetics of the SR[34–36] suggest that ethanol may induce a passive leak of calcium from the SR that over time would reduce the availability of calcium sufficiently to account for a reduction of calcium transients.[38]

Actions of ethanol on myosin ATPase, which would be important in the energetics of contraction, have not been observed at relevant concentrations of ethanol.[39] By contrast, ($Na^+ + K^+$)-ATPase activity has been found to be reversibly inhibited at pharmacological concentrations of ethanol in plasma membranes obtained from guinea pig hearts[40] and at more relevant concentrations in neonatal rat myocytes.[41] However, the significance of these findings is not clear. Inhibition of this electrogenic pump should affect the resting myocardial transmembrane potential, which ethanol has not been demonstrated to do even when it changes other characteristics of the action potential[8]; inhibition of this pump, an action of digitalis, moreover, would be expected to enhance contractility rather than depress it.

Ethanol produces a depression of myocardial contractility at a concentration lower than that at which a reduction of calcium transients is observed.[33] This suggests that at least some of ethanol's myocardial depressant action occurs at the level of the myofilament, either by affecting electromechanical coupling or by a direct effect on contractile proteins. An ADP-induced association of actin and myosin, in fact, has been found to be reversibly inhibited in a dose-dependent relation by ethanol and acetaldehyde, albeit this effect has been demonstrated only in skeletal muscle and at higher ethanol concentration than that needed to produce myocardial depression or an effect on myocardial calcium transients.[42] Thus, although alcohol's myocardial depressant actions have been associated with metabolic changes and effects on the contractile process, a clear definition of the factor (or factors) producing these changes is still evolving.

3. Effects of Ethanol on Regional Blood Flow

Ethanol has regional circulatory effects that do not merely reflect its changes in cardiac output. These actions of alcohol may be a response to local metabolic effects[43,44] and therefore a response to changes in blood flow requirements, direct neurohumoral effects of ethanol and/or its metabolites,[45] the effects of ethanol on modulating local neural and endothelial influences on vascular tone,[46,47] or a direct effect of ethanol and/or its metabolites on the local vasculature.[10] Experimental studies have demonstrated that at relevant concentrations ethanol may have a direct vasodilatory action on arterioles and muscular venules and may antagonize various vasoconstrictors in some regional circulations, such as the splanchnic vasculature.[10] These findings appear to be a direct action of ethanol on the smooth muscle of these vessels, related perhaps to a reduced availability of calcium to the contractile proteins,[10] analogous to ethanol's myocardial effects. In contrast to these effects, alcohol at comparable concentrations has been found to vasoconstrict cerebral[48] and coronary[49] arteries. Moreover, ethanol has been observed to enhance neurally mediated vasoconstriction, an effect attributed to an increase of norepinephrine release by ethanol.[47] In addition, ethanol has been found to inhibit endothelium-dependent acetylcholine relaxation[46,47]; the decrease in cGMP expected with this effect has also been observed.[46] Substances that are direct nitric oxide donors (such as sodium nitroprusside) and therefore not influenced by actions that impact on nitric oxide release, however, do not appear to be affected by ethanol.[46]

Because of the complexity of the vascular responses to ethanol, findings related to regional blood flow changes have often been conflictive. At relevant blood alcohol concentrations, ethanol generally increases skin[50] and splanchnic flow[43,44,51] and reduces flow to limb muscle.[52] Studies that have assessed the effects of ethanol on the brain and coronary circulations, actions that might have important clinical implications, have produced less consistent findings.

Early investigations on brain blood flow in humans were limited by the techniques available for measurement and had important confounders. Severe intoxication, for instance, might result in respiratory depression, which could produce acidosis and hypercapnea, obscuring the direct effects of ethanol on brain blood flow.[53] In experimental studies in animals, alcohol has been demonstrated to decrease,[48] increase,[54] and produce no change[55] in brain blood flow at relevant blood alcohol concentrations. Alcohol also has been found to have an inhibitory effect on substances that vasodilate pial arterioles through release of nitric oxide.[55] In recent studies in humans at moderate blood alcohol concentrations following ingestion of alcohol, cerebral blood flow has been found to increase,[56–58] preferentially in the frontal[57,58] and temporal[57] regions. These focal changes have been found to relate well to blood acetate levels and inversely to blood ethanol levels,[58] consistent with the direct vasoconstrictive effects of ethanol on cerebral blood vessels[48] and the vasodilating effects of acetate generally observed.[10] Furthermore, the focal effects of ethanol on brain blood flow appear to be attenuated by opioid antagonists.[58] These changes in cerebral blood flow might not necessarily reflect the dynamics at other sites in the brain: In an experimental study in conscious dogs, at a time when a transient decrease cerebral blood flow was no longer evident, cerebellar blood flow as still diminished.[59]

Although concentration-dependent enhanced contractile effects of ethanol have been observed in isolated[49] and intact coronary arteries,[60] an increase in coronary blood flow was found in most studies in which ethanol was administered slowly, not associated with a fall in cardiac output, and associated with high blood ethanol concentrations (greater than 200 mg/dl).[61–63] This effect in anesthetized dogs is shown in Fig. 2. Not only do the increases

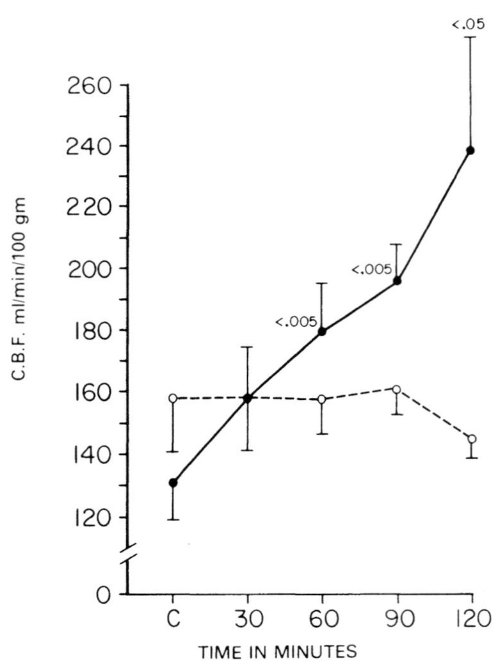

Figure 2. Effects of ethanol (●—●, $n = 8$) on coronary blood flow (CBF). During an ethanol infusion (see Fig. 1), CBF increased; saline (control, ○---○, $n = 5$) did not produce such a change. (Reprinted with permission from Friedman *et al.*[63])

in heart rate, blood pressure, and cardiac dimensions that generally occur with ethanol administration[5] result in increased myocardial oxygen requirements, but ethanol, in at least one study,[64] and its metabolites are coronary vasodilators.[10] Despite these changes, alcohol exerts an unfavorable effect on myocardial ischemia. Because the vasculature of ischemic myocardium is near-maximally dilated, the coronary vasodilatory effects of ethanol occur primarily in arterioles supplying the nonischemic myocardium, resulting in a distribution of blood flow away from the ischemic myocardium, in effect, producing a "coronary steal."[65] This phenomenon occurring in dogs with the left anterior descending artery ligated is shown in Fig. 3. Clinical studies of patients with coronary disease in which ethanol was administered have demonstrated detrimental effects consistent with these findings[66,67] (see Section 7).

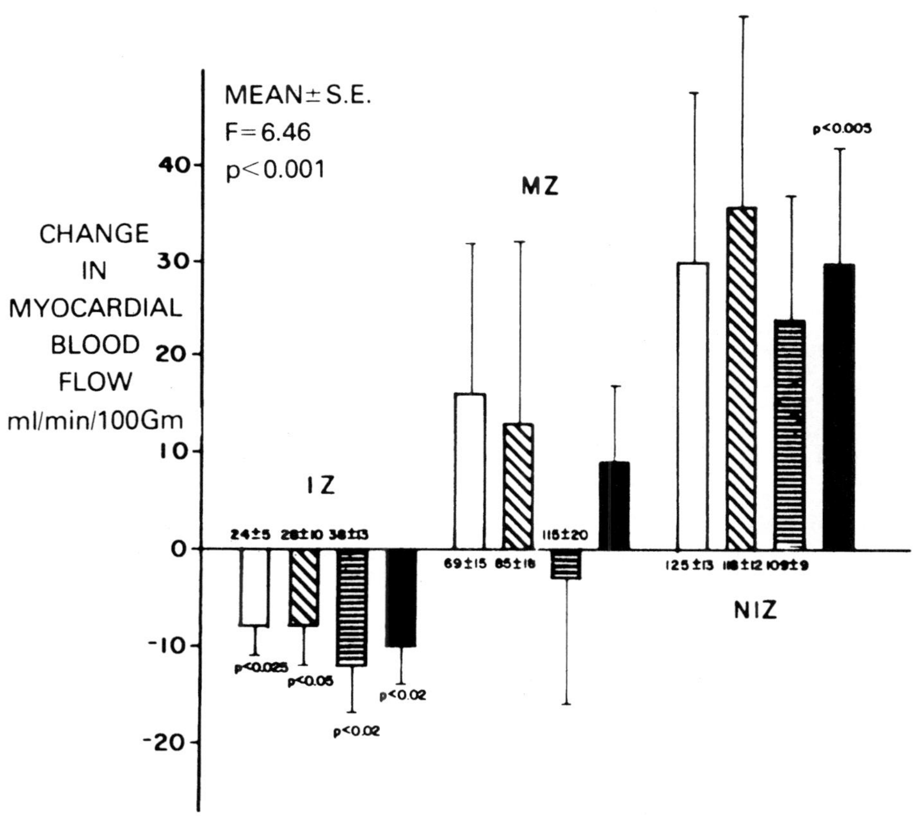

Figure 3. Redistribution of blood flow produced by ethanol. Ischemic (IZ), adjacent to ischemic (MZ) and nonischemic (NIZ) zones, and subendocardial (□), myocardial (▧), subepicardial (▤), and average transmural (■) flows are compared. Values at base of bars indicate myocardial flow after coronary ligation; bars indicate change produced by ethanol. (Reprinted with permission from Friedman *et al.*[65])

Following intravenous administration of alcohol, at relevant blood alcohol concentrations pancreatic blood flow has been found to decrease.[68–71] The use of anesthesia appears to obscure this finding, although a decrease of pancreatic capillary blood flow also has been observed in anesthetized rats.[70] When osmotic[68] or loop[70] diuretics have been administered with alcohol, this effect has become less evident or changed. Whether diuretics act by attenuating pancreatic swelling ascribed to ethanol[68,70] or by some other action still needs to be clarified. In any case, because the decrease in pancreatic blood flow is associated with a reduction in tissue oxygenation,[71] ischemia as a mechanism for acute alcohol-related pancreatitis remains a plausible hypothesis.

Thus, in humans and/or relevant animal models, acutely alcohol generally increases skin, splanchnic, and cerebral blood flow and reduces limb muscle and pancreatic flow. Although myocardial blood may also increase following alcohol administration, an unfavorable distribution of blood flow occurs under ischemic conditions. Because of the difficulties in measuring regional flow and the myriad confounding variables, the effects of ethanol on these and other regional circulations are still not entirely clear. However, such changes may indeed contribute to the injurious actions of alcohol.

4. Alcoholic Heart Disease

Alcohol abuse can result in an array of cardiac abnormalities. From a functional perspective, this ranges from a heart that is hypocontractile, has a reduced output, and is associated with an increased systemic vascular resistance—the findings of alcoholic cardiomyopathy[72]—to one that is hyperdynamic, has an increased output, and is associated with a reduced systemic vascular resistance—the findings of decompensated cirrhosis.[73,74] Even before such striking abnormalities are evident, subclinical cardiac dysfunction can be detected by noninvasive methods[75–77] and can be demonstrated by tests that measure cardiac reserve.[78] Because cardiac performance is dependent on extracardiac influences (pre- and afterloading, heart rate, and neurohumoral effects), as well as the condition of the myocardium, alcohol-related myocardial disease may be present when no obvious heart disease is evident or even when hyperdynamic cardiac function is apparent.[79] Alcoholism leads to myocardial hypertrophy, sometimes with a massive increase of heart weight (>1000 mg), four-chamber cardiac dilatation, myocardial necrosis, interstitial fibrosis, and perivascular fibrosis.[80] On electron microscopy, loss of myofibrils, dilatation of the sarcoplasmic reticulum, separation of the intercalated disk, and abnormalities of the mitochondria may be observed.[81,82] When these findings are pronounced, the clinical features of alcoholic cardiomyopathy may become manifest. Cirrhosis does not preclude cardiomyopathy, and when the two conditions are examined for the presence of the other, evidence for their coexistence is not uncommon.[83] However, because decompensated cirrhosis is associated with neurohumoral changes that have peripheral vascular effects that may "unload" the heart, underlying myocardial disease may be obscured.

4.1. Decompensated Cirrhosis

The salient cardiovascular feature of decompensated cirrhotics is a reduction of systemic vascular resistance.[73,74] The increased cardiac output that occurs is primarily a reflection of this finding, with an increased cardiac output having been observed even when left ventricular systolic shortening is not enhanced.[74] The reduced systemic vascular resistance is largely a consequence of a generalized vasodilatory response rather than to the presence of arteriovenous shunting.[84–86] Systemic vascular resistance in cirrhosis can be related directly to hepatic function (both to individual variables, such as the prothrombin time or serum bilirubin, or global estimates, like the Child–Pugh score).[74] The low urinary sodium concentration observed in decompensated cirrhosis can also be related to the reduction in systemic vascular resistance.[74] However, a reduced systemic vascular resistance may be evident even before ascites is detectable by abdominal ultrasonography,[74] but tense ascites, by impeding venous return to the heart, leads to compensatory responses that may counteract the vasodilatory effects of cirrhosis.[74,87] Because many circulating vasoactive substances (some, such as glucagon, have physiological actions that can produce a hyperdynamic circulation[88]) accumulate in cirrhosis,[84–92] several have been considered as the cause of the cardiovascular findings.[74,88] However, none has been demonstrated to explain the systemic and splanchnic vasodilatation that occurs in cirrhosis.[74,88] Moreover, substances with vasoconstrictive actions—plasma renin activity, angiotensin II, aldosterone, norepinephrine, and arginine vasopressin—are also increased in cirrhosis[93–95]; a reduced responsiveness of the vasculature to these substances must therefore also be present.[95–98] The accumulation of these vasoconstrictors have, however, been related to the abnormalities of salt and water metabolism observed in cirrhosis.[93]

The potent locally derived vasodilators, adenosine[99,100] and nitric oxide,[101–104] have also been considered as possible causes of the generalized vasodilatation in cirrhosis. Adenosine administration can replicate the hemodynamic findings of decompensated cirrhosis, and a specific adenosine receptor antagonist, 8-phenyl-theophylline, has been found to reverse the systemic and splanchnic vasodilatation in experimental cirrhosis in one study[99] but not, however, in another.[100] The evidence that nitric oxide might be the mediator for the cardiovascular findings in cirrhosis is more persuasive.[101–104] Competitive nitric oxide inhibitors of nitric oxide synthase have been shown to exert enhanced systemic and splanchnic vasoconstriction[103] and reverse *in vivo*[101] and *in vitro*[102] the hyporeactivity to vasoconstrictors in some experimental models: portal vein ligation[101,102] and carbon tetrachloride-induced.[103] In contrast, in one model of cirrhosis (biliary cirrhosis), the circulatory effects of a nitric oxide inhibitor were comparable in both control and experimental animals, and cGMP, the secondary messenger of nitric oxide, was not found to be elevated or affected by nitric oxide inhibition in the cirrhotic animals.[105] Furthermore, in another model (carbon tetrachloride-induced), an isolated mesenteric arterial bed preparation did not show a diminished response to various constrictor stimuli nor was there an exaggerated vasoconstrictor response to a nitric oxide inhibitor.[106] However, in a human study patients with decompensated alcohol-induced cirrhosis showed a greater vasoconstrictor effect in the forearm arterial bed to a nitric oxide synthase inhibitor than to norepinephrine; when the responses of the decompensated group were compared to those of a compensated group of alcohol-induced cirrhotics, greater vasoconstriction in response to the nitric oxide inhibitor and a lesser one to norepinephrine was observed, demonstrating hyporeactivity and suggesting a greater dependence on nitric oxide release in the peripheral vasculature of the decompensated patients.[104] Nevertheless, even if nitric oxide formation is increased in decompensated cirrhosis, whether this is the cause of the vasodilatory state or merely a reaction to it is not clear. Enhanced flow itself results in an increase in nitric oxide formation. If the reduced systemic vascular resistance in cirrhosis is not caused by an elevation in one or more vasoactive substance, vascular structural changes (thinning and dilatation) or functional changes (an abnormality of calcium kinetics) are other suggested possible causes.[106]

4.2. *Alcoholic Heart Muscle Disease*

For more than 40 years, alcoholic heart muscle disease has been recognized as a distinct clinical disorder in alcohol abusers who do not have any apparent nutritional deficiencies.[107] The relationship between prolonged alcohol abuse and the occurrence of a dilated, hypocontractile heart is sufficiently strong to suggest that ethanol, acetaldehyde, or some compound formed from these substances is toxic to heart muscle.[108,109] Fatty acid ethyl esters (nonoxidative metabolites of ethanol) have been suggested as possible mediators of the toxic effects of ethanol on the heart, doing so by adversely affecting mitochondrial function.[19] Also, acetaldehyde, a highly reactive compound, forms covalent bonds to cardiac protein.[110] Circulating antibodies to these cardiac protein–acetaldehyde adducts have been found in one third of alcoholics with heart muscle disease[110]; the clinical importance of these antibodies, however, is not known, particularly since antibodies of the IgM class were prevalent in the nonalcoholic control group.[110]

Nevertheless, despite numerous attempts to replicate this disorder in various animal models (mice, rats, hamsters, dogs, rhesus monkeys, turkey poults and even chicken embryos),[111] some using paired-feeding to ensure adequate nutritional control, none has adequately reproduced the clinical entity.[5] Furthermore, unlike alcoholic cardiomyopathy in humans, where reversibility following abstinence is rare,[112,113] albeit prognosis is improved,[114,115] the findings in these models tend to revert following cessation of ethanol administration.[22,116] The inability to reproduce alcoholic cardiomyopathy may relate, in part, to the apparent mild cardiotoxicity associated with alcohol abuse and therefore to an insufficient total dosage of alcohol in these experiments.[109,117] In a study of alcoholics, those who had developed cardiomyopathy were older (45 ± 8 vs. 35 ± 5 years), had a longer duration of alcoholism (24 ± 7 vs. 17 ± 4 years), and had consumed a larger total daily dosage (28 ± 13 vs. 17 ± 9 kg ethanol/kg body weight) than those with normal left ventricular dimensions and function.[117]

The occurrence of cardiomyopathy in some chronic alcoholics but not in others suggests a possible biological predisposition. In the United States, 85 to 90% of those with alcoholic cardiomyopathy are African American[114,118]; this disproportionate racial prevalence is evident in other dilated cardiomyopathies. The possibility that this disorder might have a viral immune basis has engendered study of the histocompatibility antigens. Associations between alcoholic cardiomyopathy and HLA Aw30[119] and B8[120] antigens have been reported; however, the relatively small increases in risk conferred by these factors and the lack of reproducibility suggest chance relationships.

Alternatively, the development of alcoholic cardiomyopathy may require other conditions besides alcohol abuse. Quebec beer drinker's cardiomyopathy may be the prototype of this phenomenon.[121] When cobalt was added to beer in trace amounts to stabilize the foam, a fulminant cardiomyopathy ensued in heavy beer drinkers.[121] Exaggerated myocardial damage from trypanosomal[122] and cocksackievirus B3[123] infections has also been observed in rats treated chronically with alcohol. Prolonged alcohol administration aggravates experimental isoproterenol cardiomyopathy[123]; this relationship may be particularly important because alcohol abuse is associated with increased concentrations of circulating catecholamines.[45]

Hypertension is associated with alcohol abuse,[124,125] and more than 50% of alcoholics undergoing detoxification have systemic blood pressures greater than 140/90 mmHg.[126] Individuals with transitory hypertension associated with alcohol detoxification continue to evidence abnormalities of cardiac performance 4 to 5 days after withdrawal when their blood pressure may be normal[77] (Tables I and II). Such individuals show exaggerated blood pressure,

Table I. Left Ventricular Systolic Function[a]

	Normal[b] (n = 16)	Hypertensive (n = 26)	Normotensive (n = 40)
PW in systole (cm)[c]	1.7 ± 0.07	1.5 ± 0.05*	1.4 ± 0.03*
FS (%)	37 ± 1	32 ± 1*	33 ± 1*
EF (%)	66 ± 1	61 ± 1*	61 ± 1*

[a]From Friedman *et al.*,[77] with permission.
[b]Values are mean ± standard error of the mean; *$P < 0.02$ vs. normal subjects.
[c]EF, Ejection fraction; FS, fractional shortening; PW, posterior wall.

Table II. Systolic Time Intervals[a]

	Normal[b] ($n = 16$)	Hypertensive ($n = 26$)	Normotensive ($n = 40$)
PEP[c]	86 ± 3	101 ± 3*	95 ± 2*
LVET (ms)	299 ± 5	257 ± 1*	273 ± 4*†
LVETI (ms)	418 ± 3	388 ± 4*	397 ± 3*
PEP/LVET	0.290 ± 0.01	0.398 ± 0.01*	0.350 ± 0.01*†

[a]From Friedman *et al.*,[77] with permission.
[b]Values are mean ± standard error of the mean; *$P < 0.02$ vs. normal subjects; †$P < 0.02$ vs. hypertensive patients.
[c]LVET, Left ventricular ejection time; LVETI, LVET index; PEP, preejection period.

heart rate, and plasma catecholamine increases to cold[127] and sustained handgrip[128] stimuli; this enhanced response to stressors has been shown to persist 3 to 4 weeks after alcohol withdrawal.[128] Even when blood pressure is normal following detoxification, increased left ventricular wall stress is present (Table III),[77] and individuals who had transitory hypertension demonstrate abnormal left ventricular stress–volume–mass relationships (Table III).[77] Moreover, even more exaggerated hemodynamic abnormalities would be expected during periods of inebriation. The increased left ventricular wall stress would be expected to produce myocardial hypertrophy. Because there are no pathognomonic findings in alcoholic cardiomyopathy that distinguish it from decompensated hypertensive heart disease,[129] this relationship may be particularly important. The increased left ventricular wall stresses and higher heart rates in the alcoholic would be expected to increase myocardial oxygen requirements and might even result in periods of myocardial ischemia. Of interest, despite high left ventricular wall stress, alcoholics with transitory hypertension demonstrate compensatory "hyperfunction"[77] (Table III), which has been postulated as a stage that precedes decompensation in hypertensive heart disease.[130]

Table III. Left Ventricular Stress-Volume Mass Relations[a]

	Normal[b] ($n = 16$)	Hypertensive ($n = 26$)	Normotensive ($n = 40$)
Stress (dynes·cm^{-2}·10^3)	46 ± 2	77 ± 6*	67 ± 4*
SBP/ESV[c] (mmHg/ml)	3.1 ± 0.4	3.3 ± 0.3	2.8 ± 0.2
Stress/ESV (dynes·cm^{-2}·10^3/ml)	1.3 ± 0.1	1.7 ± 0.1*	1.5 ± 0.1
Stress/mass (dynes·cm^{-2}·10^3/g/m^2)	0.5 ± 0.05	0.8 ± 0.06*	0.7 ± 0.05

[a]From Friedman *et al.*,[77] with permission.
[b]Values are mean ± standard error of the mean; *$P < 0.02$ vs. normal subjects.
[c]ESV, End-systolic volume; SBP, systolic blood pressure.

Atrial fibrillation, which can occur as a consequence of alcohol abuse (see Section 5) or as a complication of alcoholic cardiomyopathy,[114] might worsen or even produce myocardial dysfunction. The increased ventricular rates that may ensue from atrial fibrillation, an arrhythmia that can go unrecognized for prolonged periods, might itself produce a dilated, hypocontractile heart. The treatment of this disorder is particularly important because tachycardia-related cardiomyopathy is reversible and failure to treat it in timely fashion can result in persistent atrial fibrillation. Of interest, the first reported case of reversible alcoholic cardiomyopathy presented with atrial fibrillation; with abstinence and treatment, both the heart rhythm and myocardial function returned to normal.[112] Thus, although heavy alcohol consumption over 15 to 20 years may place anyone at risk for alcoholic heart muscle disease, associated conditions, such as high plasma catecholamines, hypertension, tachycardia, infection, a nutritional deficiency, or the presence of another cardiotoxin such as cocaine or cobalt, may be necessary to produce the clinical manifestations of alcoholic cardiomyopathy.

5. Holiday Heart

The association between arrhythmia and alcohol abuse in individuals not having evidence of heart disease or an electrolyte disturbance, such as hypokalemia or hypomagnesemia, abnormalities occurring frequently in alcoholics, has been termed "holiday heart."[131] Although both supraventricular[132–134] and ventricular arrhythmias[135–137] have been related to alcohol abuse, the association is particularly strong for the occurrence of paroxysmal atrial fibrillation.[132–134] Even ingesting alcohol in relatively modest amounts, resulting in blood ethanol concentrations of less than 100 mg/dl, will generally increase heart rate by five to ten beats/min.[138]

5.1. *Proarrhythmic Effects*

Paraoxysmal atrial fibrillation has been observed in individuals who drink little alcohol on a regular basis, but who develop the arrhythmia after a binge.[132] In case–control studies, atrial fibrillation also has been found to occur two to three times more frequently in individuals who drink heavily compared to light drinkers.[133,134] In contrast, the association between ventricular arrhythmias and alcohol abuse is based on case reports. Using programmed electrical stimulation, three alcohol abusers with documented paroxysmal ventricular tachycardia had their arrhythmia induced only after administration of ethanol.[135–137] In one of these patients an implantable converter/defibrillator (ICD) was inserted; episodes of ventricular tachycardia recurred during periods of alcohol intoxication but were converted to sinus rhythm by the device.

The electrophysiological basis for alcohol's proarrhythmic effects is not entirely clear. Ethanol, but not acetadehyde or acetate in relevant concentrations,[138] has been shown to reduce the duration,[8,138] amplitude,[8] and rate of rise of the myocardial action potential.[8] Although such changes would be expected to slow impulse propagation and shorten myocardial refractoriness, conditions that promote atrial fibrillation, clinical studies have not demonstrated these electrophysiological effects in the atrium following alcohol administration.[139,140] Nevertheless, atrial fibrillation can be elicited with programmed electrical stimulation following alcohol administration in alcohol abusers subject to this arrhythmia.[139,140]

Some cases considered to be holiday heart may actually be instances of alcoholic cardiomyopathy becoming first manifest as an arrhythmia. Electrophysiological studies performed in patients with alcoholic cardiomyopathy have demonstrated slowing of myocardial electrical conduction and shortening of myocardial monophasic action potentials; in those patients having atrial fibrillation, shortening of the atrial refractory period and an increase in the heterogeneity of atrial refractoriness have also been observed.[141] These electrophysiological abnormalities would favor fractionation of impulse propagation and the formation of multiple wavelets, the findings observed with isochronal mapping of the fibrillating atrium. Whether some individuals with holiday heart have preclinical alcoholic heart muscle disease with electrophysiological findings similar to those observed in alcoholic cardiomyopathy still needs to be determined.

5.2. *Antiarrhythmic Actions*

Ethanol also has been found to exert antiarrhythmic effects. These actions, however, have been seen only in experimental animals. Vulnerability to ventricular fibrillation decreases in the ischemic[142] and nonischemic[143] dog heart at blood ethanol concentrations of less than 250 mg/dl and myocardial infarction-related ventricular tachycardia in the awake dog treated with alcohol is slowed and suppressed at an average blood ethanol concentration of 125 mg/dl.[144] Ventricular tachycardia induced by digitalis toxicity also converts with alcohol administration.[145] Moreover, the duration of experimental atrial fibrillation, produced either by acetylcholine[144] or rapid electrical stimulation,[146] is shortened by ethanol infusions producing a blood concentration between 100 and 200 mg/dl. Thus, the arrhythmogenicity of alcohol is complex. Alcohol's neurohumoral sympathomimetic effects are proarrhythmic. How ethanol exerts its antiarrhythmic actions is not clear; it still has not been found to have reproducible electrophysiological properties that would allow its placement into one of the antiarrhythmic groupings.

5.3. *Sudden Death in Alcoholics*

Epidemiological studies have disclosed an increased incidence of sudden and unexpected death in alcoholics.[147–149] These deaths have been reported in individuals in their third to fifth decade of life, with a fatty liver as the only remarkable autopsy finding.[147,148] Blood ethanol concentrations generally have been found to be less than 50 mg/dl.[148] The immediate cause of death of individuals dying in this fashion is almost always due to a cardiac arrhythmia. Ventricular arrhythmias evoked by severe hypokalemia or hypomagnesemia may be responsible for some of these events. Because of the relatively low blood ethanol concentrations found in these individuals, alcohol withdrawal-related effects may be contributory. An intense sympathoadrenal reaction,[45] coronary artery spasm,[150] and small coronary artery thrombosis due to rebound hypercoaguability[151] are possible mechanisms that might lead to arrhythmia. Also, if any of these alcoholics had an automatic neuropathy,[152–154] a sympathetic imbalance (between the right and left stellate ganglia) might have occurred, resulting in left ventricular electrical inhomogeneities and the potential for lethal arrhythmia. Myocardial ischemia, from small vessel disease,[155] and arrhythmia associated with subclinical alcoholic cardiomyopathy are other possible mechanisms for sudden death.

Alcohol abuse has also been associated with sudden death in individuals with coronary artery disease. In a multivariate analysis of factors associated with sudden death in patients with coronary disease, heavy alcohol use emerged as an independent predictor of such events.[156] Also, in a 10-year follow-up study of people given a health screening examination, 46% of individuals dying suddenly from coronary disease were alcoholic, a prevalence of more than four times that in the general population.[149] Thus, alcohol abuse increases the risk of sudden death in individuals with coronary heart disease, a group already at increased risk for such events. Recognition of alcohol abuse and counseling with regard to binge drinking in this population, especially those with a history of myocardial infarction, is therefore of particular importance.

6. Hypertension

There have now been over 60 population studies worldwide that have examined the relationship between blood pressure and alcohol use.[157] These surveys have demonstrated in diverse populations that alcohol use elevates systemic blood pressure independent of the confounding influence of age, body weight, or cigarette smoking, and that hypertension is more prevalent in individuals who abuse alcohol.[5,158] The relationship between alcohol use and hypertension is evident for both systolic and diastolic pressures, although the influence appears to be greater on systolic pressure. In a recent survey of middle-aged white women, however, the relationship between alcohol use and systolic blood pressure was not present in alcoholic women but was evident in all groups of women for diastolic pressure; the effect of abstinence at the time of the blood pressure measurements might have confounded the relation between estimated quantity of *habitual* alcohol use and systolic pressure.[159] Nevertheless, the relationship appears to be stronger for men. After adjustment for age and weight, an increase of both systolic and diastolic pressure is found after one or two unit drinks per day in men, whereas an equally strong correlation is not evident with less than three drinks per day in women.[160] The biological plausibility of this difference is supported by the observation that the hypertensive effects of alcohol use in women over 50 years of age is attenuated by estrogen replacement therapy,[161] even though estrogens in nonusers of alcohol tend to elevate blood pressure.[162]

The epidemiological evidence that alcohol use has blood pressure lowering effects, as suggested by U- or J-shaped relationships, seems to be largely artifactual. When adjustments are made for weight and age, this dip tends to disappear.[163–165] Moreover, the associative decreases of blood pressure, which have been reported mainly in women, are observed with only occasional alcohol use, suggesting the presence of a hidden confounder rather than a causal effect. The positive relationship between alcohol use and blood pressure appears to be stronger in whites,[160] although residual higher blood pressure following detoxification of alcoholics is more evident in African Americans.[166]

Studies in humans[167–172] and experimental animals[10,173] have validated these associations by demonstrating a clear causal link between alcohol use and changes of blood pressure. In a study of hypertensives using moderate amounts of alcohol daily, a fall of blood pressure was demonstrated within 72 hr of stopping alcohol use; resumption of subjects' usual consumption of alcohol resulted in elevation of blood pressure within 48 hr.[169] A similar effect has been observed in normotensive, moderate drinkers who merely curtailed their use, demonstrating a decrease in supine systolic pressure that was evident within a week of changing their pattern of drinking.[170] Using the same study protocol, hypertensives averaging four to five unit drinks per day showed a reduction of both systolic and diastolic pressure after curtailment of their alcohol use by 85%.[171] These findings were also related to markers of alcohol consumption, and the reduction of blood pressure persisted after adjusting for weight change.[170,171] The effects of alcohol on blood pressure have been found to be related to both baseline blood pressure and quantity of alcohol generally used[172]: five to six drinks per day for 5 days were found to have little effect on blood pressure in normotensive, light users; elevated only standing blood pressures in hypertensive, light drinkers; but increased systolic and diastolic pressure in both standing and supine positions in hypertensive, moderate drinkers. Furthermore, prolonged alcohol administration has also been shown to elevate blood pressure and change vascular responsiveness in experimental animals.[10,173] Blood pressure elevation has been observed in rats given alcohol in their drinking water for 4 weeks,[173] and a loss of the vasodilatory response to alcohol and an increased sensitivity to vasoconstrictors have been found in these animals after 12 weeks of alcohol ingestion.[10]

Hypertension is observed frequently in alcoholics.[126,127] More than 50% of alcoholics undergoing detoxification have a blood pressure greater than 140/90 mmHg[126] and 33% have a value greater than 160/95 mmHg.[127] Figures 4 and 5 show the patterns of blood pressure changes that were observed during alcohol withdrawal in a study of hypertensive alcoholics.[127] Eighty percent of the subjects had their highest blood pressures recorded at time of admission, whereas the others demonstrated peak values on the second or third hospital day.[127] Because their average blood ethanol concentration was 79 mg/dl on admission and none had severe withdrawal symptoms at any time,[127] the chronic effects of alcohol abuse rather than the detoxification process itself would appear to have explained at least some of the blood pressure findings. Moreover, on the fourth or fifth hospital day, when these individuals were no longer hypertensive, they demonstrated an exaggerated blood pressure response to a cold pressor test compared to those alcoholics

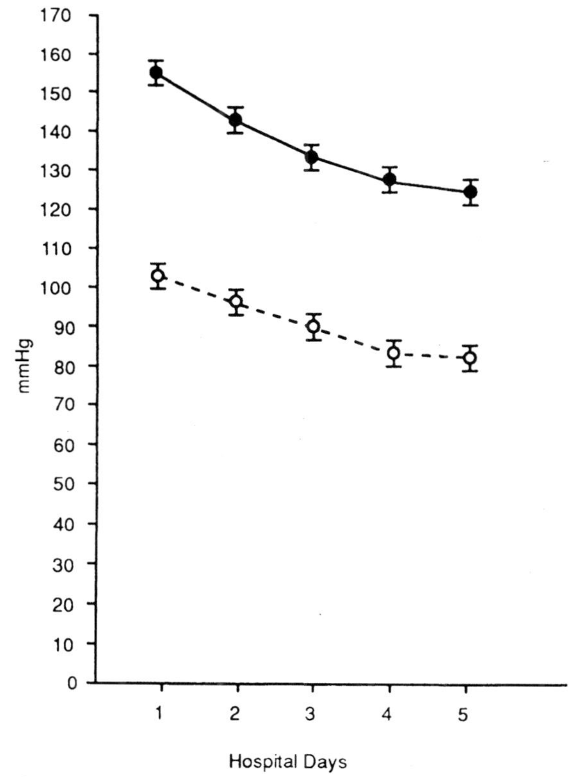

Figure 4. Average blood pressures in 48 patients with transitory hypertension, having highest blood pressures on admission with a gradual decline over 5 days. Mean ± SEM; ●—●, systolic; ○--○, diastolic. (Reprinted with permission from Clark and Friedman.[127])

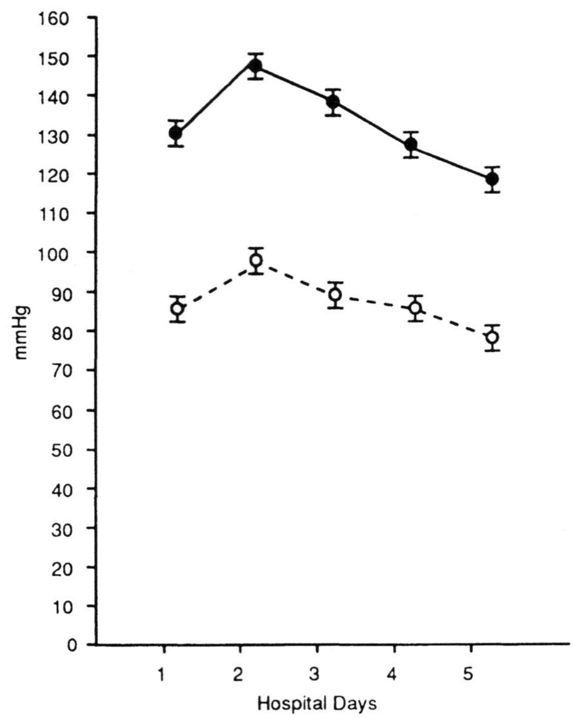

Figure 5. Average blood pressures in 12 patients with transitory hypertension, having highest blood pressures on 2nd or 3rd hospital day. Mean ± SEM; ●—●, systolic; ○--○, diastolic. (Reprinted with permission from Clark and Friedman.[127])

who had not been hypertensive (Fig. 6). A similar enhanced blood pressure response has been observed with a sustained handgrip task on the fourth or fifth day of withdrawal and also in the third or fourth week postdetoxification, when these individuals, who had had transitory hypertension, were both normotensive and abstinent.[128] Moreover, casual-adjusted (including age as a covariate) diastolic pressure measured in alcoholics abstinent for an average of 35 days has been related to the duration of their history of drinking; this correlation, however, was not significant for white women.[166]

The acute hypertensive effects of ethanol administration have been related, at least in part, to a central-nervous-system-mediated sympathoexcitatory response.[168] Muscle sympathetic nerve activity (intraneural peroneal nerve action potentials) increases following ingestion[167] or intravenous administration of alcohol,[168] and this enhanced effect is associated with an elevation of blood pressure.[167,168] Initial attempts to relate the acute transient elevation of blood pressure that generally follows the ingestion of alcohol to changes in plasma catecholamines produced what appeared to be conflicting findings.[174–176] Although increases of norepinephrine[174–176] and epinephrine[174,176] were found to occur concomitantly with the blood pressure changes, a similar catecholamine response occurred when the placebo was not water.[175,176] Because oral carbohydrate administration but not water also results in a sympathetic response,[177] the vehicle used to administer alcohol probably confounded the findings of these early investigations. However, an infusion of ethanol over 45 min, producing an average blood alcohol concentration of 63 mg/dl, increased sympathetic nerve activity but had no effect on blood pressure; following the infusion, as blood alcohol concentration decreased, sympathetic nerve activity continue to increase and blood pressure rose.[168] Both the sympathetic nerve and blood pressure responses were blocked by pretreatment with dexamethasone, whereas the blood pressure but not the sympathetic nerve effects were blocked by phentolamine.[168] Thus, alcohol appears to elevate blood pressure by an α-adrenergic effect that is mediated by sympathetic nervous system activated probably by the release of corticotrophin-releasing hormone. Although changes in epinephrine and cortisol were not reported in this study,[168] adrenal effects probably also ensue.

Alcohol ingestion also impairs the baroreceptor reflex control of heart rate.[178] Following alcohol administration to normotensive subjects, baroreceptor sensitivity (slowing of heart rate to sudden elevation of blood pressure) was impaired and the reflex reset to higher blood pressures.[178] Both

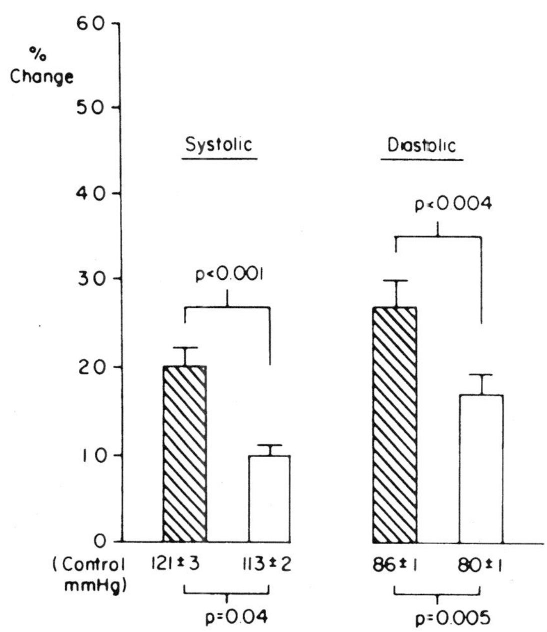

Figure 6. Percent changes of blood pressure with cold pressor test. Increment in hypertensives (▧, $n = 17$) is greater than in normotensives (□, $n = 17$); mean ± SEM. (Reprinted with permission from Clark and Friedman.[127])

changes were concentration dependent and were accompanied by an exaggerated blood response to the α-adrenergic agonist, phenylephrine.[178] The effect appears to be, at least in part, also centrally mediated.[179] The injection of alcohol into the nucleus tractus solitarius, the first central synapse of the baroreceptor reflex arc, impairs baroreceptor sensitivity, which appears to be the result of blockade of the receptor for the excitatory amino acid, *N*-methyl-*d*-aspartate.[179]

Alcoholic-associated hypertension also appears to be catecholamine mediated.[127] Eighty-six percent of hypertensive alcoholics were found to have elevations of epinephrine, whereas only 46% had elevations of plasma renin activity and 19% of norepinephrine (neither value was significantly greater than that found in nonhypertensive alcoholics).[127] Moreover, when alcoholics who had been hypertensive were given a cold pressor test on the fourth or fifth day after alcohol withdrawal, at a time their blood pressure was normal, they demonstrated an exaggerated increase in plasma norepinephrine and epinephrine[127] (Fig. 7). The increase of plasma epinephrine with a cold pressor test in alcoholics with transitory hypertension is a unique response that has

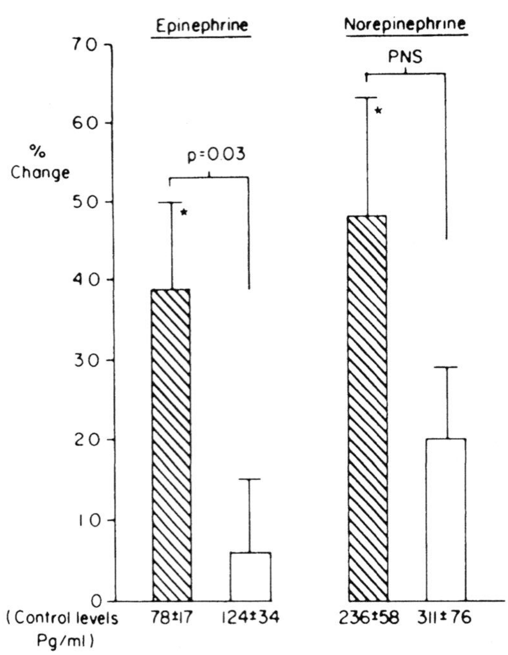

Figure 7. Percent changes of catecholamines with cold pressor test. Increment of both plasma epinephrine and norephinephrine is significant only in hypertensives; also, percentage of increment of epinephrine is greater in hypertensives (▧, $n = 5$) than in normotensives (□, $n = 5$); mean ± SEM; $^*P < 0.05$. (Reprinted with permission from Clark and Friedman.[127])

not been observed in other individuals.[180] Increased plasma norepinephrine has also been associated with alcohol-associated hypertension in rats.[181] In addition, a weak correlation between plasma cortisol and systolic pressure has been found in alcoholics undergoing detoxification.[182] The mechanisms involved in the higher blood pressures observed in moderate drinkers, however, have not been elucidated.[180] Plasma concentrations of catecholamines, cortisol, renin activity, angiotensin II, and aldosterone and the responses to various blood pressure stressors in moderate drinkers were not different than that found in nondrinkers with lower blood pressures.[180]

Thus, alcohol has divergent influences on blood pressure. Ethanol and its metabolites have an overall vasodilatory effect on the systemic circulation; however, alcohol has centrally mediated actions that stimulate the sympathetic nervous system, and probably also the adrenal cortex and medulla, and attenuate the baroreceptor reflex. Because of possible tachyphylaxis to the vasodilating actions of alcohol, chronic adaptive vascular responses, and persistent sympathoadrenal effects, blood pressure increases and resets to a higher level while alcohol use is maintained. In individuals with a defective autonomic nervous system[183] and often in the elderly,[184] the vasodilatory actions predominate and hypotension may ensue following ethanol ingestion. Although the elevations of blood pressure due to habitual use of alcohol disappear after several days of abstinence, in alcoholics there is a residual sensitivity of the sympathetic nervous system to stressors that persists for at least 3 to 4 weeks after alcohol withdrawal, and there are subtle blood pressure relationships that may last even longer.

7. Coronary Heart Disease and Stroke

Alcohol abuse is associated with an increased risk of coronary events[185] and stroke.[186,187] In contrast, moderate use of alcohol is favorably related to these disorders.[2,188–193] The associations have been demonstrated in numerous population studies and have been found to be present in both men[186–189] and women,[2,190–193] albeit with a lower dose–effect relationship in women.[194] The benefits associated with alcohol use emerge in middle age, when the risks of these diseases become sufficiently high to offset the detrimental effects of alcohol use, such as the increased incidence of accidental and violent deaths.[2,188–189,192,194]

The relationships between alcohol use and the occurrence of coronary and cerebrovascular disease largely can be explained by ethanol's effects on blood pressure, atherogenesis, and hemostasis. The development of hypertension, the leading risk factor for these diseases, resulting from alcohol abuse, would explain most of the increased incidence of cardiovascular disease in alcoholics,[185,187,195,196] whereas the favorable effects of moderate alcohol use on atherogenesis would account for most of its reduction in coronary heart disease and ischemic stroke.[4,197,198] The benefits attributable to alcohol on coronary heart disease have been related in part to its effects on the lipoprotein cholesterol fractions.[4,197,198] About 50% of the reduction related to alcohol consumption in myocardial infarction[4] and death from coronary heart disease[197] is explained by an increase in high-density lipoprotein (HDL) cholesterol. The favorable relation between moderate alcohol use and coronary heart disease is strengthened statistically by adjusting for the effects of alcohol use on systolic pressure (demonstrating the negative interaction), whereas it is weakened by an adjustment for the effects on HDL cholesterol *and* low-density lipoprotein cholesterol (demonstrating positive interactions).[198] The protective effects of moderate alcohol use on the risk of developing stable angina pectoris has been found to be comparable to that for myocardial infarction.[3] Because angina pectoris is caused by coronary atherosclerosis and myocardial infarction by both coronary atherosclerosis and thrombosis, it has been argued that the effects of alcohol consumption on atherogenesis alone accounts for its benefits in coronary heart disease.[3]

Not only does alcohol use influence the incidence of angina pectoris and myocardial infarction, but it also appears to affect outcomes in acute myocardial infarction.[199] Moderate alcohol use has been related to a reduced fatality rate in individuals without a previous history of myocardial infarction; in contrast, the same amount of alcohol use with a history of a previous myocardial infarction has been associated with a tendency toward a *worse* outcome.[199] The apparent influence of alcohol use in adversely affecting the mortality rate of an acute myocardial infarction with established cardiovascular disease[199] is consistent with the finding of an increased incidence of sudden death in alcohol abusers with coronary heart disease.[149,156]

Alcohol may affect cardiovascular disease by its hemostatic actions. Alcohol use has been found to influence coagulation, reducing plasma fibrinogen, a risk factor for coronary artery disease, by about 1% for each unit drink per day consumed.[200] The effects of alcohol on platelet aggregation, a predictor of coronary events,[201] however, is more complex.[151] In brief, alcohol consumption in moderation is associated with a dose-dependent reduction in platelet aggregation (especially to the agonist, ADP, affecting particularly the secondary peak of its aggregation curve, which has been related to coronary events).[151] This effect is exaggerated by a diet high in saturated fats.[151] In contrast, acute ingestion of alcohol produces a short-lived reduction in platelet aggregability that is followed by a more prolonged "rebound" enhancement.[151] This rebound phenomenon can be attenuated by one of the antioxidant-containing substances—tannins—present in red wine,[202] which may explain the additional cardiovascular protective effects of moderate wine consumption reported in some studies.[203] Moreover, the enhanced attenuation of platelet aggregation by alcohol in high-fat-containing diets and/or the inhibition of the platelet rebound by tannins may provide an explanation for the "French paradox," which is the relatively low incidence of coronary heart disease in France, where the diet is rich in saturated fats, smoking is prevalent, and consumption of considerable amounts of red wine is customary.[204]

Of interest also is the observation that alcohol use enhances the antiplatelet actions of aspirin.[205] This interaction may increase the risk of hemorrhage in individuals receiving aspirin for cardiovascular disease.

Although the incidence of ischemic stroke has been reported to be reduced in moderate drinkers,[206] hemorrhagic stroke has also been found to be increased.[190,206,207] Because of the substantially higher risk of ischemic stroke in most populations, the overall effect of moderate alcohol use on stroke in these studies generally has been favorable.[190,206] In addition, strokes in young men not having hypertension have been related to alcohol intoxication,[208,209] and strokes in young women are often preceded by recent alcohol use.[210] Whether these occurrences of ischemic stroke are due to cerebral thromboses resulting from rebound-enhanced platelet aggregation[151] or cerebral spasms[48] is not clear.

Despite the favorable effects of moderate alcohol use on coronary atherogenesis, such use in individuals with coronary heart disease does not have beneficial actions. Alcohol increases myocardial oxygen requirements by increasing heart rate, blood pressure, and left ventricular dimensions. Moreover, even when alcohol administration has been found to increase myocardial blood flow, blood is distributed away from ischemic muscle.[65] Clinical studies reflect these unfavorable hemodynamic effects.[67,211,212] Following ingestion of alcohol, patients with coronary heart disease perform less well on stress testing,[211,212] and ambulatory electrocardiography has disclosed an increase in the number of episodes of myocardial ischemia.[67] Moreover, these studies suggest that alcohol ingestion tends to mask angina pectoris yet worsen myocardial ischemia, creating the potentially dangerous condition of silent ischemia.[67,211] In addition, alcohol ingestion appears to evoke coronary vasospasm in individuals susceptible to this condition,[150,213,214] apparently as a rebound effect to its acute vasodilating actions. Thus, in individuals with coronary heart disease, moderate alcohol use might be detrimental.

8. Conclusion

The ingestion of one or two alcohol-containing drinks has acute effects on heart rate, blood pressure, cardiac output, myocardial contractility, and regional blood flow. Although these actions are generally not clinically important, in the presence of cardiovascular disease they might result in transient unfavorable hemodynamic changes. Habitual moderate use of alcohol might therefore have adverse effects in individuals with heart disease. Moreover, alcohol abuse can lead to cardiac arrhythmia, hypertension, cardiomyopathy, stroke, and even sudden death. Moderate alcohol use also produces changes that have an overall favorable effect on atherosclerotic-related vascular diseases. In Western society, where cardiovascular disease due to atherosclerosis is the leading cause of death, this desirable effect of alcohol use outweighs its detrimental actions resulting in favorable findings in population studies. Even though it may be reassuring for those who derive pleasure from moderate alcohol use that ethanol might have some health benefits, the body of evidence argues against any recommendation that alcohol use be encouraged for its cardiovascular medicinal value.

References

1. *Nutrition and Your Health: Dietary Guidelines for Americans.* 4th ed. US Department of Agriculture, US Department of Health and Human Services, 1995.
2. Fuchs CS, Stampfer MJ, Colditz GA, *et al:* Alcohol consumption and mortality among women. *N Engl J Med* 332:1245–1250, 1995.
3. Camargo CA, Stampler MJ, Glynn RJ, *et al:* Moderate alcohol consumption and risk for angina pectoris or myocardial infarction in US male physicians. *Ann Intern Med* 126:372–375, 1997.
4. Gaziano JM, Buring JE, Breslow JL, *et al:* Moderate alcohol intake, increased of high-density lipoprotein and its subfractions and decreased risk of myocardial infarction. *N Engl J Med* 329:1829–1834, 1993.
5. Friedman HS: Cardiovascular effects of ethanol, in Lieber CS (ed): *Medical and Nutritional Complications of Alcoholism. Mechanisms and Management.* New York, Plenum Medical, 1992, pp 359–401.
6. Nakano J, Moore SE: Effect of different alcohols on the contractile force of the isolated guinea pig myocardium. *Eur J Pharmacol* 20:266–270, 1972.
7. Gomes AL, Gimeno MF, Webb JL: Effects of ethanol on cellular membrane potentials and contractility of isolated rat atrium. *Am J Physiol* 203:194–196, 1962.
8. Richards IS, Kulkarni A, Brooks SM, *et al:* A moderate concentration of ethanol alters cellular membrane potentials and decreases contractile force of human fetal heart. *Dev Pharmacol Ther* 13:51–56, 1989.
9. Kelbaek H, Gjorup T, Hartline OJ, *et al:* Left ventricular function during alcohol intoxication and autonomic nervous blockade. *Am J Cardiol* 59:685–688, 1987.
10. Altura BM, Altura B: Microvascular and vascular smooth muscle actions of ethanol, acetaldehyde and acetate. *Fed Proc* 41:2447–2451, 1982.
11. Riff DP, Jain AC, Doyle JT: Acute hemodynamic effects of ethanol on normal human volunteers. *Am Heart J* 78:592–597, 1969.
12. Blomqvist G, Saltin B, Mitchell JH: Acute effects of ethanol ingestion on the response to submaximal and maximal exercise in man. *Circulation* 42:463–470, 1970.
13. Delgado CE, Fortuin NJ, Ross RS: Acute effects of low doses of alcohol on left ventricular function by echocardiography. *Circulation* 31:535–540, 1975.
14. Cherrick GR, Leevy GM: The effect of ethanol metabolism on levels of oxidized and reduced nicotinamide-adenine dinucleotide in liver, kidney and heart. *Biochim Biophys Acta* 107:29–37, 1965.
15. Lochner A, Cowley R, Brink AJ: Effect of ethanol on metabolism and function of perfused rat heart. *Am Heart J* 78:709–789, 1969.
16. Laposata EA, Lang LG: Presence of nonoxidative ethanol metabolism in human organs commonly damaged by ethanol abuse. *Science* 231:497–499, 1986.
17. Lang LG: Nonoxidative ethanol metabolism: Formation of fatty acid ethyl esters by cholesterol esterase. *Proc Natl Acad Sci USA* 79:3954–3957, 1982.
18. Lang LG, Sobel BE: Myocardial metabolites of ethanol. *Circ Res* 52:479–482, 1982.
19. Lang LG, Sobel BE: Mitochondrial dysfunction induced by fatty acid ethyl esters, myocardial metabolites or ethanol. *J Clin Invest* 72:724–731, 1983.
20. Segel LD, Dean TM: Acute effects of acetaldehyde and ethanol on rat heart mitochondria. *Res Commun Chem Pathol Pharmacol* 25:461–474, 1979.

21. Segel LB: Mitochondrial respiration after cardiac perfusion with ethanol or acetaldehyde. *Alcohol Clin Exp Res* 8:560–563, 1984.
22. Aufferman W, Wu S, Parmley WE, *et al:* Reversibility of acute alcohol cardiac depression: ^{31}P NMR in hamsters. *FASEB J* 2:256–263, 1988.
23. Wendt VE, Ajiuni R, Bruce TA, *et al:* Acute effects of alcohol on the human mycardium. *Am J Cardiol* 17:804–812, 1966.
24. Regan TJ, Koroxenidis G, Moschos CB, *et al:* The acute metabolic and hemodynamic responses of the left ventricle to ethanol. *J Clin Invest* 45:270–278, 1966.
25. Kako KJ, Liu MS, Thornton MJ: Changes in fatty acid composition of myocardial triglyceride following a single administration of ethanol to rabbits. *J Mol Cell Cardiol* 5:473–489, 1973.
26. Preedy VR, Peters TJ: The acute and chronic effects of ethanol on cardiac protein synthesis in the rat. *Alcohol* 7:97–102, 1989.
27. Siddiq T, Richardson PJ, Mitchell WD, *et al:* Ethanol-induced inhibition of ventricular protein synthesis *in vivo* and the possible role of acetaldehyde. *Cell Biochem Funct* 11:43–54, 1993.
28. Siddiq T, Salisbury JR, Richardson PJ, Preedy VR: Synthesis of ventricular mitochondrial proteins *in vivo:* Effect of acute ethanol toxicity. *Alcohol Clin Exp Res* 17:894–899, 1993.
29. Williams ES, Mirro MJ, Bailey JC: Electrophysiological effects of ethanol, acetaldehyde, and acetate on cardiac issues from dog and guinea pig. *Circ Res* 47:473–478, 1980.
30. Niggli E, Rudisuli A, Maurer P, Weingart R: Effects of general anesthetics on current flow across membranes in guinea pig myocytes. *Am J Physiol* 256:C273–C281, 1989,
31. Mongo KG, Vassort G: Inhibition by alcohols, halothane and chloroform of the Ca current in single frog ventricular cells. *J Mol Cell Cardiol* 22:939–953, 1990.
32. Thomas AP, Sass EJ, Tun-Kirchmann TT, Rubin E: Ethanol inhibits electrically induced calcium transients in isolated rat cardiac myocytes. *J Mol Cell Cardiol* 21:555–565, 1989.
33. Guarnieri T, Lakatta EG: Mechanism of myocardial contractile depression by clinical concentrations of ethanol. *J Clin Invest* 85:1462–1467, 1990.
34. Danziger RS, Sakai M, Capogrossi MC, *et al:* Ethanol acutely and reversibly suppresses excitation–contraction coupling in cardiac myocytes. *Circ Res* 68:1660–1668, 1991.
35. Swartz MH, Repke DI, Katz Am, Rubin E: Effects of ethanol on calcium binding and calcium uptake by cardiac microsomes. *Biochem Pharmacol* 23:2369–2377, 1974.
36. Retig JN, Kirchberger MA, Rubin E, Katz AM: Effects of ethanol on calcium transport by microsomes phosphorylated by cyclic AMP-dependent protein kinase. *Biochem Pharmacol* 26:393–396, 1977.
37. Horton JW, White DJ: Cardiac contractile and sarcoplasmic reticulum function after acute ethanol consumption. *J Surg Res* 64:132–138, 1996.
38. Thomas AP, Rozanski DJ, Renard DC, Rubin E: Effects of ethanol on the contractile function of the heart: A review. *Alcohol Clin Exp Res* 18:121–131, 1994.
39. Reddy YS, Beesley RC: Effects of acute and chronic ethanol on cardiac contractile protein ATPase activity of Syrian hamsters. *Biochem Med Metab Biol* 44:259–265, 1990.
40. Williams JW, Tada M, Katz AM, Rubin E: Effects of ethanol and acetaldehyde on the (Na^+ + K^+)-activated adenosine triphosphatase activity of cardiac plasma membranes. *Biochem Pharmacol* 24:27–32, 1975.
41. McCall D, Ryan K: The effects of ethanol and acetaldehyde on Na pump function in cultured rat heart cells. *J Mol Cell Cardiol* 19:453–463, 1987.
42. Puszkin, Rubin E: Adenosine diphosphate effect on contractility of human muscle actomyosin: Inhibition by ethanol and acetaldehyde. *Science* 188:1319–1320, 1975.
43. McKaigney JP, Carmichael FJ, Saldivia V, *et al:* Role of ethanol metabolism in the ethanol-induced increase in splanchnic circulation. *Am J Physiol* 250:G518–G523, 1986.
44. Carmichael FJ, Israel Y, Saldivia V, *et al:* Blood acetaldehyde and the ethanol-induced increase in splanchnic circulation. *Biochem Pharmacol* 36:2673–2678, 1987.
45. Ogata M, Mendelson JH, Mello NK, Majechrowicz W: Adrenal function and alcoholism. *Psychosom Med* 33:159–180, 1971.
46. Hatake K, Wakabayashi I, Hishida S: Mechanism of inhibitory action of ethanol on endothelium-dependent relaxation in rat aorta. *Eur J Pharmacol* 238:441–444, 1993.

47. Brizzolara AL, Morris, DG, Burnstock G: Ethanol affects sympathetic cotransmission and endothelium-dependent relaxation in the rat. *Eur J Pharmacol* 254:175–181, 1994.
48. Altura BM, Altura BT, Gebrewold A: Alcohol-induced spasms of cerebral blood vessels: Relation to cerebrovascular accidents and sudden death. *Science* 220:331–333, 1983.
49. Altura BM, Altura AT, Carella A: Ethanol produces coronary vasospasm: Evidence for a direct action of ethanol on vascular muscle. *Br J Pharmacol* 78:260–262, 1983.
50. Huges JM, Henry RE, Daly MJ: Influence of ethanol and ambient temperature on skin blood flow. *Ann Emerg Med* 13:597–600, 1984.
51. Shaw S, Heller EA, Friedman HS,*et al:* Increased hepatic oxygenation following ethanol administration in the baboon. *Proc Soc Exp Biol Med* 156:509–513, 1977.
52. Fewings JD, Hanna JD, Walsh JA, Whelan RF: The effects of ethyl alcohol on blood vessels of the hand and forearm in man. *Br J Pharmacol Chemother* 27:93–106, 1966.
53. Battey LL, Heyman A, Patterson JL: Effects of ethyl alcohol on cerebral blood flow and metabolism. *JAMA* 152:6–10, 1953.
54. Goldman H, Sapirstein LA, Murphy S, Moore J: Alcohol and regional blood flow in brains of rats. *Proc Soc Exp Biol Med* 144:983–988, 1973.
55. Mayhan WG, Didion SP: Acute effects of ethanol on responses of cerebral arterioles. *Stroke* 26:2097–2102, 1995.
56. Schwartz JA, Speed NM, Gross M, *et al:* Acute effects of alcohol administration on regional cerebral blood flow: The role of acetate. *Alcohol Clin Exp Res* 17:1119–1123, 1993.
57. Sano M, Wendt PE, Wirsen A, *et al:* Acute effects of alcohol on regional cerebral blood flow in man. *J Stud Alcohol* 54:369–376, 1993.
58. Tiihonen J, Kuikka J, Hakola P, *et al:* Acute ethanol-induced changes in cerebral blood flow. *Am J Psychiatry* 151:1505–1508, 1994.
59. Friedman HS, Lowery R, Archer M, *et al:* The effects of ethanol on brain blood flow in awake dogs. *J Cardiovasc Pharmacol* 6:344–348, 1984.
60. Lasker N, Sherrod TR, Killalm F: Alcohol on the coronary circulation of the dog. *J Pharmacol Exp Ther* 113:441–420, 1958.
61. Mendoza LC, Hellberg K, Rickart A, *et al:* The effect of intravenous ethyl alcohol on the coronary circulation and myocardial contractility of the human and canine heart. *J Clin Pharmacol* 7:165–176, 1971.
62. Hayes SN, Bove A: Ethanol causes epicardial coronary artery vasoconstriction in the dog. *Circulation* 78:169–170, 1988.
63. Friedman HS, Matsuzaki S, Choe SS, *et al:* Demonstration of dissimilar acute haemodynamic effects of ethanol and acetaldehyde. *Cardiovasc Res* 13:477–487, 1979.
64. Abel FL: Direct effects of ethanol on myocardial performance and coronary resistance. *J Pharmacol Exp Ther* 212:28–33, 1980.
65. Friedman HS: Acute effects of ethanol on myocardial blood flow in the nonischemic and ischemic heart. *Am J Cardiol* 47:61–67, 1981.
66. Ahlawat S, Siwach SB, Jadish: Indirect assessment of acute effects of ethyl alcohol on coronary circulation in patients with chronic stable angina. *Int J Cardiol* 33:385–392, 1991.
67. Rossinen J, Paratanen J, Koskinen P, *et al:* Acute heavy alcohol intake increases silent myocardial ischemia in patients with stable angina pectoris. *Heart* 75:563–567, 1996.
68. Horwitz LD, Myers JH: Ethanol-induced alterations in pancreatic blood flow in conscious dogs. *Circ Res* 50:250–256, 1982.
69. Friedman HS, Lowery R, Shaughnessy E, Scorza J: The effects of ethanol on pancreatic blood flow in awake and anesthetized dogs. *Proc Soc Exp Biol Med* 174:377–382, 1983.
70. Dib JA, Cooper-Vastika SA, Meirelles RF, *et al:* Acute effects of ethanol and ethanol plus furosemide on pancreatic capillary blood flow in rats. *Am J Surg* 166:18–23, 1993.
71. Foitzik T, Castillo CF, Rattner DW, *et al:* Alcohol selectively impairs oxygenation of the pancreas. *Arch Surg* 130:357–361, 1985.
72. Brigden W, Robinson J: Alcoholic heart disease. *Br Med J* 2:1283–1289, 1964.
73. Friedman HS, Fernando H: Ascites as a marker for the hyperdynamic heart of Laennec's cirrhosis. *Alcohol Clin Exp Res* 16:968–970, 1992.

74. Friedman HS, Cirillo N, Schiano F, *et al:* Vasodilatory state of decompensated cirrhosis: Relation to hepatic dysfunction, ascites and vasoactive substances. *Alcohol Clin Exp Res* 19:123–129, 1995.
75. Spodick DH, Pigott VM, Chirife R: Preclinical cardiac malfunction in chronic alcoholism. *N Engl J Med* 287:677–680, 1972.
76. Mathews E, Gardin JM, Henry W, *et al:* Echocardiographic abnormalities in chronic alcoholics with and without overt congestive heart failure. *Am J Cardiol* 47:570–576, 1981.
77. Friedman HS, Vasavada BC, Malec AM, *et al:* Cardiac function in alcohol-associated systemic hypertension. *Am J Cardiol* 57:227–231, 1986.
78. Regan TJ, Levinson GE, Oldewurtel HA, *et al:* Ventricular function in noncardiacs with alcoholic fatty liver: Role of ethanol in the production of cardiomyopathy. J Clin Invest 48:397–406, 1969.
79. Wendt VE, Wu C, Balcon R, *et al:* Hemodynamic and metabolic effect of chronic alcoholism in man. *Am J Cardiol* 15:178–184, 1965.
80. Alexander CS: Idiopathic heart disease. *Am J Med* 41:213–228, 1966.
81. Alexander CS: Electron microscopic observations in alcoholic heart disease. *Br Heart J* 29:200–206, 1967.
82. Tsiplenkova VG, Vihert AA, Cherpackenko NM: Ultrastructural and histochemical observations in human and experimental alcoholic cardiomyopathy. *J Am Coll Cardiol* 8:22A–32A, 1986.
83. Estruch R, Fernandez-Sola J, Sacanella E, *et al:* Relationship between cardiomyopathy and liver disease in chronic alcoholism. *Hepatology* 22:532–538, 1995.
84. Vorobioff J, Bredfeldt JE, Groszmann RJ: Hyperdynamic circulation in portal-hypertensive rat model: A primary factor for maintenance of chronic portal hypertension. *Am J Physiol* 244:G52–G57, 1983.
85. Sikuler E, Kravetz D, Groszmann RJ: Evolution of portal hypertension and mechanisms involved in its maintenance in a rat model. *Am J Physiol* 248:G618–G625, 1985.
86. Munzo DF, Caramelo C, Santos JC, *et al:* Systemic and splanchnic hemodynamic disturbances in conscious rats with experimental liver cirrhosis without ascites. *Am J Physiol* 249:G316–G320, 1985.
87. Kowalski HJ, Abelmann WH, McNeely WF: The cardiac output in patients with cirrhosis of the liver and tense ascites with observations on the effect of paracentesis. *J Clin Invest* 33:768–773, 1954.
88. Korthuis RJ, Benoit JN, Kvietys PR, *et al:* Humoral factors may mediate increased rat hindquarter blood flow in portal hypertension. *Am J Physiol* 249:H827–H833, 1985.
89. Marco J, Diego J, Villanueva ML, *et al:* Elevated plasma glucagon levels in cirrhosis of the liver. *N Engl J Med* 289:1107–1111, 1973.
90. Sherwin R, Joshi P, Hendler R, *et al:* Hyperglucagonemia in Laennec's cirrhosis. *N Engl J Med* 290:239–242, 1974.
91. Kravetz D, Aarderiu M, Bosch J, *et al:* Hyperglucagonemia and hyperkinetic circulation after portocaval shunt in the rat. *Am J Physiol* 252:C257–G261, 1987.
92. Hortnagl H, Singer KA, Lenz *et al:* Substance P is markedly increased in plasma of patients with hepatic coma. *Lancet* 1:480–483, 1984.
93. Bichet DG, Ban Putten VJ, Schrier RW: Potential role of increased sympathetic activity in impaired sodium and water excretion in cirrhosis. *N Engl J Med* 25:1552–1557, 1982.
94. Floras JS, Legault DL, Morali GA, *et al:* Increased sympathetic outflow in cirrhosis and ascites. Direct evidence from intraneural recordings. *Ann Intern Med* 114:373–380, 1991.
95. Bosch J, Arroyo V, Betriu A, *et al:* Hepatic hemodynamics and the renin–angotensin–aldosterone system in cirrhosis. *Gastroenterology* 78:92–99, 1980.
96. Bomson A: Vascular reactivity in liver disease, in Bomzon A, Blendis LM (eds): *Cardiovascular Complications of Liver Disease.* Boca Raton, FL, CRC Press, 1990, pp 208–220.
97. Murray B, Paller MS: Decreased pressor reactivity to angiotensin II in cirrhotic rats. *Circ Res* 57:424–431, 1985.
98. Bomzon S, Rosenberg M, Gali D, *et al:* Systemic hypotension and decreased pressor response in dogs with chronic bile duct ligation. *Hepatology* 6:595–600, 1986.

99. Lee SS, Chilton EL, Pak JM: Adenosine receptor blockade reduces splanchnic hyperemia in cirrhotic rats. *Hepatology* 15:1107–1111, 1992.
100. Champigneulle B, Braillon A, Kleber G, *et al:* Adenosine and hemodynamic alterations in cirrhotic rats. *Am J Physiol* 23:G543–G547, 1991.
101. Lee FY, Albillos A, Colombato LA, Groszmann J: The role of nitric oxide in the vascular hyporesponsiveness to methoxamine in protal hypertensive rats. *Hepatology* 16:1043–1048, 1992.
102. Sieber CC, Groszmann RJ: Nitric oxide mediates hyporeactivity to vasopressors in mesenteric vessels of portal hypertensive rats. *Gastroenterology* 103:235–239, 1992.
103. Pizcueta P, Pique JM, Fernandez M, *et al:* Modulation of the hyperdynamic circulation of cirrhotic rats by nitric oxide inhibition. *Gastroenterology* 103:1909–1915, 1992.
104. Campillo B, Chabrier PE, Pelle G, *et al:* Inhibition of nitric oxide synthesis in the forearm arterial bed of patients with advanced cirrhosis. *Hepatology* 22:1423–1429, 1995.
105. Sogni P, Moreau R, Ohsuga M, *et al:* Evidence for normal nitric oxide-mediated vasodilator tone in conscious rats with cirrhosis. *Hepatology* 16:980–983, 1992.
106. Ralevic V, Mathie RT, Moore KP, Burnstock G: Vasoconstrictor responsiveness of the rat mesenteric arterial bed in cirrhosis. *Br J Pharmacol* 118:435–441, 1996.
107. Eliaser M, Giansiracusa FJ: The heart and alcohol. *Calif Med* 84:234–236, 1956.
108. Kino M, Imamitchi H, Morigutehi M, *et al:* Cardiovascular status in asymptomatic alcoholics, with reference to the level of ethanol consumption. *Br Heart J* 46:545–551, 1981.
109. Urbano-Marquez A, Estruch R, Navarro-Lopez F, *et al:* The effects of alcoholism on skeletal and cardiac muscle. *N Engl J Med* 320:409–415, 1989,
110. Harcombe AA, Ramsay L, Kenna JG, *et al:* Circulating antibodies to cardiac protein–acetaldehyde adducts in alcoholic heart muscle disease. *Clin Sci* 88:263–268, 1995.
111. Kennedy JM, Kelly SW, Meehan JM: Ventricular mitochondrial gene expression during development and following embryonic ethanol exposure. *J Mol Cell Cardiol* 23:117–131, 1993.
112. Schwartz L, Sample B, Wigle D: Severe alcoholic cardiomyopathy reversed with abstention from alcohol. *Am J Cardiol* 36:963–966, 1975.
113. Molgaard H, Kristensen BO, Baandrup U: Importance of abstention from alcohol in alcoholic heart disease. *Int J Cardiol* 26:373–375, 1990.
114. Demakis JG, Proskey A, Rahimtoola SH, *et al:* The natural course of alcoholic cardiomyopathy. *Ann Intern Med* 80:293–297, 1974.
115. Koide T, Kato A, Takabatake Y, *et al:* Variable prognosis in congestive cardiomyopathy. Role of left ventricular function, alcoholism, and pulmonary thrombosis. *Jpn Heart J* 21:451–463, 1990.
116. Segel LD, Rendig SG, Mason DT: Alcohol-induced cardiac hemodynamic and Ca^{2+} flux dysfunction are reversible. *J Mol Cell Cardiol* 13:443–455, 1981.
117. Fernandez-Sola J, Estruch R, Grau JM, *et al:* The relation of alcoholic myopathy to cardiomyopathy. *Ann Intern Med* 120:529–536, 1994.
118. Massumi RA, Rios JC, Ticktin HE: Hemodynamic abnormalities and venous admixture in portal cirrhosis. *Am J Med Sci* 250:67/275–75/283, 1965.
119. Kachru RB, Proskey AJ, Telischi M: Histocompatibility antigens and alcoholic cardiomyopathy. *Tissue Antigens* 15:398–399, 1980.
120. Fischbein L, Sachs RN, Geay D, *et al:* Etude des antigenes A et B du systeme HLA dans les myocardiopathies dilatees liees a l'alcool. *Arch Mal Coeur* 80:1171–1175, 1987.
121. Morin YL, Foley AR, Martineau G, Roussel: Quebec beer drinkers' cardiomyopathy: Forty-eight cases. *Can Med Assoc J* 97:881–904, 1967.
122. Miller H, Abelmann WH: Effects of dietary ethanol upon experimental trypanosomal (*T. Cruzi*) myocarditis. *Proc Soc Exp Biol* 126:193–198, 1967.
123. Morin Y, Roy PE, Mohiuddin SM, Tasker PK: The influence of alcohol in viral and isoproterenol cardiomyopathy. *Cardiovasc Res* 3:363–368, 1969.
124. Dyer AR, Stamler J, OgLesby P, *et al:* Alcohol, cardiovascular risk factors and mortality: the Chicago experience. *Circulation* 64(Suppl III):20–27, 1981.

125. Kozararevic D, Vojvodic N, Dawber T, *et al:* Frequency of alcohol consumption and morbidity and mortality. *Lancet* 1:613–616, 1980.
126. Beevers DB, Bannan LT, Saunders JB, *et al:* Alcohol and hypertension. *Contrib Nephrol* 30:92–97, 1982.
127. Clark LT, Friedman HS: Hypertension associated with alcohol withdrawal: Assessment of mechanisms and complications. *Alcohol Clin Exp Res* 9:125–130, 1985.
128. King AC, Errico AL, Parsons OA, Lovallo WR: Blood pressure dysregulation associated with alcohol withdrawal. *Alcohol Clin Exp Res* 12:478–482, 1991.
129. Weiss KT, Brilla CG: Pathological hypertrophy and cardiac interstitium. *Circulation* 83:1849–1865, 1991.
130. Meerson FZ: Mechanisms of hypertrophy of the heart and experimental prevention of acute cardiac insufficiency. *Br Heart J* 33:100–108, 1971.
131. Ettinger PO, Wu CF, De La Cruz C, *et al:* Arrhythmias and the "holiday heart": Alcohol-associated cardiac rhythm disorders. *Am Heart J* 95:555–562, 1978.
132. Thornton JR: Atrial fibrillation in healthy non-alcoholic people after an alcoholic binge. *Lancet* 2:1013–1014, 1984.
133. Rich EC, Siebold C, Campion B: Alcohol-related acute atrial fibrillation: A case-control study and review of 40 patients. *Arch Intern Med* 145:830–833, 1985.
134. Cohen EJ, Klatsky AL, Armstrong MA: Alcohol use and supraventricular arrhythmia. *Am J Cardiol* 62:971–973, 1988.
135. Greenspon AJ, Stang JM, Lewis RP, Schaal SF: Provocation of ventricular tachycardia after consumption of alcohol. *N Engl J Med* 301:1049–1050, 1979.
136. Panos RJ, Sutton FJ, Young-Hyman P, Peters R: Sudden death associated with alcohol consumption. *Pace* 11:423–424, 1988.
137. Russ KC, Mower MM, Veltri EP: Life-threatening ventricular tachyarrhythmias associated with holiday heart syndrome: Treatment with the automatic implantable cardioverter defibrillator. *J Electrophysiol* 3:309–312, 1989.
138. Juchems R, Klobe R: Hemodynamic effects of ethyl alcohol in man. *Am Heart J* 78:133–135, 1969.
139. Engel TR, Luck JC: Effect of whiskey on atrial vulnerability and "holiday heart." *J Am Coll Cardiol* 1:816–818, 1983.
140. Greenspon AJ, Schaal SF: The "holiday heart": Electrophysiologic studies of alcohol effects in alcoholics. *Ann Intern Med* 98:135–139, 1983.
141. Luca C: Electrophysiological properties of right heart and atrioventricular conducting system in patients with alcoholic cardiomyopathy. *Br Heart J* 42:274–281, 1979.
142. Gilmour RF Jr, Ruffy R, Lovelace DE, *et al:* Effect of ethanol on electrogram changes and regional myocardial blood flow during acute myocardial ischaemia. Cardiovasc Res 15:47–58, 1981.
143. Kostis JB, Horstmann E, Mavrogeorgis E, *et al:* Effects of alcohol on the electrocardiogram. *Circulation* 44:558–564, 1971.
144. Madan BR, Gupta RS: Effect of ethanol in experimental auricular and ventricular arrhythmias. *Jpn J Pharmacol* 17:683–684, 1967.
145. Paradise RR, Stoelting V: Conversion of acetyl strophanthidin-induced ventricular tachycardia to sinus rhythm by ethyl alcohol. *Arch Int Pharmacodyn* 157:312–321, 1963.
146. Nguyen TN, Friedman HS, Mokraoui AM: Effects of alcohol on experimental atrial fibrillation. *Alcohol Clin Exp Res* 11:474–476, 1987.
147. Kramer K, Kuller L, Fisher R: The increasing mortality attributed to cirrhosis and fatty liver, in Baltimore (1956–1966). *Ann Intern Med* 69:273–282, 1968.
148. Randall B: Sudden death and hepatic fatty metamorphosis. *JAMA* 243:1723–1725, 1980.
149. Lithell H, Aberg H, Selinus I, Hedstrand H: Alcohol intemperance and sudden death. *Br Med J* 294:1456–1458, 1987.
150. Takizawa A, Yasue H, Omote S, *et al:* Variant angina induced by alcohol ingestion. *Am Heart J* 107:25–27, 1984.
151. Renaud SC, Ruf JC: Effects of alcohol on platelet functions. *Clin Chim Acta* 246:77–89, 1996.

152. Novak DJ, Victor M: The vagus and sympathetic nerves in alcoholic polyneuropathy. *Arch Neurol* 30:273–294, 1974.
153. Duncan G, Lambie D, Johnson R, Whiteside E: Evidence of vagal neuropathy in chronic alcoholics. *Lancet* 2:1053–1057.
154. Barter F, Tanner AR: Autonomic neuropathy in an alcoholic population. *Postgrad Med J* 63:1033–1036, 1987.
155. Factor S: Intramyocardial small-vessel disease in chronic alcoholism. *Am Heart J* 92:561–575, 1976.
156. Fraser GE, Upsdell M: Alcohol and other discriminants between cases of sudden death and myocardial infarction. *Am J Epidemiol* 114:462–476, 1981.
157. Zanchetti A, Chalmers JP, Gyarfas I, *et al:* Prevention of hypertension and associated cardiovascular disease. A 1995 statement. *Clin Exp Hypertens* 18:581–593, 1996.
158. Friedman HS: Alcohol and hypertension, in Feldman EB (ed): *Nutrition and Heart Disease.* New York, Churchill Livingstone, 1990, pp 35–50.
159. Seppa K, Laippala P, Sillanaukee P: High diastolic blood pressure: Common among women who are heavy drinkers. *Alcohol Clin Exp Res* 20:47–51, 1996.
160. Klatsky AL, Friedman GD, Armstrong MA: The relationships between alcoholic beverage use and other traits to blood pressure: A new Kaiser–Permanente study. *Circulation* 73:628–636, 1986.
161. Fortman SP, Haskell WL, Vranizan K, *et al:* The association of blood pressure and dietary alcohol: Differences by age, sex and estrogen use. *Am J Epidemiol* 118:497–507, 1983.
162. Wallace RB, Connor EB, Criqui M, *et al:* Alteration in blood pressures associated with combined alcohol and oral contraceptive use—The lipid research clinics prevalence study. *J Chron Dis* 35:252–257, 1982.
163. Cooke KM, Frost GW, Thornell IR, Stokes GS: Alcohol consumption and blood pressure. *Med J Aust* 1:65–69, 1982.
164. Milon H, Froment A, Gaspard P, *et al:* Alcohol consumption and blood pressure in a French epidemiological study. *Eur Heart J* 3:59–64, 1982.
165. MacMahon S, Blackett RB, Macdonald GJ, Hall W: Obesity, alcohol consumption and blood pressure in Australian men and women. The National Heart Foundation of Australia risk factor prevalence study. *J Hypertens* 2:85–91, 1984.
166. Yor J, Hirsch JA: Residual pressor effects of chronic alcohol in detoxified alcoholics. *Hypertension* 28:133–138, 1996.
167. Grassi GM, Somers VK, Renk WS, *et al:* Effects of alcohol intake on blood pressure and sympathetic nerve activity in normotensive humans: A preliminary report. *J Hypertens* 7:S20–S22, 1989,
168. Randin D, Vollenweider P, Tappy L, *et al:* Suppression of alcohol-induced hypertension by dexamethasone. *N Engl J Med* 332:1733–1737, 1995.
169. Potter JE, Beevers DG: Pressor effect of alcohol in hypertension. *Lancet* 1:119–122, 1984.
170. Puddey IB, Beilin IJ, Vandongen R, *et al:* Evidence for a direct effect of alcohol consumption on blood pressure in normotensive men. *Hypertension* 7:707–713, 1985.
171. Puddey IB, Beilin IJ, Vandongen R: Regular alcohol use raises blood pressure in treated hypertensive subjects: *Lancet* 1:647–662, 1987.
172. Malhotra H, Mathur D, Mehta SR, Khandelwal PD: Pressor effects of alcohol in normotensive and hypertensive subjects. *Lancet* 2:584–586, 1985.
173. Chan TCK, Sutter MC: Ethanol consumption and blood pressure. *Life Sci* 33:1965–1973, 1983.
174. Ireland MA, Vandongen R, Davidson L, *et al:* Acute effects of moderate alcohol consumption on blood pressure and plasma catecholamines. *Clin Sci* 66:643–648, 1984.
175. Howes LG, Reid JL: Changes in plasma free 3,4-dihydroxyphenylethylenen glycol and noradrenaline levels after acute alcohol administration. *Clin Sci* 69:423–428, 1985.
176. Potter JF, Watson RDS, Skan W, Beevers DG: The pressor and metabolic effects of alcohol in normotensive subjects. *Hypertension* 8:625–631, 1986.
177. Berne C, Fagius J, Niklasson F: Sympathetic response to oral carbohydrate administration. *J Clin Invest* 84:1403–1409, 1989.

178. Abdel-Rahman ARA, Merrill RH, Wolles WR: Effect of acute ethanol administration on the baroreceptor reflex control of heart rate in normotensive human volunteers. *Clin Sci* 72:113–122, 1987.
179. EL-Mas MM, Abdel-Rahman AA: Role of NMDA and non-NMDA receptors in the nucleus tractus solitarius in the depressant effect of ethanol on baroreflexes. *J Pharmacol Exp Ther* 266:602–610, 1993.
180. Arkwright PD, Beilin LJ, Vandongen R, *et al:* The pressor effect of moderate alcohol consumption in man: A search for mechanisms. *Circulation* 66:515–519, 1982.
181. Chan TCK, Wall RA, Sutter MC: Chronic ethanol consumption stress and hypertension. *Hypertension* 7:519–524, 1985.
182. Bannan LT, Potter JF, Beevers DG, *et al:* Effect of alcohol withdrawal on blood pressure, plasma renin activity, aldosterone, cortisol and dopamine B-hydroxylase. *Clin Sci* 66:659–663, 1984.
183. Chaudhuri KR, Maule S, Thomaides T, *et al:* Alcohol ingestion lowers supine blood pressure, splanchnic vasodilatation and worsens postural hypotension in primary autonomic failure. *J Neurol* 241:145–152, 1994.
184. Stott DJ, Dutton M, Murray GD, *et al:* Hemodynamic effects of a single moderate dose of alcohol in elderly subjects. *J Stud Alcohol* 52:377–379, 1991.
185. Dyer AR, Stamler J, Paul O, *et al:* Alcohol consumption and 17-year mortality in the Chicago Western Electric Company Study. *Prev Med* 9:78–90, 1980.
186. Gill JS, Zezulka AV, Shipley MJ, *et al:* Stroke and alcohol consumption. *N Engl J Med* 315:1041–1046, 1986.
187. Wannamethee SG, Shaper AG: Patterns of alcohol intake and risk of stroke in middle-aged British men. *Stroke* 27:1033–1039, 1996.
188. Doll R, Peto R, Hall E, *et al:* Mortality in relation to consumption of alcohol: 13 years' observations on male British doctors. *Br Med J* 309:911–918, 1994.
189. De Labry LO, Glynn RJ, Levenson MR, *et al:* Alcohol consumption and mortality in an American male population: Recovering the U-Shaped curve—Findings from the normative aging study. *J Stud Alcohol* 53:25–32, 1992.
190. Stampfer MJ, Colditz GA, Willett WC, *et al:* A prospective study of moderate alcohol consumption and the risk of coronary disease and stroke in women. *N Engl J Med* 319:267–273, 1988.
191. Garg R, Wagener DK, Madans JH: Alcohol consumption and risk of ischemic heart disease in women. *Arch Intern Med* 153:1211–1216, 1993.
192. Fuchs CS, Stampfer MJ, Colditz GA, *et al:* Alcohol consumption and mortality among women. *N Engl J Med* 332:1245–1250, 1995.
193. Serdula MK, Koong SL, Williamson DF, *et al:* Alcohol intake and subsequent mortality: Findings from the NHANES I follow-up study. *Alcohol* 56:233–239, 1995.
194. Klatskky AL, Armstrong MA, Friedman GD: Alcohol and mortality. *Ann Intern Med* 117:646–654, 1992.
195. Kozararevic DJ, Vojvodic N, Dawber T, *et al:* Frequency of alcohol consumption and morbidity and mortality: The Yugoslavia Cardiovascular Disease Study. *Lancet* 1:613–616, 1980.
196. Iso H, Kitamura A, Shimamoto R, *et al:* Alcohol intake and the risk of cardiovascular disease in middle-aged Japanese men. *Stroke* 26:767–773, 1995.
197. Suh I, Shaten J, Cutler JA, Kuller LH: Alcohol use and mortality from coronary heart disease: The role of high-density lipoprotein cholesterol. *Ann Intern Med* 116:881–887, 1992.
198. Langer RD, Criqui MH, Reed DM: Lipoproteins and blood pressure as biological pathways for effect of moderate alcohol consumption on coronary heart disease. *Circulation* 85:910–915, 1992.
199. Wannamethee G, Whincup PH, Shaper AG, *et al:* Factors determining case fatality in myocardial infarction "Who dies in a heart attack?" *Br Heart J* 74:324–331, 1995.
200. Meade TW, Imeson J, Stirling Y: Effects of changes in smoking and other characteristics on clotting factors and the risk of ischaemic heart disease. *Lancet* 2:986–988, 1987.

201. Elwood PC, Renaud S, Sharp DS, *et al:* Ischemic heart disease and platelet aggregation. *Circulation* 83:38–44, 1991.
202. Ruf JC, Berger JL, Renaud S: Platelet rebound effect of alcohol withdrawal and wine drinking in rats. *Arterioscler Thromb Vasc Biol* 15:140–144, 1995.
203. Gronbaek M, Deis A, Sorensen TIA, *et al:* Mortality associated with moderate intakes of wine, beer or spirits. *Br Med J* 310:1165–1169, 1995.
204. Burr ML: Explaining the French paradox. *J R Soc Health* 115:217–219, 1995.
205. Deykin D, Janson P, McMahon: Ethanol potentiation of aspirin-induced prolongation of the bleeding time. *N Engl J Med* 306:852–854, 1982.
206. Camargo CA: Case–control and cohort studies of moderate alcohol consumption and stroke.*Clin Chim Acta* 246:107–119, 1996.
207. Donahue RP, Abbott RD, Reed DM, Yano K: Alcohol and hemorrhagic stroke. *JAMA* 255:2311–2314, 1986.
208. Lee K: Alcoholism and cerebrovascular thrombosis in the young. *Acta Neurol Scand* 59:270–274, 1979.
209. Hillbom M, Kaste M: Ethanol intoxication: A risk factor for ischemic brain infarction in adolescents and young adults. *Stroke* 12:422–425, 1981.
210. Haapaniemi H, Hillbom M, Juvela S: Weekend and holiday increase in the onset of ischemic stroke in young women. *Stroke* 27:1023–1027, 1996.
211. Russek HI, Naegele CF, Regan FD: Alcohol in the treatment of angina pectoris. *JAMA* 143:355–357, 1950.
212. Orlando J, Aronow WS, Cassidy J, Prakash R: Effect of ethanol on angina pectoris. *Ann Intern Med* 84:652–655, 1976.
213. Matsuguchi T, Araki H, Nakamura N, *et al:* Prevention of vasospastic angina by alcohol ingestion: Report of two cases. *Angiology* 38:394–400, 1988.
214. Matsuguchi T, Araki H, Anan T, *et al:* Provocation of variant angina by alcohol ingestion. *Eur Heart J* 5:906–912, 1984.

II

Neuropsychiatric Consequences of Alcoholism

Edward Gottheil and Ellen F. Gottheil, Section Editors

Overview

Edward Gottheil and Ellen F. Gottheil

The 1990s have been declared to be the "Decade of the Brain." As the Human Genome Project closes in on its goal, neuropsychiatric research focuses increasingly on the brain for answers to insistent age-old questions such as: Why do people drink to excess, despite the obvious destruction they cause themselves and those around them? How can we help them to stop? How does ethanol, such a simple molecule, wreak such havoc?

A variety of exciting new research techniques and models have been developed to address persistent questions about causes and consequences of excess drinking. The five chapters that are collected within this section focus on new information about the effects of alcohol abuse within the brains of subjects considered normal, alcoholic, or ill with a coexistent psychiatric problem. These chapters provide updates on models of alcohol craving; effects of moderate alcohol intake on psychiatric and sleep disorders; executive cognitive function and behavioral self-regulation mediated by prefrontal lobes; brain-imaging studies of alcohol in the central nervous system; and interactions between alcohol, drugs, and psychiatric illness. Together, these chapters incorporate and review many of the new findings and developments emerging in relation to the important questions in this field.

It is curious that craving, variously defined and measured, and drinking often tend to be linked so closely, if not causally, despite our awareness that craving can occur without leading to drinking and that drinking may occur without being precipitated by craving. We hear many abstinent alcoholics and smokers report that once they gave it up, it never bothered them and they

Edward Gottheil • Department of Psychiatry, Jefferson Medical College, Thomas Jefferson University, Philadelphia, Pennsylvania 19107. **Ellen F. Gottheil** • Department of Psychiatry and Behavioral Sciences, University of Washington Medical School, Seattle, Washington 98195.

Recent Developments in Alcoholism, Volume 14: The Consequences of Alcoholism, edited by Galanter. Plenum Press, New York, 1998.

never thought about it again. About as many others, however, report that on each and every day, even after years or decades, they still crave a cigarette with their morning coffee, alcohol when they hear the tinkle of ice cubes, and a cigar after a good dinner. In Chapter 6, Singleton and Gorelick systematically review models of craving and their supporting evidence (92 references). They discuss the dissociation between craving and drinking and note the difficulties that models based on conditioning have in attempting to account for such dissociation. Also difficult to explain on the basis of conditioning is when an alcoholic drink, instead of reducing craving, serves as a priming dose and increases craving. Newer conceptualizations provided by the incentive sensitization model, which implicates dopamine reward system mediation, and more recent cognitive theoretical models are described as having more explanatory power and being better able to account for these observations.

As the models of craving have become more complex, so have the instruments used to measure craving. There are now multi-item, multidimensional measures based on factor analyses being employed along with the older visual analogue, single-item, or unidimensional scales. One analysis, for example, resulted in four separate and clinically meaningful factors: negative mood state, current desire and intent to drink, lack of confidence in ability to quit, and expectancy to derive the positive benefits of drinking as in the past.

Singleton and Gorelick then discuss the clinical implications of the theoretical craving models for behavioral interventions and/or pharmacotherapies based on relevant neural transmitter mechanisms. Relevant outcome studies are included in their thoughtful discussions and evaluations of the different models. The chapter ends with a set of recommendations/questions for further research. These include: the desirability of longitudinal studies of the relationship between craving and drinking in social and alcoholic drinkers; how individuals cope with craving when they resist drinking; and the use of modern imaging methods to localize brain areas associated with craving and to determine activity levels in these areas in response to the administration of putative treatment agents.

The special problems of combined alcoholism and other psychiatric disorders have become well known to clinicians and researchers alike. However, according to Castaneda and coauthors (Chapter 7), the consequences of moderate or social drinking have been largely overlooked. Even modest amounts of ethanol, often regarded as harmless if not healthy, may adversely affect individuals with psychiatric and sleep disorders whether they are taking psychotropic medications or not.

Alcohol has many widespread effects: It may be inhibiting or stimulating to the main neurotransmitter systems, depending on dose and brain area; it may dampen or activate the stress response; and, of course, it has troublesome effects on cognition, perception, impulse control, alertness, mood, and judgment. Since these are the systems and functions most commonly disturbed in psychiatric disorders, it should not be surprising if psychiatric patients were more affected by alcohol than the general population. For patients on medication, a number of other actions of alcohol become problematic: it may alter metabolic pathways by its effect on liver function; by interference with the cytochrome P450 system, it may modify the effect of many psychotropic agents such as valproate, carbamezapine, neuroleptics, antidepressants, and benzodiazepines; it may interact with other drugs and change how they act on the serotonin, dopamine, and other neurotransmitter systems; it may affect renal clearance, making it difficult to maintain lithium levels; it may increase sleep apnea and disturb sleep quality; and it may seriously affect compliance with treatment regimens.

Given all of these potential actions and interactions, the authors devote most of Chapter 7 to reviewing the effects of moderate alcohol intake on many of the specific disorders (190 references), on the need for broadening the base of treatment for alcohol problems,[1] and on opportunities for prevention efforts. They conclude by providing a summary of interactions of alcohol and psychotropic medications and their effects. The emphasis that Castaneda and coauthors place on the importance of moderate drinking as it affects psychiatric patients is very well taken, as is their call for more research on these difficult problems. We all know of the patient with a schizophrenic disorder who is admitted to the hospital, stabilized on Haldol (haloperidol), and shortly discharged. He then has a drink to celebrate, finds it more pleasant than Haldol, and so continues to drink, perhaps only a few daily, stops taking his Haldol, and is shortly returned to the hospital, hallucinating and delusional, to begin the process over again. These difficult patients are not easily entered into controlled, randomized studies. Indeed, one usually excludes drinking patients when studying schizophrenia and excludes schizophrenic patients when studying drinking. Castaneda and coauthors are to be commended for their work in this difficult but important area; one would hope that a review chapter such as theirs, in providing a basic framework, might encourage others to follow suit.

If Castaneda and coauthors contend that we have not paid enough attention to a significant population of patients, i.e., moderate drinkers, in Chapter 8, Giancola and Moss contend that we have not paid enough attention to a significant organ system, that is, the cortex of the brain, especially the prefrontal area. Many theories of dependence on alcohol and other drugs have centered on various models of reinforcement, and hence on the dopamine system of the ventral striatum, including the nucleus acumbens. This focus on the mesolimbic area as the neural substrate for the brain's reward system has tended to overlook the contribution of the prefrontal cortex, the extensive neural connections between the striatum and the prefrontal cortex, or the influence of the prefrontal cortex on the regulation of striatal dopamine release.

Alcoholic patients, for example, have been found to exhibit deficits in a variety of cognitive functions such as word fluency, visuospatial ability, memory, abstract reasoning, attention, set shifting, sequencing, hypothesis formation, and so forth. These deficits among others are included under the rubric of executive cognitive functioning (ECF), which is described as a higher-order cognitive construct involved in the self-regulation of goal-directed behavior. Since individuals with prefrontal pathology may display similar patterns of cognitive deficits, the prefrontal cortex with its subcortical connections is considered to represent the primary neurological substrate subserving ECF.

Individuals with prefrontal lesions may also display apathy, social withdrawal, restlessness, disinhibition, decreased concern with social propriety, poor judgment, inappropriate jocularity, lack of foresight, altered mood, unreliability, and so forth. These characteristics are not uncommon in individuals with antisocial personality disorder, attention-deficit–hyperactivity disorder (ADHD), and conduct disorder and many alcoholics and other substance abusers. A number of studies have shown that individuals with ADHD, delinquents, and aggressive children and adolescents have ECF deficits and are more prone to alcohol problems in adulthood. In addition to overlapping behavioral syndromes, alcoholics and antisocial personalities have been shown to have linkages in family studies, for example, alcoholics with positive family histories for alcoholism are more likely to have antisocial relatives and to exhibit antisocial behavior themselves. Also, individuals at high risk for alcoholism, that is, sons of alcoholics, have been found to have deficits in ECF.

Bringing together many threads of evidence, the authors describe a frontostriatal hypothesis of the development of alcoholism involving dysregulation of the prefrontal cortex, ECF deficits, sensation seeking, and impulsive behavior. The clinical implications of this model follow in straightforward fashion from the theory and include parenting techniques to prevent the development of ECF deficits and therapeutic approaches to modify patients' cognitive disturbances and to provide alternatives. Giancola and Moss recognize that the 185 studies they reference are not all consistent with the theory or with each other and that there are gaps remaining to be filled. Nevertheless, a great deal of relevant information is provided in a logical organization and offered in the form of a heuristic model. It suggests many research questions and opportunities to close gaps in the theory, put inconsistent findings to further test, try suggested preventive and therapeutic techniques, and evaluate the outcome results.

In Chapter 9, on brain imaging, Lyons and coauthors review developments (124 references) that have occurred in these methodologies in recent years, describe the techniques, discuss findings that have emerged, and show us the promise they hold for future contributions. Initially, computed tomography and magnetic resonance imaging (MRI) provided noninvasive methods for visualizing the anatomy of the brain in great detail, assisting in the diagnosis of various abnormalities, and following the progress of structural change as, for example, brought about by the continuing chronic ingestion of alcohol. The main focus of this chapter, however, is on the more recent developments in functional imaging, using measures of cerebral blood flow

(CBF) and energy metabolism (glucose), to assess the effects of acute and chronic alcohol intake on animals and humans.

The purposes and the particular advantages and disadvantages of employing radioactive tracers to measure CBF and glucose in conjunction with positron emission tomography (PET), single-photon emission computed tomography (SPECT), and MRI scanning are systematically described and discussed. Examining regional activity in the living brain with various combinations of these powerful methods enables study, for example, of the site and intensity of the effects of different stimuli (e.g., cocaine), pharmacological agents (e.g., naltrexone), or feelings (e.g., craving). These effects can also be observed/compared as they occur in particular populations such as women, individuals at high risk for alcoholism, or those with antisocial personalities.

Among the many new findings reported are some very interesting correlations between biological and behavioral observations. Imaging results, for example, have given new meaning, as well as understanding, to the behaviorally observed biphasic effect of going from high to low spirits while drinking. Observing brain activity reveals that there is biphasic activity by dose (low vs. high) and by time (earlier vs. later), and that the sequences also vary by specific brain region. Regarding treatment implications, in a study using SPECT, alcohol intake by normal subjects was found to result in higher metabolic activity in the prefrontal cortex, an effect prevented by pretreatment with naloxone. Especially interesting to us was the finding that neural activity differed when alcohol was ingested voluntarily than when it was passively administered. We have previously reported that patients in treatment who made voluntary public commitments to abstain while in a group session adhered to their commitments significantly more often than those whose commitments were made involuntarily.[2] Now we have the observation from imaging of the brain that when alcohol is taken voluntarily, the effects are found primarily in the brain region mediating positive reinforcement, whereas this is not the case when alcohol is administered passively. In terms of further research using these brain-imaging techniques, if we were to consider only some of the recommendations/questions emerging from the previous chapters in this section, we could think of attempting to localize and measure brain activity in different samples (e.g., age, sex, drinking pattern) associated with craving, tolerance, and various cognitive tasks, and also to determine the persistence of any significant findings over time. Indeed, the possibilities seem endless.

In Chapter 10, the final chapter of this section, Drake and Brunette review studies of the effects of alcohol and drug use disorders (127 references) on the course and management of severe mental disorders. This problem has been receiving increasing attention as the extent to which alcohol and drug addictions occur and complicate these disorders has become more apparent. Recent studies estimate that as many as 40–60% of patients with severe mental illness also have substance use disorders. Often described as *dual disorder,* the term is unfortunate in that it is frequently unclear, inaccurate, and usually serves to underestimate the complexity of the problem. It may refer, for example, to two substance use disorders, a substance use disorder with an Axis I disorder, a substance use disorder with a personality disorder, or some other combination. In reality, of course, it has become rare to find individuals with single-substance use or personality disorders. Most cases of dual disorder are more likely to have a combination of several substance use, personality, and Axis I disorders.

The main purpose of the review chapter was to examine evidence regarding the ways and the extent to which substance use adversely affects the course of severe mental illness. Empirical information was sought in the literature regarding 11 categories of purported complications (e.g., disruptive behavior, decreased functional status, family problems, relapse). The studies were categorized as correlational or prospective and longitudinal, with more weight given to the latter. On the whole, the evidence did show that substance use did complicate the course of severe mental illnesses in most but not all categories examined.

Typical of the type of studies surveyed were comparisons of rates of violence manifested by individuals with schizophrenic disorders who were abusing substances with those who were not abusing substances. Overall level of functioning was found to be lower in patients with combined disorders, and it worsened with continued substance abuse. In studies examining family relationships and residential instability, patients with combined disorders were found to have more problems, but were found to improve following dual-diagnosis treatment and decreased substance use.

Drake and Brunette noted that although psychiatrically disturbed patients had higher levels of substance abuse than the rest of the population, there was no evidence that it was helpful in any of the disorders. That is, even if abused substances were sought as a form of symptom reduction, they did not serve effectively as any true "self-medication."

The authors cautioned about the difficulty of making causal inferences. Does the substance of abuse exert a direct biological affect on the course of the psychiatric disorder? Or do psychiatric diseases result in impaired biological processing of substances of abuse? Finally, Drake and Brunette remind us that as we look within the brain for causal links, we ought not overlook the mediation of the psychosocial surround. For example, cocaine use and positive psychotic symptoms were found to be correlated and to peak at the beginning of the month, when disability checks were received and cocaine could be purchased.

In conclusion, the five chapters in Section II were well written, well organized, and well referenced. They include a great deal of information and bring to our attention a surprising wealth of new findings, new technological innovations, and new conceptualizations. Most impressive were the organized presentations of significant topics, providing useful updates for clinicians and frameworks for future research. There is a need for more prospective, controlled studies, with careful diagnostic workups, and the development of more reliable and valid measures of outcome. Clearly, we are just beginning our exploration of the neuropsychiatric frontier where biology, psychology, and sociology interact in the brain. Hopefully, we are proceeding in a direction that will at some time in the future supplant our 14 alcohol-related disorders (and subcategories) listed in the *Diagnostic and Statistical Manual of Mental Disorders*, 4th edition, with a more comprehensive theory with clear explanatory power and implications for treatment.

References

1. Institute of Medicine: *Broadening the Base of Treatment for Alcohol Problems.* Washington, DC, National Academy Press, 1990.
2. Thornton CC, Gottheil E, Gellens HK, Alterman AI: Voluntary vs. involuntary abstinence in the treatment of alcoholics. *J Stud Alcohol* 38:1740–1748, 1977.

6

Mechanisms of Alcohol Craving and Their Clinical Implications

Edward G. Singleton and David A. Gorelick

Abstract. Craving for alcohol is frequently given as a reason for drinking and is often used as a surrogate measure in studies of alcoholism and its treatment. Despite this wide use, there is little consensus on what craving for alcohol means, the best way to measure it, what mechanism accounts for the urge to drink, or what is its true relationship to alcohol use. This chapter reviews theoretical and measurement issues about the possible mechanisms involved in craving for alcohol and the clinical implications of evidence supporting them. Until recently, most instruments for assessing craving assumed it was a univariate construct and usually contained only one or a few items. Several multi-item and multidimensional rating instruments have now been developed that offer the promise of more useful assessment of clinically relevant behavior. Most models of craving have assumed that a consistent and positive relationship exists between craving and drinking. The incentive sensitization model and the cognitive theory of drug use and drug urges may account better than the older models for the frequent clinical observation of a dissociation between craving and drinking. However, no single model or theory of craving accounts for the wide variation in findings reviewed here, suggesting that multiple mechanisms may be involved. A comprehensive, multidisciplinary approach is necessary to elucidate the nature of craving for alcohol and its implications for pharmacological and psychosocial treatment of alcoholism.

1. Introduction

There is no universally recognized concept called *craving for alcohol*. Clinicians and researchers have used the term to label a variety of self-report statements,

Edward G. Singleton • Behavior Therapy Treatment Research Center, Johns Hopkins University School of Medicine, Baltimore, Maryland 21224. **David A. Gorelick** • Intramural Research Program, National Institute on Drug Abuse, National Institutes of Health, Baltimore, Maryland 21224.

Recent Developments in Alcoholism, Volume 14: The Consequences of Alcoholism, edited by Galanter. Plenum Press, New York, 1998.

including urges and desires to drink and wanting, needing, or liking alcohol. There is often discrepancy between the standard dictionary definition of craving as "a strong desire" and how persons with alcohol-related problems use the word to mean "any desire or urge, even a weak one, to use that substance."[1,2] Despite the absence of consensus on a working definition of the concept, craving is frequently given as a reason for drinking, as an explanation for relapse, and as a subjective marker for alcohol use disorders.[3,4] However, the role of craving in the development and maintenance of alcoholism remains unclear and the mechanisms through which craving operates have not been identified.[5,6] This chapter provides an overview of these issues, including (1) models and theories of craving and the evidence supporting them; (2) methods for measuring craving; and (3) the clinical implications of craving. The chapter concludes with some recommended areas for future research.

2. Theoretical Issues

2.1. *Conditioning Mechanisms*

Alcohol-related stimuli can acquire the properties of conditioned stimuli through associations and pairings with alcohol use. Most traditional accounts of alcohol craving propose that it arises from conditioning mechanisms associated with three aspects of neuroadaptation: (1) positively reinforcing (rewarding) alcohol effects, for example, euphoria or "high," (2) alcohol tolerance, and (3) aversive aspects of the alcohol withdrawal syndrome.[7,8]

2.1.1. Conditioned Incentive and Appetitive Models. These models are based on the action of alcohol in producing a subjective feeling of "high" or euphoria.[9] This experience is highly reinforcing to the user and provides a powerful incentive for reexperiencing the initial effect. Conditioned incentive and appetitive models[10,11] posit that alcohol-related cues become conditioned stimuli that elicit craving or a druglike response similar to that of acute alcohol administration. This conditioned positive reinforcement provides the catalyst for continued drinking or relapse. It is also possible for a priming dose of alcohol or positive affect to activate the appetitive motivational state.[12,13] Activation of brain dopamine systems (especially mesolimbic neural circuits) has been proposed as the neurobiological substrate for the model.[14] Appetitive models have had a dominant influence on addiction research, but have been criticized for failure to articulate the mechanisms underlying incentive motivation.[8] These models, by themselves, do not account well for drinking that occurs in the absence of conscious craving or in the presence of severe negative consequences (i.e., punishment).[15–17]

2.1.2. Conditioned Tolerance Models. With repeated drinking, neural systems adapt to and compensate for the presence of alcohol by compensatory mechanisms that are drug-opposite or counterdirectional to the alcohol effects. One such mechanism may represent learned compensatory behavior that can be precipitated by contextual cues.[18,19] For example, tolerance is maximally expressed when drinking takes place within the same context in which alcohol use previously occurred.[18,19] Such environment-dependent[19] tolerance may increase the motivational desire to drink alcohol by eliciting drug-opposite (i.e., withdrawal-like) responses in persons who use alcohol. These models assert that craving arises from conditioned negative reinforcement, that is, the desire to alleviate the aversive experience represented by the compensatory responses involved in conditioned tolerance.

2.1.3. Conditioned Withdrawal Models. Once the drug is removed, the adaptive neural changes that developed in response to repeated alcohol exposure manifest themselves as drug-opposite withdrawal effects, since there is no longer any drug present to counteract them. The aversive withdrawal effects can become conditioned to environmental or internal stimuli, which then elicit the withdrawal experience even in the absence of recent drug use. These models, similar to conditioned tolerance models, assert that craving arises from conditioned negative reinforcement, in this case to alleviate the aversive experience of conditioned withdrawal.[20,21] Some models of conditioned withdrawal predict that negative affect or other internal states resembling withdrawal may also elicit craving for alcohol.[12,13] These models, by themselves, do not account well for drinking that occurs in the absence of conscious craving or experienced withdrawal.[15–17,22]

2.1.4. Autoshaping. This model of alcohol craving is based on autoshaping,[23] a Pavlovian conditioning paradigm in which presentations of the conditioned and unconditioned stimuli are contingent on the individual's responses, while the responses themselves produce no other contingencies. In the autoshaping model, the urge to drink reflects tracking of internal and external stimuli that in the past have been reliably associated with the appearance of alcohol. Because of the powerful reinforcing properties of alcohol, there is a strong association between alcohol-related cues and actual drinking, an association that is relatively insensitive to extinction and other changes in response contingencies. A recent study of cocaine users was consistent with autoshaping, in that subjects who visually scanned an item of drug paraphernalia showed significantly smaller attentional shifts compared to users who viewed a neutral stimulus.[24] However, there is no direct evidence regarding autoshaping and alcohol craving.

2.1.5. Incentive Sensitization. In the incentive sensitization model of addiction, drug craving is defined as the conscious experience that accompanies the attribution of excessive incentive salience to drug-related stimuli or their mental representations.[15,25] Incentive salience is defined as the attractiveness or ability of external stimuli or their mental representations to attract attention. Excessive incentive salience ("wanting") is distinguished from the conscious experience of reward (pleasure or "liking"). In this model, initial exposure to a drug activates mesotelencephalic dopamine neural systems that mediate reward (incentive motivation), producing positive reinforcement and the conscious experience of pleasure, or "liking." With repeated, intermittent drug exposure, progressive and persistent hypersensitivity (sensitization) of this dopamine reward system develops, resulting in increased incentive salience. Conditioning processes lead this incentive salience to be focused on drug taking and its associated environmental or interoceptive stimuli. The model holds that this sensitized increase in incentive salience occurs outside of conscious awareness (in preconsciousness) and independently of any consciously perceived "liking" for drug. Thus, the model predicts that drug taking may occur without verbally expressible or consciously experienced drug "liking" (craving). In fact, "people may find themselves wanting particular things without knowing why, . . . [or] may not even know that they want them."[25]

The incentive sensitization model can account for some clinical phenomena relating alcohol craving and drinking that are not easily explainable by other models. It can explain the frequent reports in both naturalistic observation studies and treatment trials of a poor correlation between self-reported alcohol craving and actual drinking behavior. Craving in these studies is usually measured with an instrument that assesses conscious liking for alcohol, a phenomenon that the incentive sensitization model considers independent of the preconscious wanting for alcohol that actually drives drinking. The model also explains the frequent dissociation in alcoholics' self-report between craving and the immediate pleasurable experience of drinking ("high") or the dysphoric experience of early alcohol abstinence (withdrawal). Finally, the model can account for the observation that alcohol craving is often not reduced and may even be increased immediately after drinking that is experienced as pleasurable (e.g., the first drink that stimulates craving and precipitates relapse). These phenomena are not readily explained by straightforward conditioned incentive or appetitive or conditioned withdrawal models of craving, which would predict that the immediate pleasurable or withdrawal-suppressing effects of drinking should temporarily reduce craving (analogous to eating temporarily suppressing hunger).

While there is substantial experimental evidence supporting the incentive sensitization model for stimulant and opiate use, there is relatively little such animal or human evidence with regard to alcohol.[15,26] There is some evidence of behavioral sensitization to ethanol's locomotor-activating effect in rodents, that is, increased psychomotor stimulation in response to successive alcohol doses, especially in alcohol-preferring strains, and of the conditioning of this sensitization to environmental stimuli.[27,28] The dopamine-releasing action of alcohol has been reported to undergo sensitization in rats.[29]

2.2. *Cognitive Mechanisms*

Both anecdotal and experimental evidence indicates that responses to alcohol and to alcohol-related stimuli may be mediated by a wide range of cognitive processes,[30,31] including expectations of the positive benefits of drinking[32] (e.g., tension reduction or social disinhibition), a shift in focus from alcohol cues to internal thinking,[33] and self-efficacy or the belief in one's ability to cope with the desire to drink.[34] Several models of craving are based on these cognitive processes.

2.2.1. Cognitive–Behavioral Models. Cognitive–behavioral models of craving have emerged from cognitive and social learning theories and clinical practice. For example, craving has been defined as a subjective state that is mediated by the powerful incentive properties of positive outcome expectancies or beliefs that drugs will transform dysphoric moods into a more pleasant state of affairs.[30,32] The "anticipation of transformation" or expectation of the positive benefits of drinking will be experienced as craving, especially in high-risk situations where self-efficacy is low, that is, individuals have little confidence in their ability to resist alcohol use. Craving for alcohol appears as persons think about the positive benefits of drinking and feel that they owe it to themselves to use alcohol. The limited evidence for this model includes the demonstration that exposure to alcohol-related cues decreased confidence in the ability to resist drinking.[35]

Craving has also been defined as a strong desire for a particular experience, based on response to anhedonia (lack of pleasure) or to hedonic desires.[36] In this model, an urge is the instrumental sequel to craving, and the ultimate goal of an urge is its consummation, in this case drinking alcohol. A similar model adapts the abstinence–low frustration tolerance (LFT) pattern to include desire to drink in response to cues for drinking.[37] LFT ascribes these desires to irrational thinking or dysfunctional beliefs that adversely affect the decision not to use alcohol. Craving reduction has not been systematically investigated within the framework of either the hedonic or LFT models.

2.2.2. Cognitive Model of Drug Urges and Drug Use Behavior. This model conceptualizes urges and desires to drink as nonautomatic, cognitive responses that are distinct from but activated in parallel with automatized drinking behavior.[17] With repeated practice, the cognitive systems subserving drinking take on the character of automatic behavior, that is, the behaviors become relatively effortless, fast, and efficient, are enacted without conscious intention and awareness, and are difficult to stop or impede. In contrast, the cognitive systems subserving craving are slow, effortful, controlled, and highly dependent on attention and intention. Craving serves to activate cognitive schema, which are mental representations that support drinking action plans. If the drinking plans are blocked or impeded, craving would be experienced and urges would be linked to planning and intention to secure alcohol. The model does not assume that (conscious) craving is a direct manifestation of the motivational processes that cause drinking or relapse, and so can account for drinking that occurs in the absence of craving.

2.3. *Neurocognitive Mechanisms*

If craving is primarily a cognitive process, it should be influenced by and able to influence other cognitive processes.[17] Limited experimental evidence is consistent with this prediction. The effect on craving of thinking about alcohol has been studied, using guided imagery to simulate drinking or abstinence.[38] Results suggest that craving can be elicited and controlled through guided imagery simulations.

Craving has been found to disrupt concurrent cognitive tasks, suggesting that it operates through capacity-limited cognitive processes.[17] In a dual-task procedure, subjects were required to press a button when a hissing tone (probe stimulus) was detected, while at the same time imagining themselves in scenarios eliciting the urge to smoke.[39] Craving produced slower reaction times and increased heart rate and skin conductance level, higher ratings of negative mood, and lowered ratings of positive mood. Reaction times to auditory probe stimuli were greater in the presence of alcohol-related cues than in the presence of alcohol-neutral cues,[40] also consistent with the hypothesis of cognitive disruption. However, a study of nonproblem, heavy-drinking college students found that positive mood induction and sniffing a placebo beer failed to disrupt performance on either concurrent math or tracking tasks.[41]

Pilot studies[42,43] have found craving for alcohol positively correlated with increased general cognitive impairment and a history of neurological illness, injury, or symptomatology, as well as decreased attention, memory, and concentration and learning and academic abilities. The etiologic implications of these associations are uncertain. Implicit memory studies in adolescents using a cue–behavior association task suggest that there are strong associations in memory between certain alcohol cues and drinking behavior.[44] Responses to memory associations for alcohol reflect a pattern of activation in memory that fosters alcohol-consistent decisions and behaviors. These findings are consistent with the cognitive model prediction that the nonautomatic cognitive processes subserving craving could become automatized with long-term use.[17]

Recent human imaging studies indicate that several brain loci typically associated with affect and memory are activated during alcohol craving. A study of regional cerebral blood flow measured with single-photon emission computerized tomography (SPECT) found increased blood flow in the head of the right caudate nucleus associated with increased craving for alcohol, suggesting a functional role for the limbic striatum in the mediation of alcohol craving.[45] This is consistent with positron emission tomography (PET) studies showing metabolic activation in limbic and related brain areas in association with craving for cocaine.[46]

3. Measurement Issues

3.1. Operational Definition

There is little consensus regarding the operational definition of craving for alcohol,[47] so it is not surprising that there is wide variation in how it is measured. To further complicate the matter, there is evidence that self-reported craving may be substantially influenced by treatment setting,[48] time of day, and sociocultural factors such as age, gender, and level of education.[42] Such influences make cross-study comparisons difficult and may help explain the marked variability in findings and frequent lack of association between craving and alcohol use.

3.2. *Unidimensional Indicators*

Historically, craving has been most commonly measured as a unidimensional or single-factor variable,[49] typically associated with one or at most a few items in a Likert or visual analogue (such as a 100-cm line) scale format.[17] A unidimensional (by factor analysis) but multi-item (8 questions) instrument, the Alcohol Urge Questionnaire (AUQ) has recently been developed with questions covering a number of domains including desire for a drink, expectations of positive outcomes or effects following drinking, relief of withdrawal and negative affect following drinking, and intention to drink.[50] The AUQ has been found to be internally consistent, reliable, and psychometrically valid, but the reliability and validity of single-item, unidimensional instruments generally have been low or not evaluated at all.

There is limited experimental support for a unidimensional model of craving. A one-dimensional measure of cue responsivity was found to correlate significantly with craving for alcohol.[51] The AUQ was found to have statistically significant, albeit modest, correlations with recent drinking (number of drinks in past 30 days, $r = 0.33$) and days since last drink ($r = -0.25$).[50]

3.3. *Multidimensional Indicators*

Alcohol craving can be operationalized as a multidimensional construct. A recently developed 47-item instrument incorporated a broad range of theories of craving and its relationship to drug use: (1) desire to use, (2) intention and planning to use, (3) anticipation of positive outcome, (4) anticipation of relief from withdrawal, and (5) loss of control over use.[52] Initial validation of the full instrument [Alcohol Craving Questionnaire-Now (ACQ-Now)][52] and a 12-item short form (ACQ-Now-SF)[42] using factor analysis revealed four dimensions with moderate to high reliability or internal consistency: *emotionality* (negative mood state), *purposefulness* (desire and intent to drink right now), *compulsivity* (lack of confidence in ability to quit drinking), and *expectancy* (expected positive benefits of drinking). These findings support the hypothesis[17] that craving has multidimensional manifestations, with a prominent component being the user's intention to use alcohol.

3.4. *Obsessive–Compulsive Drinking Scale*

Phenomenological similarities between alcohol dependence (especially persistent thoughts focused on obtaining and/or drinking alcohol and loss of control over drinking behavior) and obsessive–compulsive syndromes[53] suggested to some observers that alcohol craving could be conceptualized and measured in the same way as obsessions and compulsions.[54] Modell and colleagues[55] developed a ten-item interviewer-rated instrument by adapting the Yale–Brown Obsessive Compulsive Scale (YBOCS) to specifically relate to heavy drinking. This instrument, the YBOCS for heavy drinkers, successfully discriminates patients with alcoholism from nonalcoholic control subjects, and its scores are significantly correlated with global, single-item self-ratings of alcohol craving. Anton and colleagues[56,57] further adapted the YBOCS for heavy drinkers into a 14-item self-rating scale that can be self-administered in about 5 min. This Obsessive Compulsive Drinking Scale (OCDS) assesses a subjects' thoughts about drinking, their resistance to thoughts about drinking, and the distress caused by such thoughts. Scores on the OCDS have high internal consistency and good interrater and test–retest reliability and are highly correlated with scores on the YBOCS for heavy drinkers. About 20% of the variance in OCDS scores is accounted for by alcohol intake and 40–50% of the variance is shared with standard global craving measures. This suggests that the OCDS is also measuring some other component of alcohol dependence and craving, perhaps a cognitive–behavioral component as proposed in cognitive models of craving. The OCDS has been suggested for use as an outcome measure in treatment trials. It successfully discriminated drinkers from abstainers over a 12-week medication (naltrexone) treatment trial.[54]

4. Clinical Implications

4.1. *Cognitive–Behavioral*

The clinical implications of cognitive models of craving have been very influential in the treatment of alcoholism. The dominant paradigm of relapse prevention therapy and coping skills training represents a mixture of applied cognitive–behavioral techniques. The most well-developed programs are based on Marlatt's coping skills and relapse prevention model.[30,58] The cornerstone of the program is training in cognitive strategies for coping with urges and cravings and learning problem-solving and decision-making skills. Patients are prepared in advance for the possibility of a slip or a lapse into drinking by developing coping skills that can be used in high-risk situations that trigger high levels of craving.

Other cognitive techniques for coping with craving include distraction, the use of flashcards containing coping statements, imagery (i.e., image refocusing, negative image replacement, image rehearsal, and image mastery), rational responding to urge-related automatic thoughts, activity scheduling, and relaxation training.[36] The goal of these craving reduction techniques is to replace dysfunctional beliefs with ones that involve positive control and resisting the urge to drink. Although relapse prevention and cognitive therapy have become an important adjunct to behavioral[59] and pharmacological treatments, few controlled studies of their effectiveness exist.[60] Most studies of cognitive techniques of craving reduction have been restricted to anecdotal case reports.[36]

4.2. *Cue Exposure and Cue Extinction*

Exposure to alcohol-related stimuli (cues) in experimental settings is commonly associated with measurable signs of physiological arousal (e.g., increased heart rate and skin conductance) and increased alcohol craving.[61] If such conditioned responses to alcohol-related stimuli mediate craving[61] (see Section 2.1.1), then extinction of such responses might have therapeutic benefit.[62–64] In the typical paradigm, patients are exposed to alcohol-related cues while being prevented from drinking. Cues may include the taste, sight, and smell of alcohol; situations where cravings are triggered; physical sensations associated with alcohol use; and moods, thoughts, and beliefs that precede drinking. In general, five to ten sessions of cue exposure therapy are required to reduce physiological arousal to alcohol-related stimuli. Some controlled studies suggest that persons enrolled in cue extinction therapy have higher rates of abstinence, increased use of coping strategies following treatment, and longer latency to relapse compared to controls.[65,66] Other studies have found no differences in outcome using a cue extinction component as part of treatment.[7,67] These equivocal findings question the assumption that conditioned responses to alcohol-related cues play a significant role in alcohol craving and drinking. It is possible, for example, that increased reactivity to alcohol-related stimuli actually reflects a shift of attention from environmental cues to internal thoughts and feelings,[22] a process more consistent with a cognitive than a conditioning model of craving.

4.3. *Pharmacotherapy*

A wide variety of medications have been evaluated for the treatment of alcoholism, that is, for help in initiating and/or maintaining abstinence.[68,69] None of these medications appears to act directly on alcohol's neuronal binding site, and none, except disulfiram (Antabuse), alters the pharmacokinetics of alcohol. Thus, a remaining possible mechanism of action is an influence on the mechanisms that mediate craving for alcohol.

The various models of alcohol craving described above generate hypotheses as to which neural mechanisms mediate craving and therefore which medications are likely to influence alcohol craving. The models of conditioned incentive and appetitive mechanisms suggest that medications that act on the dopamine or endogenous opiate (endorphin) brain neurotransmitter systems might reduce craving, since these neurotransmitter systems are considered to mediate positive reinforcement. The model of conditioned withdrawal suggests that medications that act on the amino acid neurotransmitter systems such as glutamate and γ-aminobutyric acid (GABA) might reduce craving, since such activity is thought to influence alcohol tolerance and withdrawal.

The sensitization model suggests that anticonvulsant medications might be useful, since they might influence the neurophysiological processes of sensitization or kindling.

Craving for alcohol is often used as a surrogate dependent variable (outcome measure) to develop and test medications for treating alcohol abuse and dependence,[54] because of the presumed link between craving and drinking. Its use is especially common in residential or short-term studies, where subjects have little or no opportunity to drink alcohol, so that drinking behavior itself is not available as an outcome measure. However, many studies of both pharmacological and psychosocial treatment have reported a poor correlation between self-reported craving and actual drinking behavior, with drinking occurring in the absence of craving and craving occurring without being followed by drinking (see, for example, ref. 16). Thus, the failure of a medication to significantly decrease craving does not necessarily imply that the medication will be clinically ineffective. In fact, at least two of the craving models described above—the incentive sensitization and cognitive—explicitly predict that drinking can occur in the absence of conscious craving for alcohol.

4.3.1. Opiates. Preclinical research suggests that the endogenous opioid systems in the brain play an important role in positive reinforcement by influencing dopaminergic reward systems, both by disinhibiting dopamine activity at the level of the ventral tegmental area (VTA) (by inhibiting GABAergic inhibitory interneurons) and by enhancing dopamine activity in the nucleus accumbens.[70] Alcohol appears to stimulate endogenous opiate systems,[71] for example, alcohol produces dose-dependent increases in plasma β-endorphin levels in people at high risk for alcoholism. Transgenic mice lacking β-endorphin have decreased spontaneous alcohol intake. These findings led to the hypothesis that blocking activity in brain opioid systems, such as by administration of the μ-opioid receptor antagonists naloxone or naltrexone, would block the reinforcing effects of alcohol, and thereby reduce alcohol self-administration.

Several recent double-blind, placebo-controlled clinical trials found that naltrexone (50 mg by mouth daily) significantly reduced drinking among alcohol-dependent outpatients also receiving psychosocial treatment (counseling).[69] Self-reported alcohol craving was also significantly reduced, and patients with greater craving at the start of treatment tended to have a better response to naltrexone. While both placebo and naltrexone patients had the same tendency to restart drinking (a slip or lapse) during treatment, naltrexone patients reported less of a "high" from these drinks and were significantly less likely to have a lapse progress into a full-blown relapse. These findings suggest that naltrexone is producing its beneficial effects at least in part by reducing the positive reinforcement created by drinking alcohol.

Another opiate antagonist, nalmefene, has recently been reported in a preliminary study to reduce relapse to drinking in alcoholic outpatients in treatment but without any change in alcohol craving.[72] Analgesic doses of nitrous oxide, which is thought to activate endogenous opioid systems, have been reported to rapidly decrease craving (within 40 min) when administered as treatment for acute alcohol withdrawal.[73,74]

4.3.2. Dopamine. Dopamine is the neurotransmitter in several central nervous system (CNS) neural circuits, for example, mesolimbic and corticostriatal, proposed as important in mediating reinforcement, including the rewarding effects of abused substances such as alcohol.[70] Animals given alcohol show increased extracellular dopamine levels in mesolimbic brain areas, presumably reflecting increased synaptic dopamine release.[75] Animals given a priming dose of alcohol or exposure to environmental stimuli previously associated with alcohol self-administration also show increased extracellular dopamine levels.[70] These findings suggest that CNS dopamine activity is relevant to the conditioned incentive and reinforcement models of alcohol craving. These models would predict that medications that block dopaminergic neurotransmission, such as dopamine receptor antagonists, might reduce alcohol craving.

Limited clinical evidence is consistent with this prediction. In an experimental setting, pretreatment with the dopamine D_2 receptor antagonist haloperidol significantly reduced alcohol craving and increased resistance to drinking following a priming dose of alcohol, as compared to a double-blind placebo.[76,77] In an outpatient setting, the dopamine D_2 receptor agonist bromocriptine significantly reduced alcohol craving, but only in subjects with the A_1 allele of the D_2 receptor gene (the allele reportedly associated with more severe alcohol dependence).[78] Bromocriptine may have been working because, at the doses used, it preferentially activated presynaptic D_2 autoreceptors, thereby down-regulating dopamine synaptic activity (functionally equivalent to blockade of postsynaptic dopamine receptors).

Dopamine neural systems may also play a role in the conditioned withdrawal model of craving. It has been suggested that frequent stimulation of dopamine reward systems by chronic, heavy substance use leads to a state of relative dopamine depletion and depressed activity when substance use temporarily stops (i.e., during early abstinence). This condition of relative dopamine inactivity is experienced as substance withdrawal and is associated with craving and increased risk for relapse.[70,71] This model predicts that medications that restore normal dopamine activity, for example, dopamine receptor agonists or amino acid precursors (e.g., tyrosine) would reduce craving. This model has received much attention in terms of treatment for cocaine addiction but relatively little with respect to alcoholism, although there is some experimental evidence for decreased mesolimbic dopamine activity during early alcohol abstinence in animals.[71]

Despite the suggestive findings of a role for dopamine in alcohol craving, clinical experience with dopaminergic medications has not been generally successful. Patients on long-term treatment with D_2 receptor antagonists (e.g., schizophrenic patients taking neuroleptics such as haloperidol) do not appear to have a lower prevalence of heavy drinking or alcoholism. Early clinical trials with bromocriptine showed promise, but later controlled clinical trials have not shown significant efficacy.[68,69] However, the finding of a differential anticraving response to bromocriptine based on D_2 receptor allelic status[78] suggests that such dopamine medications may be effective in a subgroup of alcoholic patients.

4.3.3. Serotonin. Serotonin appears to play an important role in modulating appetitive behaviors, including alcohol self-administration.[68,79] Rodent studies consistently show a significant negative (inverse) correlation between brain serotonin activity and alcohol intake. Medications that increase brain serotonin activity, such as selective serotonin uptake inhibitors (SSRIs) (e.g., fluoxetine) and amino acid precursors of serotonin (e.g., tryptophan) result in decreased alcohol self-administration. In a human experimental study, *m*-chlorophenylpiperazine hydrochloride, a partial serotonin agonist, produced alcohol-like effects and alcohol craving in recently detoxified alcoholics.[80] These findings suggest that medications that increase brain serotonin activity would reduce drinking, even if not directly influencing alcohol craving.

Clinical trials of serotonergic medications have not generally shown significant efficacy in reducing drinking, except for some short-term studies of SSRIs in early problem or heavy social drinkers.[68,69] The few SSRI studies in more dependent drinkers that showed reduced drinking did not find persistent reductions, that is, any beneficial effect dissipated after about 1 week of treatment. Even in these studies, there was no consistent relationship between decreased self-reported craving and decreased drinking, although subjects with long-term abstinence did tend to have less craving.[81] Ritanserin, a 5-HT_2 receptor antagonist, and ondansetron, a 5-HT_3 receptor antagonist, have not been found clinically effective in reducing drinking, but they do decrease craving for alcohol.[79,82] These findings suggest that whatever action serotonergic medications may have on drinking, it is unlikely to be mediated through an effect on alcohol craving.

4.3.4. Amino Acid Neurotransmitters. Amino acid neurotransmitter systems play an important role in the phenomenology of alcohol withdrawal.[71] GABA is an important inhibitory neurotransmitter whose activity is decreased during alcohol withdrawal. Medications cross-tolerant with alcohol that suppress acute alcohol withdrawal, such as benzodiazepines and barbiturates, appear to act by activating brain $GABA_A$ receptors. Thus, medications that increase brain GABA activity might work as posited in the conditioned withdrawal model of craving by suppressing the experience of alcohol withdrawal. Activity of excitatory amino acid neurotransmitter systems, for example, glutamate, is increased during alcohol withdrawal. Thus, medications that decrease glutamate activity might also decrease craving by suppressing the experience of alcohol withdrawal.

At least two medications that act on amino acid neurotransmitter systems have been found to be effective in reducing drinking in clinical trials. Acamprosate (calcium *N*-acetyl-homotaurinate) is a synthetic structural analogue of GABA that has been studied in Europe but is not yet marketed in the United

States. Several double-blind, placebo-controlled trials lasting up to 12 months have found significant decreases in alcohol intake, although not associated with significant changes in self-reported alcohol craving (using a visual analogue scale).[71,83] Acamprosate appears to act, at least in part, by decreasing glutamate activity and may also increase GABA activity. In animals, acamprosate decreases the physical signs and aversiveness of alcohol withdrawal while not influencing the positive reinforcing effects of alcohol. γ-Hydroxybutyric acid is a GABA metabolite that was effective in reducing both drinking and craving in one clinical trial.[84] These findings support the efficacy of glutamate and GABA manipulations in the treatment of alcoholism and suggest a possible dissociation between glutamate and GABA in their effects on craving mechanisms.

4.3.5. Kindling. Kindling is a neurophysiological process by which intermittent, low-intensity brain stimulation, either chemical or electrical, results in an enhanced response to later low-intensity stimulation.[68] Limbic kindling due to repeated neurophysiological trauma from episodes of acute alcohol withdrawal has been postulated as a mechanism for the severity of alcohol withdrawal[85] and as a factor in making subsequent drinking episodes more severe or relapse more likely. There is limited circumstantial evidence for the kindling hypothesis in that a significant positive correlation between number of prior alcohol withdrawal episodes and current withdrawal severity has been reported, independent of total amount and duration of alcohol intake. Alcohol-related kindling has never been directly demonstrated in humans.

Kindling may also be the neurophysiological mechanism underlying sensitization, the basis of the incentive sensitization model of craving. In either event, reductions in or cessation of drinking might result in protracted withdrawal, which has been observed in animal models and is sometimes associated with long-lasting craving for alcohol in humans.[86]

The concept of alcohol-related kindling and sensitization has led to the use of anticonvulsant medications in the treatment of alcoholism, as well as alcohol withdrawal. The rationale is that such medications would retard the development of kindling and sensitization during successive episodes of acute withdrawal, thereby reducing craving and drinking. A recent small-scale (29 subjects), double-blind, placebo-controlled clinical trial did find that carbamazepine (dose adjusted to maintain a blood concentration around 6.0 μg/ml) significantly reduced drinking over the 12-month study period,[87] consistent with this rationale. Assessments of alcohol craving were not reported. The anticonvulsant phenytoin (diphenylhydantoin, Dilantin) has been reported to reduce craving when used to treat acute alcohol withdrawal.[88]

5. Directions for the Future

Despite a variety of craving definitions and assessment instruments used in clinical research, until recently there was substantial consistency in the underlying models of craving and of its measurement. Most models of alcohol craving explicitly or implicitly assumed that there is a consistent and positive relationship between craving (the conscious urge or desire to use alcohol) and drinking behavior. Most instruments for assessing craving assumed it was a univariate construct and often included only one or a few items. More recently, several multi-item and multidimensional craving rating instruments have been developed that offer the promise of more useful assessment of clinically relevant behavior. At least two craving models have recently been proposed—incentive sensitization[15] and the cognitive theory of drug use and drug urges[17]—that explicitly reject any consistent, positive relationship between conscious craving and drinking. These models may account better than older models for the frequent clinical observation of dissociation between self-reported alcohol craving and actual drinking behavior (see, for example, ref. 16). Each model awaits validation by further clinical research; meanwhile, they generate important research and treatment implications.

Several models of alcohol craving, especially conditioned incentive, appetitive, and incentive sensitization,[15] emphasize the significant role of the mesolimbic dopamine system in mediating the reinforcing effects of alcohol. This suggests that dopaminergic manipulations might be effective in reducing alcohol craving and drinking. While clinical trials of dopamine medications have generally not been very successful, circumstantial physiological evidence does support a role for the mesolimbic dopamine system in alcohol craving.

Decreased delta and increased alpha brain wave activities have been reported in the electroencephalograms of some alcohol patients.[89,90] Biofeedback training that reduced alpha wave activity has been associated with decreased alcohol craving.[91] A main source of delta brain wave activity in humans is the medial frontal cortex, the major cortical terminus of dopamine projections from the midbrain VTA.[92] Experimentally induced alcohol craving in a group of alcohol-dependent research subjects was highly correlated with increased blood flow in the head of the right caudate nucleus,[45] a part of the limbic striatum with dopaminergic synapses. This brain region also shows increased blood flow in patients with obsessive–compulsive disorder, supporting a possible neurophysiological similarity between this condition and loss of control over alcohol use. Future research should use modern techniques of brain imaging, for example, quantitative electroencephalograms, PET scanning, and functional magnetic resonance imaging, to localize brain areas associated with the experience of alcohol craving, both in the natural state and after administration of putative treatment medications.

The cognitive model of drug use and drug urges[17] deemphasizes the role of motivational mechanisms in craving for alcohol and assigns a central role to attention, memory, and other higher-order cognitive functions.[38–46] Modern brain-imaging techniques offer a powerful new approach for exploring the neural mechanisms underlying cognitive functioning and its association with alcohol craving and alcohol dependence. The cognitive model also generates important clinical implications. It predicts that cognitive therapies targeted at relapse prevention, coping skills training, and cue extinction will be effective in reducing drinking, regardless of changes in the subjective motivational experience termed "craving." Future research should include controlled clinical trials of these cognitive therapies, as well as other potentially useful cognitive approaches that are conceptually linked to information-processing theory, such as alcohol expectancy (an individual's expectations about the consequences of drinking or abstaining) and self-efficacy (an individual's beliefs about the ability to abstain from drinking). Future studies should attend to possible subtypes or differentiating characteristics among alcoholic patients, which may be associated with differential response to treatment. There is no a priori reason why the same alcohol craving mechanisms must operate in all individuals or why craving must respond to a treatment intervention in the same way in all patients.

Because craving is still an important factor in many models of alcoholism and its treatment, and craving measures are often used to evaluate the state of the disorder and an individual's response to treatment, there is a need for a better natural history of alcohol craving. Future research should include prospective, long-term, large-scale studies that evaluate the relationship between alcohol craving and drinking behavior in both normal drinkers and alcoholic drinkers, starting before the development of problem drinking and continuing throughout treatment interventions and long-term abstinence. For example, there should be systematic inquiry into how alcoholics cope with the consequences of experiencing craving, how the desire to use alcohol influences abstinence, and how patients plan and make decisions as to what steps to take when they crave alcohol.

To allow these studies to be successful, valid and reliable means of assessing craving for alcohol are necessary. Craving measures should cover a broad range of content, yet be easy to administer and score. A major challenge is the fact that craving has multiple meanings. This points out the need for researchers and clinicians to be explicit about the definitions and measures of craving that they are using and, to the extent possible, to use comparable definitions and measures. Future research should systematically evaluate the usefulness in various settings of one-dimensional versus multidimensional measures of craving and compare verbal self-report measures with psychophysiological measures such as cue reactivity and with neuropsychological measures of cognitive processing such as reaction time.[39,40]

In summary, there appears to be little consensus in the literature on what craving for alcohol means, the best way to measure it, what mechanism accounts for the urge to drink, or what is its true relationship to alcohol use. No single model or theory of craving accounts for the wide variation in findings reviewed here, suggesting that multiple mechanisms may be involved. A comprehensive, multidisciplinary approach is necessary to elucidate the true nature of craving for alcohol and its clinical implications.

References

1. Kozlowski LT, Mann RE, Wilkinson DA, *et al:* "Cravings" are ambiguous: Ask about urges or desires. *Addict Behav* 14:443–445, 1989.
2. Kozlowski LT, Wilkinson DA: Use and misuse of the concept of craving by alcohol, tobacco, and drug researchers. *Br J Addict* 82:31–45, 1987.
3. Martin CS, Kaczynski NA, Maisto SA, *et al:* Patterns of DSM-IV alcohol abuse and dependence symptoms in adolescent drinkers. *J Stud Alcohol* 56:672–680, 1995.
4. American Psychiatric Association: *Diagnostic and Statistical Manual of Mental Disorders.* 4th ed. Washington, DC, Author, 1995, p 176.
5. Hunt WA: Neuroscience research: How it has contributed to our understanding of alcohol abuse and alcoholism? A review. *Alcohol Clin Exp Res* 17:1055–1065, 1993.
6. Anderson P, Cremona A, Paton A, *et al:* The risk of alcohol. *Addiction* 88:1493–1508, 1993.
7. Glautier S, Remington B: The form of responses to drug cues, in Drummond DC, Tiffany ST, Glautier S, *et al* (eds): *Addictive Behaviour: Cue Exposure Theory and Practice.* Chichester, England, John Wiley & Sons, 1995, pp 21–46.
8. Tiffany ST: Potential functions of classical conditioning in drug addiction, in Drummond DC, Tiffany ST, Glautier S, *et al* (eds): *Addictive Behaviour: Cue Exposure Theory and Practice.* Chichester, England, John Wiley & Sons, 1995, pp 47–74.
9. Frascella J, Brown RM: Preface. *NIDA Res Monogr* 124:v–vii, 1992.
10. Stewart J, deWit H, Eikelboom R: Role of unconditioned and conditioned drug effects in the self-administration of opiates and stimulates. *Psychol Rev* 91:251–268, 1984.
11. Stewart J, Eikelboom R: Conditioned drug effects, in Iversen LI, Iversen SD, Snyder SH (eds): *New Directions in Behavioral Pharmacology,* vol 19. New York, Plenum, 1988, pp 1–57.
12. Roshenow DJ, Niaura RS, Childress AR, *et al:* Cue reactivity in addictive behaviors: Theoretical and treatment implications. *Int J Addict* 25:957–993, 1990.
13. Roshenow DJ, Monti PM, Abrams DB: Cue exposure treatment in alcohol dependence, in Drummond DC, Tiffany ST, Glautier S, *et al* (eds): *Addictive Behaviour: Cue Exposure Theory and Practice.* Chichester, England, John Wiley & Sons, 1995, pp 169–196.
14. Markou A, Weiss F, Gold LH, *et al:* Animal models of drug craving. *Psychopharmacology* 112:163–182, 1993.
15. Robinson TE, Berridge KC: The neural basis of drug craving: An incentive-sensitization theory of addiction. *Brain Res Rev* 18:247–291, 1993.
16. Miller NS, Gold MS: Dissociation of "conscious desire" (craving) from and relapse in alcohol and cocaine dependence. *Ann Clin Psychiatry* 6:99–106, 1994.
17. Tiffany, ST: A cognitive model of drug urges and drug-use behavior: Role of automatic and nonautomatic processes. *Psychol Rev* 97:147–168, 1990.
18. Siegel S: Pharmacological conditioning and drug effects, in Goudie AJ, Emmett-Oglesby MW (eds): *Psychoactive Drugs: Tolerance and Sensitization.* Clifton, NJ, Humana Press, 1989, pp 115–180.
19. McCusker CG, Brown K: Alcohol-predictive cues enhance tolerance to and precipitate "craving" for alcohol in social drinkers. *J Stud Alcohol* 51:494–499, 1990.
20. Ludwig AM, Wikler A: Craving and relapse to drink. *Q J Stud Alcohol* 35:108–130, 1974.
21. Ludwig AM: Pavlov's "bells" and alcohol craving. *Addict Behav* 11:87–91, 1986.
22. Laberg JC: What is presented, and what prevented, in cue exposure and response prevention with alcohol dependent subjects? *Addict Behav* 15:367–386, 1990.
23. Newlin DB: A comparison of drug conditioning and craving for alcohol and cocaine, in Galanter M (ed): *Recent Developments in Alcoholism,* vol 10. New York, Plenum, 1992, pp 147–164.
24. Rosse RB, Miller MW, Hess AL, *et al:* Measures of visual scanning as a predictor of cocaine cravings and urges. *Biol Psychol* 33:554–556, 1993.
25. Berridge KC, Robinson RE: The mind of an addicted brain: Neural sensitization of wanting versus liking. *Curr Directions Psychol Sci* 4:71–76, 1995.

26. Hunt WA, Lands WEM: A role for behavioral sensitization in uncontrolled ethanol intake. *Alcohol* 9:327–328, 1992.
27. Masur J, Boerngen R: The excitatory component of ethanol in mice: A chronic study. *Pharmacol Biochem Behav* 13:777–780, 1980.
28. Cunningham CL, Noble D: Conditioned activation induced by ethanol: Role in sensitization and conditioned place preference. *Pharmacol Biochem Behav* 47:307–313, 1992.
29. Benjamin D, Grant ER, Goldstein KR, *et al:* Sensitization to the dopamine release-enhancing effects of ethanol demonstrated in male Long-Evans rats. *Soc Neurosc Abstr* 18:43, 1992.
30. Wilson GT: Cognitive studies in alcoholism. *J Consult Clin Psychol* 55:325–331, 1987.
31. Cox WM, Klinger E: A motivational model of alcohol use. *J Abnorm Psychol* 97:168–180, 1988.
32. Marlatt GA, Gordon JR: *Relapse Prevention and Maintenance Strategies in the Treatment of Addictive Behaviors.* New York, Guilford Press, 1985.
33. Laberg JC, Bjerland T, Nordby H, *et al:* Autonomic cued reactivity in alcoholics: The effect of olfactory stimuli. *Addict Behav* 20:571–584, 1995.
34. Rees VW, Heather N: Individual differences and cue reactivity, in Drummond DC, Tiffany ST, Glautier S, *et al* (eds): *Addictive Behaviour: Cue Exposure Theory and Practice.* Chichester, England, John Wiley & Sons, 1995, pp 99–118.
35. Cooney NL, Gillespie RA, Baker LH, *et al:* Cognitive changes after alcohol cue exposure. *J Consult Clin Psychol* 55:150–155, 1987.
36. Beck AT, Wright FD, Newman CD, *et al: Cognitive Therapy of Drug Abuse.* New York, Guilford Press, 1993.
37. Thombs DL: *Introduction to Addictive Behaviors.* New York, Guilford Press, 1993.
38. Sherrill TD, Douglas TE, Singleton EG, *et al:* The use of simulated conditions to identify the effects of craving among alcohol users. Baltimore, Maryland, Division of Intramural Research, National Institute on Drug Abuse, June 1994, unpublished research.
39. Cepeda-Benito A, Tiffany ST: The use of a dual-task procedure for the assessment of cognitive effort associated with cigarette craving. *Psychopharmacology* 127:155–163, 1996.
40. Sayette MA, Monti PM, Rosenhow DJ, *et al:* The effects of cue exposure on reaction time in male alcoholics. *J Stud Alcohol* 103:629–633, 1995.
41. Bradizza CM, Lisman SA, Payne DG: A test of Tiffany's cognitive model of drug urges and drug-use behavior. *Alcohol Clin Exp Res* 19:1043–1047, 1995
42. Singleton EG: Development of a questionnaire to assess human drug craving appropriate for use with African Americans and other culturally or socially defined groups. Baltimore, Maryland, Johns Hopkins University Medical School, November 1996, Unpublished manuscript.
43. Douglas TE, Singleton EG, Henningfield JE: The relationship between craving and neuropsychological functioning. *NIDA Res Monogr* 153:289, 1995.
44. Stacy AW, Ames SL, Sussman, *et al:* Implicit cognition in adolescent drug use. *Psychol Addict Behav* 10:190–203, 1996.
45. Modell JG, Mountz JM: Focal cerebral blood flow change during craving for alcohol measured by SPECT. J Neuropsychiatry Clin Neurosci 7:15–22, 1995.
46. Grant S, London ED, Newlin D: Activation of a cortical memory circuit is related to cue-elicited cocaine craving. *Proc Nat Acad Sci USA* 93:12040, 1996.
47. Pickens RW, Johanson C-E: Craving: Consensus of status and agenda for future research. *Drug Alcohol Depend* 30:127–131, 1992.
48. Newlin DB, Hotchkiss B, Cox WM, *et al:* Autonomic and subjective responses to alcohol stimuli with appropriate control stimuli. *Addict Behav* 14:625–630, 1989.
49. Kozlowski LT, Pillitteri JL, Sweeney CT, *et al:* Asking questions about urges or cravings for cigarettes. *Psychol Addict Behav* 10:248–260, 1996.
50. Bohn MJ, Krahn DD, Staeler BA: Development and initial validation of a measure of drinking urges in abstinent alcoholics. *Alcohol Clin Exp Res* 19:600–606, 1995.
51. Glautier S, Drummond DC: Alcohol dependence and cue reactivity. *J Stud Alcohol* 55:224–229, 1994.
52. Singleton EG, Tiffany ST, Henningfield JE: Development and validation of a new questionnaire to assess craving for alcohol. *NIDA Res Monogr* 153:289, 1995.

53. Caetano R: Alcohol dependence and the need to drink: A compulsion? *Psychol Med* 15:463–469, 1985.
54. Anton RF: New methodologies for pharmacological treatment trials for alcohol dependence. *Alcohol Clin Exp Res* 20(7 Suppl):3A–9A, 1996.
55. Modell JG, Glaser FB, Cyr L, *et al:* Obsessive and compulsive characteristics of craving for alcohol in alcohol abuse and dependence. *Alcohol Clin Exp Res* 16:272–274, 1992.
56. Anton RF, Moak DH, Latham P: The Obsessive Compulsive Drinking Scale: A self-rated instrument for the quantification of thoughts about alcohol and drinking behavior. *Alcohol Clin Exp Res* 19:92–99, 1995.
57. Anton RF, Moak DH, Latham PK: The Obsessive Compulsive Drinking Scale: A new method of assessing outcome in alcoholism treatment studies. *Arch Gen Psychiatry* 53:225–231, 1996.
58. Marlatt GA: Cognitive factors in the relapse process, in Marlatt GA, Gordon JR (eds): *Relapse Prevention.* New York, Guilford Press, 1985, pp 128–200.
59. Monti PM, Rohsenow DJ, Rubonis AV, *et al:* Cue exposure with coping skills treatment for male alcoholics: A preliminary investigation. *J Consult Clin Psychol* 61:1011–1019, 1993.
60. Dimeff LA, Marlatt GA: Relapse prevention, in Hester RK, Miller WR (eds): *Handbook of Alcoholism Treatment Approaches.* Boston, Allyn and Bacon, 1995, pp 176–194.
61. Childress AR, Hole AV, Ehrman RN: Cue reactivity and cue reactivity interventions in drug dependence. *NIDA Res Monogr* 137:73–95, 1993.
62. Roshenow DJ, Monti PM, Abrams DB: Cue exposure treatment in alcohol dependence, in Drummond DC, Tiffany ST, Glautier S, *et al* (eds): *Addictive Behaviour: Cue Exposure Theory and Practice.* Chichester, England, John Wiley & Sons, 1995, pp 169–198.
63. Drummond DC, Tiffany ST, Glautier S, *et al:* Cue exposure in understanding and treating addictive behaviours, in Drummond DC, Tiffany ST, Glautier S, *et al* (eds): *Addictive Behaviour: Cue Exposure Theory and Practice.* Chichester, England, John Wiley & Sons, 1995, pp 1–20.
64. Walitzer KS, Sher KJ: Alcohol cue reactivity and ad lib drinking in young men at risk for alcoholism. *Addict Behav* 15:29–46, 1990.
65. Drummond DC, Glautier SP: A controlled trial of cue exposure treatment in alcohol dependence. *J Consult Clin Psychol* 62:809–817, 1994.
66. Monti PM, Rohsenow DJ, Rubonis AV, *et al:* Alcohol cue reactivity: Effects of detoxification and extended cue exposure. *J Stud Alcohol* 54:235–245, 1993.
67. Newlin DB: Craving for alcohol and cocaine: From inside the brain to the clinic. *Alcohol Clin Exp Res* 20:45A–47A, 1996.
68. Gorelick DA: Pharmacological treatment of alcoholism, in Galanter M (ed): *Recent Developments in Alcoholism,* vol 11. New York, Plenum Press, 1993, pp 413–427.
69. Litten RZ, Allen J, Fertig J: Pharmacotherapies for alcohol problems: A review of research with focus on developments since 1991. *Alcohol Clin Exp Res* 20:859–876, 1996.
70. Van Ree JM: Endorphins and experimental addiction. *Alcohol* 13:25–30, 1996.
71. Spanagel R, Zieglgansberger W: Anti-craving compounds for ethanol: New pharmacological tools to study addictive processes. *Trends Pharmacol Sci* 18:54–59, 1997.
72. Mason BJ: Dosing issues in the pharmacotherapy of alcoholism. *Alcohol Clin Exp Res* 20(7 Suppl):10A–16A, 1996.
73. Daynes G, Gillman MA: Psychotropic analgesic nitrous oxide prevents craving after withdrawal for alcohol, cannabis and tobacco. *Int J Neurosci* 76:13–16, 1994.
74. Ojurkangas R, Gillman MA: Psychotropic analgesic nitrous oxide for treating alcohol withdrawal in an outpatient setting. *Int J Neurosci* 76:35–39, 1994.
75. Di Chiara G, Imperato A: Drugs abused by humans preferentially increase synaptic dopamine concentrations in the mesolimbic system of freely moving rats. *Proc Natl Acad Sci USA* 87:5274–5278, 1988.
76. Modell JG, Mountz JM, Glaser FB, *et al:* Effect of haloperidol on measures of craving and impaired control in alcoholic subjects. *Alcohol Clin Exp Res* 17:234–240, 1993.
77. Mountz JM, Modell JG, Beresford TP: Basal ganglia/limbic striatal and thalamocortical involvement in craving and loss of control in alcoholism. *J Neuropsychiatry Clin Neurosci* 2:123–144, 1990.

78. Lawford BR, Young RM, Rowell JA, *et al:* Bromocriptine in the treatment of alcoholics with the D2 dopamine receptor A1 allele. *Nat Med* 1:337–341, 1995.
79. Sellers EM, Higgins GA, Sobell MB: 5-HT and alcohol abuse. *Trends Pharmacol Sci* 13:69–75, 1992.
80. Krystal JH, Webb E, Cooney N, *et al:* Specificity of ethanol-like effects elicited by serotonergic and noradrenergic mechanisms. *Arch Gen Psychiatry* 51:898–911, 1994.
81. Kabel DI, Petty F: A placebo-controlled, double-blind study of fluoxetine in severe alcohol dependence: Adjunctive pharmacotherapy during and after inpatient treatment. *Alcohol Clin Exp Res* 20:780–784, 1996.
82. Naranjo CA, Poulos CX, Lanctot KL, *et al:* Ritanserin, a central 5-HT2 antagonist, in heavy social drinkers: Desire to drink, alcohol intake and related effects. *Addiction* 90:893–905, 1995.
83. Littleton J: Acamprosate in alcohol dependence: How does it work? *Addiction* 90:1179–1188, 1995.
84. Gallimberti L, Ferri M, Ferrara SD, *et al:* Gamma-hydroxybutyric acid in the treatment of alcohol dependence: A double-blind study. *Alcohol Clin Exp Res* 16:673–676, 1992.
85. Langley M: Posttraumatic stress disorder and addiction: What are the links? in Miller NS (ed): *The Principles and Practice of Addictions in Psychiatry*. Philadelphia, Saunders, 1997, pp 284–285.
86. Satel SL, Kosten TR, Schuckit MA, *et al:* Should protracted withdrawal from drugs be included in DSM-IV? *Am J Psychiatry* 150:695–704, 1993.
87. Mueller TI, Stout RL, Rudden S, *et al:* A double-blind, placebo-controlled pilot study of carbamazepine for the treatment of alcohol dependence. *Alcohol Clin Exp Res* 21:86–92, 1997.
88. Ilyuchina VA, Nikitina LI: Clinical physiological study of the therapeutic effects of phenytoin in acute alcohol withdrawal and the asthenic-autonomic syndrome in patients with chronic alcoholism. *Alcohol* 12:511–517, 1995.
89. Herning RI: Cognitive event-related potentials in populations at risk for substance abuse. *NIDA Res Monogr* 159:161–179, 1996.
90. Brigham J, Moss HB, Tarter RE, *et al:* Event-related potential differential of prepubertal sons of alcoholics and substance abusers. *Psychophysiology* 30(Suppl):21, 1993.
91. Fahrion SL, Walters ED, Coyne L, *et al:* Alterations in EEG amplitude, personality factors, and brain electrical mapping after alpha-theta brain wave training: A controlled case study of an alcoholic in recovery. *Alcohol Clin Exp Res* 16:547–552, 1992.
92. Prichep LS, Alper KR, Kowalik S, *et al:* Quantitative electroencephalographic characteristics of crack cocaine dependence. *Biol Psychiatry* 40:986–993, 1996.

7

A Review of the Effects of Moderate Alcohol Intake on Psychiatric and Sleep Disorders

Ricardo Castaneda, Norman Sussman, Robert Levy, Mary O'Malley, and Laurence Westreich

Abstract. In this chapter we discuss the effects of moderate ethanol consumption on the treatment of psychiatric and sleep disorders. A review of the literature on the interactions of ethanol with neurotransmitters and psychotropic medications suggests that although ethanol affects the clinical course of psychiatric and sleep disorders by different mechanisms, it does so principally through perturbations it causes in the balance of central nervous system neurotransmitter systems, which may modify the clinical course of primary psychiatric and sleep disorders and undermine the therapeutic response to psychotropic medications. Neurotransmitter responses may also be manifested clinically by rebound phenomena, akin to a subsyndromal withdrawal, which affect sleep and precipitate anxiety and mood symptoms. In addition, ethanol also modifies the clearance and disposition of a variety of psychotropic metabolites and interferes with their clinical effectiveness.

We recommend that most psychiatric patients, and all patients with sleep disorders, should abstain from even moderate ethanol use, as this may adversely affect their clinical course and response to treatment.

1. Introduction

Minimal attention has been paid to the clinical consequences of moderate or "social" drinking by individuals with psychiatric or sleep disorders, whether

Ricardo Castaneda, Norman Sussman, Robert Levy, Mary O'Malley, and Laurence Westreich • Department of Psychiatry, New York University School of Medicine, Bellevue Hospital Medical Center, New York, New York 10016.

Recent Developments in Alcoholism, Volume 14: The Consequences of Alcoholism, edited by Galanter. Plenum Press, New York, 1998.

they are taking psychotropic medications or not. Although general or moralistic comments are frequently offered to these patients in the hope of preventing complications such as the development of addiction or toxicity, they are largely unsubstantiated by any consensus in the field. In the treatment setting there is little discussion of the possible complications of moderate alcohol use resulting from its ability to alter both brain functioning and the metabolism of prescribed medications.[1]

The body's responses to ethanol vary according to the intensity and frequency of ethanol consumption. Moderate use of ethanol is accepted as a healthy or at least harmless practice. Individuals with psychiatric and sleep disorders, however, may experience adverse clinical consequences from even modest alcohol ingestion. These effects reflect the process of adaptation to the influence of ethanol on a wide range of neurotransmitter and other body systems. Acute alcohol ingestion depresses some neurotransmitters and stimulates others, and there is abundant evidence that psychiatric disorders, particularly those involving mood and anxiety disturbances, are associated with underlying dysfunction of one or more neurotransmitter system.[2] Thus, it is reasonable to expect that psychiatric patients, compared with the general population, would display more extreme or unpredictable responses to the effects of ethanol on the central nervous system (CNS).

Alcohol is just one of numerous factors, external and internal, that affects the course of psychiatric disorders. For example, certain exogenous agents such as alcohol, nicotine, over-the-counter cold preparations, cannabis, and cocaine, and habits such as sleep deprivation, diet, exercise, and hyperventilation, as well as life stressors, all seem capable of eliciting panic symptoms,[3] and even small amounts of ethanol have been associated with the development of anxiety and mood symptoms.[4] Evidence suggests that alcohol use, even when it conforms to normal or social patterns, significantly complicates the clinical course and treatment of mood and anxiety disorders and warrants very specific attention by clinicians.[5,6]

While occasional ethanol and marijuana do not induce next-day behavioral problems among healthy asymptomatic individuals,[4] clinical observation confirms that increased quantities of alcohol consumed per drinking occasion are associated with increased symptoms of depression and anxiety in the sober state.[5] The acute influence of alcohol on the CNS elicits adaptive mechanisms, such as an increase in excitatory neurotransmitters,[7] that counteracts ethanol's mostly depressant effects. Even a single dose of ethanol may influence the CNS after blood ethanol levels have significantly decreased. In all likelihood, these CNS adaptive changes outlive the presence of ethanol in the system.

Ethanol-induced cognitive disruption may also impair otherwise successful coping mechanisms and initiate the development of psychiatric symptoms.[5] Some alterations of brain functions such as alertness, judgment, impulse control, decision making, and mood, which result from recent ethanol consumption, could conceivably be wrongly interpreted by the patient as proof of a relapse of primary psychiatric symptoms, paradoxically precipitating the formation of symptoms.

Normal and pathological consumption of ethanol may influence the clinical course of psychiatric disorders by several mechanisms. These include, particularly, ethanol's effects on neurotransmitter systems and on the pharmacology and pharmacokinetics of other drugs, including antianxiety agents, antidepressants, hypnotics, antipsychotics, and mood stabilizers. Ethanol modifies the clearance and disposition of many psychotropic metabolites, which interferes with the acute clinical course of primary psychiatric disorders.

Clinical observations suggest that neurotransmitter alterations may also underlie a rebound phenomena, akin to a subsyndromal withdrawal state. Adaptive changes in the level of activity of excitatory neurotransmitters may affect sleep, cognition, and alertness and may precipitate behavioral, mood, psychotic, and anxiety symptoms. Also, symptoms that are a direct consequence of recent alcohol use may alter the subjective interpretation of the patient's "internal milieu," causing confusion and eliciting reactive psychopathology.[6]

Chronic alcohol use and alcoholism, on the other hand, are associated with massive alterations in brain functioning and cause both morphological and biochemical changes, contributing severe mood symptomatology of their own.

What follows is a discussion of the effects of moderate alcohol use on the CNS and on several disorders including schizophrenia, anxiety and mood disorders, depression, sleep disorders, personality, attention deficit disorders, and dementia. In addition, a review of pharmacokinetics and pharmacodynamics of ethanol and psychotropics closes the chapter.

2. Central Nervous System

The diverse phenomena involved in the CNS response to acute alcohol ingestion, as well as the development of craving, tolerance, and dependence to chronic alcohol consumption, are only partially understood. Yet the brain responses to acute consumption of ethanol among different neurotransmitter systems are generally different from those observed in states associated with chronic use, such as dependence and withdrawal. The fact is that alcohol abusers react differently to alcohol than moderate drinkers.

Dopamine turnover, for example, although increased during initial exposure to alcohol, is decreased during chronic administration.[8] Initially, ethanol facilitates the transmission of γ-aminobutyric acid (GABA) and inhibits glutamatergic function, but tolerance associated with chronic ethanol consumption leads to a reduced GABAergic and increased glutamatergic function.[9,10] It should be noted that profiles of neurotransmission associated with genetic loading for risk for alcoholism differ from controls, presumably including those at risk for other psychiatric disorders. For example, reduced blood

GABA-like activity is found among adults with alcoholic fathers when compared to controls.[11] Decreases in glutamate binding to *N*-methyl-D-asparate (NMDA) receptor in the hippocampus have been found in both male rats subjected to 5 days of ethanol administration and in the brains of alcoholics.[12] Ethanol-preferring rats have fewer dopamine D_2 receptors in the limbic system,[13] and males at high risk for alcoholism display reduced serum prolactin levels following ethanol administration as compared with controls.[14] Furthermore, studies of genetic animal models of withdrawal suggest that genes influencing the severity of alcohol withdrawal are different from those mediating sensitivity and tolerance.[15]

The phenomena associated with CNS responses to ethanol range from genetic factors influencing predisposition to alcohol abuse and dependence to neurochemical adaptive mechanisms in various neuronal receptor systems, including the norepinephrine and the dopaminergic neurons, GABA receptor-coupled chloride channel, the NMDA receptor-gated ion channel, the serotonin 5-HT_3 receptor-coupled potassium channels, and the stimulatory G-protein, Gs.[16] Other systems such as those governing calcium channel flux[17] and arginine vasopressin (AVP)[18] are also affected by ethanol. Specific interactions with ethanol have been reported for the major neurotransmitters such as glutamate,[19] norepinephrine,[7] dopamine,[8] serotonin,[20] GABA,[21] and others, and for signal transduction systems such as adenylate cyclase and consequently, cyclic adenosine 3′, 5′-monophosphate (cAMP).[22] Dopaminergic and noradrenergic mechanisms and the endogenous opiate systems appear to affect the reinforcing effects of ethanol. The serotonergic system, in turn, seems to mediate negative reinforcement of compulsive use. Several ligands of the dopaminergic, serotonergic, and opioidergic receptors involved in ethanol consumption-related behaviors reduce preference for ethanol and modify the expression of the syndrome of withdrawal. The central cholinergic systems plays a noteworthy role only among alcoholics, probably underlying the detrimental effects of ethanol on learning and memory.[23] It seems that the sedative and anxiolytic effects of ethanol may be mediated by the GABA–benzodiazepine receptor complex.[24] Ethanol also alters ligand binding to μ and δ receptors and may increase endogenous opiate system activity, either by increasing enkephalin levels or by producing opiatelike alkaloids from acetaldehyde.[22,25,26] Such widespread effects are likely to influence not only the course of psychiatric disorders but also the putative effects of psychotropics on neurotransmitters systems in the brain.

Profiles of genetic expression that likely determine the patterns of neurotransmission and predisposition to psychiatric disorders,[2] such as alcoholism, mood, or psychotic disorders, are also likely to determine the nature of an individual's response to ethanol. Individuals genetically predisposed to developing alcoholism, for example, may go on to display compulsive patterns of drinking upon repeated exposure to ethanol.[27] Such a behavioral response probably occurs in the context of a specific neurotransmission profile. It may be that, in the same way that repeated exposure to ethanol evokes compulsive drinking among individuals at risk for alcoholism, ethanol may also provoke specific behavioral responses among individuals who are genetically predisposed to other psychiatric disorders.

Even less is known about the neurobiology associated with personality disorders. Alterations in serotonergic neurotransmission have been reported among psychopathic individuals,[28] and damage or anomalies of specific brain structures have been implicated in behavioral abnormalities and aggression. Damage to the dorsal convexity, for example, results in a diminution of long-term planning and a state of apathy or indifference, which in turn leads to impairment of problem-solving abilities.[29] It also is well known by now that damage to the orbital undersurface of the frontal lobe results in a character change marked by irresponsibility and superficial, reflexive emotional responses to the environment.[30]

Even in small amounts ethanol has widespread effects on the body. Although its impact on cell membranes and lipids has been recognized since the beginning of this century,[31,32] its effects on membrane proteins[16] and specific neurotransmitters have been identified more recently.[8]

Ethanol affects the function of most body organs because of its effects on the CNS and its disruption of the cellular milieu as ethanol freely diffuses across cell membranes and body fluids. CNS phenomena associated with ethanol include ethanol's direct pharmacological effects such as behavioral excitation, incoordination, sedation, and ataxia and the withdrawal syndrome characterized by CNS hyperexcitability, reflecting neuroadaptation to ethanol's depressant effects.[33] Ethanol's neuroendocrine effects, however, are also noteworthy, particularly since they are different in populations at risk for alcoholism. Acute ethanol ingestion in sons of alcoholics, for example, results in lower plasma levels of adrenocorticotropin hormone (ACTH) than in sons of nonalcoholics.[34] These findings would suggest that changes in cortisol activity associated with drinking include responses by the pituitary as well as the adrenal glands. Whether cortisol responses to ethanol are related to subsequent risk of alcoholism, however, is unclear. Recent studies have found no differences in ACTH and cortisol response to ovine corticotropin-releasing hormone and ethanol among sons of alcoholics and controls.[35] Nevertheless, any ethanol-related increases in cortisol activity are likely to significantly contribute to the overall profile of neuroadaptation to ethanol ingestion. The course of alcohol withdrawal, which to a large extent reflects a neurological rebound from abrupt reduction of ethanol intake, is influenced by the relative activity of different neurotransmitters.[33] Stimulant withdrawal, for example, recently has been demonstrated to reduce the severity of concurrent alcohol withdrawal,[36] a finding that probably reflects the contrasting neurotransmitter changes associated with the chronic abuse of each substance.

3. Schizophrenia

A growing body of evidence suggests that chronic substance abuse may induce psychosis. Boutros and Bowers[37] report that use of illicit drugs [particularly phencyclidine (PCP), amphetamines, and lysergic acid diethylamide (LSD)] can produce a persistent drug-induced psychotic state, which may be difficult to distinguish from idiopathic schizophrenia. They noted that drug-induced psychosis correlated with three factors: dosage, frequency of use, and genetic vulnerability. The final factor raises the question of whether substance abuse precipitated or hastened the onset of schizophrenia in biologically susceptible individuals. In one longitudinal study of PCP abusers, after 8 years, 80% were still on neuroleptics and 60% were officially diagnosed with undifferentiated or residual schizophrenia. In a 1986 study, 10% of individuals with history of chronic, heavy amphetamine abuse developed a chronic psychotic disorder lasting more than 6 months after assertion of amphetamine use.[37]

These data are related to patients who consume alcohol, both because of neurochemical similarities between the effects of ethanol and those of certain recreational drugs and because of the observation that alcohol may also produce chronic psychotic symptoms, such as alcohol hallucinosis. Unfortunately, most studies of substance use in schizophrenia have included both drugs and alcohol, the latter generally in substantial quantities. Noordsy *et al.*[38] have looked at moderate alcohol use as well as alcohol use disorders in schizophrenia; however, they cite a 14 to 51% comorbidity rate between schizophrenia and alcohol abuse in various studies, which have also associated alcohol use disorders in schizophrenia with exacerbation of delusions, depressive symptoms, disruptive behaviors, assaultiveness, impaired judgment, and homelessness. In their study of rural schizophrenics, many of whom used alcohol only moderately, there appeared to be an equal likelihood of exacerbation or amelioration of psychotic symptoms by ethanol. A majority of the patients they interviewed cited improvements in social anxiety, tension, dysphoria, apathy, and sleep disturbance associated with alcohol use,[38] but the reliability and insightfulness of the respondents are open to question.

With chronic alcohol use there is eventually a loss of the increase in dopamine synthesis (although there is no tolerance to the inhibition of dopamine reuptake), in addition to the supersensitization of dopamine receptors. Cessation of chronic drinking may increase dopamine levels in the frontal cortex during withdrawal. Based on these ethanol-induced changes in dopaminergic function in the CNS, it may come as no surprise that an increase in central dopaminergic activity and an alteration in receptor sensitivity have been reported in alcohol hallucinosis.[39]

Tsai *et al.*[10] describe that chronic use of alcohol may induce changes in the striatum, thalamus, and hippocampus that compensate for the inhibition of glutamatergic transmission. Thus, prolonged inhibition of the NMDA receptor by ethanol results in the development of supersensitivity, with an increase in the NMDA receptors through which calcium cations can enter the cell. The up-regulation of glutamate receptors in the locus ceruleus can enhance the noradrenergic system's activity and may account for the autonomic instability, agitation, and psychosis seen in alcohol withdrawal states (along with the increase in glutamatergic stimulation of dopaminergic neurons also seen following alcohol cessation). Finally, alcohol can inhibit long-term potentiation in the hippocompus via this inhibitory effect on NMDA receptors, an effect it has in common with PCP.[10]

These glutamatergic effects of alcohol are of particular interest when considered in light of findings regarding glutamate receptor dysfunction in schizophrenia. Krystal *et al.*[40] reported that ketamine and PCP, both NMDA antagonists, produce behavior similar to positive and negative symptoms of schizophrenia, including paranoia, loosening of associations, tangentiality, concreteness, referential thinking, unusual thought content, changes in bodily perception, auditory hallucinations (at high dosages), emotional withdrawal, affective blunting, psychomotor retardation, and impairment of thought and speech. The observations that ketamine and PCP could induce these symptoms in normal controls and that PCP can produce a protracted exacerbation of symptoms in schizophrenics have been a source of support for the glutamatergic hypothesis of schizophrenia. Moreover, ketamine administration to normal controls was found to replicate the neuropsychiatric impairments characteristic of schizophrenia, including impaired vigilance, verbal fluency, and executive functions, such as those measured in the Wisconsin Card-Sorting Test, while performance on the Mini-Mental Status Examination was unchanged, consistent with a clear sensorium. Interestingly, individuals who were administered ketamine likened the sensation to alcohol intoxication.[40]

In view of this PCP and ketamine data and studies of rat brains, Olney and Farber[41] have proposed a model that posits NMDA receptor hypofunction as a means to explain the development of positive and negative symptoms of schizophrenia, the latency period prior to the onset of psychotic symptoms, and the cognitive deterioration often associated with the disease. They suggest that glutamate, acting through NMDA receptors on GABAergic and neuradrenergic neurons, maintains tonic inhibitory control over excitatory pathways present in the posterior cingulate gyrus. By means of inhibitory input from these GABAergic and neuradrenergic tracts and from a recurrent collateral feedback inhibitory circuit, which is also GABAergic, the outflow to corticolimbic brain regions is limited. They suggest that with hypofunction of the NMDA receptors, there is a loss of this inhibitory filter, which permits unmodulated stimulatory activity to flood corticolimbic brain regions, producing psychotic symptoms if this hypofunction is present in some of the pathways and structural brain damage if it is present in all of the pathways. Dopamine may also be involved, because dopaminergic hyperactivity could also result in excess suppression of glutamate release at NMDA receptors.[41]

Benes[42] extends this model to the anterior cingulate gyrus as well and emphasizes that this hyperdopaminergic state in schizophrenia could be referable to glutamatergic dysfunction or to the loss or impairment of GABAergic interneurons. An understanding of the foregoing is necessary to appreciate the manner in which ethanol's capacity to antagonize glutamatergic transmission and bolster dopaminergic transmission can potentially exacerbate the underlying pathophysiological abnormalities in schizophrenia, which lead not only to positive and negative symptoms, but also to cognitive deterioration and potentially to structural brain damage.

The possible involvement of NMDA receptor dysfunction causing an increase in control dopaminergic activity in the development of alcohol hallucinosis[39,43] is of particular interest because of the controversy about whether hallucinosis is a unique reflection of ethanol's neurotoxicity or it may share common features with schizophrenia. Sohya[44] notes that both syndromes include auditory hallucinations, referential thinking, chronicity, and the presence of a clear sensorium. Schizophrenia, however, is associated with an earlier onset, a poorer prognosis, and the presence of a greater degree of ego dysfunction. In addition, there seems to be a clear demarcation between these two syndromes when family pedigrees are examined.[44] However, Horrbin *et al.*[45] noted an additional similarity between alcohol hallucinosis and schizophrenia, namely, the measurement of essential fatty acids in red cell membrane phospholipids, which was comparable between these two groups and significantly different from alcoholics without hallucinosis. Additional evidence suggesting a difference between these two syndromes has come from the observation that increased lymphocyte spiperone binding capacity, thought to be a marker for schizophrenic vulnerability, is rarely found in patients with alcohol-induced psychosis,[46] and from the observation that piracetam, a novel compound that is a GABA analogue with structural similarities to vasopressin, was effective in treating alcohol-related psychotic symptoms.[47]

While there may be mechanistic differences between the alcoholic induction of chronic psychotic symptoms and the etiology of schizophrenia, there is clearly an overlap in the means by which alcohol produces alterations in the brains of nonschizophrenic individuals and the pathophysiological processes that underlie schizophrenia. Thus, while there is little research directly linking moderate ethanol consumption to exacerbation in schizophrenic patients, there are underlying similarities between ethanol's neurochemical effects and the neurochemical hypotheses involved in discussions of schizophrenia. In fact, it may be appropriate to advise schizophrenic patients that even moderate alcohol intake may be deleterious and that alcohol may share with other substances, such as PCP and amphetamine, a capacity to provoke symptom relapse or exacerbation. Moreover, as alcohol has the capacity to alter absorption or metabolism of psychotropic medications such as chlorpromazine, it may also destabilize the schizophrenic patient through its pharmacokinetic effects.

Regarding pharmacokinetics, short-term alcohol consumption may decrease the clearance of medications by glucuronidation and oxidative metabolism and increase clearance by *N*-acetylation, whereas long-term alcohol consumption may increase clearance by oxidative metabolism.[48,49] These effects can have significant implications for a variety of patients maintained on psychotropic medications and should be considered when the risk–benefit ratio of alcohol consumption is discussed with patients. For example, alcohol ingestion was found to produce a significant drop in neuroleptic blood levels in patients maintained on a stable fluphenazine decanoate dosage.[50] This may be a factor in the finding that comorbid alcohol use is associated with higher-dose antipsychotic regimens.[51]

4. Anxiety and Mood Disorders

According to a recent review by the National Institute on Alcoholism,[52] about 70% of American adults drink alcohol at least occasionally and 10% drink every day. The review also points out that nearly 3000 prescription drugs and 2000 over-the-counter drugs are available in the United States, a situation that creates considerable potential for alcohol–medication interactions. This is supported by the finding that about 50% of the population has experienced one or more adverse alcohol-related event, as defined in the *Diagnostic and Statistical Manual of Psychiatric Disorders,* 4th edition (DSM-IV).[53] Of all mental disorders, anxiety and depressive illnesses represent the most common potential for interactions involving alcohol and drugs, because antidepressants and anxiolytics represent the most widely used psychotropic drugs and are among the most widely prescribed of all types of drugs. Alcohol, anxiety, depression, and psychotropic drugs can interact in several ways: pharmacokinetically, pharmacodynamically, and psychosocially. The latter interaction—commonly overlooked—can take the form of behavioral disinhibition.

Alcohol use produces numerous pharmacological effects through its interactions with various neurotransmitters and neuromodulators that have been implicated in the pathophysiology of mood and anxiety disorders.[54–59] In addition to some of the examples mentioned earlier, nitric oxide recently has been found to play a major role in CNS activity and has in fact been described as a nonconventional neurotransmitter.[60] Studies have shown that ethanol can inhibit nitric oxide production *in vivo.*[61]

The comorbidity of alcoholism and anxiety disorders is well documented. It has been found that between 23 and 70% of patients in treatment for alcoholism have an anxiety disorder.[9] Among the known factors leading to comorbidity of anxiety and alcoholism are being female, being alcohol-dependent rather than an alcohol abuser, and having phobic disorders rather than generalized anxiety disorder. It is not known to what extent this comorbidity reflects a causal relationship between the disorders or a common underlying etiology.[62] Thus, the relationship between alcoholism and anxiety is complex. Alcohol use in times of anxiety, particularly in anticipation of phobic situations, is quite common. Patients with anxiety disorders, particularly with social phobia, develop a binge pattern of alcohol consumption.[63] Concentrations of homovanillic acid (HVA), a dopamine metabolite, are also reduced during alcohol withdrawal, suggesting decreased dopamine turnover.[64] Various dopamine agonist have been shown to lessen the intensity of some of the symptomatology of alcohol withdrawal.[65] It seems that ethanol consumption in rats is associated with a subsequent increase in the release and synthesis of dopamine.[66] Chronic ethanol administration results in enhanced cholinergic brain activity in rodents, probably reflecting the reciprocally balancing interaction between the dopamine and cholinergic systems. The cholinergic response to ethanol varies in different brain regions, but it seems clear that alcohol induces adaptive changes in the cholinergic system.[67] How these changes may affect cognitive and emotional performance is unclear.

The negative effects of alcohol use on the clinical course of mood and anxiety disorders among alcoholic patients have been recognized.[68,69] Alcohol is not used consistently among depressed alcoholic populations,[70] but it is clear that alcoholics without depression are as likely to report drinking in response to depressive symptoms as depressed alcoholics.[71] Empirical studies of the self-medication hypothesis in different diagnostic populations confirm that subjective effects of alcohol on primary psychiatric symptoms are inconsistent.[72–74] Still, depressive symptoms in alcoholics resemble those seen in major depressive disorder.[68] There are some commonalities between the symptomatology of both disorders. Both alcoholism and major depression, for example, decrease natural killer cell cytotoxicity[75] and disrupt sleep by increasing sleep latency and reducing rapid eye movement (REM) latency.[76]

4.1. *Depression*

Researchers[68,77] and clinicians[78] have long documented the correlation between alcohol dependence and depressive symptoms, and now delve into this association with increasingly sophisticated methods including validated psychological measurement instruments.[79] Less studied is the connection between moderate drinking—the use of alcohol without obvious biopsychosocial consequences—and alcohol's putative depressogenic effects.[80] Although the scientific literature concentrates on the effects of frank alcohol dependence and its effects on mood, alcoholism and depression exist along a spectrum of expression, and interactions between the two fluctuate with the intensity of each condition.

In an influential 1990 report,[81] the Institute of Medicine noted that from a theoretical perspective alcohol problems in the general population vary along a range from nonexistent to culminating in the most severe and life-threatening conditions. From a public policy point of view, prospective treatments should run the gamut from primary prevention for those unaffected by alcoholism to specialized treatment for those whose lives are being destroyed by their alcohol dependence. In regard to these overall epidemiological issues, the report concluded, commonsensically, that "most people have no alcohol problems, many people have some alcohol problems, and a few people have many alcohol problems" (p. 28).

Research on the subtle effects of moderate alcohol use on mood focuses on three main categories: clinical correlations between alcohol use of any kind and decrements in mood, the "self-medication" hypothesis, and the biological connections between alcohol use and depression that have been discussed earlier.

Clinicians and alcohol users commonly note the dysphoria and mild cognitive deficits that occur even after the ingestion of seemingly innocuous amount of alcohol. Because of its subtlety, documentation of this affective response occurs often by proxy, or as an incidental finding in research focusing on more distinct phenomena. In one such study of a classification of the chronic depressive condition known as dysthymia,[82] two of the four subtypes of major depression had statistically significant rates of alcohol abuse/dependence scores that differentiated them from the remaining two categories of chronic depression. Interestingly, the alcohol abuse/dependence scores as measured by the Structural Clinical Interview for DSM-III (SCID) were 1.7 and 2.4 in a range from 0 to 4, suggesting an alcohol use pattern that did not meet criteria for dependence. The subjects in these two categories of chronic depression had alcohol ingestion, but not necessarily dependence, associated with their depressive condition.

One early study[83] on the correlation between alcoholism and depressive symptoms tested a household sample of 515 adults over the age of 19 using the Research Diagnostic Criteria for mental illness and addiction. The study cast a "wide net" for alcoholics and defined them as "probable and definite cases," with a 6.7% lifetime prevalence of alcoholism broadly defined in this manner. The authors noted that the 34 alcoholics in their sample had a high rate of lifetime psychiatric diagnosis (71%), mostly different forms of depression. Many of the subjects diagnosed under these inclusive criteria were likely problem drinkers, demonstrating the high prevalence of depressive disorder even in this population. More recent epidemiological studies[84] use stricter and more scientific criteria for defining alcohol dependence, but with this improved specificity comes the loss of surveillance for alcoholism that does not meet criteria for frank alcohol dependence.

The self-medication hypothesis[85] holds that addicted persons use particular substances to alleviate painful feeling states, and that understanding this process can lead to recovery from the addiction. The alcohol-dependent person uses the sedative effects of alcohol to escape a disturbing internal reality, while a cocaine-addicted person might take advantage of the stimulant effects of cocaine to "treat" an internal lethargy or lack of motivation. Although this hypothesis has been attacked on empirical grounds,[72–74,86] the undeniable reality of "happy hour" is that the addition of alcohol to a social occasion is perceived by most as a way to lift the mood of those present. In the individual vulnerable to depressive symptoms, this socially acceptable drinking pattern can lead to the opposite effect: a measurable decrement in mood state.

4.2. *Bipolar Disorder*

A large body of literature has confirmed the comorbidity of bipolar disorder and substance abuse. Bipolar patients who abuse alcohol or drugs are likely to have an earlier onset of illness and a worse longitudinal course. As described by Brady and Sohne,[87] patients are also more likely to experience irritable and dysphoric mood states, to require hospitalizations, and to develop treatment resistance. Comorbid alcohol abuse in bipolar patients is also a strong predictor of lethality in suicide attempts, especially in males.[88(pp210–226)]

In the studies reviewed by Goodwin and Jamison,[88] rates of alcohol abuse and alcoholism in bipolar patients ranged from 11 to 75%, with an estimated average of 35%. This figure is strikingly different from the 6 to 7% cited in the general population. The alcohol use was most strongly associated with the manic state, with an intermediate rate of usage associated with hypomanic and mixed states, and a lower rate in depressed states cited in the majority of the studies reviewed. The incidence of alcohol usage was comparable in type I and type II bipolar males, but was higher in type II bipolar females than in type I females.[88(pp210–226)] Bipolar patients with high anxiety scores were more likely to present with comorbid alcohol abuse.[89]

Most of the study data reviewed above relate to comorbid alcohol abuse or alcoholism; little has been written about the effects of moderate alcohol use on bipolar patients. Given the profound pharmacological and pharmacokinetic effects of alcohol, it is likely that even acute, moderate alcohol intake may significantly affect patients with bipolar disorder.

The serotonergic effects of acute alcohol intake have proved to be complex, with evidence of decreased whole blood serotonin concentration 45 min after drinking[90] and of lowered circulating tryptophan concentration and availability in the brain. The latter finding may be due to enhancement of hepatic tryptophan pyrolase activity and might impair brain serotonin synthesis. The resulting serotonin depletion in susceptible individuals could then induce aggressive behavior and dysphoria following alcohol consumption.[91] This capacity of acute, as well as chronic, alcohol intake to decrease serotonergic function in the brain is of particular concern in patients with bipolar disorder. One of the neurochemical models for this illness postulates a serotonergic hypofunction, with the loss of the serotonergic dampening effects on other neurotransmitter systems. In this "permissive hypothesis," the hyposerotonergic state is a precondition for the induction of mania or depression by perturbations in the catecholamine systems.[88(pp421–423)] Thus, the consumption of even moderate amounts of alcohol would seem to have the potential to exacerbate underlying neurochemical abnormalities in bipolar patients.

Consumption of small amounts of alcohol can also produce an initial increase in norepinephrine release, reflected in an acute increase in 3-methoxy-4-hydroxyphenylethylene glycol (MHPG) levels. This is followed by a decrease in neuradrenergic turnover. With more chronic ethanol ingestion, there are alterations in the pathways of catecholamine catabolism, an increase in noradrenergic turnover, and a decrease in β-adrenergic receptors. Heavy alcohol consumption can produce increased activity of noradrenergic neurons, and withdrawal states can then produce a rebound respond in β-adrenergic receptors.[7,92] Thus, alcohol possesses a range of noradrenorganic effects, depending on dosage and duration of use. Disturbances in the noradrenergic system have been associated with both the manic and the depressive phase of bipolar illness, and this system is influenced both by antidepressants and by mood stabilizers such as lithium. In one formulation, noradrenergic overactivity has been linked to the euphoria and grandiosity seen in hypomania.[88(pp416–421)]

Ethanol's acute effects on the dopaminergic system are of concern in bipolar patients as well because of dopamine's hypothesized role in the switching mechanism and because of its involvement in the hyperactivity and psychosis that characterize more severe manics states. Moreover, other agents which bolster dopaminergic transmission, such as L-dopa and amphetamine, frequently induce hypomania.[88(pp416–421)]

Although these neurotransmitters are relevant individually, bipolar disorder may be better understood as a product of the interaction between these systems, rather than as a perturbation in any one system. In light of this view, alcohol's range of effects on these neurochemical systems, both directly and indirectly through its glutamatergic action, would seem likely to have a profound effect on bipolar patients. Even moderate consumption of alcohol may influence bipolar patients both through its effects on sleep, discussed in Section 5, and its depressant medication, which may prompt the addiction of the antidepressant effect, altering the course of the disorder. Finally, repeated ethanol administration may have a kindling effect, which could be involved in switching phenomena noted in rapid cycling. Thus, the evolution in the clinical presentation of bipolar disorder, with psychotic and dysphoric and dysphoric mania replacing grandiose, euphoric mania, may be due in part to the use of alcohol and drugs by mood-disorder patients.[88(pp210–226)]

Ethanol's pharmacokinetic effects are a cause of concern in bipolar patients. As Decker and Ries[93] point out, alcohol may interfere with the action of psychotropic medications in a variety of ways, including altering their metabolism, their clearance or excretion, and the brain neurotransmitters or receptors upon which these medications act, and inducing medical or psychiatric syndromes when taken in combination. Regarding the first mode of interference, ethanol can interfere with the cytochrome P450 system, which is involved in the metabolism of a variety of medications used to treat bipolar patients, including valproate, carbamazepine, neuroleptics, antidepressants, and benzodiazepines.[93] Acute ingestion can also impair the hepatic extraction of tricyclic antidepressants, resulting in larger amounts reaching the heart and brain and the possibility of toxicity. In addition, fluid load and diuretic effect of alcohol consumption can alter the renal absorption of lithium, increasing its clearance and altering serum lithium levels.[94] Alcohol may also potentiate the sedative or anticholinergic effects of psychotropic agents when the two are taken together. Finally, alcohol use has been implicated as a factor in poor medication compliance.[93]

5. Sleep Disorders

Alcohol is one of the oldest folk remedies used to facilitate sleep. However, since the advent of standardized sleep recordings, it has become clear that alcohol actually worsens sleep quality and disrupts many aspects of sleep-related physiology. The result of small doses of alcohol (0.25 to 1.0 g/kg; 1 to 3 oz.) consumed shortly before bedtime is an enhancement of slow-wave sleep and suppression of REM sleep early in the night.[95–100] These effects of alcohol on sleep electroencephalogram (EEG) are different than those elicited by benzodiazepine receptor agonists,[101] although the subjective reports of alcohol's initial sedative and anxiolytic effects probably occur in part through a GABA–benzodiazepine receptor mechanism.[102] However, as the alcohol is metabolized throughout the night, a rebound increase in sympathetic tone results in a heightened arousal state with relative tachycardia, tachypnea, and increased wakenings 2 to 3 hr after alcohol levels have reached zero. REM sleep rebound also occurs in the second half of the sleep period, which may become manifest as intense, vivid dreaming or nightmares.[105] With nightly use, tolerance may develop to many of these effects, but when alcohol consumption is discontinued a rebound of decreased slow-wave, increased REM and fragmentation will occur.[1,104] Clearly, alcohol is a poor choice for optimizing sleep quality and duration.

Alcohol can also have profound effects on the body's physiology during sleep. Moderate intoxication decreases hypoxic and hypercapnic ventilatory responses, even during wakefulness.[105,106] In addition, alcohol has direct and indirect depressant effects on the pharyngeal muscles necessary to maintain a patent airway.[107,108] Normal sleepers consuming a single large alcoholic drink can develop snoring and even obstructive sleep apneas, intervals of obstructed airflow despite efforts to breathe, with resulting blood oxygen desaturations.[109–111] Chronic snorers are likely to develop frank obstructive sleep apneas, especially in the first hours of sleep when blood alcohol levels are the highest.[112] In people with obstructive sleep apnea syndrome, even modest amounts of alcohol can greatly increase the frequency and severity of hypoxic apneas during sleep[113] Alcohol can also markedly worsen the oxygen saturation during sleep of patients with chronic obstructive pulmonary disease,[114] which may result in increased ventricular ectopy.[115]

Alcohol use has also been associated with movement disorders that disturb sleep. One study found that people who consumed two or more alcoholic drinks per day had a two- to threefold increase in leg movements that fragmented their sleep.[116] Furthermore, women who consumed two or more drinks were more likely to report sensations of restlessness, leading to a diagnosis of restless legs syndrome. Sleepwalking (somnambulism) in adults also has been associated with the use of alcohol. Sleepwalking is a disorder of impaired arousal from sleep that commonly occurs in the first half of the night during transitions from slow-wave to lighter stages of sleep. It is a common, mostly benign, disorder in childhood, which less commonly persists into adulthood. When this disorder develops during adulthood, it is often symptomatic of an underlying psychiatric or medical disorder. However, sleepwalking is occasionally elicited by the use of psychotropic medications, especially the sedative-hypnotics.[117] Alcohol has been reported to provoke sleepwalking when taken in combination with methylphenidate, diphenhydramine, amitriptyline and ethchlorvynol.[118] Because it carries a genuine risk of injury, patients with psychiatric disorders should be cautious about the combination of alcohol with medications, especially if there is a childhood history of sleepwalking.

A number of endocrine systems may also be affected by alcohol consumption prior to sleep. The pineal hormone melatonin has been shown to play a critical role in the regulation of the circadian rhythms of humans and other species.[119,120] In healthy normal volunteers, low to moderate amounts of alcohol (0.5 to 1.0 g/kg) ingested 4 hr before bedtime significantly inhibited nocturnal melatonin secretion in a dose-dependent manner.[121] This inhibition occurred after alcohol intake despite increased catecholamine levels that might be expected to stimulate melatonin. The mechanism of this inhibition is thought to be mediated by alcohol-induced central GABAergic activity, which has been shown to reduce nighttime melatonin secretion.[122] The impact of this suppression of melatonin is unclear, but suggests that even social drinking may interfere with human endogenous rhythms.

Other aspects of nocturnal pituitary function may also be altered by moderate alcohol intake. Growth hormone (GH) is normally released in a single major pulse in the first hours of sleep.[123] GH, or somatomedin, is known to be necessary for pubertal development and somatic maturation and may have a significant role in maintaining the health of aging tissues. Moderate alcohol intake has been shown to significantly suppress GH secretion during sleep in humans,[124] perhaps by suppression of GH-releasing hormone release. This finding is potentially of concern, given the number of adolescents who electively consume large amounts of alcohol during critical periods of growth. The implication for mature adults is that by reducing the protective effect of GH, alcohol may accelerate the aging of body tissues, but this hypothesis remains to be evaluated. Interestingly, recent work has demonstrated that nocturnal GH release is also blunted during major depressive episodes,[125–127] as a result of impaired serotonergic function.[128] It is possible that alcohol's depressant effects reflect this common mechanism.

Because of sleep disturbances provoked by nocturnal alcohol consumption, those who use alcohol as a sleep aid are more tired and show impairment in their daytime alertness compared with people who abstain from alcohol at night.[129] Worsened daytime performance compounds psychosocial difficulties and leads to increased utilization of health services. Perhaps more serious is the risk of moderate alcohol use in a chronically sleep-deprived population. Individuals likely to be chronically sleep-deprived, such as shiftworkers and teenagers, show greatly increased rates of fatal traffic accidents due to falling asleep at the wheel,[130] especially during the early morning hours and late afternoon, when circadian rhythms cue for sleep. As little as one ounce of alcohol markedly increases sleepiness in sleep-deprived individuals, and increases the risk of work- and driving-related accidents.[131] For many tasks where sustained vigilance is essential, aggravation of sleepiness by consumption of low to moderate doses of alcohol has potentially lethal consequences.

Unfortunately, the consequences of disrupted sleep may be difficult to differentiate from many of the signs and symptoms of psychiatric disorders. Poor sleep can manifest as early morning wakenings, lethargy, fatigue, decreased concentration, and depressed mood, complicating psychiatric diagnosis and monitoring of affective symptoms. Moreover, sleep problems often exacerbate primary psychiatric symptoms.[132] It is essential to understand that even moderate use of alcohol before bedtime perpetuates insomnia symptoms rather than ameliorating them, which in turn may provoke anxious and obsessional overconcern with sleep that continues in a vicious cycle. The habitual use of alcohol to treat anxiety and insomnia symptoms is a form of alcohol abuse defined as alcohol-dependent sleep disorder.[133] This pattern of self-medication is an underrecognized risk to the development of chronic alcohol dependence, as the recurrence of insomnia symptoms is a powerful inducement to the continued nightly use of alcohol. Effective treatment requires eliminating the use of alcohol as a sedative-hypnotic and addressing the anxiety and sleep complaints with more appropriate psychotropic medications in combination with cognitive–behavioral strategies.[134,135] It is important to educate patients about the disruptive effects of alcohol on sleep and to teach good sleep habits, including relaxation and stress reduction techniques.

6. Personality Disorders

Moderate use of alcohol influences the expression of personality (defined as the individual's unique qualities and traits) and can also affect the course of frank personality disorders. The well-known effects of alcohol on mentation account for most instances of driving under the influence (DUI) charges and instances of disinhibition, sedation, and depressive symptoms in people who are neither alcohol dependent nor diagnosed with any Axis I or Axis II psychiatric disorder.

One study of "social drinkers" and alcoholics demonstrated a clear continuum of deficits on neuropsychological testing among the diagnosed alcoholics.[136] By evaluating 60 male alcoholics between the ages of 24 and 60 with a broad range of psychological tests, the investigators correlated increasing maximum quantity frequency of alcohol with greater and greater neuropsychological deficits. In a similar study of "social drinkers" alone, Jones-Saumty and Zeiner[137] found that among the 80 undergraduates they assessed, those diagnosed as "heavy social drinkers" were more similar to alcohol-dependent persons on the Beck Depression Scale, the Shipley Institute for Living Scale, and the Self-Rating Depression Scale than they were to "light social drinkers." These studies demonstrate the spectrum of alcohol's effect on behavior.

Nolan and co-workers[138] assessed personality style in 200 DUI arrestees using the Hogan Personality Inventory and compared these results to several other groups, including 30 social drinkers and 30 alcoholics. Although hampered by methodological problems (the diagnostic rubric for alcoholism is undefined), the study did find that the impulsive–extravert and normal personality types were similar to social drinkers. Most provocatively, the authors recommend a sophisticated personality assessment "as a basis for tailoring therapeutic treatments to different types of DUI offenders" (p. 33).

Few studies in the literature examine the interaction between moderate alcohol use and Cluster A personality disorders as defined by the DSM-IV. One study by McGlashan[139] peripherally addressed this issue. In a long-term follow-up of persons diagnosed with DSM-III-R schizotypal personality disorder, ten such patients were followed up after 15 years and compared to control groups of schizophrenics and borderline personality disorder patients and to mixed groups of schizotypal/schizophrenic patients and schizotypal/borderline personality disorder patients. Schizotypal personality disorder was evaluated as more related to schizophrenia than to borderline personality disorder. The schizotypal personality disorder subjects shared low rates of alcohol use with the schizophrenic patients; borderline personality disorder, either alone or in a mixed picture, was correlated with heavier alcohol use.

Contrary to Cluster A, the relationship between the DSM-IV Cluster B personality disorder and alcohol has engendered much curiosity and research. Antisocial Personality Disorder is the best example of the "dramatic" personality disorders that are correlated with alcohol. In *The Mask of Sanity,* Cleckley's[140] seminal book on the idea of sociopathy, he wrote that "The major point about the psychopath and his relation to alcohol can be found in the shocking, fantastic, uninviting, or relatively inexplicable behavior which emerges when he drinks—*sometimes only when he drinks only a little*" (italics mine) (p. 407). A more quantitative study[141] done in the prison system examined 1149 male prison inmates using the Diagnostic Interview Schedule and found that "substance abuse appears to magnify antisocial personality symptomatology." This observation has been strengthened by epidemiological studies that have noted the association between alcohol dependence/abuse and antisocial personality disorder in household[142] and treatment-seeking[143] populations.

Type I alcoholics, as defined by Cloninger *et al.*,[144] have anxious personality traits, rapid development of tolerance, and a binge-drinking pattern. Type II alcoholics, by contrast, start drinking at a young age, drink continuously and manifest antisocial traits. Although some investigations have failed to replicate these findings,[145,146] biological hypotheses about the basis of the apparent connection abound. In a study of genetic links in addiction and antisocial personality disorder (ASPD), Gabel *et al.*[147] evaluated levels of HVA and the enzyme dopamine-β-hydroxylase (DBH) in 65 young people in a treatment facility for youth with behavior problems. The subjects with addicted fathers had significantly greater HVA levels than the sons of nonaddicted fathers, and boys younger than 12 years old with non-ASPD fathers had markedly lower DBH activity than the offspring of fathers with ASPD, demonstrating a theoretic neurochemical link between ASPD and addiction.

Using a retrospective chart review of all patients discharged from a suburban New York hospital, Loranger[148] found the Cluster C condition dependent personality disorder to be the admission diagnosis in 342 patients (4.2% of all psychiatric admission). Compared with patients admitted with other personality disorders, "dependent" patients had significantly fewer alcohol-use disorders (21 vs. 26.6%). As with many studies, however, the author did not differentiate between alcohol dependence and abuse and did not address the presence or absence of "nonpathologic alcohol use," an important question because these patients struggle with social inhibition and are at least theoretically vulnerable to using alcohol as a social lubricant.

7. Attention Deficit Disorders

A genetic association has also been established between attention deficit disorder (ADD) and increased risk for alcoholism[149,150]; maternal alcohol abuse has been clearly implicated among several etiologic factors for childhood ADD.[151] The effects of moderate ethanol consumption on the symptomatology of residual ADD in adults, however, have not been studied. Current understanding of the biological factors underlying the relationship between ADD and alcoholism is limited. Although available research findings on the neurochemistry of ADD are inconsistent, most studies suggest that ADD is associated with underactivity of the dopaminergic or phenethyl aminergic systems.[152,153] Adults with ADD also have been found to display lower total cerebral glucose metabolism in positron emission tomographic studies than controls,[154] and Giedd *et al.*[155] have reported frontal lobe abnormalities in magnetic resonance imaging studies on ADD adults.

In light of these findings and given its effects on the dopamine system and brain functioning in general, ethanol would be expected to influence the symptomatology of ADD. Anecdotal reports and clinical speculations suggest that alcohol may be consumed in order to self-medicate the mood changes frequently associated with ADD (e.g., the "downs").[156] In our own sample of 16 adults with ADD who have never met DSM-IV criteria for alcohol abuse/dependence, we have not found that moderate alcohol consumption either aggravates or improves their mood symptoms.

Surprisingly, our limited experience suggests that small amounts of ethanol do not aggravate these patients' cognitive functioning. In fact, eight patients asserted that consuming two to three drinks actually improved their concentration. Furthermore, their spouses and relatives not only confirmed these reports, but they also claimed that for at least a couple of hours after two drinks these patients were more easily engaged socially and they seemed more capable of carrying out tasks that required focus and attention than before drinking. The ability of these patients to accurately recognize and report any ethanol-induced alterations in their cognition and affective state has not been assessed. However, to corroborate our preliminary observations it may be necessary to assess the relevance of ethanol-induced stimulation of the dopamine system on ADD patients who, after all, are known to improve when treated with dopaminergic agents such as stimulants like amphetamines and methylphenidate.[156,157] In any event, further research is needed to clarify the relationship between ethanol and ADD.

8. Dementia

Alcohol use by older adults must be considered in any assessment of their psychiatric and medical symptoms, especially when considering the diagnosis and treatment of dementia. Although age does not affect the rate of absorption or elimination of alcohol, there is a greater dose-related effect in the elderly because of their decreased total body water. Thus, moderate drinking for an elderly person is no more than one drink per day. Low to moderate alcohol intake in the healthy older population may have some health benefits such as stimulation of appetite and regular bowel function and reduced risk of myocardial injury.[158] As long as individuals are properly cautioned about the potential for alcohol-induced sleep disturbances and interactions with prescription and nonprescription medications, there are no absolute contraindications for occasional alcohol use in the elderly population.

On the other hand, alcohol use among the elderly population is frequently underestimated, and regular use represents a significant health problem, especially for individuals with early dementing illness. Alcohol use and abuse are often not easily separated from other factors as a cause of cognitive deficits. Individuals who start to abuse alcohol only late in life may present initially for evaluation of atypical dementia, sleep disturbance, confusion, or self-neglect.[159–161] One survey found significant alcohol consumption present in 25% of cognitively impaired patients presenting for geriatric assessment.[162] Given these issues, a careful assessment of alcohol intake is essential in the geriatric population.

Alcohol's effects on cognitive performance have been mostly studied in young, healthy adults. Fewer studies have evaluated the effect of alcohol on older, nonalcoholic adults and adults with dementia. Low-dose alcohol has been demonstrated to enhance simple tasks of verbal memory in young adults,[163] but it impairs a number of other cognitive functions including planning, verbal fluency, memory, and complex motor control.[164] The capacity to divide and sustain attention is impaired even by low doses of alcohol in healthy young adults (blood alcohol concentration levels of 0.02 to 0.03%), especially during periods of sleepiness.[165] Tasks that place greater demands on visual–spatial attention are also easily disrupted by alcohol.[166] Moderate alcohol doses (0.05% blood alcohol concentration) significantly slow reaction time in driving skills paradigms,[167] and higher doses begin to impair motor skills directly. Given the decreases in cognitive reserve and heightened sensitivity to alcohol that occur with age, it would not be surprising to find that cognitive tasks are more sensitive to the effects of alcohol in older individuals. This is the case for some, but not all, of the cognitive performance measures studied so far.[168] In fact, performance under the influence appears to depend more on baseline abilities when sober and the degree of intoxication rather than age itself.[169] Interestingly, the selective serotonin reuptake inhibitors fluvoxamine and paroxetine appear to antagonize acute alcohol-induced cognitive impairments to a limited extent in elderly patients,[170,171] although this does not imply this combination is safe to recommend.

Alcoholism is the third most frequent cause of organic cerebral dementia, as a consequence of liver failure, thiamine deficiency, or other illnesses.[172] It is unclear, through, whether there is a form of dementia attributable to the direct toxic effects of alcohol on the brain.[173] Neuropsychological deficits including dementia in some alcoholics may potentially result from progressive, submicroscopic loss of muscarinic cholinergic and benzodiazepine receptors in the absence of morphological lesions or alcohol-induced illnesses.[174] The degree of cognitive impairment resulting from such receptor losses may depend on the individual's cognitive reserve, as manifested on the cellular level by spare receptors.

Although the neurotoxic mechanisms remain unclear, alcohol appears to place an additional burden on the progression of dementing illnesses. A large meta-analysis involving case–control studies of Alzheimer's disease found that alcohol intake of any level does not seem to increase the risk of developing dementia of the Alzheimer's type.[175] However, in individuals already diagnosed with Alzheimer's disease, alcohol use leads to significantly faster rates of cognitive decline as well as higher mortality rates.[176,177] It has been suggested that alcohol-induced loss of muscarinic and benzodiazepine receptors is a contributing factor in the accelerated dementia in these patients.[178] Alcohol abuse also significantly worsens the effect of human immunodeficiency virus disease on frontal cortex function,[179] perhaps by a similar mechanism.

Given the potential risks of alcohol use on the mental health in the aging population, accurate screening methods to detect regular alcohol use should be included in the assessment of older adults. Most screening tests focus on high levels of alcohol use, abuse, and dependence. They may not provide useful information about potentially hazardous consumption of low to moderate amounts of alcohol alone or in combination with medications.[180] Further research is necessary to develop and utilize the diagnostic tools necessary to distinguish alcohol-related from age-related problems.

9. Pharmacokinetics and Pharmacodynamics of Ethanol and Psychotropics

Specific interactions between ethanol and a variety of psychotropics have been reported. Several drugs have little or no significant clinical interaction with ethanol. Among currently marketed antidepressants in the United States and Canada, fluoxetine, maprotiline, moclobemide, and fluvoxamine do not seem to affect the phamacokinetics of alcohol.

Acute alcohol consumption potentiates the sedative effects of antipsychotic drugs, increasing risk of both psychomotor impairment and respiratory distress. Ethanol's influence on the treatment of anxiety and mood disorders extends to its multiple pharmacokinetic interactions in the CNS and liver. In the brain, ethanol induces the isoenzyme of cytochrome P4502E1.[48,181] Outside the brain, ethanol affects the disposition of these drugs by influencing a variety of mechanisms, including drug clearance, volume of distribution, and plasma protein binding, which in turn determine the qualitative differences in ethanol interactions with drugs of low and high hepatic extraction ratio.

The duration of alcohol consumption also impacts differently on several types of drug metabolism such as oxidation, acetylation, and glucuronidation. Long-term alcohol consumption increases drug clearance by induction of oxidative metabolism, while short-term consumption may decrease the clearance of the same drug, and ethanol clearly increases clearance by *N*-acetylation. Single doses of alcohol, on the other hand, decrease clearance of some drugs by conjugation to glucuronic acid.[182]

The frequent association of alcoholism and depression results in the risk of drug–alcohol interactions. Among the possible consequences are increased sedative effects and impaired mental and motor skills. For example:

- Ethanol increases benzodiazepine levels in the brain.
- Tyramine, found in beer and wine, can interact with monoamine oxidase inhibitors to produce a potentially lethal increase in blood pressure.
- Ethanol increases the rate of fluvoxamine absorption and the T_{max} of trazodone.
- Both trazodone and amitriptyline increase the symptoms of ethanol-induced CNS depression and choice reaction time.
- Ethanol minimally influences blood levels of triazolam and estazolam, yet it significantly decreases their brain concentrations.
- Ethanol slightly increases the brain concentration of diazepam.
- Ethanol hardly alters the brain concentration of chlordiazepoxide.[183]
- Trazodone and amitriptyline increase ethanol-induced aggression and disinhibition.[184]
- Diazepam has addictive and synergistic effects to those of ethanol.[185]
- Flurazepam with alcohol can increase sleep movements.

- Alprazolam has been noted to greatly increase aggression among moderate alcohol drinkers.[186]
- Imipramine and amitriptyline have been reported to aggravate ethanol-induced sedation and decrease reaction time.
- Amitriptyline with alcohol augments ethanol euphoria.
- Clomipramine increases the effects of alcohol on body sway, prolongs reaction time, and diminished the alcohol-induced memory impairment in one study.
- Nefazodone, although sedating, has not been found to potentiate the effects of alcohol.[182,187]
- Paroxetine has been shown to have no effect on psychomotor performance and cognitive functioning after moderate ethanol consumption.[188]
- Mirtazapine, while not having any pharmacokinetic interactions with alcohol, does increase sedation when used while drinking.
- Bupropion can lower the seizure threshold, resulting in seizures. This is true not only if used during alcohol withdrawal but also when part of a pattern of moderate binge drinking.
- Buspirone, with no known clinically significant pharmacokinetic or pharmacodynamic interactions with ethanol,[189] is the drug of choice for patients who require medication for chronic generalized anxiety and who insist on continuing to drink socially.

References

1. Mino Y, Tsuda T, Aoyama H, Ohara H: Relationship between alcohol use and depressive/anxiety symptoms among a general population: A review of literature. *Arukoru Kenkyuto Yakabutsu Ison* [Jpn J Alcohol Stud Drug Depend] 27(3):242–253, 1992.
2. Hyman SE, Nestler EJ: *The Molecular Foundations of Psychiatry*. Washington, DC, American Psychiatric Press, 1993.
3. Golding JM, Burnam MA, Wells KB, Benjamin B: Alcohol use, depressive symptoms, and cultural characteristics in two Mexican-American samples. *Int J Addict* 28(5):451–476, 1993.
4. Haack MR, Harford TC, Parker DA: Alcohol use and depression symptoms among female nursing students. *Alcohol Clin Exp Res* 12(3):365–367, 1988.
5. Chait LD, Perry JL: Acute and residual effects of alcohol and marijuana, alone and in combination, on mood and performance. *Psychopharmacology* 115(3):340–349, 1994.
6. Castaneda R, Sussman N, Westreich L, *et al:* A review of the effects of moderate alcohol intake on the treatment of anxiety and mood disorders. *J Clin Psychiatry* 57:207–212, 1996.
7. Ogata M, Mendelson JH, Mello NK, Majchroxicz E: Adrenal function and alcoholism *Psychosom Med* 33:159–180, 1971.
8. Hoffman PL, Tabakoff B: Ethanol's action on brain biochemistry, in Tarter RE, van Thiel DH, Edwards KL (eds): *Alcohol and the Brain: Chronic Effects*. New York, Plenum, 1985, pp 19–68.
9. Martin D, Swartzwendler HS: Ethanol inhibits release of excitatory amino acids from slices of hippocampal area CAI. *Eur J Pharmacol* 219:469–472, 1992.
10. Tsai G, Gastfriend DR, Coyle JT: The glutamatergic basis of human alcoholism. *Am J Psychiatry* 152:332–340, 1995.

11. Sillanaukee P, Lf K, Harlin A, Martensson O: Plasma GABA-like activity in response to ethanol challenge in men at high risk for alcoholism. *Biol Psychiatry* 27(6):617–625, 1990.
12. Cummins JT, Sack M, von Hungren K: The effect of chronic ethanol on glutamate binding in human and rat brains. *Life Sci* 47(10):877–882, 1990.
13. Stefanini E, Frau M, Garau MG, Garau B: Alcohol-preferring rats have fewer dopamine D_2 receptors in the limbic system. *Alcohol Alcohol* 27(2):127–130, 1992.
14. Schuckit M, Parker DC, Rossman LR: Ethanol-related prolactin responses and risk for alcoholism. *Biol Psychiatry* 18(10):1153–1159, 1983.
15. Grabbe JC, Merrill CM, Kim D, Belkap JK: Alcohol dependence and withdrawal: A genetic animal model. *Ann Med* 22(4):259–263, 1990.
16. Miller RJ: Multiple calcium channels and neuronal function. *Science* 235:46–52, 1987.
17. Hoffman PL: Central nervous system effects of neurohypophyseal peptides, in Smith CS (ed): *The Peptides*. New York, Academic Press, 1987, pp 239–295.
18. Meyer HH: Zur Theorie der Alkoholnarkose:III. Der Einfluss wechselnder Temperature auf Wirkungesstarke und Teilunskoeffizient der Narkotica. *Naunyn Scmiedebergs Arch Exp Pathol Pharmacol* 46:338–346, 1990.
19. Lovinger DM, White G, Weight FF: Ethanol inhibits NMDA-activated ion current in hippocampal neurons. *Science* 243:1721–1724, 1989.
20. Nutt D, Glue P: Monoamines and alcohol. *Br J Addict* 8:327–338, 1986.
21. Nestoros JN: Ethanol specifically potentiates GABA-mediated neurotransmission in feline cerebral cortex. *Science* 209:708–710, 1980.
22. Tabakoff B, Hoffman PL: Alcohol interactions with brain opiate receptors. *Life Sci* 32:197–204, 1983.
23. Nevo I, Hamon M: Neurotransmitter and neuromodulatory mechanisms involved in alcohol abuse and alcoholism. *Neurochem Int* 26(4):305–336, 1995.
24. Suzdak PD, Glowa JN, Schwartz RD, *et al:* A selective imidazobenzodiazepine antagonist of ethanol in the rat. *Science* 234:1243–1247, 1986.
25. Khatami S, Hoffman PL, Shibuya T, Salafsky B: Selective effects of ethanol on opiate receptors subtypes in the brain. *Neuropharmacology* 26:1503–1507, 1987.
26. Davis VE, Walsh MJ: Alcohol, amines and alkaloids: A possible biochemical basis for alcohol addiction. *Science* 167:1005–1007, 1970.
27. Vaillant GE: Natural history of male psychological health: VIII. Antecedent of alcoholism and "orality." *Am J Psychiatry* 137(2):181–186, 1980.
28. Brown GL, Goodwin FK: Human aggression: A biological perspective, in Reid WH, Dorr D, Walker JI, Bonner JW (eds): *Unmasking the Psychopath*. New York, Norton, 1986, pp 55–61.
29. Stuss DT, Benson DF: *The Frontal Lobes*. New York, Raven Press, 1986.
30. Blumer D, Benson DF: Personality changes with frontal and temporal lobe lesions, in Benson DF, Blumer D (eds): *Psychiatric Aspects of Neurologic Disease*. New York, Grune & Stratton, 1975, pp 116–128.
31. Goldstein DB, Chin JH: Interaction with biological membrane. *Fed Proc* 40:1073–1076, 1981.
32. Tabakoff B, Hoffman PL: Biochemical pharmacology of alcohol, in Meltzer HY (ed): *Psychopharmacology: The Third Generation of Progress*. New York, Raven Press, 1987, pp 1521–1526.
33. Castaneda R, Cushman P Jr: Alcohol withdrawal: A review of clinical management. *J Clin Psychiatry* 50(8):278–283, 1989.
34. Schuckit MA, Risch SC, Gold EO: Acute ethanol ingestion in sons of alcoholics results in lower plasma levels of ACTH than in sons of non-alcoholics. *Am J Psychiatry* 145(11):1391–1395, 1988.
35. Waltman C, McCaul ME, Wand GS: Adrenocorticotropin responses following administration of ethanol and ovine corticotropin-releasing hormone in the sons of alcoholics and control subjects. *Alcohol Clin Exp Res* 18(4):826–830, 1994.
36. Castaneda R, Lifshutz H, Westreich L, Galanter M: Concurrent cocaine withdrawal is associated with reduced severity of alcohol withdrawal. *Compr Psychiatry* 36(6):441–447, 1995.
37. Boutros NN, Bowers MB Jr: Chronic substance-induced psychotic disorders: State of the literature. *J Neuropsychiatry Clin Neurosci* 8:262–269, 1996.

38. Noordsy DL, Drake RE, Teague GB, *et al:* Subjective experiences related to alcohol use among schizophrenics. *J Neurons Mental Dis* 179(7):410–414, 1991.
39. Fadda F, Mosca E, Columbo G, Gessa G: Effect of spontaneous ingestion of ethanol on brain dopamine metabolism. *Life Sci* 44:281–287, 1989.
40. Krystal JH, Kerper LP, Seibyl JP, *et al:* Subanesthetic effects of the NMDA antogonist ketamine in human. *Arch Gen Psychiatry* 51:199–214, 1994.
41. Olney JAW, Farber NB: Glutamate receptor dysfunction and schizophrenia. *Arch Gen Psychiatry* 52:988–1007, 1995.
42. Benes FM: Altered glutamatergic and GABAergic mechanisms in the cingulate cortex of the schizophrenic brain. *Arch Gen Psychiatry* 52:1015–1017, 1995.
43. Sohya M: Pathophysiological mechanisms possibly involved in the development of alcohol hallucinosis. *Addiction* 2:292–290, 1990.
44. Sohya M: Psychopathological characteristics in alcohol hallucinosis and paranoid schizophrenia. *Acta Psychiatr Scand* 81(3):255–259, 1990.
45. Horrobin DF, Mark MS, Hilman H, *et al:* Fatty acid levels in the brains of schizophrenics and normal controls. *Biol Psychiatry* 30:795–805, 1991.
46. Sohya M, Bondje B, Peuker B, Achenheil M: Spiperone binding capacity in lymphocytes of patients with alcohol and drug induced psychosis: Preliminary results. *J Stud Alcohol* 55(4):503–507, 1994.
47. Kabes J, Shondia V, Maholdivak K, Sosnom Z: Piracetam effective in alcohol psychosis: Double-blind, crossover, placebo-controlled comparison. *Activats Nervosa Superior* 27(1):66–67, 1985.
48. Anandatheerthavarada HK, Shankar SK, Bhamre S, *et al:* Induction of brain cytochrome P-450 111E1 by chronic ethanol treatment. *Brain Res* 601:279–285, 1993.
49. Lane EA, Guthrie S, Linnoila M: Effects of ethanol on drug and metabolite pharmacokinetics. *Clin Pharmacokinet* 10(3):228–247, 1985.
50. Sonic SD, Bamrah JS, Krska J: Effects of alcohol on serum fluphenazine levels in stable chronic schizophrenics. *Hum Psychopharmacol* 6(4):301–306, 1991.
51. D'Mello DA, Boltz MK, Msibi B: Relationship between concurrent substance abuse in psychiatric patients and neuroleptic dosage. *Am J Drug Alcohol Abuse* 21(2):257–265, 1995.
52. National Institute on Alcoholism: *Alcohol Alert*. No 27 PH355. Washington, DC, author, 1995.
53. American Psychiatric Association: *Diagnostic and Statistical Manual of Mental Disorders*. 4th ed. Washington, DC, author, 1994.
54. Herz A: Endogenous opioid systems and alcohol addiction. *Psychopharmacology* 129:99–111, 1997.
55. Schildkraut JJ: The cathecholamine hypothesis of depression: A review of supporting evidence. *Am J Psychiatry* 122:509–522, 1965.
56. Costa E: Benzodiazepines and neurotransmitters. *Arzneimittel-Forschung* 30:858–861, 1980.
57. Carroll BJ, Feinberg M, Greden JF, *et al:* A specific laboratory test for the diagnosis of melancholia: Standardization, validation, and clinical utility. *Arch Gen Psychiatry* 38:15–22, 1981.
58. Nishikawa T, Scatton B: Neuroanatomical site of the inhibitory influence of anxiolytic drugs on central serotonergic transmission. *Brain Res* 371:123–132, 1986.
59. Charney DS, Bremmer JD, Redmond E Jr: Noradrenergic neural substrates for anxiety and fear: Clinical associations based on preclinical research, in Bloom FE, Kupfer DJ (eds): *Psychopharmacology: The Fourth Generation of Progress*. New York, Raven Press, 1995, pp 387–395.
60. Calapai G, Mazzaglia G, Sautebin L, *et al:* Inhibition of nitric oxide formation reduces voluntary alcohol consumption in the rat. *Psychopharmacology* 125:398–401, 1996.
61. Persson MG, Gustafsson LE: Ethanol can inhibit nitric oxide production. *Eur J Pharmacol* 224:99–100, 1992.
62. Merikangas KR, Angst J, Eaton W, Canino G, Rubio-Stipec M, Wacker H, *et al:* Comorbidity and boundaries of affective disorders with anxiety disorders and substance misuse: Results of an international task force. *Brit J Psych* 30(Suppl): 58–67, 1996.

63. Wells JC, Tien AY, Garrison R, Eaton WW: Risk factors for the incidence of social phobia as determined by the Diagnostic Interview Schedule in a population-based study. *Acta Psychiatr Scand* 90:84–90, 1994.
64. Major LF, Ballenger JC, Goodwin FK, Brown GL: Cerebrospinal fluid homovanillic acid in male alcoholics: Effects of disulfiram. *Biol Psychiatry* 12:635–642, 1977.
65. Borg S, Weinholdt T: Bromocriptine in the treatment of the alcohol withdrawal syndrome. *Acta Psychiatr Scand* 65:101–111, 1982.
66. Mereu G, Fadda F, Gessa GL: Ethanol stimulates the firing rate of nigral dopaminergic neurons in unanesthetized rats. *Brain Res* 292:63–69, 1984.
67. Hoffman PL, Tabakoff B: Ethanol's action on brain biochemistry, in Tarter RE, van Thiel DH, Edwards KL (eds): *Alcohol and the Brain: Chronic Effects.* New York: Plenum Press, 1985, pp 19–68.
68. Schuckit MA: Alcohol and depression: A clinical perspective (review). *Acta Psychiatr Scand* 377(Suppl):28–32, 1994.
69. Hasin DS, Glick H: Depressive symptoms and DSM-III-R alcohol dependence: General population results. *Addiction* 88(10):1431–1436, 1993.
70. Golding JM, Burnam MA, Wells KB, Benjamin B: Alcohol use, depressive symptoms, and cultural characteristics in two Mexican-American samples. *Int J Addict* 28(5):451–476, 1993.
71. Liebenluft E, Fiero PL, Bartko JJ, Rosaenthal NE: Depressive symptoms and the self-reported use of alcohol, caffeine, and carbohydrates in normal volunteers and four groups of psychiatric outpatients. *Am J Psychiatry* 150(2):294–301, 1993.
72. Castaneda R, Galanter M, Franco H: Self-medication among addicts with primary psychiatric disorders. *Compr Psychiatry* 30(1):80–83, 1989.
73. Castaneda R, Galanter M, Lifshutz H, Franco H: Effects of drugs abuse on psychiatric symptoms among schizophrenics. *Am J Drug Alcohol Abuse* 17(3):313–320, 1991.
74. Castaneda R, Lifshutz H, Galanter M, Franco H: An empirical assessment of the self-medication hypothesis. *Compr Psychiatry* 2:180–184, 1994.
75. Irwin M, Caldwell C, Smith TL, Brown S: Major depressive disorder, alcoholism and reduced natural killer cell cytotoxicity: Role of severity of depressive symptoms and alcohol consumption. *Arch Gen Psychiatry* 47(8):713–719, 1990.
76. Moeller FG, Gillin JC, Irwin M, Golshan S: A comparison of sleep EEGs in patients with primary major depression and major depression secondary to alcoholism. *J Affect Disord* 27(1):39–42, 1993.
77. Powell BJ, Penick EC, Othmer E, *et al:* Prevalence of psychiatric syndromes among male alcoholics. *J Clin Psychiatry* 43:404–407, 1982.
78. Rank DH: Subsyndromal symptomatic depression may include sleep disorders (letter). *Psychiatry* 56:329, 1995.
79. Brown SA, Inaba RK, Gillin C, *et al:* Alcoholism and affective disorder: Clinical course of depressive symptoms. *Am J Psychiatry* 152:45–52, 1995.
80. Castaneda R, Sussman N, Westreich L, *et al:* A review of the effects of moderate alcohol intake on the treatment of anxiety and mood disorders. *J Clin Psychiatry* 57:207–212, 1996.
81. Institute of Medicine: *Broadening the Base of Treatment for Alcohol Problems.* Washington DC, National Academy Press, 1990.
82. Schrader GD: An attempt to validate Akiskal's classification of chronic depression using cluster analysis. *Compr Psychiatry* 36:344–352, 1995.
83. Weissman MM, Myers JK: Clinical depression in alcoholism. *Am J Psychiatry* 137:372–373, 1980.
84. Regier DA, Farmer ME, Rae DS, *et al:* Comorbidity of mental illness with alcohol and other drug abuse: Results from the epidemiologic catchment area (ECA) study. *JAMA* 264:2511–2518, 1990.
85. Khantzian EJ: The self-medication hypothesis of addictive disorders: Focus on heroin and cocaine dependence. *Am J Psychiatry* 142:1259–1264, 1985.
86. Surman OS: Limits to the self-medication hypothesis of addictive disorders. *Am J Psychiatry* 142:1488, 1985.

87. Brady KT, Sohne SC: The relationship between substance abuse and bipolar disorder. Symposium on optimizing treatment in forms of biopolar disorder. *J Clin Psychiatry* 56(13):19–24, 1995.
88. Goodwin FK, Jamison KR: *Manic–Depressive Illness.* New York, Oxford University Press, 1990.
89. Young LT, Cooke RG, Robb JC, *et al:* Anxious and non-anxious bipolar disorder. *J Affect Disord* 29(1):49–52, 1993.
90. Pietraszek MH, Urano T, Sumioshik, *et al:* Alcohol induced depression: Involvement of serotonin. *Alcohol Alcohol* 26(2):155–159, 1991.
91. Badawy AAB, Morgan CJ, Lovett JWT, *et al:* Decrease in circulating tryptophan to the brain after acute ethanol consumption by normal volunteers: Implications for alcohol-induced aggressive behavior and depression. *Pharmacopsychiatry* 28(2):93–97, 1999.
92. Borg S, Kvande H, Mossberg D, Valerious P, Sedvall G. Central nervous system noradrenaline metabolism and alcohol consumption in man. *Pharmcol Biochem Behav* 18:375–378, 1998.
93. Decker KP, Ries RK. Differential diagnosis and psychopharmacology of dual disorders. *Psychiatr Clin North Am* 16(4):703–718, 1993.
94. Presskorn SH, Goodwin DW: Medical management of the depressed alcoholic patient. *Int J Psychiatry Med* 17(2):117–131, 1987.
95. Yules RB, Freedman DX, Chander KA: The effect of ethyl alcohol on man's electroencephalographic sleep cycle. *Neurophysiology* 20:109–111, 1966.
96. Yules RB, Lippman ME, Freedman DX: Alcohol administration prior to sleep. The effect of EEG sleep stages. *Arch Gen Pyschiatry* 19:94–97, 1967.
97. Greenberg R, Perlman C: Delirium tremens and dreaming. *Am J Psychiatry* 124:133–142, 1967.
98. Lester BK, Runder OH, Cowden LC, Williams HL: Chronic alcoholis, alcohol and sleep. *Adv Exp Med Biol* 35:261–279, 1972.
99. Johnson LC, Burdick JA, Smith J: Sleep during alcohol intake and withdrawal in the chronic alcoholic. *Arch Gen Psychiatry* 22:406–418, 1970.
100. Zarcone VP, Schreier L, Mitchell G, *et al:* Sleep variables, cyclic AMP and biogenic amine metabolites after one day ethanol ingestion. *J Stud Alcohol* 41:318–324, 1980.
101. Dijk DJ, Brunner DP, Aeschbach D, *et al:* The effects of ethanol on human sleep: EEG power spectra differ from those benzodiazepine receptor agonist. *Neuropsychopharmacology* 7(30):225–232, 1992.
102. Suzdak PD, Glowa JN, Schwartz RD, *et al:* A selective imidazobenzodiazepine antagonist of ethanol in the rat. *Science* 167:1005–1007, 1970.
103. Zarcone VP: Sleep and alcoholism, in Weitzman ED (ed): *Sleep Disorders: Intersections of Basic and Clinical Research.* Vol 8. New York, Spectrum Press, 1982, pp 319–326.
104. Roth T, Roehrs T, Zorick F, Conway W: Pharmacological effects of sedative-hypnotics, narcotic analgesics, and alcohol during sleep. *Med Clin North Am* 69:1281–1288, 1985.
105. Sahn SA, Lakshminarayan S, Pierson DJ, *et al:* Effects of ethanol on ventilatory responses to oxygen and carbon dioxyde in men. *Clin Sci Mol Med* 49:33–38, 1975.
106. Johnstone RE, Reier CE: Acute repiratory effects of ethanol in man. *Clin Pharmacol Ther* 14:501–508, 1973.
107. Bonora M, Sheilds G, Kauphs S, *et al:* Selective depression by ethanol of upper airwave respiratory motor activity in cats. *Am Rev Respir Dis* 130:156–161, 1984.
108. Krol RC, Knuth SL, Bartlett D: Selective reduction of genioglossal muscle activity by alcohol in normal human subjects. *Am Rev Respir Dis* 129:247–250, 1984.
109. Block AJ, Hellard DW, Slayton PC: Effect of alcohol ingestion on breathing of asymptomatic subjects. *Arch Intern Med* 147:1145–1147, 1987.
110. Mitler MM, Dawson A, Henriksen SJ, *et al:* Bedtime ethanol increases resistance of the upper airways and produces sleep apneas in asymptomatic snorers. *Alcohol Clin Exp Res* 12:801–805, 1988.
111. Scrima L, Hartman PG, Thomas EE, *et al:* Sleep disordered breathing in non-obese 50-69-year-old male snorers and non-snorers: Effects of three alcohol doses. *Sleep Res* 21:263, 1992.

112. Issa FG, Sullivan CE: Alcohol, snoring, and sleep apnea. *J Neurol Neurosurg Psychiatry* 45:353–359, 1982.
113. Scrima L, Broudy M, Nay KN, *et al:* Increased severity of obstructive sleep apnea after bedtime alcohol ingestion: Diagnostic potential and proposed mechanism of action. *Sleep* 5:318–328, 1982.
114. Easton PA, West P, Meatherall RC, *et al:* The effect of excessive ethanol ingestion on sleep in severe COPD. Sleep 10:224–233, 1987.
115. Dolly FR, Block AJ: Increased ventricular ectopy and sleep apnea following ethanol ingestion in COPD patients. *Chest* 83(3):9–72, 1993.
116. Aldrich MS, Shipley JE: Alcohol use and periodic limb movements of sleep. *Alcohol Clin Exp Res* 17(1):192–196, 1993.
117. Ruela, LM: Zolpidem and sleepwalking [letter]. *J Clin Psychopharmacol* 14(2):150, 1994.
118. Berlin RM, Qayyum U: Sleepwalking: Diagnosis and treatment through the life cycle. *Psychosomatics* 27(11):755–760, 1986.
119. Reiter RJ: 1991 melatonin: The chemical expression of darkness. *Mol Cell Endocrinol* 69:C153–C158, 1991.
120. Nicholson AN, Spencer MB, Pascoe PA, Stone BM: Sleep after transmeridian flights. *Lancet* 2:1205–1208, 1986.
121. Ekman AC, Leppaluoto J, Huttunen P, *et al:* Ethanol inhibits melatonin secretion in healthy volunteers in a dose-dependent randomized double blind cross-over study. *J Clin Endocrinol Med* 77(3):780–780, 1993.
122. Kabuto M, Namura I, Saitoh Y: Nocturnal enhancement of plasma melatonin could be suppressed by benzodiazepines in humans. *Endocrinol Jpn* 33:405–414, 1986.
123. Moore-Ede MC, Czeisler CA, Richardson GS: Circadian timekeeping in health and disease. *N Engl J Med* 309:469–476, 1983.
124. Valimaki M, Tuominen JA, Huhtanienmi I, Ylikakri R: The pulsatile secretion of gonadotrophins and growth hormone, and the biological activity of luteinizing hormone in men acutely intoxicated with ethanol. *Alcoholism* 14:928–931, 1990.
125. Anand A, Charney DS, Delgado PL, *et al:* Neuroendocrine and behavioral responses to intravenous *m*-chlorophenylpiperazine (mCPP) in depressed patients and healthy comparison subjects. *Am J Psychiatry* 151:1626–1630, 1994.
126. Jarrett DB, Kupfer DJ, Miewald JM, *et al:* Sleep-related growth hormone secretion is persistently suppressed in women without recurrent depression: A preliminary longitudinal analysis. *J Psychiatr Res* 28:211–223, 1994.
127. Fiasche R, Fideleff HL, Moisezowicz J, *et al:* Growth hormone neurosecretory dysfunction in major depressive illness. *Psychoneuroendocrinology* 20:727–733, 1995.
128. Cowen PJ, Power AC, Ware CJ, Anderson IM: 5-HT_{1A} receptor in major depression. A neuroendocrine study with buspirone. *Br J Psychiatry* 154:372–379, 1994.
129. Roehrs T, Claiborue D, Knox M, Roth T: Residual sedating effects of ethanol. *Alcohol Clin Exp Res* 18(4):831–834, 1994.
130. Pack AI, Pack AM, Todgman E, *et al:* Characteristics of crashes attributed to the driver having fallen asleep. *Accid Anal Prev* 27:769–775, 1995.
131. Zwyghuizen-Doorenbos A, Roehrs T, Lamphere J, *et al:* Increased daytime sleepiness enhances ethanol's sedative effects. *Neuropsychopharmacology* 1:279–286, 1988.
132. Bliwise NG: Factors related to sleep quality in healthy elderly women. *Psychol Aging* 7(1):83–88, 1992.
133. American Sleep Disorders Association: *International Classification of Sleep Disorders: Diagnostic and Coding Manual.* Rochester, MN, American Sleep Disorders Association, 1990.
134. Spielman AJ, Caruso LS, Glovinsky PB: A behavioral perspective on insomnia treatment. *Psychiatry Clin North Am* 10(4):541–553, 1987.
135. Erman MK: Insomnia. *Psychiatry Clin North Am* 10(4):525–539, 1987.
136. Schaeffer KW, Parsons OA: Drinking practices and neuropsychological test performance in sober male alcoholics and social drinkers. *Alcohol* 3:175–179, 1986.

137. Jones-Saumty DJ, Zeiner DJ: Psychological correlates of drinking behavior in social drinker college students. *Alcohol Clin Exp Res* 9:158–163, 1985.
138. Nolan Y, Johnston JA, Pincus AL: Personality and drunk driving: Identification of DUI types using the Hogan Personality Inventory. *Psychol Assess* 6:33–40, 1994.
139. McGlashan TH: Schizotypal personality disorder: Long-term follow-up perspectives. Chestnut Lodge follow-up study: VI. *Arch Gen Psychiatry* 43:329–334, 1986.
140. Cleckley H: *The Mask of Sanity*. St. Louis, C.V. Mosby, 1964.
141. Collins JJ, Schlenger WE, Jordan BK: Antisocial personality and substance abuse disorders. *Bull Am Acad Psychiatry Law* 16:187–198, 1988.
142. Helzer JE, Pryzbeck TR: The co-occurrence of alcoholism with other psychiatric disorders in the general population and its impact on treatment. *J Stud Alcohol* 49:219–224, 1988.
143. Ross HE, Glaser FB, Germanson T: The prevalence of psychiatric disorders in patients with alcohol and others drugs problems. *Arch Gen Psychiatry* 45:1023–1031, 1988.
144. Cloninger CR, Sigvardsson S, Gilligan SB, *et al:* Genetic heterogeneity and the classification of alcoholism. *Adv Alcohol Substance Abuse* 7:3–16, 1988.
145. Irwin M, Schuckit M, Smith TL: Clinical importance of age at onset in type 1 and type 2 primary alcoholics. *Arch Gen Psychiatry* 47:320–324, 1990.
146. Lamparski DM, Roy A, Nutt DJ, Linnoila M: The criteria of Cloninger *et al.* and Van Knorring *et al.* for subgrouping alcoholics: A comparison in a clinical population. *Acta Psychiatr Scand* 84:497–502, 1991.
147. Gabel S, Stadler J, Bjorn J, Shindledecker R: Homovanillic acid and dopamine-beta-hydroxylase in male youth: Relationships with paternal substance abuse and antisocial behavior. *Am J Drug Alcohol Abuse* 21:363–378, 1995.
148. Loranger AW: Dependent personality disorder. *J Nerv Ment Disord* 184:17–21, 1995.
149. DeObaldia R, Parsons OA, Yohman R: Minimal brain dysfunction symptoms claimed by primary and secondary alcoholics: Relation to cognitive functioning. *Int J Neurosci* 20:173–182, 1983.
150. DeObaldia R, Parsons OA: Relationship of neuropsychological performance to primary alcoholism and self-reported symptoms of childhood minimal brain dysfunction. *J Stud Alcohol* 45:386–392, 1984.
151. Jones KL, Smith DW, Ulleland CN, Streissguth AP: Pattern of malformation in offspring of chronic alcoholic mothers. *Lancet* 1:1267–1271, 1973.
152. Reimherr FW, Wender PH, Wood DR: Cerebrospinal fluid homovanillic acid and 5-hydroxyindole acetic acid in adults with attention deficit disorder, residual type (ADD,RT). *Psychiatry Res* 11:71–78, 1984.
153. Shaywitz SE, Cohen DJ, Bowers MB: CSF monoamine metabolites in children with minimal brain dysfunction: Evidence for alteration of brain dopamine. *J Pediatr* 90:67–71, 1977.
154. Zametkin AJ, Nordahl TE, Gross M, *et al:* Cerebral glucose metabolism in adults with hyperactivity of childhood onset. *N Engl J Med* 323:1361–1366, 1990.
155. Giedd JN, Castellanos X, Casey BJ, *et al:* Quantitative morphology of the corpus callosum in attention deficit hyperactivity disorder. *Am J Psychiatry* 151:665–669, 1994.
156. Wender PH: *Attention Deficit Hyperactivity Disorder in Adults*. New York, Oxford University Press, 1995.
157. Wood DR, Reimherr FW, Wender PH, Johnson GE: Diagnosis and treatment of minimal brain dysfunction in adults. *Arch Gen Psychiatry* 33:1533–1460, 1976.
158. Dufour MC, Archer L, Gordis E: Alcohol and the elderly. *Clin Geriatr Med* 8(1):127–141, 1992.
159. Wattis JP: Alcohol problems in the elderly. *J Am Geriatr Soc* 29(3):131–134, 1981.
160. Iliffe S, Haines A, Gallivan S, *et al:* Assessment of elderly people in general practice. *Br J Gen Pract* 41(342):9–12, 1991.
161. Miller NS, Belkin BM, Gold MS: Alcohol and drug dependence among the elderly: Epidemiology, diagnosis, and treatment. *Compr Psychiatry* 32(2):153–165, 1991.

162. Rains VS, Ditzler TF: Alcohol use disorders in cognitively impaired patients referred for geriatric assessment. *J Addict Dis* 12(1):55–64, 1993.
163. Tyson PD, Schirmuly M: Memory enhancement after drinking ethanol: Consolidation, interference, or response bias? *Physiol Behav* 56(5):933–937, 1994.
164. Peterson JB, Rothfleisch J, Zelazo PD, Pihl RO: Acute alcohol intoxication and cognitive functioning. *J Stud Alcohol* 51(2):114–122, 1990.
165. Elega HA: Alcohol and vigilance performance: A review. *Psychopharmacology* 118:233–249, 1995.
166. Post RB, Lott LA, Maddock RJ, Beede JI: An effect of alcohol on the distribution of spatial attention. *J Stud Alcohol* 57:260–266, 1991.
167. West R, Wilding J, French D, *et al:* Effect of low and moderate doses of alcohol on driving hazard perception latency and driving speed. *Addiction* 88:527–532, 1993.
168. Tupler LA, Hege S, Ellinwood EH Jr: Alcohol pharmacodynamics in young-elderly adults contrasted with young and middle-aged subjects. *Psychopharmacology* 118(4):460–470, 1995.
169. Yesavage JA, Dolhert N, Taylor JL: Flight simulator performance of younger and older aircraft pilots: Effects of age and alcohol. *J Am Geriatr Soc* 42(6):577–582, 1994.
170. Van Harten J, Stevens LA, Raghoebar M, *et al:* Fluvoxamine does not interact with alcohol or potentiate alcohol-related impairment of cognitive function. *Clin Pharmacol Ther* 52(4):427–435, 1992.
171. Kerr JS, Fairweather DB, Mahendran R, Hindmarch I: The effects of paroxetine, alone and in combination with alcohol on psychomotor performance and cognitive function in the elderly. *Int Clin Psychopharmacol* 7(2):101–108, 1992.
172. Carlen PL, McAndrews MP, Weiss RT, *et al:* Alcohol-related dementia in the institutionalized elderly. *Alcohol Clin Exp Res* 18(6):1330–1334, 1994.
173. Victor M: Alcoholic dementia. *Can J Neurol Sci* 21(2):88–99, 1994.
174. Freund G, Ballinger WE: Loss of synaptic receptors can precede morphologic changes induced by alcoholism. *Alcohol* 1(Suppl):385–391, 1991.
175. Graves AB, van Duijn CM, Chandra V, *et al:* Alcohol and tobacco consumption as risk factors for Alzheimer's disease: A collaborative re-analysis of case–control studies. EURODEM Risk Factors Research Group. *Int J Epidemiol* 20(Suppl)2:S48–57, 1991.
176. Teri L, Hughes JP, Larson EB: Cognitive deterioration in Alzheimer's disease: Behavioral and health factors. *J Gerontol* 45(2):P58–63, 1990.
177. Jagger C, Clarke M, Stone A: Predictors of survival with Alzheimer's disease: A community-based study. *Psychol Med* 25(1):171–177, 1995.
178. Freund G, Ballinger WE Jr: Alzheimer's disease and alcoholism: Possible interactions. *Alcohol* 9(3):233–240, 1992.
179. Fein G, Biggins CA, MacKay S: Alcohol abuse and HIV infection have additive effects on frontal cortex function as measured by auditory evoked potential P3A latency. *Biol Psychiatry* 37(3):183–195, 1995.
180. Fink A, Hays RD, Moore AA, Beck JC: Alcohol-related problems in older persons: Determinants, consequences, and screening. *Arch Intern Med* 156(11):1150–1156, 1996.
181. Mereu 6, Faddle F, Oessa GL: Ethanol stimulates the firing rate of migral dopaminergic neurons in unanesthetized rats. *Brain Res* 292:63–69, 1984.
182. Lane EA, Guthrie S, Linnoila M: Effects of ethanol on drug and metabolite pharmacokinetics. *Clin Pharmacokinet* 10(3):228–247, 1985.
183. Warrington SJ, Ankier SI, Turner P: An evaluation of possible interactions between ethanol and trazodone or amitriptyline. *Br J Clin Pharmacol* 18(4)549–597, 1984.
184. Salvadori C, Ward C, Defrance R, Hopkins R: The pharmacokinetics of the antidepressant Tianeptine and its main metabolite in healthy humans—influence on alcohol coadministration. *Fundament Clin Pharmacol* 4(1):115–125, 1990.
185. Linnoila MI: Benzodiazepines and alcohol. *J Psychiatr Res* 2(Suppl 24):121–127, 1990.
186. Bond AJ, Silveira JC: The combination of alprazolam and alcohol on behavioral aggression. *J Stud Alcohol* 11(Suppl):30–39, 1993.

187. Frewer LJ, Lader M: The effects of nefazodone, imipramine and placebo, alone and combined with alcohol in normal subjects. *Int Clin Psychopharmacol* 8:13–20, 1993.
188. Kerr JS, Fairweather DB, Mahendran R, Hindmarch I: The effects of paroxetine, alone and in combination with alcohol on psychomotor performance and cognitive function in the elderly. Int Clin Psychopharmacol 7(2):101–108, 1992.
189. Sussman N: *Buspirone: A Review of the Literature.* Princeton, NJ, Excerpta Medica, 1995.

8

Executive Cognitive Functioning in Alcohol Use Disorders

Peter R. Giancola and Howard B. Moss

Abstract. Executive cognitive functioning (ECF) has been identified as an important determinant in the etiology of alcoholism. ECF represents a "higher-order" cognitive construct involved in the self-regulation of goal-directed behavior. The prefrontal cortex and its subcortical connections represent the primary neurological substrate that subserves ECF. Both alcoholics and individuals at high risk for alcoholism exhibit a mild dysfunction in ECF. However, this deficit appears to be significantly stronger in alcoholics with a comorbid diagnosis of an antisocial personality disorder. Individuals with other disorders that are also highly comorbid with alcoholism, such as attention deficit hyperactivity disorder and conduct disorder, also demonstrate deficits in ECF. As such, compromised ECF may not be specific to alcoholism, but instead, might be a potential underlying etiologic substrate for a number of disorders of behavioral excess–disinhibition.

Subsequent to reviewing the literature implicating ECF deficits in alcoholism and comorbid disorders, the authors present a heuristic cognitive–neurobehaivoral model of alcoholism implicating the frontostriatal system. Finally, recommendations for the prevention and treatment of alcoholism, based on this model, are discussed.

1. Introduction

Alcoholism is a devastating disorder both at the level of the individual and society. Findings from large epidemiological studies have shown that between 13.5 and 23.5% of Americans qualify for a lifetime diagnosis of an alcohol use disorder.[1,2] Alcoholism carries with it a legion of undesirable consequences. In 1990, the total economic costs associated with alcohol abuse

Peter R. Giancola and Howard B. Moss • Western Psychiatric Institute and Clinic, Department of Psychiatry, University of Pittsburgh School of Medicine, Pittsburgh, Pennsylvania 15213.

Recent Developments in Alcoholism, Volume 14: The Consequences of Alcoholism, edited by Galanter. Plenum Press, New York, 1998.

were estimated at 98.6 billion dollars, a 40% increase from just 5 years prior.[3] Alcoholism decreases work productivity and the probability of being employed,[4] while increasing work-related injuries and absenteeism.[5] Finally, alcoholism also engenders a myriad of socially destructive effects such as firearm assaults, sexual assaults, homicides, and motor vehicle fatalities,[6] to say nothing of its harmful medical and health-related concomitants.[7]

Clearly, the need for effective treatment and prevention efforts for this insidious and destructive disorder is paramount. However, the etiology of alcoholism encompasses multiple determinants from genetic to social influences, and these influences interact in a variety of highly complex ways that reflect the developmental pathways to an alcohol use disorder. At present, these developmental trajectories are not well understood, thus hampering the advancement of effective intervention efforts. As we have learned from the history of medicine, the development of an efficacious treatment for a particular disease requires a firm understanding of the etiology of that particular disease. Unfortunately, alcoholism is not immune to this maxim. Although there is a clear and present need for effectual clinical interventions for alcoholism and other forms of drug abuse, as researchers we must focus on increasing our understanding of the structure of the underlying etiologic mechanisms of these disorders before we can espouse useful intervention strategies that are expected to have lasting and positive effects.

Research has shown that one potentially important etiologic determinant of alcoholism is a deficit in cognitive functioning, in particular, executive cognitive functioning (ECF). ECF can be broadly defined as a "higher-order" cognitive construct involved in the self-regulation of goal-directed behavior.[8,9] ECF involves the ability to create a strategic goal-oriented plan, initiate it at the proper time, self-monitor the execution of that plan, attend to its aftereffects, and finally, the ability to use internal and external feedback to further modify the plan in order to successfully achieve the desired goal. The cognitive abilities subsumed within this construct include attentional control, strategic goal planning, abstract reasoning, cognitive flexibility, hypothesis generation, temporal response sequencing, as well as the ability to organize and adaptively utilize information in working memory.[10,11] The purpose of this chapter is to review direct and indirect research evidence linking alcoholism to a deficit in ECF and to present an heuristic cognitive–neurobehavioral model indicating how impaired ECF may contribute to the genesis of alcoholism.

2. Neural Substrate

Prior to reviewing the data supporting an association between a deficit in ECF and alcoholism, it is necessary to describe the neuroanatomical underpinnings of this cognitive construct.

2.1. *Prefrontal Cortex*

It is consensually recognized that the prefrontal cortex represents the primary neural substrate involved in governing ECF.[8,11,12] The prefrontal cortex designates the large portion of neural expanse that extends anterior to the precentral gyrus and superior to the lateral fissure.[13] This region is the site of numerous interconnections and feedback loops between the major sensory, limbic, and motor systems, thereby integrating all components of behavior at the highest level.[8,14] For clinical purposes, the prefrontal cortex can be divided into three distinct neuroanatomical regions: the dorsolateral convexity, the medial aspect, and the basal–orbital concavity.[15] Dysfunction of the prefrontal cortex may be conceptualized as disrupting the reciprocal relations between the major functional systems: the sensory system of the posterior cortex; the limbic–memory system with its interconnections to subcortical areas involved in arousal, affective, and motivational states; and the effector components of the motor system.[12] Although the neuroanatomic differentiation of the prefrontal cortex is not complete, primate research has suggested that specific anatomic regions of the prefrontal cortex serve different roles in the regulation of cognition and behavior.[16,17]

2.2. *Frontal–Subcortical Circuits*

Five frontal–subcortical circuits have been described that originate in different parts of the prefrontal cortex (e.g., dorsolateral, orbital, and medial prefrontal cortex), which then project to the corpus striatum (either caudate or nucleus accumbens), connect to the globus pallidus–substantia nigra, link with specific thalamic nuclei (either medial dorsal or ventral anterior), and finally project back to the prefrontal cortex.[18] Lesions in these subcortical pathways may produce neurobehavioral syndromes identical to those observed with prefrontal pathology.[19] Thus, these subcortical circuits may be as important as prefrontal structures as the neural substrate for behavioral self-regulation.

3. Behavioral Sequela following Damage to the Prefrontal Cortex

As noted above, substantial evidence links different aspects of human behavioral self-regulation with an underlying neural substrate localized either in the prefrontal cortex or the frontal–subcortical circuitry. Much of this evidence comes from neuropsychological and neurobehavioral investigations of individuals who have acquired focal lesions or neurodegenerative disorders in the frontal regions of the brain. Clinical syndromes resulting from orbitofrontal and dorsolateral prefrontal cortical damage are the best-characterized prefrontal cortical syndromes in the neuropsychological literature.

Harlow's[20] famous analysis of the case of Phineas Gage provided early evidence that anterior brain structures probably represent the neural substrate governing the capacity to plan and execute socially appropriate goal-directed behavior (i.e., ECF). Gage, a well-regarded railroad construction foreman, suffered a traumatic injury when an explosion propelled an iron tamping bar through his skull and frontal brain region. As a consequence of his injury to his medial prefrontal lobes, Gage underwent a profound change in affect and behavior. Although his intellectual capacity appeared unchanged by the accident, he lost respect for social conventions, began using extensive profanity in his speech, lost all sense of responsibility, and could no longer be relied on to honor his commitments.[21] In essence, he lost his prosocial disposition and became antisocial.

A variety of behavioral syndromes are documented as being associated with prefrontal cortical lesions. As catalogued by Stuss and colleagues,[22] individuals with frontal lobe damage may display behavioral variations that include altered mood, decreased concern with social propriety, apathy, automaticity, incontinence, restlessness, exuberance, euphoria, inappropriate jocularity, lack of initiative, lack of judgment, diminished reliability or foresight, disinhibition, anxiety, social withdrawal, irritability, inertia, a lack of social restraint, slowness in thinking, impulsivity, distractibility, egocentricity, and grandiosity. Many of these descriptors are associated with orbitofrontal lesions or pathology.

Prefrontal pathology may also produce deficits in ECF.[16] These include difficulties with concentration, planning, temporal sequencing, problem solving, cognitive flexibility, abstract reasoning, working memory, maintaining attention and self-awareness, resisting interfering stimuli, and the ability to effectively carry out goal-directed behaviors. In contrast to those noted above, these deficits have typically been associated with damage to the dorsolateral region of the prefrontal cortex.[23–25]

The cognitive and behavioral sequela of pathological and accidental damage to the prefrontal cortex are interesting with respect to alcoholism because alcoholics appear to exhibit a mild but similar neurobehavioral profile as individuals who have experienced prefrontal damage. This discovery was one of the main catalysts that prompted researchers to study prefrontal cortical functioning–ECF in alcoholics.

4. Executive Cognitive Functioning in Alcoholics

Alcoholics exhibit deficits in a variety of cognitive functions.[26,27] These include verbal skills,[28,29] visuospatial abilities,[30,31] cognitive efficiency,[32] and long- and short-term memory.[33] However, the research literature indicates that a disturbance in ECF is one of the most consistent and predominant deficits in this group of individuals. Alcoholics show deficits in abstract reasoning, set shifting, and set persistence.[34,35] These deficits are even more pronounced given a longer duration of drinking history.[35] Alcoholics also show difficulties with allocating attentional resources for information processing,[36] verbal fluency,[37] category word fluency,[38] concept generation,[39] persistence,[40] temporal organization, sequencing,[41] motor control,[42] hypothesis formation–testing, and cognitive flexibility.[29,43]

Nevertheless, these data must be interpreted with caution. Whereas a cognitive deficit may be, in part, a causal factor for the development of alcoholism, it is also possible that it may be a result of the disorder. It is well known that alcohol has deleterious effects on all body systems including neural tissue.[44] Postmortem studies have shown that alcoholics have lower neuronal cell counts, especially in the prefrontal cortex compared to nonalcoholic controls.[45,46] Therefore, the typical profile of cognitive deficits seen in alcoholics may simply be the result of the deleterious effects of chronic alcohol abuse on the brain. Furthermore, given the well-known relation between alcoholism and aggression, the cognitive deficits seen in this group may also be due to head injuries incurred from increased physical violence.

5. The High-Risk Paradigm

One manner of extricating cause from consequence with regard to the role of ECF in alcohol use disorders is to employ the high-risk paradigm. Instead of studying seasoned alcoholics, the high-risk paradigm involves investigating nonalcoholic individuals at heightened risk for the development of alcoholism. Typically, such individuals are defined by having at least one biological parent, usually the father, who is an alcoholic. By studying persons who are at high risk, one avoids the limitations inherent in studying alcoholics, because their nonalcoholic offspring have either not yet begun to consume alcohol or have consumed so little as to have negligible, if any, lasting effects on cognitive functioning.

The research data on cognitive functioning in individuals at high-risk for alcoholism suggest that, like alcoholics, these individuals also suffer from a mild deficit in ECF. Sons of alcoholics show deficits in problem solving, attention, working memory,[47–52] categorization, organization, temporal sequencing, associative learning, response perseveration, motor control,[43,47,53–57] strategic planning, and abstracting ability.[47–49,55,58,59]

Again, although these data provide support for a mild ECF deficit in children of alcoholics, they should be interpreted with caution. Children of alcoholics are significantly more likely to suffer perinatal complications, physical abuse, and severe head trauma by virtue of the environments in which they are reared. As with alcoholics, researchers must be careful to rule out these possibilities, since the existence of head trauma can invalidate any inferences made about inherited cognitive deficits as predisposing factors for alcoholism. Moreover, studies that do not exclude high-risk subjects on the basis of having an alcoholic mother should be scrutinized carefully, given the possibility that the cognitive deficits seen in these children may be the result of fetal alcohol syndrome.

Nevertheless, there have been some negative findings indicating no or limited cognitive differences between sons of alcoholics and controls.[50,60–63] However, many of these findings have been attributed to methodological difficulties in these studies.[64]

One interesting alternative possibility for some of these negative findings is that the cognitive deficits seen in alcoholics and children of alcoholics may actually be due to antisocial behavior. One study found neuropsychological deficits in men with a family history of alcoholism, but only if they also had a comorbid diagnosis of an antisocial personality disorder (ASPD).[65] Another study showed that alcoholics with a diagnosis of ASPD had greater neuropsychological impairments compared to non-ASPD alcoholics.[66] Furthermore, a diagnosis of ASPD in these individuals was still related to cognitive deficits even when controlling for length of drinking history.[66] Parenthetically, bolstering these data on alcoholics, substance abusers with ASPD have also been shown to have more cognitive deficits compared to their non-ASPD counterparts.[67] These data are supported by studies indicating that alcohol use disorders tend to be preceded by antisocial and aggressive behavior.[68–70] Together, these findings suggest that the cognitive deficits seen in alcoholics and those at risk for alcoholism may be secondary to antisocial/disinhibited behavior.

6. Executive Cognitive Functioning in Psychiatric Disorders Characterized by Disinhibited and Antisocial Behavior

One of the major behavioral concomitants of alcoholism is antisocial behavior.[29,61] Alcoholics with a family history of alcoholism are more antisocial than alcoholics without such a history[71,72] and are more likely to have antisocial relatives.[73] The association between antisocial behavior and alcohol use also extends to childhood. Alcohol use occurs more often in hyperactive, impulsive, conduct-disordered, antisocial, aggressive, and violent children.[74–79] Retrospective accounts also indicate that adult alcoholics report externalizing, delinquent, antisocial, and aggressive behaviors as children.[29,80,81] Furthermore, two longitudinal studies have demonstrated that academic failure, running away from home, truancy, delinquency, thievery, and high school dropout rates are predictive of adult alcohol abuse.[82,83] Not surprisingly, psychiatric disorders characterized by antisocial, impulsive, and disinhibited behavior have all been linked to deficits in ECF.

6.1. *Studies with Children*

Chelune *et al.*[84] found that children with attention-deficit–hyperactivity disorder (ADHD) did not differ from controls on most tests of general intellectual ability; however, they did perform worse on tests of ECF, reflecting problems in attentional skills, cognitive flexibility, response inhibition, and goal-directed behavior. Another study corroborated these results by demonstrating that inattentive–overactive children performed at a lower level than controls on various tests of ECF.[85] Nevertheless, two other studies were unable to detect group differences in ECF between children with ADHD and controls.[86,87]

Yeudall *et al.*[88] administered comprehensive neuropsychological examinations to a sample of juvenile delinquents who committed both violent and nonviolent crimes. Results indicated that the delinquent group performed poorly in comparison to the nondelinquent group on a number of tests of ECF. Skoff and Libon[89] also detected impaired ECF in a sample of incarcerated male juvenile delinquents. Deficits were noted in the areas of mental planning, initiating and preserving a mental set, set shifting, and mental control. In addition, Shapiro *et al.*[90] found that undersocialized, aggressive, conduct-disordered (CD) males exhibited more maladaptive response perseveration behavior compared to normal controls. Another study found that, compared to controls, CD adolescent males performed poorly on a variety of neuropsychological tests of ECF; however, there were no group differences on tests measuring "non-ECF" functions.[91] Similarly, others have shown that physically aggressive boys demonstrate poorer ECF capacity compared to their nonaggressive counterparts.[92] These boys have also been shown to exhibit greater deficits in ECF compared to other neuropsychological functions. Moreover, Moffitt and colleagues investigated neuropsychological functioning in a large New Zealand sample of adolescent delinquents and nondelinquents. Results from one report indicated that compared to controls, delinquent girls had poorer ECF capacity; however, this finding was not seen in delinquent boys.[93] Findings from two other reports demonstrated compromised ECF only in boys with comorbid diagnoses of CD and ADHD.[94,95] Last, other researchers assessed adolescent CD males and normal controls on the nine Lurian tests of prefrontal cortical functioning.[96] Results demonstrated that the CD group performed poorly compared to controls. However, this difference disappeared when language comprehension was controlled.

6.2. *Studies with Adults*

A study by Gorenstein[97] assessed ECF in a sample of ASPD males. Results indicated that these individuals performed poorly compared to psychiatric and normal controls. As noted above, other studies found that compared to alcoholics[66] and substance abusers[67] without ASPD, those with ASPD demonstrated significantly more deficits in ECF. Pertinently, two recent studies with ASPD males found reductions in the electrical amplitude of the P300 event-related potential, particularly in the frontal scalp region.[98,99] The P300 is thought to reflect attentional processes[100] and is believed to originate in the prefrontal cortex.[101,102] In addition, a reduced frontal P300 amplitude has been linked to poor performance on neuropsychological tests of ECF.[103,104]

Nevertheless, there are studies that have been unable to replicate findings of decreased ECF in men with ASPD.[105–108]

7. Integration and Possible Explanations

It has been noted that one possibility for the contradictory findings in demonstrating an ECF deficit in individuals with ADHD, CD, and ASPD is because the relation between ECF and these disorders may be better accounted for by physical aggression.[109] Physical aggression has been strongly related to deficits in ECF.[110–112] Giancola[109] has provided a heuristic model detailing the manner in which a deficiency in ECF may foster physical aggression given a sufficiently provoking context. For example, impaired self-monitoring, abstract reasoning, and attentional skills may compromise the ability to correctly interpret potentially ambiguous social cues during interpersonal interactions, which may lead to misattributions in the perception of threat or hostility in conflict situations. In addition, ineffectual hypothesis generation, poor concept formation, and cognitive inflexibility along with poor judgment may undermine the ability to generate and implement alternative nonaggressive behavioral responses in anger-provoking situations. Moreover, inadequate planning, temporal sequencing, and organization capacities may interfere with the ability to execute a series of responses in the proper order and manner to avoid an aggressive interaction. Finally, compromised cognitive control over behavior may allow hostile cognitions and negative affective states to manifest themselves as overt aggression.

Physical aggression is not a paramount feature in the diagnostic taxonomy of ADHD, CD, and ASPD. Specifically, ASPD and CD comprise a variety of diagnostic features only one of which is physical aggression. Further, although children with ADHD are sometimes aggressive, physical aggression is not a symptom of ADHD according to standard classification schemes. Moreover, according to Hare's Revised Psychopathy Checklist, physical aggression is not explicitly mentioned in any of the 20 diagnostic criteria for psychopathy.[113] Consequently, the absence of physical aggression in an individual does not preclude a diagnosis of any of these disorders, and therefore it would appear that such individuals may not be optimal groups to test if one is interested in assessing deficits in ECF. In fact, a close examination of the studies reviewed above (and others) on ECF in CD males indicates that the investigations with positive results likely employed more aggressive samples than those demonstrating negative findings.[109]

8. A Heuristic Cognitive–Neurobehavioral Model for Psychological Dependence on Alcohol

Existing theoretical models of dependence on alcohol and other drugs include those that incorporate conceptualizations of addiction that are driven by either negative (e.g., tension reduction hypothesis[114]; stress response dampening[115]) or positive reinforcement (e.g., psychomotor stimulant theory[116]). Recently, Robinson and Berridge[117] synthesized an incentive sensitization theory of addiction that is consistent with both views. They posit that the neural substrate for incentive salience is the dopamine system of the ventral striatum including the nucleus accumbens, an essential aspect of the brain's reward system subsumed by the mesolimbic dopaminergic pathway. Sensitization of these structures through repeated administration of alcohol and other drugs is posited to increase the incentive salience of alcohol-associated stimuli, as well as the enhancement of stereotypic drug-seeking motivation and behavior.

However, this conceptualization, while comprehensive in several respects, does not recognize a role for the functional status of the prefrontal cortex in this process of acquisition of addictive behaviors, nor does it take into account the substantial neural connections between the striatum and the prefrontal cortex. Specifically, the mesolimbic dopaminergic reward pathway extends from the ventral tegmental area beyond the ventral striatum (and nucleus accumbens), passes through the anterior cingulate gyrus, ultimately leading to innervate the prefrontal cortex. Other dopaminergic tracts also originate in the ventral tegmental area and take a more direct route to the prefrontal cortex. Importantly, there is good evidence for extensive reciprocal innervation between the ventral striatum and the prefrontal cortex.[118] Moreover, the medial prefrontal cortex also appears to play an important role in the regulation of striatal dopamine release.[119]

Consequently, we have extended Robinson and Berridge's[117] theory to incorporate the current research on the direct effects of alcohol and other drugs on the prefrontal cortex, as well as their sensitizing propensities on the ventral striatum. The behavioral role of the prefrontal–striatal relation is addressed by employing aspects of Shallice's[120] cognitive "information-processing" model that was originally designed to predict behavioral changes produced by specific brain lesions.

Shallice's model proposes two cognitive systems of behavioral activation: the contention scheduling system (CSS) and the supervisory attentional system (SAS). The CSS is posited to reside in the corpus striatum and is activated by environmental demands for routine behavior. Consistent with Robinson and Berridge,[117] sensitization of this system by alcohol and other drugs could result in high-incentive stereotypic drug-taking behavior. On the other hand, the SAS is posited to reside in the prefrontal cortex and is activated when new environmental demands require novel and flexible adaptive behavioral responses. Coping, problem solving, abstract reasoning, responses to novelty, and the planning and initiation of behavior all fall under the rubric of the SAS. As such, it would appear that in order to function properly, the SAS must draw on functions that fall under the purview of ECF. Consequently, a selective lesion of the prefrontal cortex would impair the functioning of the SAS while permitting the CSS to continue functioning with a specific set of routinized behaviors becoming dominant.

Acute alcohol intoxication has been demonstrated to be associated with significant decreases in glucose metabolism in the prefrontal cortex,[121] with a relative sparing of the basal ganglia, in effect, producing a selective pharmacological prefrontal "lesion."

These data are corroborated with neuropsychological studies indicating that acute alcohol intoxication disrupts abstracting,[122] attentional shifting,[123] set shifting,[124] and working memory abilities.[125] In addition, alcohol has also been found to produce the greatest amount of cognitive disruption on the performance of neuropsychological tests of ECF compared to non-ECF tests. Research has shown that alcohol disrupts word fluency, strategic planning, perceptual organization, abstract reasoning, attention, and the organization of information in working memory, whereas it does not, or only minimally, affect vocabulary, general intelligence, visuospatial and spatial orientation functions, and the encoding and retrieval of information into/from long-term memory.[112,126–128] Further supportive evidence comes from postmortem studies indicating that the brains of chronic alcoholics exhibit a higher degree of loss of cortical neurons in the prefrontal cortex compared to other brain regions.[45,46] These alcoholics also have fewer prefrontal neurons compared to age and sex matched controls.[45,46] Therefore, under alcohol intoxication, it can be argued that the CSS is to some extent preserved while the SAS is impaired. The resultant cognitive–behavioral picture is that of a diminished capacity to plan, problem solve, attend to novel stimuli, resist distraction, and regulate goal-directed behavior with a concomitant unimpaired ability and uninhibited motivation to engage in routinized behaviors (drinking), given the proper environmental cues.

A heuristic frontostriatal alcohol addiction model is graphically represented in Fig. 1. Here, both direct pharmacological effects of alcohol and alcohol associated-stimuli activate a sensitized ventral striatum either directly via the dopaminergic reward pathway beginning in the ventral tegmentum or through input from cortical association areas. This stimulates the CSS (ventral tegmentum), resulting in stereotypic and overlearned alcohol-taking behaviors. Simultaneously, dopaminergic innervation from the ventral tegmentum inhibits the prefrontal cortex. Additional prefrontal inhibition is produced by the direct pharmacological actions of alcohol on the prefrontal cortex and the SAS (ECF). Chronic alcohol exposure further disrupts prefrontal physiology via a loss of neurons in the prefrontal cortex,[129] diminished frontal–cortical regional cerebral blood flow,[130,131] and reduced frontal metabolism.[121,132] This alteration in the physiological functioning of the prefrontal cortex could be associated with a significant diminution in the capacity to respond to alcohol-related stimuli with novel and adaptive coping behaviors, while concurrent sensitization of the CSS could account for the stereotypic and overlearned alcohol-seeking behaviors and motivational cognitions associated with compulsive drinking and craving. Generally, the behavioral consequences of this scenario appear consistent with the clinical syndrome of psychological dependence on alcohol.

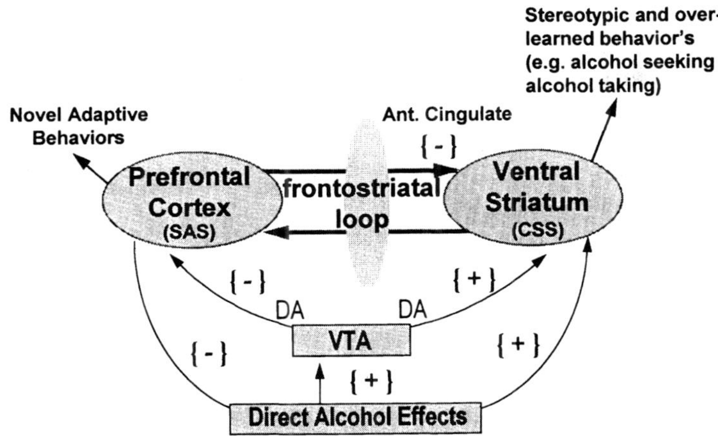

Figure 1. Schematic representation of the frontostriatal hypothesis of alcoholism using the information-processing model of Shallice[120] (SAS, supervisory attentional system; CSS, contention scheduling system). The CSS is posited to reside in the ventral region of the corpus striatum (including the nucleus accumbens) and is responsible for the emanation of routine, overlearned behaviors. The sensitization of the CSS system by repeated administration of alcohol and other drugs could result in high-incentive stereotypic drug-seeking, drug-taking behavior consistent with the model of Robinson and Berridge.[117] Effects of alcohol on the ventral tegmental area (VTA) would also stimulate the CSS via the mesolimbic dopaminergic pathways. The SAS is posited to reside in prefrontal cortex and is activated when environmental demands require new and flexible adaptive behavioral responses. These include coping, problem solving, responses to novelty, and the planning and initiation of new behaviors. The two systems are in balance with the SAS, exerting inhibitory tone on the CSS, while the CSS stimulates the SAS. A constitutive dysfunction or selective lesion of the prefrontal cortex would impair the capacity of the SAS, thereby permitting the CSS schema to dominate the behavioral repertoire through the generation of specific sets of routinized behaviors. Thus, individuals with antisocial personality disorder, conduct disorder, or other disorders of executive functioning may be more susceptible to developing alcohol-associated stereotypic and overlearned behaviors consistent with views of psychological dependence. Alcohol effects on the prefrontal neural substrate of the SAS appear to be inhibitory through dopaminergic inhibition at the level of the VTA, as well as through direct inhibitory effects mediated by the GABA interneurons associated with the dopaminergic neurons in prefrontal cortex.[118] Thus, under the chronic influence of alcohol, the CSS is sensitized while the SAS is impaired, leading to an unopposed emergence of overlearned alcohol-associated behaviors.

9. The Frontostriatal Model and the Etiology of Antisocial Alcoholism

The research literature suggests that there may be a common diathesis localized in the prefrontal cortex for both persistent dyssocial behavior and the antisocial variant of alcoholism that has been referred to as type 2[133] or type B[134] alcoholism. The most prevalent adult psychiatric disorder occurring comorbidly with alcoholism is ASPD.[2] Antisocial adults show impulsive, aggressive, and disinhibited behavior similar to that seen among human and subhuman primates with lesions in prefrontal cortical regions.[135] These same features of dysregulated behavior frequently have been shown to predispose to psychoactive substance use disorders.[136] Although similarity in behavior does not necessarily imply commonality in underlying mechanisms, as noted above, numerous investigations have suggested that CD in adolescence and ASPD in adulthood are associated with a dysfunction of the prefrontal cortex–ECF.[109,137] In fact, in one study, ASPD adults performed as poorly on neurpsychological tests sensitive to prefrontal lobe functioning as would patients with prefrontal lesions.[47]

Evidence from prospective research suggests that there is substantial developmental continuity for CD at the syndromal and phenomenological level.[138] For example, dispositional aggressivity [a feature of CD in the *Diagnostic and Statistical Manual of Mental Disorders*, 4th ed.[139] (DSM-IV)] has been demonstrated to be nearly as stable as IQ across the lifespan.[140] Importantly, aspects of this ipsative developmental continuity include later adult antisociality and substance use.[137,141,142]

The frontal–striatal hypothesis presented herein is heuristic in terms of understanding how diminished ECF capacities due to variations in prefrontal functioning could be important in the etiology of some types of alcohol and other drug use disorders. As noted above, research suggests that children of alcoholic and substance-abusing parents frequently display impairments in ECF attributable to variations in prefrontal functioning.[47,53,143] Such children also demonstrate problems with inattention, aggressivity, and impulsivity.[144] Longitudinal research has suggested that aggressivity and impulsivity are robust predictors of alcoholism and other forms of drug abuse.[68–70,82,145] Consistent with these findings is prospective research from the Ontario Child Health Study. In keeping with the studies described earlier demonstrating that ASPD likely accounts for deficits in ECF in alcoholics and substance abusers, this investigation revealed that, even when controlling for ADHD, the only syndromal psychiatric disorder that predicted substance abuse in either early or late adolescence was CD.[146,147] Importantly, as noted above, neuropsychological investigations of CD youth have revealed a pattern of cognitive impairments on tests of prefrontal cortical functioning.[138,148] However, to define this position even further, it has been suggested that physical aggression may be the component of CD that is most strongly related to prefrontal–ECF deficits.[109]

9.1. *Autonomic Reactivity to Stress*

Consistent with the frontostriatal hypothesis is the observation of similarity in autonomic reactivity to stress among individuals at risk for alcoholism, other forms of substance abuse, and those with ASPD. Lykken[149] first demonstrated that psychopathic individuals showed a reduced skin conductance response to anticipated shock. Subsequently, Hare[150] found that psychopathic individuals undergoing a similar anticipated threat procedure not only showed less palmar sweating and skin conductance than normals, but also displayed greater cardiac acceleration than normals. As recently noted by Lykken,[149] these psychophysiological variations among psychopathic individuals that were initially observed by Lykken and subsequently by Hare have been repeatedly replicated by other investigators.

In related research, Eslinger and Damasio[151] reported about a patient, EVR, who, like Gage, was a well-socialized, intelligent, and hard-working individual premorbidly, became dyssocial following the surgical ablation of his ventromedial frontal cortices. Interestingly, EVR performed fairly normally on standard neuropsychological tests. However, in the psychophysiological laboratory, EVR showed a marked failure to generate electrodermal responses to passive viewing of stressful pictures depicting social disasters, mutilation, or nudity. When he was required to actively respond to these stimuli, his skin conductance responses were normal. This single-case observation was later confirmed in a study of several individuals with bilateral frontal damage whereby stressful social stimuli again failed to elicit an autonomic response.[152] Thus, attenuated skin conductance responses to stressful stimuli may be acquired as a consequence of frontal brain damage, and as a result, provide a noteworthy degree of commonality between psychopathic individuals and individuals with prefrontal lesions. Relatedly, another study by these investigators found that neurologically intact individuals generated increased anticipatory skin conductance responses prior to making risky decisions, whereas those with frontal lesions did not demonstrate this response profile.[153] Findings from these studies are supported by research indicating that the prefrontal cortex mediates skin conductance responsivity.[154]

Psychophysiological studies of individuals at familial risk for alcoholism also provide some convergence of evidence concerning autonomic reactivity to stress and liability status. For example, sober adult sons of alcoholics have been shown to manifest increased heart rate, frontal skull muscle tension, and decreased digital blood flow in anticipation of shock.[155–157] These results are similar to those reported by Hare[150] in psychopathic individuals. Findings with respect to skin conductance responses to shock in high-risk individuals are less consistent. One study demonstrated that compared to controls, high-risk men exhibited an exaggerated response,[157] whereas another study demonstrated the opposite finding.[158] Post-hoc examinations attempting to determiner whether the hyporeactivity in skin conductance responses in the latter study could be accounted for by diagnoses of ASPD in the high-risk sample were not conclusive due to limited statistical power.[158]

Findings appear to be more consistent with regard to the acute effects of alcohol on responsivity to stress in individuals at high risk for alcoholism. Research has shown greater reductions in stress after alcohol consumption in individuals at high risk for alcoholism compared to controls on measures of heart rate, digital blood flow, pulse transmission time, and skin conductance.[155–161] These findings suggest that, compared to controls, individuals at high risk for alcoholism may experience greater physiological reinforcement from alcohol when under stress. Nevertheless, the mechanism underlying this stress response dampening (SRD) effect in high-risk individuals is unclear. However, one study has found a strong negative relation between the SRD effect of alcohol and ECF, thus suggesting that a prefrontal deficit may be involved in hyperreactivity to stress and alcohol SRD.[56] This interpretation is consistent with data suggesting that the prefrontal cortex is involved, in part, in the regulation of autonomic arousal.[154,162]

Interestingly, Sher and Levenson[160] have demonstrated that high-risk individuals with increased aggressivity, impulsivity, and extroversion (traits that may reflect impaired ECF and diminished prefrontal capacities) are most sensitive to the physiological SRD effects of alcohol. This finding again corroborates previous results indicating that antisociality may be a better predictor of risk for alcoholism than a family history of the disorder and that deficits in ECF–prefrontal cortical functioning may be an underlying etiologic determinant of pathological alcohol consumption.

At the level of neural systems, what might occur when individuals with diminished prefrontal capacities are exposed to the ubiquity of alcohol in the environment? Under the frontal–striatal hypothesis, a constitutive imbalance between the reduced functioning of the SAS (localized in the prefrontal cortex) and a preserved CSS (localized in the ventral striatum) might predispose such individuals toward greater behavioral sensitization and more stereotypic responses toward alcohol and alcohol-related stimuli without the benefit of a highly functional countervening system for eliciting novel and well-regulated behavioral responses. Moreover, under this hypothesis, dysregulation in psychophysiological responsivity to stress either in the sober or in the intoxicated state would be secondary to complications to the SAS. Data indicating a relation between ECF and autonomic reactivity[56] and data from patients such as EVR[151] would support this interpretation. As such, given that individuals with ASPD, and especially those exhibiting excessive aggressive behavior, tend to show more severe deficits with ECF, such persons may also experience greater levels of autonomic dysregulation, and therefore be at higher risk for the development of alcoholism.

While alcohol exposure in normal individuals has an adverse impact on prefrontal functioning, one could posit that those who have an a priori disruption of prefrontal physiology might experience an even more profound detrimental impact (especially those with ASPD and/or aggressive tendencies). Consequently, these individuals could be more susceptible to the development of psychological dependence on alcohol as manifested by greater incentive salience, a narrowed behavioral repertoire in response to alcohol stimuli due to an unopposed sensitization of the CSS in the ventral striatum, and dysregulated autonomic arousal while under stress. These responses may therefore set the stage for the psychological dependence component of an alcohol use disorder.

10. A Developmental Psychopathology Perspective and Its Implications for the Prevention and Treatment of Alcoholism

Several specific dispositional propensities have been linked to a heightened risk for alcoholism and other substance use disorders. These include deficits in ECF,[47] sensation seeking,[163] impulsivity,[70,164] and aggression.[47] Each of these propensities implicating behavioral disinhibition is common across persons with anterior cortical pathology injury. Grafman *et al.*[165] investigated the effects of lateralized orbitofrontal and dorsolateral prefrontal injuries on mood regulation. Lesions of the right orbitofrontal region were associated with increased irritability, anxiety, and depression, while left dorsolateral lesions were associated with greater anger and hostility. These affective characteristics have been implicated to presage psychoactive substance use disorders.[68,69,166] Sensation-seeking or risk-taking behavior has also been linked to reduced behavioral inhibitor capacity. Associated with this behavioral characteristic is impulsivity. This propensity, like sensation seeking, has been frequently related to substance use disorders[167] and is manifest following an anterior cerebral injury.[168] Offspring of alcoholics not only exhibit these latter propensities but also display a pattern of evoked potential abnormalities that have been interpreted to reflect functional developmental retardation localized to the anterior cerebral region.[94,104,169]

Others have also hypothesized that the presence of a putative delay (or dysfunction) in the chronological attainment of stages of cerebral maturation is characteristic of subgroups of youth at high risk for psychoactive substance abuse disorders.[170] From the perspective of neural development, there is now substantial evidence that during normal human brain maturation, both synaptogenesis and synaptic elimination are critically important developmental phenomena.[171–174] Neurons in the deep layers of the frontal poles mature at about 1 year of age[175] and an excess number of synapses have been observed at the end of the first year. The process of synaptic elimination (sometimes called "synaptic pruning") has been demonstrated to occur in the maturing human prefrontal cortex from about age 8 through late adolescence.[176] Human positron emission tomography studies have shown that prefrontal glucose metabolism, although elevated from birth to 8 months, subsequently follows a prolonged period of decline through maturation that parallels a decline in synaptic density.[177,178]

Are there specific factors associated with this process of prefrontal neural development? Both synaptogenesis and synaptic pruning appear to be manifestations of synaptic plasticity that is activity dependent. During the process of synaptic pruning, the selection of retained neural circuits is based on both activation of specific circuits and the integration of those functions into ongoing patterns of behavior.[179] In humans, experiential stimuli seem to be critically important in influencing the maturation of the prefrontal cortex.[180] Early stresses may condition or sensitize developing neural networks to produce effects manifested in later life.[181] Socialization and attachment behavior may also influence the maturation of the prefrontal cortex.[182] In fact, it has been argued that the prefrontal cortex is the brain region most influential in inculcating societal mores into socially appropriate behavior. Importantly, it is in the experience-dependent physiological maturation of the prefrontal cortex that genetic and environmental factors may readily interact in producing the neural substrate for subtle executive deficits, dysregulated behaviors, and substance abuse risk.[181]

If socializing childhood experiences are essential components for the normative maturation of the prefrontal cortex and normative maturation is associated with enhanced behavioral self-regulation, it stands to reason that more effective alcoholism prevention strategies could be timed to those critical developmental periods in the maturation of the prefrontal cortex. From birth to the end of the first year of life is one such critical period. Through social contact and perhaps attachment processes, synaptogenesis of the prefrontal region goes into high gear.[182] Thus, the experience of stimulating social interactions with parents and other caregivers enhances the development of this critical brain region. However, in disruptive alcoholic or antisocial families, both parenting skills and parent–child bonding may be limited or irregular, thereby decreasing the intensity or duration of the child's critical experiential stimulation. Thus, prevention strategies that promote parenting skills and parent–child bonding could be effective interventions to offset subsequent behavioral dysregulation through stimulation of prefrontal synaptogenesis.

The other critical developmental interval for maturation of the prefrontal cortex is between the ages of 8 and 18. Here too, experience and salience of stimulation is associated with the process of synaptic elimination and the strengthening of remaining neural connections. Again, this process is highly activity dependent. Passive learning experiences will do little to mold synaptic plasticity, while active and relevant interventions will have greater impact on the maturing prefrontal cortex. Therefore, parental skill in socializing offspring may be a critical factor in molding childhood behavior to be prosocial and resilient. In fact, preliminary research has suggested that having a substance-abusing father increases a boy's risk for externalizing and internalizing problem behaviors only when the paternal substance use disorder extends beyond the child's sixth year into the period of prefrontal synaptic elimination.[183]

Moreover, given that a deficit in ECF has been highlighted as a risk factor for the development of alcoholism and because activity-dependent interventions are favored over passive learning approaches, another potential prevention and possibly treatment strategy would be to strengthen ECF capacity. This may be accomplished by training high-risk or affected individuals through the use of neurocognitive tasks designed to increase and strengthen their attentional, strategic planning, abstract reasoning, hypothesis generation, cognitive flexibility, and self-monitoring capacities. In fact, Barkley[184] has suggested that hyperactive children may benefit from intervention techniques aimed at increasing cognitive skills. Such cognitive techniques may be particularly effective in increasing ECF capacity, as others have demonstrated that behavior therapy for obsessive–compulsive disorder alters brain activity in neural circuits involving the prefrontal cortex.[185,186] As deficits in ECF have been related to behavioral dysregulation, strengthening these cognitive functions may be helpful in producing more regulated and controlled drinking patterns or an improved ability to maintain abstinence.

11. Summary and Conclusions

The literature reviewed in this chapter suggests that alcoholics and children at high risk for the develpment of alcoholism suffer from a mild dysfunction of the prefrontal cortex. This biological deviation is manifested psychologically, in part, as a deficit in ECF capacity. A frontostriatal model of alcoholism was advanced in which it was theorized that a deficit in ECF is associated with an inability of the prefrontal cortex to regulate and inhibit high-incentive stereotypic drug-taking messages from the ventral striatum. Consequently, from a prevention perspective, it could be argued that fostering maximal development of the prefrontal cortex in high-risk children would be a useful strategy leading to an enhanced ability to adaptively regulate drug-taking messages. This can be accomplished by exposing the child to a variety of positive experiential stimuli and through close parent–child socialization and attachment interactions. In addition to this, more direct methods of bolstering prefrontal development in high-risk children would involve teaching them to effectively use ECF skills, most likely through the use of specialized neuropsychological tasks.

Despite recommendations for prevention and treatment, as stated earlier, the etiology of alcoholism is not well understood. Current etiologic models of alcoholism either speak beyond the available empirical data or are impossible to test, given current assessment and diagnostic technologies. Although the authors recognize the immediate need for efforts directed toward the prevention and treatment of alcoholism, effective interventions cannot be developed without continued research into the etiology of this disorder. Such information will come from high-risk studies, longitudinal studies, and behavioral pharmacology studies.

References

1. Kessler RC, McGonagle KA, Zhao S, *et al:* Lifetime and 12-month prevalence of DSM-III-R psychiatric disorders in the United States: Results from the national comorbidity survey. *Arch Gen Psychiatry* 51:8–19, 1994.
2. Regier DA, Farmer ME, Rae DS, *et al:* Comorbidity of mental disorders with alcohol and other drug abuse: Results from the epidemioloc catchment area (ECA) study. *JAMA* 264:2511–2518, 1990.

3. Rice DP: The economic cost of alcohol abuse and alcohol dependence: 1990. *Alcohol Health Res World* 17:10–11, 1993.
4. Mullahy J, Sindelar J: Effects of alcohol on labor market success: Income, earnings, labor supply, and occupation. *Alcohol Health Res World* 16:134–139, 1992.
5. Podolsky DM, Richards D: Investigating the role of substance abuse in occupational injuries. *Alcohol Health Res World,* Summer, 42–45, 1985.
6. Murdoch D, Pihl R, Ross D: Alcohol and crimes of violence: Present issues. *Int J Addict* 25:1065–1081, 1990.
7. Sands BF, Knapp CM, Ciraulo DA: Medical consequences of alcohol–drug interactions. *Alcohol Health Res World* 17:316–320, 1993.
8. Luria A: *Higher Cortical Functions in Man.* New York, Basic Books, 1980.
9. Milner B, Petrides M, Smith M: Frontal lobes and the temporal organization of memory. *Hum Neurobiol* 4:137–142, 1985.
10. Milner B, Petrides M: Behavioural effects of frontal-lobe lesions in man. *Trends Neurosci* November, 403–407, 1984.
11. Stuss D, Benson D: Neuropsychological studies of the frontal lobes. *Psychol Bull* 95:3–28, 1984.
12. Lezak M: *Neuropsychological Assessment,* 3rd ed. New York, Oxford University Press, 1995.
13. Kolb B, Whishaw I: *Fundamentals of Human Neuropsychology,* 3rd ed. New York, W.H. Freeman & Co, 1990.
14. Luria A: *The Working Brain: An Introduction to Neuropsychology.* New York, Basic Books, 1973.
15. Walsh K: *Neuropsychology: A Clinical Approach,* 2nd ed. New York, Churchill Livingstone, 1987.
16. Fuster J: *The Prefrontal Cortex: Anatomy, Physiology, and Neuropsychology of the Frontal Lobe,* 2nd ed. New York, Raven Press, 1989.
17. Goldman-Rakic PS: Topography of cognition: Parallel distributed networks in primate association cortex. *Annu Rev Neurosci* 11:137–156, 1988.
18. Cummings J: Frontal–subcortical circuits and human behavior. *Arch Neurol* 50:873–880, 1993.
19. Degos JD, da Fonseca N, Gray F, *et al:* Severe frontal syndrome associated with infarcts of the left anterior cingulate gyrus and the head of the right caudate nucleus: A clinicopathological case. *Brain* 116:1541–1548, 1993.
20. Harlow JM: Recovery after severe injury to the head. *Pub Mass Med Soc* 2:327–346, 1968.
21. Damasio H, Grabowski T, Frank R, *et al:* The return of Phineas Gage: Clues about the brain from the skull of a famous patient. *Science* 264:1102–1105, 1994.
22. Stuss DT, Gow CA, Hetherington CR: "No longer Gage": Frontal lobe dysfunction and emotional changes. *J Consult Clin Psychol* 60:349–359, 1992.
23. Duffy J, Campbell J: The regional prefrontal syndromes: A theoretical and clinical overview. *J Neuropsychiatry Clin Neurosci* 6:379–387, 1994.
24. Malloy P, Richardson E: Assessment of frontal lobe functions. *J Neuropsychiatry Clin Neurosci* 6:399–410, 1994.
25. Petrides M, Alivisatos B, Evans A, *et al:* Dissociation of human mid-dorsolateral from posterior dorsolateral frontal cortex in memory processing. *Proc Natl Acad Sci USA* 90:873–877, 1993.
26. Hesselbrock V, Hesselbrock M, Stabenau J: Alcoholism in men patients subtyped by family history and antisocial personality. *J Stud Alcohol* 46:59–64, 1985.
27. Parsons O: Neuropsychological measures and event-related potentials in alcoholics: Interrelationships, long-term reliabilities, and prediction of resumption of drinking. *J Clin Psychol* 50:37–46, 1994.
28. Yohman J, Parsons O: Verbal reasoning deficits in alcoholics. *J Nerv Ment Dis* 175:219–223, 1987.
29. Glenn S, Errico A, Parsons O, *et al:* The role of antisocial, affective, and childhood behavioral characteristics in alcoholics, neuropsychological performance. *Alcohol Clin Exp Res* 17:162–169, 1993.

30. Errico A, Parsons O, King A: Assessment of verbosequential and visuospatial cognitive abilities in chronic alcoholics. *Psychiol Assess* 3:693–696, 1991.
31. O'Mahony J, Doherty B: Patterns of intellectual performance among recently abstinent alcohol abusers on WAIS-R and WMS-R sub-tests. *Arch Clin Neuropsychol* 8:373–380, 1993.
32. Nixon S, Tivis R, Parsons O: Behavioral dysfunction and cognitive efficiency in male and female alcoholics. *Alcohol Clin Exp Res* 19:577–581, 1995.
33. Brandt J, Butters N, Ryan C, *et al:* Cognitive loss and recovery in long-term alcohol abusers. *Arch Gen Psychiatry* 40:435–442, 1983.
34. Tarter R: An analysis of cognitive deficits in chronic alcoholics. *J Nerv Ment Dis* 157:138–147, 1973.
35. Tarter R, Parsons O: Conceptual shifting in chronic alcoholics. *J Abnorm Psychol* 77:71–75, 1971.
36. Smith M, Oscar-Berman M: Resource-limited information processing in alcoholism. *J Stud Alcohol* 53:514–518, 1992.
37. Cutting J: Specific psychological deficits in alcoholism. *Br J Psychiatry* 133:119–122, 1978.
38. Hewett L, Nixon S, Glenn S, *et al:* Verbal fluency deficits in female alcoholics. *J Clin Psychol* 47:716–719, 1991.
39. Beatty W, Katzung V, Nixon S, *et al:* Problem-solving deficits in alcoholics: Evidence from the California Card Sorting Test. *J Stud Alcohol* 54:687–692, 1993.
40. Cynn V: Persistence and problem-solving skills in young male alcoholics. *J Stud Alcohol* 53:57–62, 1992.
41. Alterman A, Tarter R, Petrarulo E, *et al:* Evidence for inpersistence in young adult male alcoholics. *Alcohol Clin Exp Res* 8:448–450, 1984.
42. Parsons O, Tarter R, Edelberg R: Altered motor control in chronic alcoholics. *J Abnorm Psychol* 80:308–314, 1972.
43. Braun C, Richer M: A comparison of functional indexes derived from screening tests of chronic alcoholic neurotoxicity in the cerebral cortex retina and peripheral nervous system. *J Stud Alcohol* 54:11–16, 1993.
44. Lehman L, Pilich A, Andrews N: Neurological disorders resulting from alcoholism. *Alcohol Health Res World* 17:305–309, 1993.
45. Harper C, Kril J, Daly J: Are we drinking our neurones away? *Br Med J* 294:534–536, 1987.
46. Kril J, Harper C: Neuronal counts from four cortical regions of alcoholic brains. *Acta Neuropathol* 79:200–204, 1989.
47. Giancola P, Martin C, Tarter R, *et al:* Executive cognitive functioning and aggressive behavior in preadolescent boys at high risk for substance abuse/dependence. *J Stud Alcohol* 57:352–359, 1996.
48. Harden PW, Pihl RO: Cognitive function, cardiovascular reactivity, and behavior in boys at high risk for alcoholism. *J Abnorm Psychol* 104:94–103, 1995.
49. Schaeffer K, Parsons O, Yohman J: Neuropsychological differences between male familial and nonfamilial alcoholics and nonalcoholics. *Alcohol Clin Exp Res* 8:347–351, 1984.
50. Sher K, Walitzer K, Wood P, *et al:* Characteristics of children of alcoholics: Putative risk factors, substance use and abuse, and psychopathology. *J Abnorm Psychol* 100:427–448, 1991.
51. Tarter R, Hegedus A, Goldstein G, *et al:* Adolescent sons of alcoholics: Neuropsychological and personality characteristics. *Alcohol Clin Exp Res* 8:216–222, 1984.
52. Tarter R, Jacob T, Bremer D: Cognitive status of sons of alcoholic men. *Alcohol Clin Exp Res* 13:232–235, 1989.
53. Drejer K, Theilgaard A, Teasdale T, *et al:* A prospective study of young men at high risk for alcoholism: Neuropsychological assessment. *Alcohol Clin Exp Res* 9:498–502, 1985.
54. Giancola P, Peterson J, Pihl R: Risk for alcoholism, antisocial behavior, and response perseveration. *J Clin Psychol* 49:423–428, 1993.
55. Knop J: Premorbid assessment of young men at high risk for alcoholism, in Galanter M (ed): *Recent Developments in Alcoholism,* vol 3. New York, Plenum Press, 1985, pp 53–64.
56. Peterson J, Finn P, Pihl R: Cognitive dysfunction and the inherited predisposition to alcoholism. *J Stud Alcohol* 53:154–160, 1992.

57. Whipple S, Parker E, Noble E: An atypical neurocognitive profile in alcoholic fathers and their sons. *J Stud Alcohol* 49:240–244, 1988.
58. Alterman A, Bridges K, Tarter R: Drinking behavior of high risk college men: Contradictory preliminary findings. *Alcohol Clin Exp Res* 10:305–310, 1986.
59. Hegedus A, Alterman A, Tarter R: Learning achievement in sons of alcoholics. *Alcohol Clin Exp Res* 8:330–333, 1984.
60. Alterman A, Searles J, Hall J: Failure to find differences in drinking behavior as a function of familial risk for alcoholism: A replication. *J Abnorm Psychol* 98:50–53, 1989.
61. Hesselbrock V, Stabenau J, Hesselbrock M: Minimal brain dysfunction and neuropsychological test performance in offspring of alcoholics, in Galanter M (ed): *Recent Developments in Alcoholism,* vol 3. New York, Plenum Press, 1985, pp 65–82.
62. Reed R, Grant I, Adams K: Family history of alcoholism does not predict neuropsychological performance in alcoholics. *Alcohol Clin Exp Res* 11:340–344, 1987.
63. Workman-Daniels K, Hesselbrock V: Childhood problem behavior and neuropsychological functioning in persons at risk for alcoholism. J Stud Alcohol 48:187–193, 1987.
64. Pihl R, Peterson J, Finn P: Inherited predisposition to alcoholism: Characteristics of sons of male alcoholics. *J Abnorm Psychol* 99:291–301, 1990.
65. Gillen R, Hesselbrock V: Cognitive functioning, ASP, and family history of alcoholism in young men at risk for alcoholism. *Alcohol Clin Exp Res* 16:206–214, 1992.
66. Malloy P, Noel N, Rogers S, *et al:* Risk factors for neuropsychological impairment in alcoholics: Antisocial personality, age, years of drinking and gender. *J Stud Alcohol* 50:422–426, 1989.
67. Malloy P, Noel N, Longabaugh R, *et al:* Determinants of neuropsychological impairment in antisocial substance abusers. *Addict Behav* 15:431–438, 1990.
68. Kandel D, Simcha-Fagan O, Davies M: Risk factors for delinquency and illicit drug use from adolescence to young adulthood. *J Drug Issues* 60:67–90, 1986.
69. Kellam S, Stevenson D, Robinson B: *How Specific Are the Early Predictors of Teenage Drug Use?* vol 43. Washington, DC, National Institute on Drug Abuse Research Monograph, 1983.
70. McCord W, McCord J, Gudeman J: *Origins of Alcoholism.* Palo Alto, CA, Stanford University Press, 1960.
71. Alterman A: Patterns of familial alcoholism severity and psychopathology. *J Nerv Met Dis* 176:167–175, 1988.
72. Latcham R: Familial alcoholism: Evidence from 237 alcoholics. *Br J Psychiatry* 147:54–57, 1985.
73. Cook B, Winokur G: A family study of familial positive vs. familial negative alcoholics. *J Nerv Ment Dis* 173:175–178, 1985.
74. August G, Stewart M, Holmes C: A four-year follow-up of hyperactive boys with and without conduct disorder. *Br J Psychiatry* 143:192–198, 1983.
75. Gittelman R, Mannuzza S, Shenker R, *et al:* Hyperactive boys almost grown up: Psychiatric status. *Arch Gen Psychiatry* 42:937–947, 1985.
76. Hechtman L, Weiss G: Controlled prospective fifteen year follow-up of hyperactives as adults: Non-medical drug and alcohol use and anti-social behaviour. *Can J Psychiatry* 31:557–567, 1986.
77. Hechtman L, Weiss G, Perlman T: Hyperactives as young adults: Past and current substance abuse and antisocial behavior. *Am J Orthopsychiatry* 54:415–425, 1984.
78. Mannuzza S, Klein R, Bonagura N, *et al:* Hyperactive boys almost grown-up: Replication of psychiatric status. *Arch Gen Psychiatry* 48:77–83, 1991.
79. Milin R, Halikas J, Meller J, *et al:* Psychopathology among substance abusing juvenile offenders. *J Am Acad Child Adolesc Psychiatry* 30:569–574, 1991.
80. Andreasson S, Allebeck P, Brandt L, *et al:* Antecedents and covariates of high alcohol consumption in young men. *Alcohol Clin Exp Res* 16:708–713, 1992.
81. Goodwin D, Schulsinger F, Hermansen L, *et al:* Alcoholism and the hyperactive child syndrome. *J Nerv Ment Dis* 160:349–353, 1975.

82. Robins LN: *Deviant Children Grown Up: A Sociological and Psychiatric Study of Sociopathic Personality*. Baltimore, Williams & Wilkins, 1966.
83. Robins L, Murphy G, Breckenridge M: Drinking behavior of young urban negro men. *Q J Stud Alcohol* 29:657–684, 1968.
84. Chelune GJ, Ferguson W, Koon R, *et al:* Frontal-lobe disinhibition in attention deficit disorder. *Child Psychiatry Hum Dev* 16(4):223–234, 1986.
85. Gorenstein EE, Mammato CA, Sandy JM: Performance of inattentive–overactive children on selected measures of prefrontal-type function. *J Clin Psychiatry* 45(4):619–632, 1989.
86. Fischer M, Barkley RA, Edelbrock CS, *et al:* The adolescent outcome of hyperactive children diagnosed by research criteria: II. Academic, attentional, and neuropsychological status. *J Consult Clin Psychol* 58(5):580–588, 1990.
87. Loge DL, Staton RD, Beatty WW: Performance of children with ADHD on tests sensitive to frontal lobe dysfunction. *J Am Acad Child Adolesc Psychiatry* 29(4):540–545, 1990.
88. Yeudall LT, Fromm-Auch D, Davies P: Neuropsychological impairment of persistent delinquency. *J Nerv Ment Dis* 170(5):257–265, 1982.
89. Skoff B, Libon D: Impaired executive functions in a sample of male juvenile delinquents. *J Clin Exp Neuropsychol* 9:60, 1987.
90. Shapiro SK, Quay HC, Hogan AE, *et al:* Response perseveration and delayed responding in undersocialized aggressive conduct disorder. *J Abnorm Psychol* 97(3):371–373, 1988.
91. Lueger RJ, Gill KJ: Frontal-lobe cognitive dysfunction in conduct disorder adolescents. *J Clin Psychol* 46(6):696–705, 1990.
92. Seguin J, Pihl R, Harden P, *et al:* Cognitive and neuropsychological characteristics of physically aggressive boys. *J Abnorm Psychol* 104:614–624, 1995.
93. Moffitt T: Neuropsychology and self-reported early delinquency in an unselected birth cohort: A preliminary report from New Zealand, in Moffitt T, Mednick S (eds): *Biological Contributions to Crime Causation*. Boston, Martinus Nijhoff, 1988, pp 93–117.
94. Moffitt T, Henry B: Neuropsychological assessment of executive functions in self-reported delinquents. *Dev Psychopathol* 1:105–118, 1989.
95. Moffitt T, Silva P: Self-reported delinquency, neuropsychological deficit, and history of attention deficit disorder. *J Abnorm Child Psychol* 16:553–569, 1988.
96. Linz T, Hooper S, Hynd G, *et al:* Frontal lobe functioning in conduct disordered juveniles: Preliminary findings. *Arch Clin Neuropsychol* 5:411–416, 1990.
97. Gorenstein E: Frontal lobe functions in psychopaths. *J Abnorm Psychol* 91:368–379, 1982.
98. Bauer L, Hesselbrock V, O'Connor S, *et al:* P300 differences between non-alcoholic young men at average and above-average risk for alcoholism: Effects of distraction and task modality. *Prog Neuropsychopharmacol Biol Psychiatry* 18:263–277, 1994.
99. O'Connor S, Bauer L, Tasman A, *et al:* Reduced P3 amplitudes are associated with both a family history of alcoholism and antisocial personality disorder. *Prog Neuropsychopharmacol Biol Psychiatry* 18:1307–1321, 1994.
100. Polich J: On the clinical application of the P300. *Biol Psychiatry* 31:647–649, 1992.
101. Alexander J, Porjesz B, Bauer L, *et al:* P300 hemispheric amplitude asymmetries from a visual oddball task. *Psychophysiology* 32:467–475, 1995.
102. Yamaguchi S, Knight R: Anterior and posterior association cortex contributions to the somatosensory P300. *J Neurosci* 11:2039–2054, 1991.
103. Brigham J, Giancola P, Moss H: Event-related potentials and executive cognitive function in preadolescent males. Presented at the annual meeting of the Cognitive Neuroscience Society, April 2, 1996, San Francisco, CA.
104. Hesselbrock V, Bauer L, O'Connor S, *et al:* Reduced P300 amplitude in relation to family history of alcoholism and antisocial personality disorder among young men at risk for alcoholism. *Alcohol Alcohol Suppl* 95–100, 1993.
105. Hare R: Performance of psychopaths on cognitive tasks related to frontal lobe function. *J Abnorm Psychol* 93:133–140, 1984.
106. Sutker P, Allain A: Cognitive abstraction, shifting, and control: Clinical sample comparisons of psychopaths and nonpsychopaths. *J Abnorm Psychol* 96:73–75, 1987.

107. Hoffman J, Hall R, Bartsch T: On the relative importance of "psychopathic" personality and alcoholism on neuropsychological measures of frontal lobe dysfunction. *J Abnorm Psychol* 96:158–160, 1987.
108. Smith S, Arnett P, Newman J: Neuropsychological differentiation of psychopathic and nonpsychopathic criminal offenders. *Pers Indiv Differences* 13:1233–1243, 1992.
109. Giancola P: Evidence for dorsolateral and orbital prefrontal cortical involvement in the expression of aggressive behavior. *Aggressive Behav* 21:431–450, 1995.
110. Giancola P, Zeichner A: Neuropsychological performance on tests of frontal-lobe functioning and aggression in human males. *J Abnorm Psychol* 103:832–835, 1994.
111. Lau M, Pihl R, Peterson J: Provocation, acute alcohol intoxication, cognitive performance, and aggression. *J Abnorm Psychol* 104:150–155, 1995.
112. Hoaken PNS, Assaad JM, Pihl RO: Cognitive performance and the inhibition of alcohol-induced aggression. *J Studs Alcohol*, in press.
113. Hare R, Hart S, Harpur T: Psychopathy and the DSM-IV criteria for antisocial personality disorder. *J Abnorm Psychol* 100:391–398, 1991.
114. Conger JJ: Reinforcement theory and the dynamics of alcoholism. *Q J Stud Alcohol* 17:296–305, 1956.
115. Sher K: Stress response dampening, in Blane H, Leonard K (eds): *Psychological Theories of Drinking and Alcoholism*. New York, Guilford Press, 1987, pp 227–271.
116. Wise RA, Bozarth MA: A psychomotor stimulant theory of addiction. *Psychol Rev* 94:469–492, 1987.
117. Robinson TE, Berridge KC: The neural basis of drug craving: An incentive sensitization theory of addiction. *Brain Res Rev* 18:247–291, 1993.
118. Groenewegen HJ, Berendse HW: Anatomical relationships between prefrontal cortex and the basal ganglia in the rat, in Thierry AM, Glowinski J, Goldman-Rakic PS, Christen Y (eds): *Motor and Cognitive Functions of the Prefrontal Cortex*. New York, Springer-Verlag, 1993, pp 51–77.
119. Taber MT, Fibiger HC: Electrical stimulation of the medial prefrontal cortex increases dopamine release in the striatum. *Neuropsychopharmacology* 9:271–275, 1993.
120. Shallice T: Specific impairments of planning. *Phil Trans R Soc London* 298:199–209, 1982.
121. Volkow N, Hitzemann R, Wang G, *et al:* Decreased brain metabolism in neurologically intact healthy alcoholics. *Am J Psychiatry* 149:1016–1022, 1992.
122. Parker E, Alkana R, Birnbaum I, *et al:* Alcohol and the disruption of cognitive processes. *Arch Gen Psychiatry* 31:824–828, 1974.
123. Post R, Lott L, Maddock R, *et al:* An effect of alcohol on the distribution of spatial attention. *J Stud Alcohol* 57:260–266, 1996.
124. Lyvers M, Maltzman I: Selective effects of alcohol on Wisconsin card sorting test performance. *Br J Addict* 86:399–407, 1991.
125. Parker E, Birnbaum I, Noble E: Alcohol and memory: Storage and state dependency. *J Verbal Learn Verbal Behav* 15:691–702, 1976.
126. Lex B, Breenwald N, Lukas S, *et al:* Blood ethanol levels, self-rated ethanol effects and cognitive–perceptual tasks. *Pharmacol Biochem Behav* 29:509–515, 1988.
127. Peterson J, Rothfleisch J, Zelazo P, *et al:* Acute alcohol intoxication and cognitive functioning. *J Stud Alcohol* 51:114–122, 1990.
128. Tharp V, Rundell O, Lester B, *et al:* Alcohol and information processing. *Psychopharmacologia* 40:12–33, 1974.
129. Harper C, Kril J: Neuropathology of alcoholism. *Alcohol Alcohol* 25:207–216, 1990.
130. Melgaard B, Henriksen L, Ahlgren P, *et al:* Regional cerebral blood flow in chronic alcoholics measured by single photon emission computerized tomography. *Acta Neurol Scand* 82:87–93, 1990.
131. Nicolas JM, Catafau AM, Estruch R, *et al:* Regional cerebral blood flow-SPECT in chronic alcoholism: Relation to neuropsychological testing. *J Nucl Med* 34:1452–1459, 1993.
132. Adams KM, Gilman S, Koeppe RA, *et al:* Neuropsychological deficits are correlated with

frontal hypometabolism in positron emission tomography studies of older alcoholic patients. *Alcohol Clin Exp Res* 17:205–210, 1993.
133. Cloninger C: Neurogenetic adaptive mechanisms in alcoholism. *Science* 236:410–416, 1987.
134. Babor TF, Hofman M, DelBoca FK, *et al:* Types of alcoholics, I: Evidence for an empirically derived typology based on indicators of vulnerability and severity. *Arch Gen Psychiatry* 49:599–608, 1992.
135. Pribram KH: The primate frontal cortex—Executive of the brain, in Pribram KH, Luria AR (eds): *Psychophysiology of the Frontal Lobes.* New York, Academic Press, 1973, pp 293–314.
136. Gorenstein EE, Newman JP: Disinhibitory psychopathology: A new perspective as a model for research. *Psychol Rev* 87:301–315, 1980.
137. Moffitt TE: The neuropsychology of conduct disorder. *Dev Psychopathol* 5:135–151, 1993.
138. Moffitt T: Adolescence-limited and life-course-persistent antisocial behavior: A developmental taxonomy. *Psychol Rev* 100:674–701, 1993.
139. American Psychiatric Association: *Diagnostic and Statistical Manual of Mental Disorders,* 4th ed. Washington, DC, Author, 1994.
140. Olweus D: The stability of aggressive reaction patterns in human males: A review. *Psychol Bull* 85:852–875, 1979.
141. Loeber R: Natural histories of conduct problems, delinquency, and associated substance use, in Lahey B, Kazdin A (eds): *Advances in Clinical Child Psychology,* vol 11. New York, Plenum Press, 1988, pp 73–124.
142. Farrington DP: Antisocial personality from childhood to adulthood. *Psychol Bull Br Psychol Soc* 4:389–394, 1991.
143. Tarter R, Edwards K: Antecedents to alcoholism: Implications for prevention and treatment. *Behav Ther* 17:346–361, 1986.
144. Martin CS, Earleywine M, Blackson TC, *et al:* Aggressivity, inattention, hyperactivity, and impulsivity in boys at high and low risk for substance abuse. *J Abnorm Child Psychol* 22:177–203, 1994.
145. Brook JS, Whiteman M, Finch S: Childhood aggression, adolescent delinquency and drug use: A longitudinal study. *J Genet Psychol* 153:369–383, 1992.
146. Boyle MH, Offord DR, Racine YA, *et al:* Predicting substance use in late adolescence: Results the Ontario Child Health Study Follow-up. *Am J Psychiatry* 149:761–767, 1992.
147. Boyle MH, Offord DR, Racine YA, *et al:* Predicting substance use in early adolescence based on parent and teacher assessments of childhood psychiatric disorder: Results from the Ontario Child Health Study Follow-up. *J Child Psychol Psychiatry* 34:535–433, 1993.
148. Kandel E, Freed D: Frontal-lobe dysfunction and antisocial behavior: A review. *J Clin Psychol* 45:404–413, 1989.
149. Lykken DT: A study of anxiety in the sociopathic personality. *J Abnorm Soc Psychol* 55:6–10, 1957.
150. Hare RD: Temporal gradient of fear arousal in psychopaths. *J Abnorm Soc Psychol* 70:442–445, 1966.
151. Eslinger PJ, Damasio AR: Severe disturbance of higher cognition after bilateral frontal lobe ablation: Patient EVR. *Neurology* 35:1731–1741, 1985.
152. Damasio AR, Tranel D, Damasio H: Individuals with sociopathic behavior caused by frontal damage fail to respond autonomically to social stimuli. *Behav Brain Res* 41:81–94, 1990.
153. Bechara A, Damasio H, Tranel D, *et al:* Deciding advantageously before knowing the advantageous strategy. *Science* 275:1293–1295, 1997.
154. Raine A, Reynolds G, Sheard C: Neuroanatomical correlates of skin conductance orienting in normal humans: A magnetic resonance imaging study. *Psychophysiology* 28:548–558, 1991.
155. Finn P, Pihl R: Men at high risk for alcoholism: The effect of alcohol on cardiovascular response to unavoidable shock. *J Abnorm Psychol* 96:230–236, 1987.
156. Finn P, Pihl R: Risk for alcoholism: A comparison between two different groups of sons of alcoholics on cardiovascular reactivity and sensitivity to alcohol. *Alcohol Clin Exp Res* 12:742–747, 1988.

157. Finn P, Zeitouni N, Pihl R: Effects of alcohol on psychophysiological hyperreactivity to nonaversive and aversive stimuli in men at high risk for alcoholism. *J Abnorm Psychol* 99:79–85, 1990.
158. Finn P, Kessler D, Hussong A: Risk for alcoholism and classical conditioning to signals for punishment: Evidence for a weak behavioral inhibition system? *J Abnorm Psychol* 103:293–301, 1994.
159. Levenson R, Oyama O, Meek P: Greater reinforcement from alcohol for those at risk: Parental risk personality risk and sex. *J Abnorm Psychol* 96:242–253, 1987.
160. Sher K, Levenson R: Risk for alcoholism and individual differences in the stress-response-dampening effect of alcohol. *J Abnorm Psychol* 91:350–367, 1982.
161. Sher K, Walitzer K: Individual differences in the stress-response-dampening effect of alcohol: A dose-response study. *J Abnorm Psychol* 95:159–167, 1986.
162. Gray J: *The Neuropsychology of Anxiety: An Enquiry into the Functions of the Septohippocampal System.* New York, Oxford University Press, 1982.
163. Zuckerman M: Drug usage as one manifestation of a "sensation seeking trait," in Keup W (ed): *Drug Abuse: Current Concepts and Research.* Springfield, IL, Charles C. Thomas, 1972, pp 154–163.
164. Jones MC: Personality correlates and antecedents of drinking patterns in adult males. *J Consult Clin Psychol* 32:2–12, 1968.
165. Grafman J, Vance SC, Weingarter H, *et al:* The effects of lateralized frontal lesions on mood regulation. *Brain* 109:1127–1148, 1986.
166. Jaffe JH, Babor TF, Fishbein DH: Alcoholics, aggression and antisocial personality. *J Stud Alcohol* 49:211–218, 1988.
167. Cadoret R, Troughton E, O'Gorman T, *et al:* An adoption study of genetic and environmental factors in drug abuse. *Arch Gen Psychiatry* 43:1131–1136, 1986.
168. Mattson AJ, Levin HS: Frontal lobe dysfunction following closed head injury. A review of the literature. *J Nerv Ment Dis* 178:282–291, 1990.
169. Hill S, Steinhauer S, Park J, *et al:* Event-related potential characteristics in children of alcoholics from high-density families. *Alcohol Clin Exp Res* 14:6–16, 1990.
170. Hudspeth WJ, Pribram KH: Psychophysiological indices of cerebral maturation. *Int J Psychophysiol* 12:19–29, 1992.
171. Huttenlocher PR, deCourten C, Garey LJ, *et al:* Synaptogenesis in human visual cortex: Evidence for synaptic elimination during normal development. *Neurosci Lett* 33:247–252, 1982.
172. Purves D, Lichtman JW: Elimination of synapses in the developing nervous system. *Science* 210:153–157, 1980.
173. Rakic P, Riley KP: Overproduction and elimination of retinal axons in the fetal rhesus monkey. *Science* 219:1441–1444, 1983.
174. Cowan WM, Fawcett JW, O'Leary DDM, *et al:* Regressive events in neurogenesis. *Science* 225:1258–1265, 1984.
175. Rabinowicz T: The differential maturation of the human cerebral cortex, in Falkner F, Tanner JM (eds): *Human Growth,* vol 3, *Neurobiology and Nutrition.* New York, Plenum Press, 1979, pp 97–103.
176. Huttenlocher PR: Synaptic density in human frontal cortex-developmental changes and effects of aging. *Brain Res* 163:195–205, 1979.
177. Chugani HT, Phelps ME: Maturational changes in cerebral function in infants determined by 18FDG positron emission tomography. *Science* 231:840–843, 1986.
178. Chugani HT, Phelps ME, Mazziotta JC: Positron emission tomography study of human brain functional development. *Ann Neurol* 22:487–497, 1987.
179. Singer W: Activity-dependent self-organization of synaptic connections as a substrate of learning, in Changeux J-P, Konishi M (eds): *The Neural and Molecular Bases of Learning.* London, John Wiley & Sons, 1987, pp 301–336.
180. Greenough WT, Black JE, Wallace CS: Experience and brain development. *Child Dev* 58:539–559, 1987.

181. Cicchetti D, Tucker D: Development and self-regulatory structures of the mind. *Dev Psychopathol* 6:533–549, 1994.
182. Schore AN: The experience-dependent maturation of a regulatory system in the orbital prefrontal cortex and the origin of developmental psychopathology. *Dev Psychopathol* 8:59–87, 1996.
183. Moss HB, Clark D, Kirisci L: Timing of paternal substance use disorder cessation and the effects on problem behaviors in sons. *Am J Addict* 6:30–37, 1997.
184. Barkley R: *Hyperactive Children: A Handbook for Diagnosis and Treatment.* New York, Guilford Press, 1981.
185. Baxter L, Schwartz J, Bergman K, *et al:* Caudate glucose metabolic rate changes with both drug and behavior therapy for obsessive–compulsive disorder. *Arch Gen Psychiatry* 49:681–689, 1992.
186. Schwartz J, Stoessel P, Baxter L, *et al:* Systematic changes in cerebral glucose metabolic rate after successful behavior modification treatment of obsessive–compulsive disorder. *Arch Gen Psychiatry* 53:109–113, 1996.

9

Brain Imaging

Functional Consequences of Ethanol in the Central Nervous System

David Lyons, Christopher T. Whitlow, Hilary R. Smith, and Linda J. Porrino

Abstract. In recent years, sophisticated methods have been developed to view structure and function within the living brain. Functional imaging methods are used to visualize dynamic chemical processes that are linked to brain activity. Increased neural activity, for example, leads to greater glucose and oxygen consumption and greater regional rates of blood flow to meet elevated energy demands. Mapping these changes provides quantitative visual descriptions of localized changes in brain activity that result from behavioral or pharmacological manipulations. This chapter first describes several current methods and how they are used to study the effects of alcohol on brain function. In the second part, the effects of acute intoxication are discussed with emphasis on the complex nature of alcohol's effects in the central nervous system, which depend on dose, time since administration, and environmental context. In the final part, the functional consequences of long-term exposure to alcohol as well as diseases associated with chronic alcoholism are reviewed.

1. Introduction

Over the past 25 years, a number of new methods have been developed that permit scientists to visualize the structure and function of the brain. These methods are powerful tools for studying the effects of a wide variety of

David Lyons, Christopher T. Whitlow, Hilary R. Smith, and Linda J. Porrino • Department of Physiology and Pharmacology, Wake Forest University School of Medicine, Winston-Salem, North Carolina 27157.

Recent Developments in Alcoholism, Volume 14: The Consequences of Alcoholism, edited by Galanter. Plenum Press, New York, 1998.

pharmacological, physiological, and psychological stimuli, and they have given us new insights into the way the brain works.

Many of these techniques, like computed tomography and magnetic resonance imaging, depict the structure of the living brain. Each of these methods allows the anatomy of the brain to be visualized in great detail. As *in vivo* techniques they are particularly important tools for the diagnosis of the results of lesions and diseases that alter brain structure. Structural imaging methods also have been applied to research questions and have provided insights into the abnormalities that accompany neurodegenerative diseases as well as the deleterious effects of chronic alcohol exposure.

Although the methods mentioned above provide a view of the living brain, this view is static. They cannot tell us whether these structural abnormalities also affect brain function. In contrast, functional imaging methods permit the visualization of dynamic neurochemical processes within the brain. Measurements of cerebral blood flow and energy metabolism in the brain are sensitive indicators of brain function. These measures derive from the fact that discrete brain regions with increased neural activity use more glucose and oxygen and have higher rates of blood flow in order to deliver metabolic substrates. Local energy metabolism and blood flow then, are closely correlated with the level of local functional activity.

The value of the use of imaging methods, both structural and functional, in investigations of the central nervous system (CNS) comes from the fact that the brain, unlike many other organs such as the liver or muscle, is highly heterogenous in its organization. It consists of a broad variety of cell types organized and connected into a mass of nuclei and complex circuits that can function quite independently from one another. Imaging permits localization of effects to specific brain circuits, regions, and even cells. This is of particular importance because many other methods are limited in that they can be applied only to one brain region at a time. Imaging methods, on the other hand, can examine the entire CNS simultaneously. This allows effects to be demonstrated in brain regions other than where predicted or expected. It also permits the visualization of entire circuits and networks in which functional activity is altered by experimental or pathological states even when those circuits span large portions of the brain.

The administration of any psychoactive drug to an organism produces a variety of pharmacological actions that may include both central and peripheral effects. These physiological and behavioral responses are unlikely to result from a single action in a single brain region, but are more likely to be the product of multiple processes at a number of distinct anatomical sites. In addition, most drugs, particularly when administered over a broad range of doses, may act not only on one neurotransmitter system or receptor subtype, but on some combination thereof. These issues are particularly pertinent when the effects of compounds such as alcohol are investigated. Ethanol is a substance that has complex physiological, behavioral, and biochemical actions. The consequences of ethanol administration change dramatically depending on factors of dose and time. A time line describing the hypothetical change in CNS activity during various stages of ethanol exposure is depicted in Fig. 1. The diversity of ethanol's neurochemical and behavioral effects can complicate the identification of the subtrates of its effects in the CNS. In order to localize the neuroanatomical substrates of the effects of a drug like ethanol, it is necessary to measure neural events in circuits and pathways throughout the brain.

Therefore, imaging methods such as those described in this chapter are ideal strategies with which to achieve a better understanding of the loci within the CNS through which alcohol mediates its effects. These imaging methods allow neuroscientists not only to make a systematic evaluation of the changes in brain function that accompany the acute effects of alcohol, but also to determine how brain function is altered by the chronic use of alcohol. The precise localization of these changes in brain function provides important pieces of information in our understanding of the basic effects of alcohol and also provides insights into the ways in which alcoholism and the effects of chronic alcohol exposure can be treated effectively.

In this chapter, functional imaging studies are reviewed, many of which have utilized measures of cerebral blood flow and glucose metabolism to

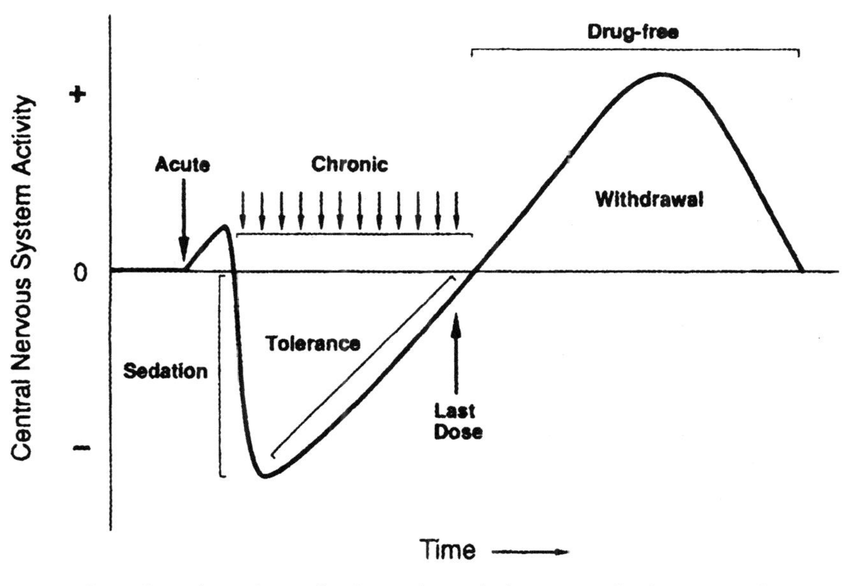

Figure 1. Time line describing the hypothetical change in CNS activity during various stages of ethanol exposure. Acute administration can lead to increased levels of functional activity that are followed by CNS depression. Following chronic treatment, tolerance to the effects of ethanol may develop. Upon cessation of ethanol exposure, CNS hyperactivity associated with withdrawal may follow until homeostatis is regained. (Reprinted with permission from Metten and Crabbe.[116])

assess the acute and chronic effects of ethanol intake in both animals and humans. The response in the CNS to acute ethanol administration is reviewed and an attempt is made to provide a better understanding of the complexity of this response as a function of both dose and time after administration. Studies of chronic exposure are also reviewed, and this section of the chapter attempts to relate the results of imaging studies of ethanol to different aspects of long-term exposure: continued use, withdrawal, and recovery. In addition, the fairly substantial literature that describes functional deficits in patients with Wernicke–Korsakoff's syndrome is discussed. First, however, a brief description of current and developing imaging methods is presented to provide a foundation for the rest of the chapter.

2. Overview of Functional Imaging Methods

2.1. Imaging in Animals

2.1.1. Regional Cerebral Blood Flow. To function properly, the brain must be supplied continuously with nutrients. In contrast to other organs, the brain cannot store sufficient nutrients and therefore depends on a constant supply delivered by the blood. Brain regions that are more active require more nutrients, and regional rates of blood flow within the brain are modulated to keep pace with the changing demands. These characteristics form the basis for the measurement of regional cerebral blood flow (RCBF).[1,2]

To detect changes in RCBF, a radiotracer is injected intravenously and deposited in brain tissue in accordance with the regional distribution of blood flow. A variety of tracers are used for this purpose; these compounds are chemically inactive, dissolve quickly in the blood, are slowly metabolized, and readily cross the blood–brain barrier. Shortly after the injection (usually after 1 min), the animal is killed and its brain is quickly removed and frozen. Brain tissue sections are collected in a cryostat, dried, and apposed to X-ray film. Brain areas that are active and have a high rate of blood flow accumulate a greater quantity of radioactive material and are visible as dark areas on the film. Less active regions that accumulate less radioactivity produce lighter signals on the film. The particular advantage of RCBF over other functional imaging methods is the short time window during which blood flow is determined. This method does not require a steady-state condition and allows researchers to investigate highly dynamic brain processes that change rapidly over time. This method was applied, for example, to evaluate changes in brain function that occurred during the rise and fall of blood ethanol levels along the time course of a single administration of ethanol to several groups of rats.[3]

2.1.2. Local Cerebral Glucose Metabolism. The quantitative 2-[^{14}C]deoxyglucose(2-[^{14}D]-DG) method developed by Louis Sokoloff and co-workers in the late 1970s is an autoradiographic measure of brain function that determines local rates of glucose utilization. The 2-[^{14}C]-DG method employs carbon-14-labeled 2-deoxyglucose, which is chemically similar to glucose. Unlike glucose, 2-[^{14}C]-DG is only partially metabolized during glycolysis, stopping after its conversion to deoxyglucose-6-phosphate, at which time it is effectively trapped within the cell. The rationale for this method is based on the fact that approximately 80% of the energy consumed by neurons is used for the transmission of nerve signals (i.e., the mechanism by which information is transferred in brain) and only 20% serves to maintain the cells' basal metabolism.[4] Furthermore, glucose is virtually the only energy source for the brain; therefore, a rise in glucose utilization in a particular brain area indicates increased neural activity in that region. As energy requirements increase, cells of localized brain regions take up more glucose, and thus more 2-[^{14}C]-DG for metabolism through glycolysis and cellular respiration. Forty-five minutes after 2-[^{14}C]-DG administration, the brain is rapidly extracted and frozen for sectioning. Thin brain slices are developed on X-ray film and imaged using quantitative densitometry. Darker areas indicate increased uptake of 2-[^{14}C]-DG and therefore greater cerebral activity. Because intact tissue slices are used, captured images preserve the complex spatial arrangement of the brain. In addition, the direct contact of brain slices with film allows for higher resolution than similar *in vivo* methods, such as positron and single-photon emission tomography, which are discussed in Sections 2.2.1 and 2.2.2. The assessment of local rates of cerebral metabolism has been effectively used, for example, to demonstrate the dose–response relationship of functional activity in specific neural systems to ethanol administration in rats.[5]

2.1.3. Cytochrome Oxidase. Cytochrome oxidase is the terminal enzyme complex of the electron transport chain, a key component of cellular respiration, the process by which oxygen is utilized for the generation of energy-laden adenosine-triphosphate (ATP) molecules. All eukaryotes express a form of cytochrome oxidase embedded in their mitochondrial membrane. The brains of mammals principally rely on aerobic respiration; consequently, levels of activity of this enzyme are closely linked to neural activity and have been determined histochemically in animal tissue for the purpose of identifying patterns of functional activity.[6] Additional efforts have been made to establish a quantitative histochemical method for assessing cytochrome oxidase activity.[7]

Alterations in cytochrome oxidase activity involve synthesis or degradation of the enzyme with measurable changes occurring only after hours or days. This activity is quite different from local cerebral glucose metabolism (LCGM), for example, which changes in minutes. Both of these techniques are in fact linked to neuronal activity; however, changes in cytochrome oxidase activity reflect longer-term alterations. Thus, this technique may be particularly useful in studies where regions of brain take on new functions, as in the case of early development, response to trauma, and, potentially, chronic drug exposure. More recently, this technique has been extended by the use of *in situ* hybridization histochemistry (ISHH) to evaluate changes in the production of mRNAs for specific subunits of the cytochrome oxidase complex.[8] Like the enzyme itself, a message for the subunits is tightly linked to functional activity in brain. Furthermore, because ISHH involves the use of a radiolabeled probe that is readily quantified in tissue, this procedure provides a straightforward means for quantitatively determining long-term regional changes in function activity. Although this method has not yet been applied to study the consequences of alcohol exposure, it has been used to study other neuropathological conditions and their treatment. Using a primate model of parkinsonism,[9] for example, monkeys treated with 1-methyl-4-phenyl-1,2,3,6-tetrahydropyridine (MPTP) had elevated levels of mRNA expression for cytochrome oxidase subunit I in the globus pallidus and the substantia nigra. Based on the known role of the basal ganglia and related structures in Parkinson's disease, these findings were as expected. Treatment with levodopa, an effective treatment for some of the motor symptoms of Parkinson's disease, returned these levels to normal. Used in a similar manner, these methods may prove to be useful for the identification of the neural circuits that are influenced by long-term ethanol exposure, as well.

2.1.4. Immediate Early Genes. ISHH is a relatively recent addition to the selection of tools available to the alcohol researcher. ISHH allows visualization and quantification of levels of endogenous messenger RNA in tissue sections by hybridizing the RNA to detectable nucleic acid probes. Immediate early genes code for nuclear transcription factors that specifically influence the expression of other genes. Therefore, changes in levels of immediate early genes indicate alterations in functional activity within the CNS. The probes may be labeled chemically, so that a colored reaction product is indicative of hybridization, or more commonly, they are labeled with radioactive isotopes such as [^{35}S] or [^{32}P]. The tissue sections may be apposed to X-ray film, thereby generating an autoradiographic image that can be analyzed for regional changes in mRNA levels. Furthermore, the sections may be dipped directly into emulsion or apposed to emulsion-dipped cover slides. When slides are developed, the presence of hybridized probe is indicated by silver grains on the tissue itself, providing localization of mRNA at the cellular level.

As an example, one study evaluated the ability of ethanol to attenuate the release of adrenocorticotropin (ACTH) in rodents.[10] Ethanol alone had no effect on ACTH release, but it did attenuate the release of ACTH induced by the intracerebroventricular administration of the cytokine, interleukin-1β. To test if alcohol blunted this release by altering functional activity in the region of the hypothalamus that is responsible for interleukin-induced ACTH release, levels of the intermediate early gene *c-fos* were determined in the hypothalamus of rats pretreated with ethanol and then administered interleukin-1β. Ethanol, which had no effect alone, did in fact attenuate the interleukin-induced changes in c-*fos* within the hypothalamus, indicating that the mechanism responsible for this effect of ethanol involved altered activity within the CNS.

2.2. *Imaging in Humans*

2.2.1. Positron Emission Tomography. Positron emission tomography (PET) is an imaging method that determines the three-dimensional distribution of specific molecular tracers in the living human brain. When it is used in conjunction with biological markers, this technique provides quantified information about activity in the brain. Currently, investigators use PET to generate tomographic images of the regional distribution of cerebral metabolism, blood flow, and receptor availability.

The radiotracers used in PET contain positron-emitting isotopes with a biological marker molecule that is injected intravenously into the patient. A positron, or positively charged electron, travels only a few millimeters before it encounters an electron, which results in annihilation of both the positron and electron and the emission of two gamma rays in nearly opposite directions. The gamma rays are detected with a PET camera, or scanner, which surrounds the patient. Referred to as "coincidence detection," the source of the emission is determined to reside along a single line by the simultaneous detection of the emissions on opposite sides of the ring of detectors. PET is sensitive enough to detect the source of the radioactivity within 4–10 mm of surrounding tissue and can detect picomolar changes in tracer distribution. These isotopes have very short half-lives, on the order of minutes or hours, that allow for only a brief window in which to administer the tracer and record its distribution. Radioisotopes are therefore most frequently generated on site immediately prior to the PET procedure using a cyclotron, which accelerates protons into the nucleus of an atom to create a positron-emitting isotope.

Fluorine-18-labeled deoxyglucose ([^{18}F]-DG) has been extensively used to investigate cerebral metabolism in the same manner that 2-[^{14}C]-DG has been used autoradiographically. Water labeled with oxygen 15 is also commonly used to study cerebral blood flow. Volkow and colleagues[11,12] investigated the effects of acute ethanol intake on both of these parameters. In this work, the cerebellum was identified as a site where functional activity was readily diminished, whereas increases in functional activity were found in frontal and temporal regions. This means that alcohol's effects in the living human brain are complex and heterogeneous with respect to both the direction of change and the spatial distribution of change. Because ethanol is pharmacologically complex, it is likely to affect disparate systems in the brain, which may in turn interact in unexpected ways. This potential for complexity plays into the strengths of these imaging methods because the real power of functional imaging lies in its ability to identify unique regional distributions of altered activity throughout the entire brain.

Because the radioactive half-life of the PET tracer is so short, individuals can undergo several scans, sometimes within just minutes. Consequently, PET studies can utilize within-subject designs, allowing the investigator to study changes over several PET sessions within a single individual. Furthermore, brain function can be directly related to specific stimuli or cognitive activity when subjects are evaluated during the completion of various tasks. For example, if a functional circuit involving temporal cortex that is suspected of subserving memory was found, imaging studies of individuals performing memory tasks under the influence of alcohol could be conducted to test this specific hypothesis.

2.2.2. Single-Photon Emission Computed Tomography. Single-photon emission computed tomography (SPECT) is similar to PET but uses tracers that emit single gamma rays, such as ^{133}xenon or ^{99m}Tc-hexamethylpropyleneamine oxime (Tc-HMPAO) to assess blood flow and ^{123}I-containing compounds to evaluate receptor availability. Several SPECT tracers are available commercially and their longer half-life removes the necessity of on-site generation, which may be the chief advantage of SPECT compared to PET. As in the case of conventional computerized tomographic (CT) scanning, a camera for detecting radiation circles the head; but unlike CT, which intercepts X rays projected through the head from an external source, SPECT intercepts the emission of radioactive decay from the tracer within the brain or other organs. Thus, three-dimensional tomographic images are generated.

In SPECT, the localization of the radioactive source along a single line is accomplished by collimation, a process whereby individual detectors sit at the end of a column so that only those emissions along the sight of each column are detected. The resulting sensitivity of SPECT is somewhat less than PET, because collimation is less efficient than coincidence detection for localizing a radioactive source. Nonetheless, SPECT has proved very useful in study of alcohol. For instance, Tiihonen *et al.*[13] tested the ability of the opiate antagonist naloxone to alter the acute effects of alcohol on cerebral blood flow. Naloxone is very similar to another opiate antagonist, naltrexone, which has been recently approved in the United States for the treatment of alcoholism. In this study, the acute intake of alcohol in normal individuals leads to increased rates of cerebral metabolism in the right prefrontal cortex. Pretreatment with naloxone in the same subjects prevented these changes. These data illustrate how the assessment of functional activity is important for demonstrating not only the effects of alcohol in the living human brain but also in the assessment of potential treatments for alcoholism.

2.2.3. Magnetic Resonance Imaging. Magnetic resonance imaging (MRI) is most frequently used to determine the structure of tissues including brain. In brief, this method is based on the fact that nuclei of atoms with an odd atomic weight align themselves in a strong magnetic field and can be sent off this alignment in response to a pulse of radio waves. When the pulse ceases, the misaligned nuclei become realigned (relaxation) in a fashion specific to the nuclei and its local environment. Realignment results in the emission of radio waves that are detected and used to construct the tomographic image. In this manner, various tissues, such as gray matter, white matter, and cerebrospinal fluid, can be identified in three-dimensional space. The resolving power of this method is impressive (ca 1 mm) and allows for straightforward recognition of specific cortical and subcortical sites. Along with CT, MRI technology has been very useful, for example, in demonstrating cortical atrophy in alcoholics and its subsequent improvement during abstinence.[14] A modification of this technique is also being used to determine changes in brain function by assessing blood flow and oxygenation (for review of method see Cohen and Bookheimer[13]).

In the first publication describing this approach, changes in blood volume were detected with the aid of a synthetic contrast agent.[15]

More recently, ultrafast echo planar imaging has been gaining popularity. This method is completely noninvasive and determines changes in oxygenation by taking advantage of important differences in the magnetic susceptibility of oxyhemoglobin and deoxyhemoglobin. The potential for functional MRI (fMRI) to contribute to our understanding of cerebral processes is great because of its superb spatial (<1 mm) and time (<1 sec) resolution.

2.2.4. Electroencephalography. Electroencephalography (EEG) measures electrical currents in the brain using electrodes strategically placed on the scalp. The EEG signal is transmitted to a computer, which quantifies it and identifies unique electrical patterns characteristic of various brain states. The EEG output can be combined with spectral techniques to give a two-dimensional image that represents the distribution of particular frequencies and amplitudes over the surface of the brain. The temporal resolution of EEG is on the order milliseconds, so that changes in brain activity can be very precisely linked to the presentation of specific stimuli. Because specific stimuli evoke a characteristic response, these event-related potentials (ERP) can be evaluated for specific changes under pharmacological or pathological conditions. The EEG and ERP can generally differentiate the alcoholic from the nonalcoholic.[16,17] One method for doing this involves the so-called oddball task in which subjects attend to a unique stimulus amid a series of repeated stimuli. In response to the unique stimuli, one particular normal peak in this response, the P300, is diminished in amplitude in alcoholics as compared to nonalcoholics.

2.3. *Summary*

There are several useful methods for examining brain function in the living brain. Continued use of these methods in humans will provide information about the essential functional features of the response to alcohol in both the short and long term among various human populations, for example, nonalcoholics, alcoholics, men, women, individuals with or without a family history of alcoholism, and so forth. In addition, specific cognitive functions related to alcohol use will be ascribed to specific brain regions in people. Human research, however, is often limited by numerous factors that cannot be easily controlled, including, for example, varied drug and alcohol histories, nutritional status, genetic makeup, and comorbid psychiatric disorders. Animal studies can effectively control many of these confounds and allow researchers to ascribe changes in brain function specifically to the action of alcohol.[18] Moreover, the spatial resolution of *in vivo* techniques that can be performed in animals is currently far better than that which can be accomplished in humans. Therefore, both human and animal functional imaging research have their useful place and will continue to increase our understanding of the effects of alcohol in the CNS.

3. Acute Intoxication

3.1. Dose Dependency

There are numerous factors that determine the behavioral response to a pharmacologically complex drug such as alcohol. Clearly, one of the most important of these is dose. At low doses alcohol can act as a stimulant, activating spontaneous locomotor activity in rodents, while at higher doses alcohol can have predominantly sedative effects. The dose-dependent nature of alcohol's actions are evident in humans, as well. Low doses can have euphorigenic properties, while the ingestion of higher doses can result in motor and sensory impairments. Determining the substrates of varying doses of alcohol, therefore, has been an important focus of a number of imaging studies in both rodents and humans.

Early work was highly inconsistent, with no clear picture emerging regarding the neuroanatomical basis of alcohol's effects. In many of these studies, although cerebral blood flow and glucose metabolism were measured, there were no attempts to localize function. Rather these studies focused on overall or global effects on these processes, considering the brain as a whole. Both increases and decreases were observed in rodents[19–29] and humans.[30–35] It is difficult to evaluate these studies because of the large differences in the dose ranges employed and differences in routes of administration, measurement methods, and environmental contexts. The greatest difficulty, however, is the fact that any regional effects of alcohol would have to be rather large to be detected when whole brain measures are used.

A clearer picture of the dose-dependent effects of alcohol has emerged more recently. The ability to examine regional changes in brain function has been the key to this understanding. The administration of low doses of alcohol to human subjects, doses that produce mild levels of intoxication (0.5–1.0

g/kg), increased cerebral blood flow in specific regions.[12,13,36–39] The prefrontal and temporal cortices were frequently activated in this low dose range.[12,13,38] The frontal cortex appears to be most sensitive. Increased functional activity was found at the lowest doses (0.5–0.7 g/kg), whereas only slightly higher doses decreased levels of activity or had no effect.[12,38] Functional activity in the prefrontal cortex contrasts with activity in temporal cortex, where moderately higher doses (1.0–1.5 g/kg) were required to increase the level of activity. Since the dose–response relationship appears to be different in these cortices, each region may play a unique role in the response to ethanol within the CNS. These studies are important because they not only demonstrate that alcohol in low doses can increase functional activity, but they also demonstrate that the effects of alcohol in this dose range are in fact heterogeneous and clearly regionally specific. Furthermore, these cortical regions must function in concert with other brain regions under normal conditions and in response to alcohol intake. What is needed now are studies that take these data one step further and identify more components of the circuits at both a cortical and subcortical level. Once the circuits are identified, the role that these regions play will become more apparent, and it will also allow more direct testing of specific functions.

At higher doses, a rather different picture emerges. High doses of ethanol (>1.5 g/kg) decrease CBF and LCGU throughout the brain in humans.[11,12,40] It does appear, however, that the cerebellum may be particularly sensitive to the effects of ethanol that reduce functional activity (1.0 g/kg).[11,12] At this time, functional imaging studies in humans have clearly found that the functional response of the CNS to ethanol is biphasic, in parallel with behavioral work. It also appears thus far that portions of prefrontal and temporal cortex may play a role in the activating effects of ethanol following low doses, and the cerebellum may be involved in the depressant action of higher doses. Future work that can localize activation to specific circuits within these regions will surely advance our knowledge of ethanol's action in the human CNS.

Many of the inconsistencies in human studies derive from the differences in the subject samples under study, as well as variability in the behavioral context. In animal studies, these factors more easily can be controlled. For example, it is possible to study the effects of alcohol in animal subjects that have never received any other pharmacological agents. The effects can be attributed directly to alcohol without any confounds of past history of alcohol use or use of other psychoactive substances such as nicotine, caffeine, and so forth. Although there have not been a large number of studies, the results to date closely parallel the effects noted in humans. When low doses are administered, alcohol can increase functional activity in forebrain regions, whereas when higher doses are administered, functional activity is reduced.

In the animal literature, there are only a few studies that have examined the brain regions affected by different alcohol doses in detail.[5,41–44] Eckardt and co-workers[41] found that ethanol at high doses decreased rates of cerebral metabolism in most affected sites (auditory system, cerebellum, vestibular nucleus, and median raphe nucleus), yet the lowest dose increased LCGU in at least two sites: the dentate gyrus of the hippocampus and the superior olivary nucleus. In the first study by Williams-Hemby and Porrino,[5] three doses of ethanol (0.25, 0.5, and 1.0 g/kg, intraperitoneally) were administered to alcohol-naive rats, and radiolabeled deoxyglucose was injected at approximately the peak of the blood ethanol curve. As illustrated in Fig. 2, the patterns of LCGU among brain structures depended on the alcohol dose. The 0.25-g/kg dose of alcohol increased neural activity, most prominently in brain structures of the mesocorticolimbic system. The 1.0-g/kg alcohol dose, in contrast, caused a distinctly different pattern of decreased activity in the thalamus, hippocampus, and locus ceruleus. First, these data demonstrate

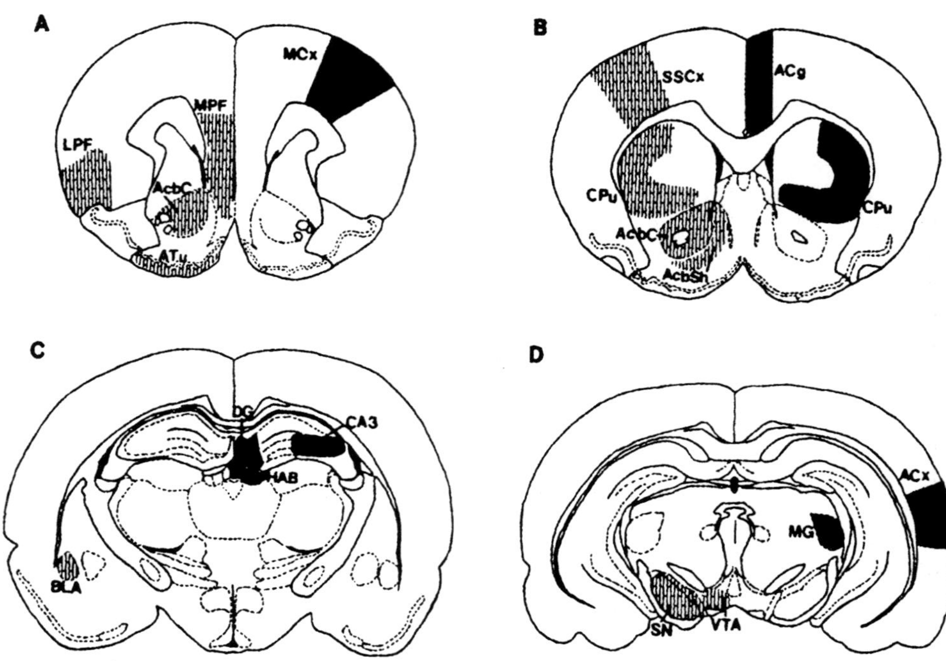

Figure 2. Schematic representation of the effects of ethanol dose on LCGU at various brain levels. Stippled areas (left) represent increases in LCGU at the low ethanol dose (0.25 g/kg, ip). The black areas (right) represent decreases in LCGU at the higher ethanol dose (1.0 g/kg). (Reprinted with permission from Williams-Hemby and Porrino[5]) AcbC, Core of the nucleus accumbens; AcbSh, shell of the nucleus accumbens; ACg, anterior cingulate; ACx, auditory cortex; ATu, anterior olfactory tubercle; BLA, basolateral amygdala; CPu, caudate/putamen; DG, dentate gyrus; HAB, habenula; LPF, lateral prefrontal cortex; MCx, motor cortex; MG, medial geniculate; MPF, medial prefrontal cortex; SN, substantia nigra; SSCx, somatosensory cortex; VTA, ventral tegmental area.

the dose-dependent nature of the functional response to acute ethanol. Second, the brain structures in which changes in functional activity were detected are consistent with the observed behavioral changes induced by alcohol. The low alcohol dose led to a widespread increase in brain activity in areas related to the behaviorally arousing and rewarding effects, whereas the moderate alcohol dose suppressed brain function and had more suppressive and sedating effects on behavior.

In a second study by Williams-Hemby and Porrino,[43] it was reported that when 0.25, 1.0, or 2.0 g/kg of ethanol was administered, all doses tested increased rates of cerebral metabolism in various structures, most prominently in the mesocorticolimbic system. Since this study determined functional activity during the period when the blood levels were rapidly rising, these data show not only that ethanol increases the level of functional activity in brain but also that the dose of ethanol is not the only determinant of the functional effects. Time after ingestion is another critical variable, which is discussed in more detail in Section 3.2.

Several additional imaging studies have examined higher doses of ethanol that lead to motor behavior impairment. Like the human work, these animal studies indicate that the cerebellum is a site where functional activity is frequently reduced following the administration of relatively high doses of ethanol. Other regions where high-dose alcohol diminishes functional activity include auditory structures, which have some of the highest levels of basal activity in the brain, the hippocampus, and portions of the thalamus.[45–50] At present, high-dose ethanol appears to alter function in a number of brain regions; but aside from the auditory system, a clear picture of the specific circuits being affected has not been shown following the administration of high doses of ethanol.

Careful manipulation of experimental environment and context is likely to be the key for ascribing altered function to circumscribed brain systems. Under conditions of rest or free, undirected activity, there is no control for perceptual or cognitive function. During *in vivo* studies, animals may have differing levels of anxiety or be engaged in different behaviors, for example, exploration, grooming, or sleep, resulting in increased variability in rates of brain activity. Other pharmacological treatments such as cocaine, for example, have powerful effects on behavior, increasing locomotor activity severalfold, and thus provide a behavioral control by the simple administration of the drug. This may be one reason that imaging studies of cocaine and other psychostimulants have yielded clearer results.[51,52] The behavioral effects of ethanol, especially of low to moderate doses, are often more subtle and therefore are likely to be more strongly influenced by environmental factors. Testing under specific task conditions, for example, tests of motor activity, or memory or perceptual tasks, may be useful for identifying impairment of specific neural systems. In this way, behavioral and brain activity may be better focused and controlled, leading to more definitive findings in future imaging studies of the acute effects of ethanol in the CNS.

3.2. Time Dependency

Another important factor that is involved in determining the behavioral response to alcohol is the time since ingestion. Here too the effects of alcohol have been shown to be biphasic. Alcohol's effects on behavior and brain functioning depend not only on the amount consumed but also on the time that has elapsed since alcohol ingestion. Following high doses (1.5–6.0 g/kg in rodents), responsiveness is often decreased and may be replaced several hours later by a rebound phenomena of hyperresponsiveness. This has been shown to occur on various measures including, for example, seizure activity, pain thresholds, and motor activity.[53] Following low to moderate doses of ethanol, by contrast, there may be a brief period of behavioral stimulation and euphoria that is replaced later with sedation.[54–59] This early period of euphoria is particular interesting because it may be responsible for the positive reinforcement associated with ethanol intake that is critical for ethanol-seeking behavior.

Acute tolerance to the effects of ethanol is another important time-dependent phenomena. This form of tolerance occurs during the course of a single exposure to ethanol and is classically described as a greater effect on the ascending limb of the blood alcohol curve than the one found on the descending limb at the same blood alcohol concentration.[53,60–62] Acute tolerance to the effects of ethanol has been clearly demonstrated in a number of motor, sensory, and cognitive tasks,[61,63] and has also been demonstrated to occur within the CNS itself.[57,64–71]

One of the first studies to address the time-dependent nature of alcohol's effects was conducted by Hadji-Dimo *et al.*[21] in cats. These investigators demonstrated that following the administration of ethanol, there was an initial increase in CBF and EEG frequency index, which was later replaced with decreases in these measures. Friedman *et al.*[45] examined CBF in awake dogs and found that 30 min after the initiation of repeated ethanol infusion blood flow was decreased in cortex, cerebellum, brain stem, and white matter, whereas only a small but significant change in CBF could be found in the cerebellum at 90 min. This occurred despite the fact that blood ethanol levels were considerably higher at 90 min (106 mg/gl at 30 min; 231 mg/dl at 90 min); this study may serve as an example of acute tolerance to ethanol's effect on the CNS using techniques that assess function.

To investigate whether brain activity reflects these behavioral observations of acute tolerance, Porrino and colleagues[72] analyzed the effects of a moderate alcohol dose (0.5 g/kg) on the brain function of rats at 10 and 40 min after alcohol administration, using the 2-[^{14}C]-DG method. These time points were chosen so that measurement of LCGU coincided with rising (10 min) and falling (40 min) blood alcohol levels. In a portion of the ventral striatum, the olfactory tubercle, LCGU was increased at the early time point and returned to normal by the late time point. In a second study, Lyons and co-workers[3] first demonstrated that a 1.0-g/kg dose of ethanol (intraperitoneally) increased RCBF in various sites in rat brain, including the olfactory tubercle, 5 min after administration. These changes were no longer detectable at 15 min after administration, despite significant blood alcohol levels at both times. This early activation and later disappearance of RCBF changes were seen even when blood alcohol levels were held constant across time. Given that the rewarding aspects of alcohol intake appear to predominate early and the known role of the ventral striatum in altering mood, the selective effects of ethanol found in the olfactory tubercle suggest that this region plays a role in the processing of ethanol's reinforcing effects much like it does with other drugs of abuse.[73,74]

Comparison of two studies conducted by Williams-Hemby and Porrino[5,43,44] further indicate that the rapid change from initial increases in functional activity to a return to normal values or an actual decrease in activity is not limited to the olfactory tubercle. When alcohol levels reached peak, the effects on cerebral metabolism were highly dose dependent. When functional activity was assessed during the ascending limb of the blood alcohol curve, however, even relatively high doses of ethanol (1.0–2.0 g/kg) were found to increase rates of metabolism in a variety of structures including the basal ganglia, thalamus, and hippocampus.

3.3. *Behavioral Context*

One particularly significant determinant of the response to a pharmacological agent such as alcohol is the behavioral context of the presentation. There are a number of studies that have shown that the pharmacological effects of a drug are distinctly different, depending on whether the drug is voluntarily self-administered or passively administered by the experimenter. For example, Dworkin and colleagues[75] have shown that if animals are chronically administered cocaine passively at a rate and in a pattern identical to that followed by rats self-administering the drug, cocaine can have lethal effects. This, despite the fact that the self-administering rats find the effects sufficiently reinforcing to respond for the drug avidly and suffer no untoward effects from its presentation. This distinction between self-administration and passive administration has also been seen with alcohol. Alcohol that is voluntarily ingested by rats decreases thresholds for electrical brain stimulation reward, while similar amounts of alcohol passively administered have no effect on thresholds.[76] It is of importance, therefore, to consider the neural correlates of alcohol when it is consumed voluntarily. It is these effects that have the most relevance to models of human alcohol consumption.

Porrino and colleagues have recently used metabolic mapping methods to identify the neural substrates of the effects of voluntarily consumed alcohol. In this study rats were trained to ingest alcohol using a modification of the sucrose fading method developed by Samson.[77] Once alcohol consumption stabilized, the 2-[^{14}C]-DG method was applied to rats immediately following a drinking session. Rats drank 0.5 g/kg during the session. Brain maps were compared to those obtained from rats consuming either water or a sucrose solution in similar paradigms. Rates of cerebral glucose utilization were significantly increased throughout portions of the mesocorticolimbic system including the nucleus accumbens, medial prefrontal cortex, and basolateral amygdala when compared to either water or sucrose controls. This pattern of activation is considerably different from that obtained following the passive intraperitoneal administration of a similar dose of ethanol. This again emphasizes the importance of the context of administration. When ingested voluntarily, the effects of alcohol appear to be restricted to brain regions that are critical to the mediation of positive reinforcement.[78] This is in clear contrast to its effects when administered passively, where effects are evident predominantly in the hippocampus and in sensory systems.[5] Although a number of factors differ in the two paradigms, the rate of administration and the behavioral history, for instance, the behavioral context of administration appears to be an important factor in determining the nature of the pattern of brain activation produced by alcohol.

3.4. *Summary*

Although short-lived, the initial increases in functional activity that result from alcohol administration are found in many specific regions of brain and following a variety of doses. Thus, although only a relatively few studies have fully utilized functional imaging methods to study the effects of alcohol to date, the results show that the neuroanatomical substrates of the effects of alcohol are the result of the interaction of both dose and time since ingestion. Because of their ability to examine the entire brain simultaneously, imaging methods may be invaluable tools for a closer investigation of the neurobiological underpinnings of the effects of alcohol.

4. Long-Term Exposure to Alcohol

Two studies by Rogers and co-workers emphasize the importance of understanding the neurobiological consequences of the habit of drinking alcohol. Using the ^{133}xenon inhalation technique in a large study of 218 social drinkers, these investigators first found that global rates of CBF were negatively correlated with the average level of alcohol consumption over the past 5 years[79]: the greater the alcohol intake, the lower the level of CBF. This study provided a solid foundation for the assertion that alcohol intake has long-term effects on human brain function even in the unimpaired social drinker. It also begs the question of whether there are concomitant changes in cognitive ability as well. In a second study, this time of severe chronic alcoholics, these investigators found that global CBF improved between the first test after initial detoxification (postwithdrawal) and a retest 3–13 weeks into a period of continued abstinence.[80] In contrast to the first experiment, these results demonstrated the dramatic recovery in cerebral perfusion that can occur during abstinence. Together, this work indicates that alcohol-related changes in brain function are likely to exist in a sizable portion of the current population, and that these changes are clearly not limited to populations of alcoholics. Yet, the degree to which brain function is altered by alcohol intake is also highly fluid, showing remarkable improvement when abstinence is sustained, even in those among us who are likely to be the most impaired. Nonetheless, recovery of function is often not complete, which means that there are in fact permanent consequences of ethanol use on brain activity. At this point it is not clear to what degree these deficits in functional activity contribute to long-term behavioral impairment and who is at risk for these persistent deficits. Given the pervasiveness of the practice of alcohol drinking, clearly it is in our long-term best interests to use imaging methods to understand better how brain function is influenced by this common indulgence.

4.1. *Animal Studies*

Animal models of chronic alcohol exposure are useful because they eliminate confounding factors that are difficult to control in a population of chronic drinkers. These factors are varied and include, for example, ethanol intake history, nutrition, and comorbid psychiatric disorders. Using animals instead, direct evidence can be obtained regarding the long-term pharmacological consequences specifically attributable to ethanol exposure. In addition, the spatial resolution of autoradiographic techniques currently surpasses that of *in vivo* imaging and makes more careful study of the involved neuroanatomical circuits possible. Since defining circuitry is one of the primary goals of this research approach, imaging of animals is capable of providing much more detailed anatomical descriptions of the functional consequences of chronic alcohol intake.

There are a number of means for obtaining animals with long-term ethanol exposure. Repeated injections have been used; however, since the preferred method of administration of alcohol in humans is by ingestion, a better animal model of human drinking involves intragastric intake. This can be accomplished by intragastric gavage, which entails the insertion of a feeding tube through the mouth and down to the stomach, although this method only partially models human drinking. Ethanol can be added to the diet or to drinking water. Perhaps the best animal model involves the free self-administration of ethanol. These techniques involve a period of training where animals acclimate to freely drinking ethanol. Rodents initially avoid drinking ethanol solutions presumably because of the unpleasant taste. Once the animals have regular exposure, however, ethanol can maintain drinking on its own. One approach to training such animals, the so-called sucrose fading technique, involves initially providing animals with ethanol solutions sweetened with sucrose[77] and then systematically removing the amount of sucrose over time. Much like in humans, ethanol intake in rodents appears to be an acquired taste.

Rodent studies of chronic alcohol exposure have either evaluated high-doses for short periods of time, usually on the order of days,[22,81] or low doses in the diet or drinking water for periods of a few weeks,[47,50,82] or a period of months to years.[83,84] Short-term experiments using the intra-arterial xenon method or the deoxyglucose method found that rats became tolerant after 3 to 4 days of nearly continuous intoxication to the effects of ethanol on CBF and cerebral metabolic rates for oxygen utilization, that is, fewer structures were affected by an acute dose of ethanol and to a lesser degree.[22,81] Repeated ethanol dosing also blunted the hypercapnic response, suggesting that cerebrovascular reactivity is compromised following repeated ethanol exposure.[22] Similar findings of tolerance to ethanol-induced changes in function after prolonged ethanol exposure have been reported after 3 or 8 weeks of daily ethanol intake in the diet.[47,50] Denays *et al.*[82] assessed levels of high-energy phosphates, ATP, and phosphocreatinine among others, using ^{31}P phosphorus nuclear magnetic resonance (^{31}P-NMR) following 3 weeks of dietary ethanol. These investigators found indications of reduced high-energy phosphate consumption and by inference reduced cerebral metabolism after both acute and chronic exposure to ethanol. They also found differences between animals treated acutely and those treated chronically. There was evidence of altered levels of phosphodiesters in chronically treated animals, indicating adaptation to chronic exposure in the form of increased breakdown of membrane phospholipids. Together, these data show that relatively short-term chronic treatment on the order of a few days to a few weeks can lead to tolerance.

Three studies have examined the functional consequences of ethanol administered via the diet for periods of 2 months or more, and each study found evidence of altered function in portions of the Papez circuit, which is a circular network within the limbic system that comprises the mammillary bodies, anterior thalamus, cingulate cortex, and the hippocampus. Pietrzak *et al.*[85] evaluated rats, within a few hours of removing access to ethanol, that had consumed ethanol for 7 months and found increased rates of cerebral metabolism, possibly due to withdrawal. Unlike other studies of withdrawal following much shorter chronic regimens, however, this study found the greatest changes in LCGU in the cingulate cortex–mammillary body–anterior thalamus pathway as well as amygdala and septum. In another study, after at least 70 days of daily intake under schedule-induced polydipsia, rates of LCGU in rats immediately following a session of ethanol intake were found to be depressed in the hippocampal complex, habenula, anterior ventral thalamus, and mammillary bodies and increased in the nucleus accumbens.[84] In the third study, Bontempi *et al.*[83] showed that residual functional deficits persist long after alcohol exposure has stopped by determining functional activity 7 weeks after the termination of ethanol intake. These researchers also controlled for the residual effects of withdrawal by removing the concentration of ethanol in a stepwise fashion to prevent overt withdrawal symptoms. It was found that 6 months of ethanol intake in these mice had little effect on the uptake of deoxyglucose, whereas 12 months of exposure decreased uptake in the lateral mammillary body and anterior thalamus and 18 months of exposure affected all of the mammillary body, more of the thalamus, and portions of the hippocampus. Overall, these findings are strikingly consistent with findings in humans with the Wernicke–Korsakoff's syndrome (addressed in Section 4.3). Future use of this animal model may be effective for studying the mechanism responsible for the diencephalic pathology found in Papez circuit in some alcoholics. In addition, there is an absence of data on alcohol-induced changes on frontal lobe function in the rodent, leaving us without an animal model for the frontal lobe pathology frequently found in human drinkers (discussed in Section 4.2). The establishment of such a model and subsequent imaging studies would surely advance our understanding of this particular aspect of alcohol-related dysfunction, as well.

4.2. Long-Term Ethanol Intake in Humans

It has been known since at least the 1950s that heavy alcohol consumption can lead to a reduction in cortical volume as determined by postmortem studies of human brain.[14,86] CT and MRI have been used subsequently to demonstrate that this cortical atrophy is in fact present in the living brain of heavy drinkers. Large ventricles and wide cortical and cerebellar sulci can be present and subcortical atrophy of hippocampus and mammillary bodies have been reported, even in non-Korsakoff alcoholics. It is also important that although atrophy can be seen throughout the brains of heavy drinkers, the changes in prefrontal cortex may be more pronounced.[86] This cortical atrophy is not necessarily permanent; ventricular size and sulcal width have been shown to at least partially recover during abstinence. Efforts thus far to link specific structural changes in the brain with changes in cognitive function of alcoholics have met with only limited success.[14,87] One hope of studying the functional consequences of chronic alcohol intake, therefore, is to identify functional deficits in specific brain regions that are responsible for this cognitive impairment in a way that structural imaging has not.

The smaller tissue volume in some alcoholics poses a particular problem for imaging studies, because apparent decreases in functional activity may simply be the result of normal activity in less tissue. Nonetheless, there is good evidence that functional activity is diminished in the frontal lobes of alcoholics.[88–95] Using SPECT technology, Melgaard *et al.*[96] found that the magnitude of the decreased RCBF in the medial prefrontal cortex of alcoholics was greater than that found in periventricular regions, where cortical atrophy appears to be greatest. These authors reasoned therefore that the changes in prefrontal cortex were likely to be functional. Furthermore, alcoholics without atrophy also had diminished RCBF in frontal cortex. Erbas *et al.*[97] compared RCBF and atrophy determined by CT in alcoholics. Here, RCBF was normalized to whole slice CBF, which partially compensated for cortical atrophy (to the degree that atrophy is equally distributed throughout the slice). In alcoholics, frontal RCBF was lower and significant cortical atrophy was evident; however, RCBF and cortical atrophy were not significantly correlated in this study, which suggests that these variables may function independently at least to some degree. Furthermore, since reduced RCBF is found in alcoholics without atrophy,[90,97,98] these structural and functional forms of alcoholic pathology can be differentiated.

Two studies compared neuropsychological function and RCBF, and both found that hypoperfusion was significantly correlated with poor task performance in alcoholics who otherwise appeared to be unimpaired.[96,98] Nicolas *et al.*[98] reported that 18 of 29 alcoholics without detectable atrophy were found to have frontal hypoperfusion. Furthermore, 17 of the 18 alcoholics with frontal hypoperfusion (but not atrophy) presented with cognitive impairment, whereas only 1 of 11 alcoholics without atrophy or altered frontal perfusion was neuropsychologically impaired. These data demonstrate that RCBF is a sensitive measure of function in alcoholics and that it was a better predictor of performance than the degree of atrophy. Furthermore, in alcoholics that abstained from alcohol for 2 months, those without atrophy had normal frontal perfusion. Those with atrophy improved but did not return to normal levels, which suggests that the prognosis for cognitive recovery may be better in nonatrophic alcoholics. It appears then, that regardless of the degree to which these structural and functional methods may be independent, they both retain an important relationship with cognitive impairment.

Reduced LCGU in the frontal cortex of alcoholics has also been correlated with poor performance on tests of frontal lobe function, including the Symbol Digit Modalities written test[93] and the Wisconsin Card Sorting Test.[88] As shown in Fig. 3, Wang *et al.*[93] also found that frontal LCGU in alcoholics was positively correlated with performance on the Weschler Memory Scale. Weingartner and co-workers[94] reported that the recognition of whether a word had been provided by the subject or the experimenter during test sessions 2 days earlier was impaired in their alcoholic population and that performance on this task further correlated with reduced metabolism in left prefrontal, temporal, and posterior orbitofrontal cortex. Here again, strong evidence has been provided, this time assessing cerebral metabolism, that poor cognitive performance and regional functional deficits concentrated in the frontal lobe are found in alcoholics. At this point, however, we do not know how long this relationship lasts in the sober, recovering alcoholic because functional activity can recover during abstinence.[96] These changes in function may in fact be the consequence of recent drinking, since altered functional activity has been correlated with the amount of recent alcohol intake,[98] the number of days since last use,[91] and the severity of alcoholism.[96] Future work is therefore needed to differentiate between these relatively short-lived residual changes in brain function associated with recent ethanol use and more permanent functional deficits.

In summary, functional deficits in cerebral blood flow and metabolism have been demonstrated clearly in chronic alcoholics, and the majority of this work indicates that dysfunction can be found in the frontal lobes. These deficits are at least partially independent of cortical atrophy and are apparent in alcoholics with demonstrable cognitive impairment and in those that appear neurologically intact. Furthermore, abstaining from alcohol leads to improvements in functional activity in these populations, although whether complete recovery can be attained by all alcoholics remains to be determined.

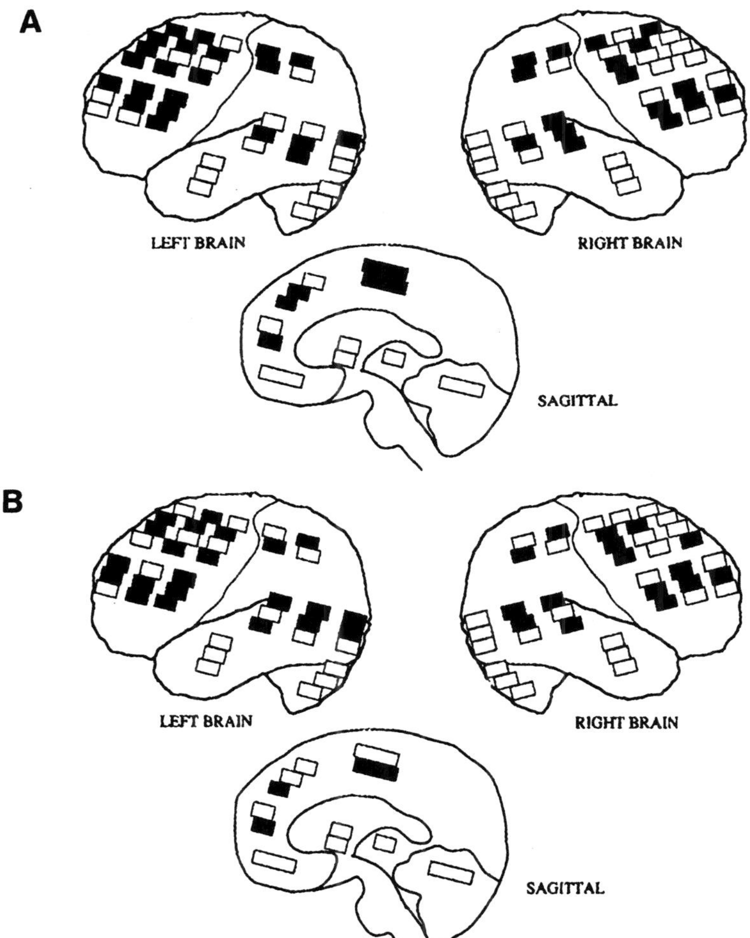

Figure 3. Schematic representations of brain regions in which metabolism was significantly correlated with (A) Symbol Digit Modalities test written score and (B) total score on Wechsler Memory Scale (in both alcoholic and control subjects). Black regions, $P \leq 0.01$; white regions, not significant. (Reprinted with permission from Wang *et al.*[93])

4.3. Wernicke–Korsakoff's Syndrome

Wernicke–Korsakoff's syndrome, the alcohol amnestic disorder, or Korsakoff's disease (KD) is a devastating short-term memory disorder. In developed countries, poor nutrition in the context of severe chronic alcoholism is the leading cause of this disease.[99] The primary clinical symptom is profound recent memory loss and an ensuing anterograde amnesia. KD is often preceded by acute Wernicke's encephalopathy, which is a clinical state consisting of ataxia, incoordination, ocular disturbances, and mental confusion resulting from a nutritional thiamine deficiency. Lesions have been identified in these patients with KD in midline brain structures including the mammillary bodies and portions of the thalamus, as well in the hippocampus and other structures.[100] This "mesial" amnestic syndrome can be differentiated from other syndromes of recent memory loss such as herpetic encephalitis, for example, that results from relatively circumscribed medial temporal lesions.[101]

Relatively early studies found that during the acute stages of Wernicke's encephalopathy and during the initial presentation of KD, functional activity as determined by global measures was reduced[102–104] or unchanged.[105,106] Hunter *et al.*[107] found that cerebrovascular transit time was greater in patients with Korsakoff's psychosis, which also suggests that rates of blood flow were decreased. In a later study, these same researchers also attempted to localize changes in blood flow by determining regional rates in patients with KD using SPECT methodology.[108] A trend toward decreased RCBF in frontal cortex of Korsakoff's patients was noted, and the rates of frontal lobe perfusion were significantly correlated with performance on neuropsychological tests of frontal lobe function.

Martin and co-workers[109] first examined ten alcoholics, seven of whom had Wernicke–Korsakoff's syndrome and three who had alcoholic dementia. In the ten alcoholics, significantly diminished RCBF values, normalized to slice mean values, were found in left cerebellar, left parietal, and right anterior temporal regions. Trends toward reduced LCGU could also be found in a number of regions of interest in the frontal cortex of alcoholics in this study. In a subsequent study by the same group,[110] more definitive differences were found between a group of ten patients with Wernicke–Korsakoff's syndrome and ten age-matched controls. The use of improved methodology and an alcoholic group consisting only of patients with KD distinguishes these studies. Since atrophy is a common feature in brains of these patients and cortical atrophy was demonstrated by CT in these Korsakoff's patients, cortical atrophy was used as a covariate in the statistical analysis. Although absolute rates of LCGU did not differ across groups, when structures were normalized to slice means, several brain regions were found to have diminished cerebral metabolism in amnestics. Under these conditions, the anterior and posterior portions of the cingulate gyrus and the precuneate region in the parietal lobe were shown with good statistical confidence to have diminished glucose utilization in Korsakoff patients. Furthermore, the majority of amnestic patients in this study had abstained from alcohol use for a year or more, indicating that the diminished functional activity in these regions may in fact be permanent.

Fazio and co-workers[111] evaluated 11 so-called "pure" amnestics (patients with marked memory loss without other changes in cognitive function), two of whom had KD, and found that absolute values of LCGU were bilaterally decreased in the cingulate gyrus, basal forebrain, hippocampus, and thalamus when compared to normal controls. These investigators interpreted these results as implicating the Papez circuit in the generation of memories, which is clearly consistent with known neuropathology found in KD.

There are additional studies that are also worth mentioning. Moffoot *et al.*[112] tested the effect of clonidine to alter RCBF in 19 patients with Korsakoff's psychosis, based on the hypothesis that this population manifests a noradrenergic impairment.[112,113] Clonidine treatment significantly improved verbal fluency in the Korsakoff patients, although the saline-treated group also improved. Nonetheless, better performance was significantly correlated with increased RCBF in the left dorsolateral prefrontal cortex of amnestics. Increased RCBF was also noted in the posterior cingulate following clinidine treatment. These data appear promising; however, a clear demonstration of the ability of clonidine to improve performance in Korsakoff's patients has not yet been provided.[114]

There is also a recent case report that describes a patient who was first evaluated during the early stages of Wernicke–Korsakoff's syndrome when she was exhibiting the common feature of confabulation, that is, providing fabricated descriptions of the recent past.[115] She was then tested 4 months later when confabulation had ceased, but the amnestic disorder remained. Initially, RCBF was low in ventral and medial prefrontal regions corresponding to orbitofrontal and cingulate cortices. After 4 months, blood flow had improved in these regions, while RCBF in mesial subcortical sites in thalamus remained relatively poor, implicating these frontal sites in confabulation and mesial sites again in amnesia.

In summary, patients with KD are subject to disturbances in functional activity in midline brain structures as expected based on the known histopathology of the disease. Since these functional deficits can be detected in living brain, imaging provides a means for more careful examination of the interaction between the functional and behavioral deficits associated with KD and for understanding the neurobiological basis of memory formation in general. Furthermore, like non-Korsakoff alcoholics, frontal lobe dysfunction is also present in KD, which implies that cognitive deficits of planning, organization, and memory processes known to be supported by dorsolateral prefrontal cortex may exist along side the main amnestic features of KD.

4.4. *Withdrawal*

One of the hallmarks of physical dependence is the phenomenon of withdrawal on cessation of drug intake. Physical symptoms of ethanol withdrawal include anxiety, hallucinations, seizures, irritability, nausea, vomiting, insomnia, tremor, hypothermia, hyperventilation, and tachycardia.[116] The study of withdrawal is important for at least two reasons. First, in the severe chronic alcoholic, withdrawal can be severe and may require medical intervention. A clearer understanding of the functional basis of withdrawal and the current treatments that alleviate it will likely lead to more rational treatment strategies. Second, it is not known whether withdrawal leads to residual deficits in brain function. Since cognitive deficits occur in alcoholics, the role withdrawal plays, if any, in the establishment of alcohol-related impairment needs to be determined. The studies reviewed below are the initial attempts to investigate the functional consequences of withdrawal, and they describe the regional changes in the brains of humans and animals during the early stages of abstinence from alcohol.

The functional consequences of withdrawal in humans appear to be regionally heterogeneous, leading to increased activity in some areas while decreasing it others. Eisenberg[117] first reported a change in functional activity in humans suffering from delirium tremens and found general reductions in CBF. Berglund and Risberg[118] and Caspari *et al.*[119] later found increased functional activity in portions of the temporal cortex in at least some of their withdrawing subjects, while at the same time decreased activity was found in other portions of temporal cortex or in parietal cortical regions. The increased temporal lobe activity was associated with greater levels of agitation.[118] As might be expected, increased functional activity was also found in the temporal and occipital lobes of patients experiencing auditory and visual hallucinations in the context of alcoholic withdrawal.[118] In an interesting case study, a highly circumscribed region of decreased RCBF was found at the junction of the frontal, temporal, and parietal lobes in the left hemisphere of a patient undergoing withdrawal associated with chronic alcohol and diazepam abuse.[120] Although more work is needed, these data suggest that increased functional activity predominately in or around the temporal lobe can be found in withdrawing patients, and this change may be most closely identified with agitation and auditory hallucinations. Decreased functional activity in other nearby regions is also a feature of withdrawal, and the extent of these decreases has been correlated to the length of the preceding binge.[118] Given that chronic alcohol exposure diminishes functional activity in and of itself, the decreased functional activity found during withdrawal may be more related to factors associated with the length of chronic abuse rather than to the magnitude of the acute episode of withdrawal.

There are reports that withdrawal leads to marked increases in functional activity as assessed using global[121] or local[48,122] measures. Figure 4 illustrates the dramatic increase in functional activity that can accompany withdrawal. Global increases have also been found in animal subjects that did not display overt withdrawal symptoms in one study in which animals voluntarily consumed ethanol for a minimum of 70 days (2.2 ± 1.0 g/kg ethanol for 14 days prior to the experimental procedure).[84]

Other studies have found localized changes in function in withdrawing animals. Campbell *et al.*[123] reported distinct patterns of increased glucose uptake in withdrawing animals that had received 8–11 g/kg of ethanol over 3 to 4 days. These functional CNS increases were localized to frontal–sensorimotor cortex, globus pallidus, several thalamic nuclei, parts of the cerebellum, genu of corpus callosum, and internal capsule. Eckardt *et al.*,[81] using a similar procedure, also reported a variety of changes in glucose utilization in a study of withdrawing animals; this time a group of intoxicated ethanol-

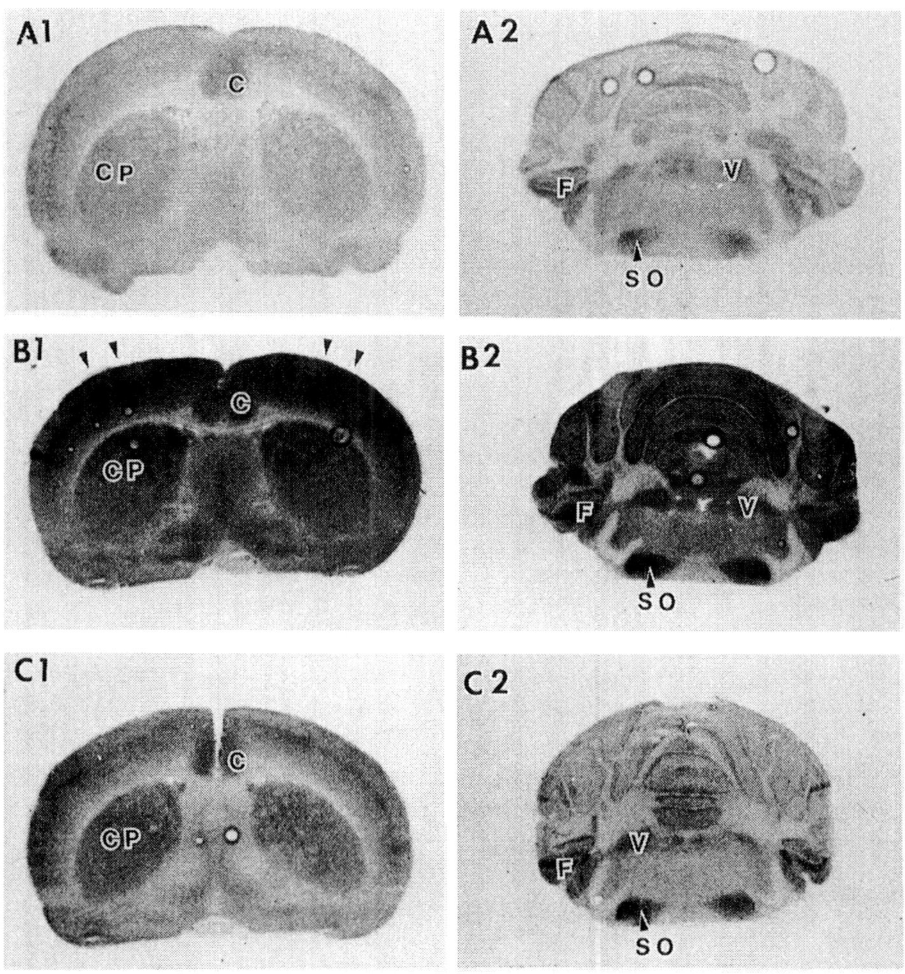

Figure 4. Effects of overt ethanol withdrawal and postwithdrawal on uptake of 2-deoxyglucose. Photographs of autoradiographs of brain sections for (A) control, (B) withdrawing, and (C) postwithdrawing rats. 1, Level of the caudate-putamen (CP), at the optic chiasm, showing light and dark cortical columnar regions (arrows) in overt withdrawal; 2, level of the cerebellum showing flocculus (F), vestibular nuclei (V), and superior olivaris nucleus (SO). The darkness of the autoradiographs indicates a relative increase of ^{14}C-labeled tracer. (Reprinted with permission from Eckardt *et al.*[122])

dependent animals was included. Besides a major trend of decreased glucose utilization in both acute and chronic treatment groups and a corresponding increase in glucose utilization in withdrawing animals, some cortical structures showed a decrease in glucose utilization during intoxication, with no corresponding change when undergoing withdrawal. This suggests that certain brain structures are less likely to exhibit increased functional activity than others, despite their sensitivity to the acute effects of ethanol. These structures included parts of the cerebellum and various limbic regions. Yet another group of brain structures showed increased glucose utilization during withdrawal without the characteristic decrease during intoxication. These structures included sensorimotor areas, sensory systems, cingulate cortex, and the habenula. Future work that investigates functional changes in animals that are treated with a range of doses for varying time periods may provide a clearer picture of the discrete patterns of regional change in the CNS during ethanol abstinence.

5. Conclusions

This growing body of work has clearly demonstrated the utility of imaging studies in the field of alcohol research. Discrete anatomically localized changes in functional activity are now being directly associated with particular structural and cognitive deficits in the living human brain. Animal studies have begun to identify specific neural circuitry associated with various consequences of ethanol exposure. We are only beginning to learn to use these methodologies effectively and to master their application in the investigation of the effects of alcohol on the brain. If imaging research is to drive our understanding of the neurobiological basis of alcohol's effects in the future, specific cortical and subcortical circuits related to alcohol use must be identified. Current and developing imaging methods can accomplish this. Special statistical analysis of PET data can identify clusters of brain structures whose activity varies as a unit, even when those changes are small. Functional MRI can provide resolution in human brain at a level that permits examination of subcortical structures and subregions of cortex that has not been possible with emission-based methods before.[124] In addition, animal studies can have a unique impact by relating structure and function at the regional and cellular level. There is every reason to believe therefore that imaging research will continue to provide tangible advances toward a better understanding of the neurobiological consequences of ethanol exposure.

ACKNOWLEDGMENT. This work was supported by a grant from the National Institutes on Alcohol Abuse and Alcoholism, AA09291.

References

1. Sakurada O, Kennedy C, Jehle J, *et al:* Measurement of local cerebral blood flow with iodo[^{14}C]antipyrine. *Am J Physiol* 234:H59–H66, 1978.

2. Sokoloff L: Cerebral circulation, energy metabolism, and protein synthesis: General characteristics and principles of measurement, in Phelps M, Mazziotta J, Shelbert H (eds): *Positron Emission Tomography and Autoradiography: Principles and Applications for the Brain and Heart.* New York, Raven Press, 1986, pp 1–71.
3. Lyons D, Miller MD, Crane AM, *et al:* Time-dependent effects of acute ethanol administration on regional cerebral blood flow in the rat. *Soc Neurosci Abstr* 21:1703, 1995.
4. Kurumaji A, Dewar D, McCulloch J: Metabolic mapping with deoxyglucose autoradiography as an approach for assessing drug action in the central nervous system, in London ED (ed): *Imaging Drug Action in the Brain.* Boca Raton, FL, CRC Press, 1993, pp 219–245.
5. Williams-Hemby L, Porrino LJ: Low and moderate doses of ethanol produce distinct patterns of cerebral metabolic changes in rats. *Alcohol Clin Exp Res* 18:982–988, 1994.
6. Wong-Riley MT: Cytochrome oxidase: An endogenous metabolic marker for neuronal activity. *Trends Neurosci* 12:94–101, 1989.
7. Gonzalez-Lima F, Jones D: Quantitative mapping of cytochrome oxidase activity in the central auditory system of the gerbil: A study with calibrated activity standards and metal-intensified histochemistry. *Brain Res* 660:34–49, 1994.
8. Hevner RF, Wong-Riley MT: Neuronal expression of nuclear and mitochondrial genes for cytochrome oxidase (CO) subunits analyzed by *in situ* hybridization: Comparison with CO activity and protein. *J Neurosci* 11:1942–1958, 1991.
9. Vila M, Levy R, Herrero M-T, *et al:* Consequences of nigrostriatal denervation on the functioning of the basal ganglia in human and nonhuman primates: An *in situ* hybridizaiton study of cytochrome oxidase subunit I mRNA. *J Neurosci* 15:765–773, 1997.
10. Lee S, Rivier C: Prenatal alcohol exposure alters the hypothalamic–pituitary–adrenal axis response of immature offspring to interleukin-1: Is nitric oxide involved? *Alcohol Clin Exp Res* 18:1242–1247, 1994.
11. Volkow ND, Hitzemann R, Wolf AP, *et al:* Acute effects of ethanol on regional brain glucose metabolism and transport. *Psychiatry Res* 35:39–48, 1990.
12. Volkow ND, Mullani N, Gould L, *et al:* Effects of acute alcohol intoxication on cerebral blood flow measured with PET. *Psychiatry Res* 24:201–209, 1988.
13. Tiihonen J, Kuikka J, Hakola P, *et al:* Acute ethanol-induced changes in cerebral blood flow. *Am J Psychiatry* 151:1505–1508, 1994.
14. Rosenbloom MJ, Pfefferbaum A, Sullivan EV: Structural brain alterations associated with alcoholism. *Alcohol Health Res World* 19:266–272, 1995.
15. Belliveau JW: Functional mapping of the human visual cortex by magnetic resonance imaging. *Science* 254:716–719, 1991.
16. Chorlian DB, Porjesz B, Cohen HL: Measuring electrical activity of the brain: ERP mapping in alcohol research. *Alcohol Health Res World* 19:315–320, 1995.
17. Porjesz B, Begleiter H: Event-related potentials in cognitive function in alcoholism. *Alcohol Health Res World* 19:108–112, 1995.
18. Lyons D, Porrino LJ, Hiller-Sturmhofel S: Visualizing neural pathways affected by alcohol in animals. *Alcohol Health Res World* 19:300–305, 1995.
19. Barbour RL, Gebrewold A, Altura BM: Optical spectroscopy and cerebral vascular effects of alcohol in the intact brain: Effects on tissue deoxyhemoglobin, blood content, and reduced cytochrome oxidase. *Alcohol Clin Exp Res* 17:1319–1324, 1993.
20. Flock EV, Tyce GM, Owen CA Jr: Effects of ethanol on glucose utilization in rat brain. *Proc Soc Exp Biol Med* 135:325–333, 1970.
21. Hadji-Dimo AA, Ekberg R, Ingvar DH: Effects of ethanol on EEG and cortical blood flow in the cat. *Q J Stud Alcohol* 29:828–838, 1968.
22. Hemmingsen R, Barry DI: Adaptive changes in cerebral blood flow and oxygen consumption during ethanol intoxication in the rat. *Acta Physiol Scand* 106:249–255, 1979.
23. Hemmingsen R, Barry DI: Cerebral oxygen consumption in the rat: Pharmacological stimulation and suppression, role of catecholaminergic mechanisms. *Eur Neurol* 20:215–218, 1981.
24. McQueen JD, Sklar FK, Posey JB: Autoregulation of cerebral blood flow during alcohol infusion. *J Stud Alcohol* 39:1477–1487, 1978.
25. Rawat AK: Effects of ethanol on brain metabolism. *Adv Exp Med Biol* 56:165–177, 1975.

26. Roach MK, Reese WN Jr: Effect of ethanol on glucose and amino acid metabolism in brain. *Biochem Pharmacol* 20:2805–2812, 1971.
27. Thomas CB: The cerebral circulation: Effect of alcohol on cerebral vessels. *Arch Neurol Psychiatry* 38:321–339, 1937.
28. Veech RL, Harris RL, Mehlman MA: Brain metabolite concentrations and redox states in rats fed diets containing 1,3-butanediol and ethanol. *Toxicol Appl Pharmacol* 29:196–203, 1974.
29. Veloso D, Passonneau JV, Veech RL: The effects of intoxicating doses of ethanol upon intermediary metabolism in rat brain. *J Neurochem* 19:2679–2686, 1972.
30. Battey LL, Heyman A, Patterson JL: Cerebral effects of ethyl alcohol on cerebral blood flow and metabolism. *JAMA* 152:6–10, 1953.
31. Goldfarb W, Bowman KM, Wortis J: The effect of alcohol on cerebral metabolism. *Am J Psychiatry* 97:384–387, 1940.
32. Hine CH, Shick AF, Margolis L: Effects of alcohol in small doses and tetraethylthiuramdisulphide (Antabuse) on cerebral blood flow and cerebral metabolism. *J Pharmacol Exp Ther* 106:253–260, 1952.
33. Loman J, Myerson A: Alcohol and cerebral vasodilation. *N Engl J Med* 227:439–441, 1942.
34. Miyazaki M: Circulatory effect of ethanol with special refernce to cerebral circulation. *Jpn Circ J* 38:381–385, 1974.
35. Sutherlund VC, Burbridge TN, Adams JE: Cerebral metabolism in problem drinkers under the influence of alcohol and chlorpromazine hydrochloride. *J Appl Physiol* 15:189–196, 1960.
36. Mathew RJ, Wilson WH: Regional cerebral blood flow changes associated with ethanol intoxication. *Stroke* 17:1156–1159, 1986.
37. Newlin DB, Golden CJ, Quaife M, *et al:* Effect of alcohol ingestion on regional cerebral blood flow. *Int J Neurosci* 17:145–150, 1982.
38. Sano M, Wendt PE, Wirsen A, *et al:* Acute effects of alcohol on regional cerebral blood flow in man. *J Stud Alcohol* 54:369–376, 1993.
39. Schwartz JA, Speed NM, Gross MD, *et al:* Acute effects of alcohol administration on regional cerebral blood flow: The role of acetate. *Alcohol Clin Exp Res* 17:1119–1123, 1993.
40. De Wit H, Metz J, Wagner N, *et al:* Behavioral and subjective effects of ethanol: Relationship to cerebral metabolism using PET. *Alcohol Clin Exp Res* 14:482–489, 1990.
41. Eckardt MJ, Campbell GA, Marietta CA, *et al:* Acute ethanol administration selectively alters localized cerebral glucose metabolism. *Brain Res* 444:53–58, 1988.
42. Hoffman WE, Miletich DJ, Albrecht RF: Dose and time dependent cerebrovascular and metabolic effects of ethanol. *Alcohol* 3:23–26, 1986.
43. Williams-Hemby L, Porrino LJ: Functional consequences of orally administered ethanol in rats as measured by the 2-[^{14}C]deoxyglucose method. *Alcohol Clin Exp Res* 21:1573–1580, 1997.
44. Williams-Hemby L, Porrino LJ: Functional consequences of orally administered ethanol in rats as measured by the 2-[^{14}C]deoxyglucose method: The contribution of dopamine. *Alcohol Clin Exp Res* 21:1581–1591, 1997.
45. Friedman HS, Lowery R, Archer M, *et al:* The effects of ethanol on brain blood flow in awake dogs. *J Cardiovasc Pharmacol* 6:344–348, 1984.
46. Goldman H, Sapirstein LA, Murphy S, *et al:* Alcohol and regional blood flow in brains of rats. *Proc Soc Exp Biol Med* 144:983–988, 1973.
47. Grunwald F, Schrock H, Biersack H, *et al:* Changes in local cerebral glucose utilization in the awake rat during acute and chronic administration of ethanol. *J Nucl Med* 34:793–798, 1993.
48. Hemmingsen R, Barry DI, Hertz MM, *et al:* Cerebral blood flow and oxygen consumption during ethanol withdrawal in the rat. *Brain Res* 173:259–269, 1979.
49. Ligeti L, Hines K, Dora E, *et al:* Cerebral blood flow and metabolic rate in the conscious freely moving rat: The effects of hypercapnia, and acute ethanol administration. *Alcohol Clin Exp Res* 15:766–770, 1991.
50. Vina JR, Salus JE, DeJoseph MR, *et al:* Brain energy consumption in ethanol-treated, Long-Evans rats. *J Nutr* 121:879–886, 1991.
51. Porrino LJ, Domer FR, Crane AM, *et al:* Selective alterations in cerebral metabolism within

the mesocorticolimbic dopaminergic system produced by acute cocaine administration in rats. *Neuropsychopharmacology* 1:109–118, 1988.
52. Porrino LJ, Pontieri FE: Metabolic mapping of the effects of psychomotor stimulants in rats, in London ED (ed): *Imaging Drug Action in the Brain.* Boca Raton, FL, CRC Press, 1993, pp 247–263.
53. Pohorecky LA: Biphasic action of ethanol. *Biobehav Rev* 1:231–240, 1977.
54. Ekman GM, Frankenhaeuser M, Goldberg L, *et al:* Subjective and objective effects of alcohol as functions of dosage and time. *Psychopharmacology* 6:399–409, 1964.
55. Lewis MJ, June HJ: Neurobehavioral studies of ethanol reward and activation. *Alcohol* 7:213–219, 1990.
56. Lukas SE, Mendelson JH, Woods BT, Mello NK, Teoh SK: Topographic distribution of EEG alpha activity during ethanol-induced intoxication in women. *J Stud Alcohol* 50:176–185, 1989.
57. Lukas SE, Mendelson JH, Benedikt RA, *et al:* EEG alpha activity increases during transient episodes of ethanol-induced euphoria. *Pharmacol Biochem Behav* 25:889–895, 1986.
58. Portans I, White JM, Staiger PK: Acute tolerance to alcohol: Changes in subjective effects among social drinkers. *Psychopharmacology* 97:365–369, 1989.
59. Risinger FO, Cunningham CL: Ethanol produces rapid biphasic hedonic effects. *Ann NY Acad Sci* 654:506–508, 1992.
60. Kalant H, LeBlanc AE, Gibbins RJ: Tolerance to, and dependence on, some non-opiate psychotropic drugs. *Pharmacol Rev* 23:135–191, 1971.
61. Le AD, Mayer JM: Aspects of alcohol tolerance in humans and experimental animals, in Deitrich RA, Erin VG (eds): *Pharmacological Effects of Ethanol on the Nervous System.* Boca Raton, FL, CRC Press, 1996, pp 251–268.
62. Mellanby E: Alcohol: Its absorption into and disappearance from blood under different conditions (Abstract) Great Britain Medical Research Council, Special Report Series No. 31, 1919.
63. Goldberg L: Quantitative studies on alcohol tolerance in man. *Acta Physiol Scand* 5:1–26, 1943.
64. Campanelli C, Le AD, Khanna JM, *et al:* Effect of raphe lesions on the development of acute tolerance to ethanol and pentobarbital. *Psychopharmacology* 96:454–457, 1988.
65. Durand D, Corrigall WA, Kujtan P, *et al:* Effect of low concentrations of ethanol on CA1 hippocampal neurons *in vitro. Can J Physiol Pharmacol* 59:979–984, 1981.
66. Givens BS, Breese GR: Electrophysiological evidence that ethanol alters function of medial septal area without affecting lateral septal function. *J Pharmacol Exp Ther* 253:95–103, 1990.
67. Grover CA, Frye GD, Griffith WH: Acute tolerance to ethanol inhibition of NMDA-mediated EPSPs in the CA1 region of the rat hippocampus. *Brain Res* 642:70–76, 1994.
68. Mullin MJ, Dalton TK, Hunt WA, *et al:* Actions of ethanol on voltage-sensitive sodium channels: Effects of acute and chronic ethanol treatment. *J Pharmacol Exp Ther* 242:541–547.
69. Noldy NE, Carlen PL: Acute, withdrawal, and chronic alcohol effects in man: Event-related potential and quantitative EEG techniques. *Ann Med* 22:333–339, 1990.
70. Pohorecky LA, Newman B: Effect of ethanol on dopamine synthesis in rat striatal synaptosomes. *Drug Alcohol Depend* 2:329–334, 1977.
71. Sinclair JG, Lo GF, Tien AF: The effects of ethanol on cerebellar Purkinje cells in naive and alcohol-dependent rats. *Can J Physiol Pharmacol* 58:429–432, 1980.
72. Porrino LJ: The application of metabolic mapping methods to the identification of the neural substrates of the effects of alcohol, in Zakhari S, Witt E (eds): *Imaging in Alcohol Research.* Rockville, MD, US Department of Health and Human Services, 1992, pp 375–388.
73. Hammer RP Jr, Cooke ES: Gradual tolerance of metabolic activity is produced in mesolimbic regions by chronic cocaine treatment, while susequent cocaine challenge activates extrapyramidal regions of rat brain. *J Neurosci* 14:4289–4298, 1994.
74. Kornetsky C, Huston-Lyons D, Porrino LJ: The role of the olfactory tubercle in the effects of cocaine, morphine and brain-stimulation reward. *Brain Res* 541:75–81, 1991.

75. Dworkin SI, Goeders NE, Grabowski J, *et al:* The effects of 12-hour limited access to cocaine: Reduction in drug intake and mortality. *NIDA Res Monogr* 76:221–225, 1987.
76. Moolten M, Kornetsky C: Oral self-administration of ethanol and not experimenter-administered ethanol facilitates rewarding electrical brain stimulation. *Alcohol* 7:221–225, 1990.
77. Samson HH: Initiation of ethanol reinforcement using a sucrose-substitution procedure in food- and water-sated rats. *Alcohol Clin Exp Res* 10:436–442, 1986.
78. Koob GF, Bloom FE: Cellular and molecular mechanisms of drug dependence. *Science* 242:715–722, 1988.
79. Rogers RL, Meyer JS, Shaw TJ: Reductions in regional cerebral blood flow associated with chronic consumption of alcohol. *J Am Geriatr Soc* 31:540–543, 1983.
80. Ishikawa Y, Meyer JS, Tanahashi N, *et al:* Abstinence improves cerebral perfusion and brain volume in alcoholic neurotoxicity without Wernicke–Korsakoff syndrome. *J Cerebr Blood Flow Metab* 6:86–94, 1986.
81. Eckardt MJ, Campbell GA, Marietta CA, *et al:* Ethanol dependence and withdrawal selectively alter localized cerebral glucose utilization. *Brain Res* 584:244–250, 1992.
82. Denays R, Chao SL, Mathur-Dere R, *et al:* Metabolic changes in the rat brain after acute and chronic ethanol intoxication: A ^{31}P-NMR spectroscopy study. *Magn Reson Med* 29:719–723, 1993.
83. Bontempi B, Beracochea D, Jaffard R, *et al:* Reduction of regional brain glucose metabolism following different durations of chronic ethanol consumption in mice: A selective effect on diencephalic structures. *Neuroscience* 72:1141–1153, 1996.
84. Williams-Hemby L, Grant KA, Gatto GJ, *et al:* Metabolic mapping of the effects of chronic voluntary ethanol consumption in rats. *Pharmacol Biochem Behav* 54:415–423, 1996.
85. Pietrzak ER, Wilce PA, Shanley BC: The effect of chronic ethanol consumption on [14C]deoxyglucose uptake in rat brain *in vivo. Neurosci Lett* 100:181–187, 1989.
86. Courville CB: *Effects of Alcohol in the Nervous System in Man.* Los Angeles, San Lucas Press, 1955.
87. Parsons O: Neuropsychological consequences of alcohol abuse: Many questions—Some answers, in Parsons O, Butters N, Nathan P (eds): *Neuropsychology of Alcoholism: Implications for Diagnosis and Treatment.* New York: Guilford Press, 1987, pp 153–175.
88. Adams KM, Gilman S, Koeppe RA, *et al:* Neuropsychological deficits are correlated with frontal hypometabolism in positron emission tomography of older alcoholics patients. *Alcohol Clin Exp Res* 17:205–210, 1993.
89. Sachs H, Russell JA, Christman DR, *et al:* Alteration of regional cerebral glucose metabolic rate in non-Korsakoff chronic alcoholism. *Arch Neurol* 44:1242–1251, 1987.
90. Samson Y, Baron J, Feline A, *et al:* Local cerebral glucose utilisation in chronic alcoholics: A positron tomography study. *J Neurol Neurosurg Psychiatry* 49:1165–1170, 1986.
91. Volkow ND, Hitzemann R, Wang GJ, *et al:* Decreased brain metabolism in neurologically intact healthy alcoholics. *Am J Psychiatry* 149:1016–1022, 1992.
92. Wang G, Volkow ND, Hitzemann R, *et al:* Brain imaging of an alcoholic with MRI, SPECT, and PET. *Am J Imag* 3:194–198, 1992.
93. Wang GJ, Volkow ND, Roque CT, *et al:* Functional importance of ventricular enlargement and cortical atrophy in healthy subjects and alcoholics as assessed with PET, MR imaging, and neuropsychologic testing. *Radiology* 186:59–65, 1993.
94. Weingartner HJ, Andreason PJ, Hommer DW, *et al:* Monitoring the source of memory in detoxified alcoholics. *Biol Psychiatry* 40:43–53, 1996.
95. Wik G, Borg S, Sjogren I, *et al:* PET determination of regional cerebral glucose metabolism in alcohol-dependent men and healthy controls using ^{11}C-glucose. *Acta Psychiatr Scand* 78:234–241, 1988.
96. Melgaard B, Henriksen L, Ahlgren P, *et al:* Regional cerebral blood flow in chronic alcoholics measured by single photon emission computerized tomography. *Acta Neurol Scand* 82:87–93, 1990.
97. Erbas B, Bekdik C, Erbengi G, *et al:* Regional cerebral blood flow changes in chronic alcoholism using Tc-99m HMPAO SPECT comparison with CT parameters. *Clin Nucl Med* 17:123–127, 1992.

98. Nicolas JM, Catafau AM, Estruch R, *et al:* Regional cerebral blood flow-SPECT in chronic alcoholism: Relation to neuropsychological testing. *J Nucl Med* 34:1452–1459, 1993.
99. Meyer JS, Tanahashi N, Ishikawa Y, *et al:* Cerebral atrophy and hypoperfusion improves during treatment of Wernicke–Korsakoff syndrome. *J Cerebr Blood Flow Metab* 5:376–385, 1985.
100. Victor M, Adams RD, Collins GH: The Wernicke–Korsakoff syndrome. A clinical and pathological study of 245 patients, 82 with post-mortem examinations. *Contemp Neurol Ser* 7:1–206, 1971.
101. Walsh KW: *Understanding Brain Damage: A Primer of Neuropsychological Evaluation.* New York, Churchill Livingstone, 1985.
102. Headlund S, Kohler V, Nylin G: Cerebral circulation in dementia. *Acta Psychiatr Scand* 40:77–106, 1964.
103. Kruger G, Haubitz I, Weinhardt F, *et al:* Brain oxidative metabolism and blood flow in alcoholic syndromes. *Subst Alcohol Actions Misuse* 1:295–307, 1980.
104. Shimojyo S, Scheinberg P, Reinmuth O: Cerebral blood flow and metabolism in the Wernicke–Korsakoff syndrome. *J Clin Invest* 46:849–854, 1967.
105. Berglund M, Ingvar DH: Cerebral blood flow and its regional distribution in alcoholism and in Kosakoff's psychosis. *J Stud Alcohol* 37:586–597, 1976.
106. Simard D, Olesen J, Paulson OB, *et al:* Regional cerebral blood flow and its regulation in dementia. *Brain* 94:273–288, 1971.
107. Hunter R, Merrick MV, Ferrington C, *et al:* Cerebral vascular transit time in alzheimer's disease and Korsakoff's psychosis and its relation to cognitive function. *Br J Psychiatry* 154:790–796, 1989.
108. Hunter R, McLuskie R, Wyper D, *et al:* The pattern of function-related regional cerebral blood flow investigated by single photon emission tomography with ^{99m}Tc-HMPAO in patients with presenile Alzheimer's disease and Korsakoff's psychosis. *Psychol Med* 19:847–855, 1989.
109. Martin PR, Rio D, Adinoff B, *et al:* Regional cerebral glucose utilization in chronic organic mental disorders associated with alcoholism. *J Neuropsychiatry* 4:159–167, 1992.
110. Joyce EM, Rio DE, Ruttimann UE, *et al:* Decreased cingulate and precuneate glucose utilization in alcoholic Korsakoff's syndrome. *Psychiatry Res* 54:225–239, 1994.
111. Fazio F, Perani D, Gilardi MC, *et al:* Metabolic impairment in human amnesia: A PET study of memory networks. *J Cerebr Blood Flow Metab* 12:353–358, 1992.
112. Moffoot A, O'Carroll RE, Murray C, *et al:* Clonidine infusion increases uptake of ^{99m}Tc-Exametazime in anterior cingulate cortex in Korsakoff's psychosis. *Psychol Med* 24:53–61, 1994.
113. McEntee WJ, Mair RG: The Korsakoff syndrome: A neurochemical perspective [published erratum appears in *Trends Neurosci* 1990 13(11):446]. *Trends Neurosci* 13:340–344, 1990.
114. O'Carroll R: Neuropsychological and neuroimaging aspects of latent hepatic encephalopathy (LHE). *Alcohol Alcohol Suppl* 2:191–195, 1993.
115. Benson DF, Djenderedjian A, Miller BL, *et al:* Neural basis of confabulation. *Neurology* 46:1239–1243, 1996.
116. Metten P, Crabbe JC: Dependence and withdrawal, in Deitrich RA, Erwin VG (eds): *Pharmacological Effects of Ethanol on the Nervous System.* Boca Raton, FL, CRC Press, 1996, pp 269–290.
117. Eisenberg S: Cerebral blood flow and metabolism in patients with delirium tremens. *Clin Res* 16:17, 1968.
118. Berglund M, Risberg J: Regional cerebral blood flow during alcohol withdrawal. *Arch Gen Psychiatry* 38:351–355, 1981.
119. Caspari D, Trabert W, Heinz G, *et al:* The pattern of regional cerebral blood flow during alcohol withdrawal—A single photon emission tomography study with 99mTc-HMPAO. *Acta Psychiatr Scand* 87:414–417, 1993.
120. Shih WJ, Hyatt M: Volume and surface three-dimensional displays of Tc-99m HMPAO brain SPECT imaging in a chronic hypnosedative abuser. *Clin Nucl Med* 18:506–509, 1993.

121. Newman LM, Hoffman WE, Miletich DJ, *et al:* Regional blood flow and cerebral metabolic changes during alcohol withdrawal and following midazolam therapy. *Anesthesiology* 63:395–400, 1985.
122. Eckardt MJ, Campbell GA, Marietta CA, *et al:* Cerebral 2-deoxyglucose uptake in rats during ethanol withdrawal and postwithdrawal. *Brain Res* 366:1–9, 1986.
123. Campbell GA, Eckardt MJ, Majchrowicz E, *et al:* Ethanol-withdrawal syndrome associated with both general and localized increases in glucose uptake in rat brain. *Brain Res* 237:517–522, 1982.
124. Cohen MS, Bookheimer SY: Localization of brain function using magnetic resonance imaging. *Trends Neurosci* 17:268–277, 1994.

10

Complications of Severe Mental Illness Related to Alcohol and Drug Use Disorders

Robert E. Drake and Mary F. Brunette

Abstract. In this chapter we review research on the relationships between substance use disorder and 11 domains of adjustment for people with severe mental illness. Studies are divided into correlational research and prospective, longitudinal research, with greater weight given to those in the latter category. The weight of the evidence indicates that substance abuse severely complicates severe mental illness in the following domains: relapse of psychiatric illness, hospitalization, disruptive behavior, familial problems, residential instability, decreased functional status, HIV infection, and medication noncompliance. We discuss the limits of causal inference in these studies and the possible mechanisms that relate substance abuse to various complications.

1. Introduction

Rates of substance use disorder are extremely high in persons with severe mental illnesses such as schizophrenia and bipolar disorder. Recent clinical studies indicate tht 40–60% of patients with severe mental illness have co-occurring substance use disorders.[1–6] The Epidemiologic Catchment Area (ECA) study[7] showed that people with schizophrenia in the community had a 10.1 times greater rate of alcohol use disorders and a 7.6 times greater rate of other drug use disorders than nonschizophrenic individuals.[8] The three most commonly abused substances in this population are alcohol, cannabis, and cocaine.[1,4,5,9,10]

Robert E. Drake and Mary F. Brunette • Psychiatric Research Center, Dartmouth Medical School, Lebanon, New Hampshire 03766.

Recent Developments in Alcoholism, Volume 14: The Consequences of Alcoholism, edited by Galanter. Plenum Press, New York, 1998.

Concern over the problem of dual diagnosis stems not only from increasing awareness of the high rates of comorbidity but also from beliefs about the ways in which substance abuse adversely affects the course of severe mental illness. The purpose of this chapter is to review the empirical evidence for these adverse effects. We reviewed the research on substance abuse-related complications in 11 areas: psychiatric symptoms and relapse; disruptive behavior, aggression, and violence; criminal behavior; suicidal behavior; problems with families; residential instability and homelessness; functional status; general medical problems; neuropsychological problems; diminished treatment response; and medication noncompliance. We excluded case reports and included studies of ten or more patients with severe mental illness. The predominant diagnoses in all studies were schizophrenia, schizoaffective disorder, and severe mood disorders. We classified studies as correlational if patients were assessed cross-sectionally or retrospectively and as prospective if they were assessed in a prospective, longitudinal fashion.

1.1. *Psychiatric Symptoms and Relapse*

Schizophrenia is of course defined in part by the presence of positive and negative symptoms of psychosis. Depressive symptoms are also common in schizophrenia and are even more common in schizoaffective disorder and severe mood disorders. Several types of studies have examined the relationships between psychoactive substance use and these symptoms. This review focuses on correlational and prospective studies. We have omitted self-reports of subjective experiences because patients are often aware of only immediate effects. We have also omitted laboratory studies of administration of psychoactive drugs because these studies have not examined the major drugs of abuse: alcohol, cannabis, and cocaine. See Dixon *et al.*[11] for a review of these latter two types of studies.

Among correlational studies, eight studies[12–19] found an association between substance abuse and some positive psychotic symptoms of schizophrenia, while 15 studies[5,6,20–32] reported no correlations. Similarly, six studies[19,24,25,29,33,34] found that patients who abused alcohol and other substances had lower levels of negative symptoms of schizophrenia than nonabusers, and ten studies[5,13–15,21,27,30,31,35,36] found no relationship between negative symptoms of schizophrenia and substance abuse. With regard to dysphoric mood, 14 studies[1,14,18,20,22–24,28–30,37–40] found an increase in depressive or anxiety symptoms associated with substance abuse, while seven studies[5,17,19,21,31,36,41] found no differences and two studies[33,35] found fewer depressive symptoms associated with substance abuse.

Number of hospital admissions offers an indirect measure of symptomatic relapse. Ten correlational studies[16,20,31,37,39,42–46] reported more previous admissions and/or time in hospital in those with alcohol or substance use, whereas five studies[6,25,26,29,47] reported no correlation between substance use disorder and previous admissions or time in hospital; one study[5] reported fewer hospitalizations in those who abused cannabis and no differences in those who abused alcohol and other drugs.

A small number of studies have examined substance abuse and psychiatric symptoms prospectively. Linszen and colleagues[36] found that heavy cannabis users showed intermittent increases in positive psychotic symptoms over 1 year compared to mild and nonusers, whereas negative symptoms did not vary between the groups over time. Based on 1-year follow-up data from the ECA study, Cuffel and Chase[48] found no correlation between substance use and psychotic symptoms for individuals with schizophrenia and co-occurring substance use disorder (primarily alcohol and cannabis); however, individuals who developed active substance abuse over the year had increases in depression, while those whose substance abuse remitted experienced decreases in depression. In a 15-week prospective study, Shaner and colleagues[49] found that cocaine use was correlated with increases in positive symptoms of psychosis. Cocaine use peaked at the beginning of the month when patients received their disability checks, indicating that drug use triggered exacerbations of psychosis rather than the reverse. In a 4-week prospective study of hospital admissions, cocaine-abusing patients with schizophrenia initially had higher anxiety and depression, but after detoxification these levels decreased and became similar to those without substance abuse.[29]

Using the dependent variable of relapse or hospitalization, eight prospective studies of patients with severe mental illness found higher rates of relapse[31,36,50] and/or rehospitalization[17,31,49–53] among the substance abusers.

Khantzian[54] suggested that patients with severe mental illness might use substances to "self-medicate" their symptoms of illness. In a single prospective study of the self-medication hypothesis, Hamera and colleagues[55] used a pooled time series analysis to examine the relationships between day-to-day fluctuations of schizophrenic symptoms and levels of substance use over time and found no evidence for increased alcohol or cannabis use following increases in positive, negative, or dysphoric symptoms.

In summary, the correlational evidence regarding psychiatric symptoms and substance abuse is inconsistent. Undoubtedly some of the inconsistency is due to differences in diagnostic composition, types of drugs of abuse, and timing and settings of assessment. The few available prospective studies suggest that cannabis and cocaine abuse worsen psychotic symptoms and that alcohol abuse is associated with increased depression, consistent with known effects of the drugs. The evidence is much stronger that substance abuse leads to higher rates of relapse and hospitalization. The association with hospitalization could of course be related to several factors in addition to symptomatic relapse. As reviewed in subsequent sections, substance-abusing patients have multiple difficulties, including suicidal and aggressive behavior, that could precipitate hospitalization.

1.2. *Disruptive Behavior, Aggression, and Violence*

For this overview, we combined studies of hostility, disruptive or aggressive behavior, and violence, all of which are common problems in persons with schizophrenia. Ten correlational studies[1,15,37,56–62] and three prospective studies[63–65] have found that patients with dual diagnoses had higher rates of disruptive behaviors, aggression, or violence than those without substance use disorders. To cite one representative study, Swanson and colleagues,[61] using ECA data, found that rates of violence were much higher in persons with schizophrenia who abused substances (30.3%) compared to those who did not (8.3%).

Although the research in this area is consistent, the mechanism linking substance abuse and disruptive behavior is unclear. Substance abuse disinhibits aggressive behavior, but other factors, such as past violence, anxiety, aggression, and psychotic symptoms, are often stronger predictors of aggressive behavior.[57,66,67] Additionally, substance abuse could be linked with violent behavior through other factors such as medication noncompliance and comorbid antisocial personality disorder.[56,68]

1.3. *Criminal Behavior*

Several studies[69–72] have found high rates of substance abuse among patients with severe mental illness who exhibited criminal behavior. Two correlational studies[1,45] showed that substance abuse was correlated with criminal behavior or convictions in those with severe mental illness, but one study[17] found no correlation with incarceration. Two prospective studies[66,73] showed that substance abuse was a predictor of criminal activity.

Like the relationship between substance abuse and violence, the connection between substance abuse and crime appears to be complex. Only a minority of criminal activity is directly related to substance abuse, for example, intoxication or possession[74] or obtaining money to pay for substances.[75] More generally, substance abuse could be linked to criminal behavior through the same factors that presumably mediate violence, such as severity of psychotic symptoms, disinhibition, medication noncompliance, comorbid antisocial personality disorder, and exposure to a dangerous environment and lifestyle.[56,66,68,76,77]

1.4. *Suicidal Behavior*

Persons with schizophrenia have a rate of completed suicide of approximately 10%, and many more exhibit less extreme suicidal behavior.[78] Nine correlational studies[1,46,63,79–84] found that substance use disorder and suicidal behavior were related in patients with severe mental illness, while two studies[24,85] reported that substance abuse was correlated with suicide attempts in males but not in females and six other studies[15,17,86–89] found no relationship.

In a 13-year prospective study of patients with schizophrenia, Westermeyer and colleagues[90] showed that those who completed suicide were more likely to have had co-occurring drug abuse (but not alcohol abuse) than patients who did not complete suicide. Thus, there is mixed evidence for a correlation between suicide and substance abuse in patients with severe mental illness. Moreover, even when correlations are present, other factors, such as depression and hopelessness, may be better predictors of suicidal behavior.[80,81,87]

1.5. *Problems with Families*

Clark and Drake[91] documented that families provided substantial amounts of time and money to support their relatives with dual disorders. Three of four correlational studies[37,47,92] showed that substance abuse among patients with severe mental illness was associated with greater family problems, while one correlational study[17] found no relationship. Two prospective treatment studies[93,94] showed that patients who received dual-disorders treatment for 18 months reported improvements in the quality of their relationships with families. Thus, the few available empirical studies suggest that substance abuse complicates family relationships for patients with severe mental illness and that relationships tend to improve over time with dual-disorders treatment.

1.6. *Residential Instability and Homelessness*

Approximately 10–20% of homeless persons suffer from co-occurring severe mental illness and substance use disorder.[95] Six correlational studies[46,52,96–99] found that comorbid substance abuse among patients with severe mental illness was associated with low-quality housing, residential instability, prior homelessness, or current homelessness. For example, Drake and Wallach[52] found that patients discharged from the state hospital with dual disorders had three times the rate of residential instability as those with single disorders. Four prospective studies[100–103] found that patients with dual disorders were more likely to become homeless or to fail to achieve stable housing than those with severe mental illness alone. For example, in a 2-year prospective study of homeless persons with severe mental illness, Hurlburt *et al.*[103] found that those with alcohol problems were only half as likely to become stably housed and those with other drug problems were only one third as likely to achieve residential stability as those without substance abuse. Two additional prospective studies[93,94] found that patients in dual-disorders treatment were likely to achieve residential stability or independent housing over time. Furthermore, in the Drake *et al.*[93] study, achieving residential stability was predicted by making progress toward recovery from substance abuse earlier in the study period.[104]

Thus, the evidence very consistently indicates that residential instability among patients with psychiatric disorders is correlated with and predicted by co-occurring substance abuse. Moreover, the available studies show that participation in dual-disorders treatment or progress toward recovery from substance abuse is associated with attaining residential stability. The mechanism by which substance abuse leads to unstable housing and homelessness probably involves a process in which problematic behaviors, loss of familial supports, inability to manage finances, and periodic institutionalizations lead to housing losses and erode the good will of landlords.

1.7. Functional Level

Diminished functional status is a core feature of schizophrenia and other severe mental disorders. Five correlational studies[37,44,52,59,82] found that substance abuse and functional status were significantly related in patients with severe mental illness, although most of the studies examined several domains of functioning and did not find significance in every area. For example, Drake and Wallach[52] found that substance abusers had greater difficulty than nonabusers with maintaining regular meals, managing their finances, maintaining stable housing, and maintaining a daily activity, but did not differ in social relationships or work. Across studies, substance abuse was most frequently related to inability to meet basic skills of independent living, such as managing finances. One study[17] found no relationships between substance abuse and measures of functional status.

Four prospective studies[49,93,94,105] examined functional status in relation to substance abuse. Each of these studies demonstrated some relationships between substance abuse status and areas of functioning over time. In one analysis, Shumway *et al.*[105] examined substance abuse status and functional level at 3-month intervals throughout an 18-month prospective study. Stochastic modeling showed that occurrences of substance abuse often preceded decreases in functional level, while the reverse was not found. Furthermore, substance abusers differed more from the nonabusers over time, suggesting that the detrimental effects of substance abuse increased over time.[106]

Thus, although the data are not entirely consistent with regard to specific domains of functioning, the correlational studies support the interpretation that substance abuse status is related to functional status, and the prospective studies are consistent with the proposition that changes in substance abuse are related to changes in functional status. Although the mechanisms are not entirely clear, substance abuse probably undermines adaptive functioning via all of the effects on symptoms, behavior, and supports previously discussed.

1.8. General Medical Problems

Correlational studies have examined three types of medical problems in relation to dual diagnosis: general medical health, neurological side effects of medications, and human immunodeficiency virus (HIV) infection. Two studies[17,52] found that chronic medical problems among patients with severe mental illnesses were not correlated with substance abuse. In separate studies of medication side effects, substance abuse was correlated with extrapyramidal symptoms[15] and with tardive dyskinesia.[107] In a third study,[19] alcohol abuse among schizophrenic patients was negatively correlated with extrapyramidal side effects and uncorrelated with tardive dyskinesia. Finally, the prevalence of HIV infection among patients with severe mental illness is estimated at 4–23%, which is 13 to 76 times greater than those in the general population.[108] At least four studies[109–112] in New York City have found that HIV infection among patients with severe mental disorders was related to intravenous drug use.

Thus, there have been few consistent findings related to medical problems, except that patients who inject intravenous drugs in New York have higher rates of HIV infection. Most of the studies of medical conditions were not controlled for age, and the two studies of chronic medical conditions were based on case managers' ratings alone. A serious confound in the studies of medical conditions is that psychiatric patients are often unaware of their medical illnesses.

1.9. Neuropsychological Problems

Tracy *et al.*[113] reviewed the separate literatures on neuropsychiatric impairments found in mental disorders and in substance use disorders and suggested that studies of comorbid patients were needed. In one available study, Cleghorn *et al.*[13] found no associations between 60 measures of neurocognitive impairment and history of drug abuse in schizophrenic patients. Thus, there is little evidence on this issue, and the single available study found no relationships.

1.10. Diminished Medication Response

Since drugs of abuse affect dopamine pathways, several studies have examined response to antipsychotic medications among schizophrenic patients. Three studies[114–116] found that substance abuse prior to hospitalization was associated with diminished response to medications. For example, Seibyl *et al.*[115] found that cocaine-abusing schizophrenic patients who were hospitalized received higher neuroleptic doses by the fifth and sixth weeks of hospitalization compared with their own non-cocaine-associated hospitalizations and with nonusing patients. However, one study[33] found no differences in medication response between schizophrenic substance abusers and nonabusers, and another study[35] found that the substance abusers experienced greater symptom reduction on equivalent doses of antipsychotic medications. Methodological differences among the studies may account for the different findings. The Buckley *et al.* study,[33] for example, contained mostly past substance abusers and examined their response to the atypical drug clozapine. Thus, the results of these few studies are mixed.

1.11. Medication Noncompliance

Medication noncompliance is a common problem in schizophrenia, affecting over half of patients followed prospectively for 1 year following a relapse.[117] The correlation between medication noncompliance and substance abuse has been examined in both outpatient and acute care settings. Seven outpatient studies[6,14,17,47,50,59,118] found relationships between substance abuse and medication noncompliance among patients with severe mental illness. The exact findings varied considerably. Kashner *et al.*[47] found a 13-fold difference in noncompliance between abusers and nonabusers, while Warner *et al.*[6] found that "alcohol use to the point of intoxication," but not other measures of substance abuse, was related to medication noncompliance.

In an emergency room study, Barbee *et al.*[12] found no differences between substance-abusing and nonabusing schizophrenic patients in self-reports of taking medications as prescribed during the week prior to emergency room visit. In an inpatient study, Pristach and Smith[119] also found no relationship between substance abuse and medication noncompliance, but they noted that patients often reported that they stopped using medications while they were using drugs just prior to hospitalization. Two additional inpatient studies[120,121] found no relationship between substance abuse and medication refusal while in the hospital. The findings in emergency and hospital settings could differ from the outpatient results because of selection factors in the acute care settings, which serve only patients who are in crisis or relapse.

Thus, the available research indicates that there is a relationship between substance abuse and medication noncompliance for outpatients with schizophrenia, but not for inpatients. One explanation for poor medication compliance in the community may be poor adherence with treatment in general. Two studies[53,59] found that schizophrenic patients with substance abuse in the community were less likely to be receiving aftercare services than those without comorbid substance abuse, and one prospective study[31] found that schizophrenic patients with comorbid substance abuse had a greater rate of missed appointments. This problem may be overcome in service systems that offer assertive aftercare that includes daily monitoring of medications.[6,17,106]

2. Discussion

Although the research reviewed here suggests that substance use disorder complicates the course of severe mental illness by producing adverse consequences in multiple areas of adjustment, several caveats warrant discussion. First, most of the studies are correlational. These studies often assume that the substance-abusing and non-substance-abusing groups of psychiatric patients are otherwise equivalent and that the direction of causality is obvious. Both assumptions are probably erroneous. For example, many studies[122] show that patients with severe mental illness who abuse substances are more likely to be young and male than those who do not. Since males with schizophrenia have more difficulties with social functioning[123] and more frequent hospitalizations,[124] gender may confound the results in these studies. Additionally, studies also suggest that patients who abuse substances may be different premorbidly. Specifically, they appear to have better premorbid social adjustment,[125] more familial substance abuse,[126] and higher rates of conduct disorder and antisocial personality disorder.[68]

Associations between substance abuse and poor adjustment may not be due to the effects of substances. In some cases, poor adjustment, such as greater symptoms of anxiety or residential instability, could lead to higher rates of substance abuse. Even more problematic is the confounding role of underlying third variables. For example, factors such as medication noncompliance and treatment resistance may be related to both substance abuse and symptomatic relapse. Obviously, more prospective studies that involve statistical modeling or time series analysis would help to understand the causal relationships that are impossible to clarify in correlational studies.

Another problem is that measures of substance abuse in most studies suffer from poor reliability and validity. Using standard self-report measures in this population typically produces low sensitivity in the range of 65 to 70%.[127] In most studies, therefore, about one third of the substance abusers are misclassified as nonabusers.

Other common problems include diagnostic heterogeneity of both severe mental illness and substance use disorder, failure to report negative results, low base rates of some adverse consequences such as incarceration, small sample sizes, and the small number of studies of most consequences. For example, when study groups contain individuals who are heterogeneous for type of mental illness and for type and severity of substance abuse, relationships between a specific drug and a specific diagnosis could be obscured.

Because of these problems, we have attempted to review the empirical evidence by giving more weight to studies that are prospective, to those that control for some of the potentially confounding variables, to those that utilize time series designs, and to areas in which there exist large numbers of consistent studies.

3. Conclusions

Substance use disorder is an extremely common comorbidity in patients with severe mental illness. The research evidence indicating that substance abuse complicates the course of severe mental illness is voluminous, but most of the available studies are correlational and limited by methodological difficulties. The prospective studies are generally more consistent and do support several relationships that are suggested by the correlational studies. Specifically, substance abuse appears to lead to relapse and rehospitalization, disruptive behavior, familial problems, residential instability, decreased functional status, HIV infection, and medication noncompliance. The evidence in other areas is too inconsistent or weak to draw conclusions. Further, there is virtually no evidence that substance use might be helpful in ameliorating any aspect of poor adjustment among persons with severe mental illness. The mechanisms by which substance abuse complicates severe mental illness are diverse and probably include direct destabilization of mental illness; disruption of social, financial, and housing supports; medication noncompliance; and the addition of aggressive disinhibition to the usual problematic behaviors of mental illness.

ACKNOWLEDGMENT. This work was supported by US Public Health Service grant #MH-00839 from the National Institute of Mental Health.

References

1. Barry K, Fleming M, Greenley J, *et al:* Characteristics of persons with severe mental illness and substance abuse in rural areas. *Psychiatric Serv* 47:88–90, 1996.
2. Comtois K, Ries R, Armstrong H: Case manager ratings of the clinical status of dually diagnosed outpatients. *Hosp Commun Psychiatry* 45:568–573, 1994.
3. Lehman AF, Myers C, Corty E, *et al:* Prevalence and patterns of "dual diagnosis" among psychiatric inpatients. *Compr Psychiatry* 35:106–112, 1994.
4. Mueser KT, Yarnold P, Bellack A: Diagnostic and demographic correlates of substance abuse in schizophrenia and major affective disorder. *Acta Psychiatr Scand* 85:48–55, 1992.
5. Mueser KT, Yarnold P, Levinson D, *et al:* Prevalence of substance abuse in schizophrenia: Demographic and clinical correlates. *Schizophr Bull* 16:31–56, 1990.
6. Warner R, Taylor D, Wright J, *et al:* Substance use among the mentally ill: Prevalence, reasons for use, and effects on illness. *Am J Orthopsychiatry* 64:30–39, 1994.
7. Regier D, Myers J, Kramer M, *et al:* The NIMH epidemiologic catchment area study: Historical context, major objectives, and study population characteristics. *Arch Gen Psychiatry* 91:934–941, 1984.
8. Boyd J, Burke J, Gruenburg E, *et al:* Exclusion criteria of DSM-III: A study of co-occurrence of hierarchy-free syndromes. *Arch Gen Psychiatry* 41:983–989, 1984.
9. Lehman AF, Myers C, Dixon L, *et al:* Detection of substance use disorders among psychiatric inpatients. *J Nerv Ment Dis* 184:228–233, 1996.
10. Toner B, Gillies L, Prendergast P, *et al:* Substance use disorders in a sample of Canadian patients with chronic mental illness. *Hosp Commun Psychiatry* 43:251–254, 1992.
11. Dixon L, Gaas G, Weiden P, *et al:* Acute effects of drug abuse in schizophrenic patients. *Schizophr Bull* 16:69–79, 1990.
12. Barbee JG, Clark PD, Crapanzano MS, *et al:* Alcohol and substance abuse among schizophrenic patients presenting to an emergency psychiatric service. *J Nerv Ment Dis* 177:400–407, 1989.
13. Cleghorn JM, Kaplan RD, Szechtman B, *et al:* Substance abuse and schizophrenia: Effect on symptoms but not on neurocognitive function. *J ClinPsychiatry* 52:26–30, 1991.
14. Drake RE, Osher FC, Wallach MA: Alcohol use and abuse in schizophrenia: A prospective community study. *J Nerv Ment Dis* 177:408–414, 1989.
15. Duke PJ, Pantelis C, Barnes TRE: South Westminster schizophrenia survey: Alcohol use and its relationship to symptoms, tardive dyskinesia, and illness onset. *Brit J Psychiatry* 164:630–636, 1994.

16. Negrete JC, Knapp WP, Douglas DE, *et al:* Cannabis affects the severity of schizophrenic symptoms: Result of a clinical survey. *Psychol Med* 16:515–520, 1986.
17. Osher FC, Drake RE, Noordsy DL, *et al:* Correlates and outcomes of alcohol use disorder among rural outpatients with schizophrenia. *J Clin Psychiatry* 55:109–113, 1994.
18. Pulver AE, Wolyniec PS, Wagner MG, *et al:* An epidemiologic investigation of alcohol-dependent schizophrenics. *Acta Psychiatr Scand* 79:603–612, 1989.
19. Soni SD, Brownlee M: Alcohol abuse in chronic schizophrenics: Implications for management in the community. *Acta Psychiatr Scand* 84:272–276, 1991.
20. Alterman AI, Erdlen DL, Laporte DJ, *et al:* Effects of illicit drug use in an inpatient psychiatric population. *Addict Behav* 7:231–242, 1982.
21. Brunette MF, Mueser KT, Xie H, *et al:* Relationships between symptoms of schizophrenia and substance abuse. *J Nerv Ment Dis* 185:13–20, 1997.
22. Carey MP, Carey KB, Meisler AW: Psychiatric symptoms in mentally ill chemical abusers. *J Nerv Ment Dis* 179:136–138, 1991.
23. Cuffel BJ, Heithoff KA, Lawson W: Correlates of patterns of substance abuse among patients with schizophrenia. *Hosp Commun Psychiatry* 44:247–251, 1993.
24. Kovasznay B, Bromet E, Schwartz JE, *et al:* Substance abuse and onset of psychotic illness. *Hosp Commun Psychiatry* 44:567–571, 1993.
25. Lysaker P, Bell M, Beam-Goulet J: Relationship of positive and negative symptoms to cocaine abuse in schizophrenia. *J Nerv Ment Dis* 182:109–112, 1994.
26. Peralta V, Cuesta MJ: Influence of cannabis abuse on schizophrenic psychopathology. *Acta Psychiatr Scand* 85:127–130, 1992.
27. Rosenthal RN, Hellerstein DJ, Miner CR: Positive and negative syndrome typology in schizophrenic patients with psychoactive substance use disorders. *Compr Psychiatry* 35:91–98, 1994.
28. Sanguineti VR, Samuel S: Comorbid substance abuse and recovery from acute psychiatric relapse. *Hosp Commun Psychiatry* 44:1073–1078, 1993.
29. Serper MR, Alpert M, Richardson NA, *et al:* Clinical effects of recent cocaine use on patients with acute schizophrenia. *Am J Psychiatry* 152:1464–1469, 1995.
30. Sevy S, Kay SR, Opler LA, *et al:* Significance of cocaine history in schizophrenia. *J Nerv Ment Dis* 178:642–648, 1990.
31. Swofford CD, Kasckow JW, Scheller-Gilkey G, *et al:* Substance use: A powerful predictor of relapse in schizophrenia. *Schizophr Res* 20:145–151, 1996.
32. Tsuang JW, Lohr JB: Effects of alcohol on symptoms in alcoholic and nonalcoholic patients with schizophrenia. *Hosp Commun Psychiatry* 45:1229–1230, 1994.
33. Buckley P, Thompson P, Way L, *et al:* Substance abuse among patients with treatment-resistant schizophrenia: Characteristics and implications for clozapine therapy. *Am J Psychiatry* 151:385–389, 1994.
34. Kirkpatrick B, Amador XR, Flaum M, *et al:* The deficit syndrome in the DSM-IV field trial: I. Alcohol and other drug abuse. *Schizophr Res* 20:69–77, 1996.
35. Dixon LB, Haas G, Weiden PJ, *et al:* Drug abuse in schizophrenic patients: Clinical correlates and reasons for use. *Am J Psychiatry* 148:224–230, 1991.
36. Linszen DH, Dintgemans PM, Lenior ME: Cannabis abuse and the course of recent-onset schizophrenic disorders. *Arch Gen Psychiatry* 51:273–279, 1994.
37. Alterman AI, Erdlen FR, McLellan AT, *et al:* Problem drinking in hospitalized schizophrenic patients. *Addict Behav* 5:273–276, 1980.
38. Brady KT, Anton R, Ballenger JC, *et al:* Cocaine abusing among schizophrenic patients. *Am J Psychiatry* 147:1164–1167, 1990.
39. Menezes PR, Johnson S, Thornicroft G, *et al:* Drug and alcohol problems among individuals with severe mental illnesses in South London. *Br J Psychiatry* 168:612–619, 1996.
40. Tsuang MT, Simpson JC, Kronfol Z: Subtypes of drug abuse with psychosis. *Arch Gen Psychiatry* 39:141–147, 1982.
41. Alterman AI, Ayre FR, Williford WO: Diagnostic validation of conjoint schizophrenia and alcoholism. *J Clin Psychiatry* 45:300–303, 1984.

42. Gupta S, Hendricks S, Kenkel AM, *et al:* Relapse in schizophrenia: Is there a relationship to substance abuse? *Schizophr Res* 20:153–156, 1996.
43. Haywood TW, Kravitz HM, Grossman LS, *et al:* Predicting the "revolving door" phenomenon among patients with schizophrenic, schizoaffective, and affective disorders. *Am J Psychiatry* 152:856–861, 1995.
44. Kutcher S, Kachur E, Marton P, *et al:* Substance abuse among adolescents with chronic mental illnesses: A pilot study of descriptive and differentiating features. *Can J Psychiatry* 37:428–431, 1992.
45. Safer D: Substance abuse by young adult chronic patients. *Hosp Commun Psychiatry* 38:511–514, 1987.
46. Soyka M, Albus M, Kathmann N, *et al:* Prevalence of alcohol and drug abuse in schizophrenic patients. *Eur Arch Psychiatry Clin Neurosci* 242:362–372, 1993.
47. Kashner TM, Rader LE, Rodell DE, *et al:* Family characteristics, substance abuse, and hospitalization patterns of patients with schizophrenia. *Hosp Commun Psychiatry* 42:195–197, 1991.
48. Cuffel BJ, Chase P: Remission and relapse of substance use disorder in schizophrenia: Results from a one-year prospective study. *J Nerv Ment Dis* 182:342–348, 1994.
49. Shaner A, Eckman TA, Roberts LJ, *et al:* Disability income, cocaine use and repeated hospitalization among schizophrenic cocaine abusers: A government sponsored revolving door? *New Engl J Med* 333:777–783, 1995.
50. Martinez-Arevalo MJ, Calcedo-Ordonez A, Varo-Prieto JR: Cannabis consumption as a prognostic factor in schizophrenia. *Br J Psychiatry* 164:679–681, 1994.
51. Craig TJ, Lin SP, El-Defrawi MH, *et al:* Clinical correlates of readmission in a schizophrenic cohort. *Psychiatric Q* 57:5–10, 1985.
52. Drake RE, Wallach MA: Substance abuse among the chronic mentally ill. *Hosp Commun Psychiatry* 40:1041–1046, 1989.
53. Fischer EP, Owen RR, Cuffel BJ: Substance abuse, community service use, and symptom severity of urban and rural residents with schizophrenia. *Psychiatric Serv* 47:980–984, 1996.
54. Khantzian EJ: The self-medication hypothesis of addictive disorders: Focus on heroin and cocaine dependence. *Am J Psychiatry* 142:1259–1264, 1985.
55. Hamera E, Schneider JK, Deviney S: Alcohol, cannabis, nicotine, and caffeine use and symptom distress in schizophrenia. *J Nerv Ment Dis* 183:559–565, 1995.
56. Bartels SJ, Drake RE, Wallach MA, *et al:* Characteristic hostility in schizophrenic outpatients. *Schizophr Bull* 17:163–171, 1991.
57. Blomhoff S, Seim S, Friis S: Can prediction of violence among psychiatric inpatients be improved? *Hosp Commun Psychiatry* 41:771–775, 1990.
58. Cuffel BJ: Violent and destructive behavior among the severely mentally ill in rural areas: Evidence from Arkansas' community mental health system. *Commun Ment Health J* 30:495–504, 1994.
59. Kozaric-Kovacic D, Folnegovic-Smalc V, Folnegovic Z, *et al:* Influence of alcoholism on the prognosis of schizophrenic patients. *J Stud Alcohol* 56:622–627, 1995.
60. Richardson MA, Craig TJ, Haugland G: Treatment patterns of young chronic schizophrenic patients in the era of deinstitutionalization. *Psychiatric Q* 57:104–110, 1985.
61. Swanson JW, Holzer CE, Ganju VK, *et al:* Violence and psychiatric disorder in the community: Evidence from the Epidemiologic Catchment Area Survey. *Hosp Commun Psychiatry* 41:761–770, 1990.
62. Yesavage JA, Zarcone V: History of drug abuse and dangerous behavior in inpatient schizophrenics. *J Clin Psychiatry* 44:259–261, 1983.
63. Convit A, Nemes ZC, Volavka J: History of phencyclidine use and repeated assaults in newly admitted young schizophrenic men. *Am J Psychiatry* 145:1176, 1988.
64. Cuffel BJ, Shumway M, Choulijian TL, *et al:* A longitudinal study of substance abuse and community violence in schizophrenia. *J Nerv Ment Dis* 182:704–708, 1994.
65. Kay SR, Wolkenfeld F, Murrill LM: Profiles of aggression among psychiatric patients II. Covariates and predictors. *J Nerv Ment Dis* 39:547–557, 1988.

66. Link BG, Cullen FT, Andrews H: The violent and illegal behavior of mental patients reconsidered. *Am Soc Rev* 57:275–292, 1992.
67. Monahan J: Mental disorder and violent behavior: Perceptions and evidence. *Am Psychol* 47:511–521, 1992.
68. Mueser KT, Rosenberg SD, Drake RE, *et al:* Antisocial personality disorder and substance abuse in schizophrenia and major affective disorders. *J Stud Alcohol*, in press.
69. Abram KM, Teplin LA: Co-occurring disorders among mentally ill jail detainees. *Am Psychol* 46:1036–1045, 1991.
70. Chiles JA, Von Cleve E, Jemelka RP, *et al:* Substance abuse and psychiatric disorders in prison inmates. *Hosp Commun Psychiatry* 41:1132–1134, 1990.
71. Lindqvist P, Allebeck P: Schizophrenia and assaultive behavior: The role of alcohol and drug abuse. *Acta Psychiatr Scand* 82:191–195, 1989.
72. Regier DA, Farmer ME, Rae DE, *et al:* Comorbidity of mental disorders with alcohol and other drug abuse. *JAMA* 264:2511–2518, 1990.
73. Wessely SC, Castle D, Douglas AJ, *et al:* The criminal careers of incident cases of schizophrenia. *Psychol Med* 224:483–502, 1994.
74. Zitrin A, Hardesty AS, Burdock EI, *et al:* Crime and violence among mental patients. *Am J Psychiatry* 133:142–149, 1976.
75. Cohen E, Henkin I: Prevalence of substance abuse by seriously mentally ill patients in a partial hospital program. *Hosp Commun Psychiatry* 44:178–180, 1993.
76. Tardiff K, Marzuk PM, Leon AC, *et al:* Violence by patients admitted to a private psychiatric hospital. *Am J Psychiatry* 154:88–93, 1997.
77. Taylor PJ: Motives for offending among violent and psychotic men. *Br J Psychiatry* 147:491–498, 1985.
78. Drake RE, Gates C, Whitaker A, *et al:* Suicide among schizophrenics: A review. *Compr Psychiatry* 26:90–100, 1985.
79. Achte KA, Stenback A, Teravainen H: On suicides committed during treatment in psychiatric hospitals. *Acta Psychiatr Scand* 42:272–284, 1966.
80. Bartels SJ, Drake RE, McHugo G: Alcohol use, depression and suicidal behavior in schizophrenia. *Am J Psychiatry* 149:394–395, 1992.
81. Dassori AM, Mezzich JE, Keshavan M: Suicidal indicators in schizophrenia. *Acta Psychiatr Scand* 81:409–413, 1990.
82. Kay SR, Kalathara M, Meinzer AE: Diagnostic and behavioral characteristics of psychiatric patients who abuse substances. *Hosp Commun Psychiatry* 40:1061–1064, 1989.
83. Noriek K: Attempted suicide and suicide in functional psychoses. *Acta Psychiatr Scand* 52:81–106, 1975.
84. Sletten I, Brown M, Evenson R, *et al:* Suicide in mental hospital patients. *Dis Nerv Sys* 33:328–334, 1972.
85. Tardiff K, Sweillam A: Assault, suicide, and mental illness. *Arch Gen Psychiatry* 37:164–169, 1980.
86. Allebeck P, Varla A, Kristjansson E, *et al:* Risk factors for suicide among patients with schizophrenia. *Acta Psychiatr Scand* 76:414–419, 1987.
87. Drake RE, Gates CG, Cotton PG, *et al:* Suicide among schizophrenics: Who is at risk? *J Nerv Ment Dis* 172:613–617, 1984.
88. Schaffer JW, Perlin S, Schmidt CW, *et al:* The prediction of suicide in schizophrenia. *J Nerv Ment Dis* 159:349–355, 1974.
89. Siris SG, Kane JM, Frechen K, *et al:* Histories of substance abuse in patients with post-psychotic depressions. *Compr Psychiatry* 29:550–557, 1993.
90. Westermeyer JF, Harrow M, Marengo J: Risk for suicide in schizophrenia and other psychotic and nonpsychotic disorders. *J Nerv Ment Dis* 179:259–265, 1991.
91. Clark RE, Drake RE: Expenditures of time and money by families of people with severe mental illness and substance use disorder. *Commun Ment Health J* 30:193–206, 1994.
92. Dixon LB, McNary S, Lehman AF: Substance abuse and family relationships of persons with severe mental illness. *Am J Psychiatry* 152:456–458, 1995.

93. Drake RE, Yovetich NA, Bebout RR, *et al:* Integrated treatment for dually diagnosed, homeless adults. *J Nerv Ment Dis* 185:298–305, 1997.
94. Jerrell JM, Ridgely MS: Evaluating changes in symptoms and functioning of dually diagnosed clients in specialized treatment. *Psychiatr Serv* 46:233–238, 1995.
95. Drake RE, Osher FC, Wallach MA: Homelessness and dual diagnosis. *Am Psychol* 46:1149–1158, 1991.
96. Benda BB, Datallo P: Homelessness: Consequence of a crisis or a long-term process? *Hosp Commun Psychiatry* 39:884–886, 1988.
97. Drake RE, Wallach MA, Teague GB, *et al:* Housing instability and homelessness among rural schizophrenic patients. *Am J Psychiatry* 148:330–336, 1991.
98. Lamb HR, Lamb DM: Factors contributing to homelessness among the chronically and severely mentally ill. *Hosp Commun Psychiatry* 41:301–305, 1990.
99. Uehara ES: Race, gender, and housing inequality: An exploration of the correlates of low-quality housing among clients diagnosed with severe and persistent mental illness. *J Health Soc Behav* 35:309–321, 1994.
100. Belcher JR: On becoming homeless: A study of chronically mentally ill persons. *J Commun Psychol* 17:173–185, 1989.
101. Caton CL, Wyatt R, Felix A, *et al:* Follow-up of chronically homeless, mentally ill men. *Am J Psychiatry* 150:1639–1642, 1993.
102. Dickey B, Gonzales O, Latimer E, *et al:* Use of mental health services by formerly homeless adults residing in group and independent housing. *Psychiatr Serv* 47:152–158, 1996.
103. Hurlburt MS, Hough RL, Wood PA: Effects of substance abuse on housing stability of homeless mentally ill persons in supported housing. *Psychiatr Serv* 47:731–736, 1996.
104. Bebout RR, Drake RE, Xie H, *et al:* Housing status among formerly homeless, dually diagnosed adults in Washington, DC. *Psychiatr Serv* 4:936–941, 1997.
105. Shumway M, Chouljian CL, Hargreaves WA: Patterns of substance use in schizophrenia: A Markov modeling approach. *J Psychiatr Res* 28:277–287, 1994.
106. Chouljian TL, Shumway M, Balancio, *et al:* Substance use among schizophrenic outpatients: Prevalence, course, and relation to functional status. *Ann Clin Psychiatry* 7:19–24, 1995.
107. Dixon LB, Weiden PJ, Haas G, *et al:* Increased tardive dyskinesia in alcohol-abusing schizophrenic patients. *Compr Psychiatry* 33:121–122, 1992.
108. Carey MP, Weinhardt LS, Carey KB: Prevalence of infection with HIV among the seriously mentally ill: Review of the research and implications for practice. *Prof Psychol Res Prac* 26:262–268, 1995.
109. Cournois F, Empfield M, Horwath E, *et al:* HIV seroprevalence among patients admitted to two psychiatric hospitals. *Am J Psychiatry* 148:1225–1230, 1991.
110. Empfield M, Cournos F, Meyer I, *et al:* HIV seroprevalence among homeless patients admitted to a psychiatric inpatient unit. *Am J Psychiatry* 150:47–52, 1993.
111. Meyer I, McKinnon K, Cournos F, *et al:* HIV seroprevalence among long-stay patients in a state psychiatric hospital. *Hosp Commun Psychiatry* 44:282–284, 1993.
112. Silberstein C, Galanter M, Marmor M, *et al:* HIV-1 among inner city dually diagnosed inpatients. *Am J Drug Alcohol Abuse* 20:101–113, 1994.
113. Tracy JI, Josiassen RC, Bellack AS: Neuropsychology of dual diagnosis: Understanding the combined effects of schizophrenia and substance use disorder. *Clin Psychol Rev* 15:67–97, 1995.
114. Bowers MB, Mazure CM, Nelson JC, *et al:* Psychotogenic drug use and neuroleptic response. *Schizophr Bull* 16:81–85, 1990.
115. Seibyl JP, Satel SL, Anthony D, *et al:* Effects of cocaine on hospital course in schizophrenia. *J Nerv Ment Dis* 181:31–37, 1993.
116. Sokoloski KN, Cummings JL, Abrams BI, *et al:* Effects of substance abuse on hallucination rates and treatment responses in chronic psychiatric patients. *J Clin Psychiatry* 55:380–387, 1994.
117. Weiden PJ, Olfson M: Cost of relapse in schizophrenia. *Schizophr Bull* 21:419–429, 1995.
118. Owen RR, Fischer EP, Booth BM, *et al:* Medication noncompliance and substance abuse among patients with schizophrenia. *Psychiatr Serv* 47:853–858, 1996.

119. Pristach CA, Smith CM: Medication compliance and substance abuse among schizophrenic patients. *Hosp Commun Psychiatry* 41:1345–1348, 1990.
120. Miller FT, Tanenbaum JH: Drug abuse in schizophrenia. *Hosp Commun Psychiatry* 40:847–849, 1989.
121. Zito JM, Routt WW, Mitchell JE, *et al:* Clinical characteristics of hospitalized psychotic patients who refuse antipsychotic drug therapy. *Am J Psychiatry* 142:822–826, 1989.
122. Cuffel BJ: Comorbid substance use disorder: Prevalence, patterns of use, and course, in Drake RE, Mueser KT (eds): *Dual Diagnosis of Major Mental Illness and Substance Abuse,* vol 2: *Recent Research and Clinical Implications.* San Francisco, Jossey-Bass, 1996, pp 93–105.
123. Dworkin RM: Patterns of sex differences in negative symptoms and social functioning consistent with separate dimensions of schizophrenic psychopathology. *Am J Psychiatry* 147:347–349, 1990.
124. Szymanski S, Liebereman JA, Alvir JM, *et al:* Gender differences in onset of illness, treatment response, course, and biologic indexes in first episode schizophrenic patients. *Am J Psychiatry* 152:698–703, 1995.
125. Drake RE, Brunette MF, Mueser KT: Substance use disorder and social functioning in schizophrenia, in Mueser KT, Tarrier N (eds): *Handbook of Social Functioning in Schizophrenia.* Boston, Allyn and Bacon, 1998, pp 280–289.
126. Noordsy DL, Drake RE, Biesanz JC, *et al:* Family history of alcoholism in schizophrenia. *J Nerv Ment Dis* 182:651–655, 1994.
127. Wolford GL, Rosenberg SD, Oxman TE, *et al:* Evaluating current methods for detecting substance use disorder in persons with severe mental illness. submitted.

III

Economic Consequences of Alcoholism

Richard K. Fuller, Section Editor

Overview

Richard K. Fuller

This volume of *Recent Developments in Alcoholism* is devoted to the consequences of alcohol abuse and dependence. Section III discusses the economic consequences of alcohol abuse and alcoholism. Among the excellent chapters in this section are those that provide up-to-date analyses of the economic cost to society of alcohol abuse and alcoholism and the effect of problem drinking on productivity. Other chapters address such important economic issues as the effect of the price of alcohol on health-related and social consequences, including whether raising the price of alcohol would reduce these consequences, and whether the cost of alcohol treatment services is offset by a subsequent reduction in the utilization and cost of health care services in general.

The economic costs of alcohol abuse and alcoholism have been studied at various times since 1975. The most detailed estimates available before the contribution contained in the present volume were published in 1990, using 1985 data.[1] In Chapter 11, Drs. Harwood, Fountain, and Livermore now provide an updated and comprehensive review of these costs. Their review uses 1992 data and improves the existing estimation methodology by using the epidemiological literature to estimate the cost of comorbid health problems. They also provide estimates of what proportion of these costs are borne by the abuser and his or her family, government, private health and life insurance, and nonabusers.

In Chapter 12, Drs. Chaloupka, Grossman, and Saffer summarize the research done by economists to study the effect of the price of alcoholic beverages on a variety of negative consequences related to alcohol consump-

Richard K. Fuller • Division of Clinical and Prevention Research, National Institute on Alcohol Abuse and Alcoholism, Bethesda, Maryland 20892-7003.

Recent Developments in Alcoholism, Volume 14: The Consequences of Alcoholism, edited by Galanter. Plenum Press, New York, 1998.

tion. A fundamental principle of economics is that demand for a good will decrease as the price of that good increases. However, some have argued that consumption of alcohol might be an exception to the rule, theorizing that individuals who are dependent on or addicted to alcohol will buy it regardless of price. However, the authors generally conclude in their review that increases in the price of alcoholic beverage are generally associated with reductions in the consequences of alcohol abuse such as liver cirrhosis, motor vehicle accidents, and so forth. As the authors suggest, these findings may have important policy implications.

Raising taxes has the effect of raising prices, and studies have shown that alcohol taxes and prices affect both alcohol consumption and consequences from drinking.[2] Studies have shown that higher taxes on beer are associated with reduced traffic crash fatality rates[3] and some types of crime.[4] However, one study has shown that increases in price do not result in the heaviest-drinking 5% of drinkers significantly reducing their alcohol consumption.[5] Kenkel[6] has pointed out that although federal taxes have been raised, the net effect on price has declined because of inflation. In 1954, the average tax rate was 50% of the price exclusive of taxes because taxes have not kept pace with inflation. Despite increases in taxes in 1984 and 1990, the real tax rate is now slightly above 20%. Kenkel estimated an "optimal" alcohol tax, balancing losses to the economy by money spent on taxes that would have been spent on other choices with gains to the economy created as socially costly heavy drinking declines. His analysis suggested that the optimal taxation rate would be to restore the alcohol excise taxes to the 1950s levels adjusted for inflation.

In Chapter 13, Drs. Mullahy and Sindelar summarize the existing knowledge of the effects of drinking and problem drinking on productivity, drawing primarily from recent economic research. They consider such labor market variables as wages, earnings, income, labor supply, and employment. They point out that most studies have focused on the direct effects of alcohol use or abuse on these labor market variables. However, indirect effects such as the effect of drinking on educational attainment, which in turn affects earnings, may be of equal importance. These indirect effects have been less studied, and the authors urge greater research attention to them. As the authors conclude, although the findings of this review are not always consistent across studies, they are, nonetheless, intriguing.

One of the negative consequences of alcoholism is that alcoholics consume medical care at about twice the rate of nonalcoholics. In Chapter 14, Dr. Holder reviews the literature on whether health care utilization is decreased after alcoholism treatment. If so, this would be another economic benefit from alcoholism treatment in addition to productivity and improved health. Studies done in fee-for-service settings indicate that total health care utilization and costs do drop after treatment, and in 2 to 4 years they reach pretreatment levels or lower except for older alcoholics (55 years and older). Dr. Holder points out that similar analyses have to be done to see if this cost benefit of alcoholism treatment is present in a managed-care environment. Research is also needed to specify how treatment location, treatment modality, and patient characteristics are related to greater or lesser costs of treatment.

This set of chapters eloquently and clearly describes the enormous cost of alcohol abuse to our society and the potential loss of productivity. They also show that the principles of economics apply to alcoholism and that increased prices of alcoholic beverages are associated with fewer adverse consequences of abusive alcohol consumption. Last, alcoholism treatment in fee-for-service settings has the economic benefit of reducing subsequent health care costs. These analyses are not only important from an economic perspective but also have important implications for prevention research and policy deliberations.

References

1. Rice DP, Kelman S, Miller LS, Dunmeyer S: *The Economic Costs of Alcohol and Drug Abuse and mental illness: 1985.* Washington, DC, DHHS Publication (ADM) 90-1694, 1990.
2. Leung S-F, Phelps CE: "My kingdom for a drink . . .?": A review of the estimates of the price sensitivity of demand for alcoholic beverages, in Hilton ME, Bloss G (eds): *Economics and the Prevention of Alcohol-Related Problems.* Rockville, MD, National Institute on Alcohol Abuse and Alcoholism Research Monograph No. 25. NIH Publication No. 93-3513, 1993, pp 1–31.
3. Grossman M, Choate D, Arluck GM: Price sensitivity of alcoholic beverages in the United States: Youth alcohol consumption, in Holder H (ed): *Control Issues in Alcohol Abuse Prevention: Strategies for States and Communities.* Greenwich, CT, JAI Press, 1987, pp 169–198.
4. Cook PJ, Moore MJ: Economic perspectives on reducing alcohol-related violence, in Martin SE (ed): *Alcohol and Interpersonal Violence: Fostering Multidisciplinary Perspectives.* Rockville, MD, National Institute on Alcohol Abuse and Alcoholism Research Monograph No. 24. NIH Publication No. 93-3496, 1993, pp 193–212.
5. Manning WG, Blumberg L, Moulton LH: The demand for alcohol: The differential response to price. *J Health Econ* 14:123–148, 1995.
6. Kenkel DS: New estimates of the optimal tax on alcohol. *Econ Inquiry* 24:296–319, 1996.

11

Economic Costs of Alcohol Abuse and Alcoholism

Henrick J. Harwood, Douglas Fountain, and Gina Livermore

Abstract. The economic cost to society from alcohol abuse and alcoholism in the United States was an estimated $148 billion in 1992. When adjusted for inflation and population, the estimates are generally comparable with cost estimates produced over the past 20 years. The current estimates are significantly greater than the most recent detailed estimates developed for 1985—about 42% above increases due to population growth and inflation. Between 1985 and 1992, inflation accounted for about 37.5% and population growth for 7.1% increases. Changes in prevalence have been associated with a modest reduction in alcohol costs. Though crime rates did not materially change over this period, criminal justice expenditures more than doubled overall, even after adjustment for price increases. The balance of changes are due to new findings and/or methodology indicating larger impacts than previously estimated. It is estimated that 45.1% of costs are borne by alcohol abusers and/or members of their households, 38.6% are borne by government, 10.2% by private insurance, and 6.0% by victims of alcohol-related trauma (motor vehicle crashes plus crime). The costs staying in the household of the abusers may be materially incident on persons other than the abuser, e.g., spouses, children.

1. Introduction

Alcohol problems carry with them a number of specific, well-recognized sequelae that have major economic impacts. Among these are the health consequences and impacts of alcohol problems on the health care system, the role of alcohol in crime/violence, and the recognition that alcohol abusers and

Henrick J. Harwood, Douglas Fountain, and Gina Livermore • The Lewin Group, Fairfax, Virginia 22031.

Recent Developments in Alcoholism, Volume 14: The Consequences of Alcoholism, edited by Galanter. Plenum Press, New York, 1998.

alcoholics can become unable to support themselves financially and therefore end up relying on society's safety nets. It is possible to quantify the effect that alcohol disorders impose on society using the economic approach embodied in cost-of-illness studies.[1,2] A more detailed report of the methodology and findings of this work can be found in Harwood *et al.*[3]

The findings are based on a compilation of the available evidence concerning the causal role played by alcohol problems in a variety of problems. The project reviewed research evidence, analyzed databases when available (and feasible), and discussed findings with topical experts. Additional research into the causal role played by alcohol problems in the variety of problems will benefit future studies.

The most recent prior US estimates were developed by Rice *et al.*,[4] using detailed data from 1985. The opportunity and need to develop new estimates were presented not only by inflation and population change, but also by changes in the extent of alcohol and drug problems (e.g., the apparent decline in the prevalence of alcohol problems, the cocaine and human immunodeficiency virus (HIV) epidemics), and major changes in the organization and delivery of alcohol and general health services (e.g., managed care, changes in Medicaid, Medicare, and private insurance). Furthermore, there have been advances in our knowledge about the nature and impact of alcohol problems. Current data and findings have been incorporated in these estimates.

The rates of alcohol consumption and associated problems were declining throughout the 1980s, perhaps by as much as 10% between 1985 and 1992.[5,6] However, treatment data suggest that since 1985, increasing proportions of those treated for alcohol problems also have drug problems.

Apart from general inflation, the three other largest sources of increase in costs between Rice *et al.*[4] and the current study are for lost earnings due to alcohol impairment in the workplace, increases in the number of persons incarcerated, and the use of the epidemiological literature to estimate the cost of comorbid health problems. The former change is primarily due to this study's use of new analyses, and the second reflects a real and widely recognized phenomenon. As for the third material change, this current study includes higher proportions of various health problems as attributable to alcohol abuse and dependence, basing this on the current epidemiological literature. In contrast, the prior study focused on how alcohol–drug–mental health diagnosed as secondary and tertiary conditions increased the length of stay during hospital stays for nonalcohol health problems (the primary diagnosed health problems during the hospital stay).

This chapter is organized in the following manner. First, a brief review of cost of illness studies in general, and with respect to alcohol abuse, is presented. This is followed by an overview of the general approach used to develop cost estimates. The major results from the cost study are then presented, identifying different components of costs with particular comparison to how these may differ from prior estimates by Rice *et al.*[4] for 1985. These results are further compared to other, older estimates of the economic cost of alcohol problems. Finally, the chapter examines and estimates which populations and/or institutions in society actually bear the economic costs of alcohol abuse, and then projections of costs for 1995 are presented.

2. A Short History of Cost-of-Illness Studies

Several strong conclusions are drawn from a review of the relatively small literature on substance abuse cost-of-illness (COI). First, most studies build on almost 40 years of experience conducting COI studies in health care, generally using an opportunity cost framework termed the *human capital* approach. Recent studies have a common understanding of the concepts at the foundation of such efforts. Second, the specifics of how the studies have been performed differ primarily in the details. Many of the differences between studies are attributable to differences in the data that have been available to use in constructing the estimates. The specific methodology used or approach taken in developing COI estimates is often dictated by the data available to the analyst. Finally, there is almost universal agreement by the authors of the research studies that such studies are not sufficient justification for any particular social initiatives directed at substance abuse. COI estimates do provide insights to help answer questions such as:

- What types and what quantity of health services are required to treat alcohol abuse and its related health consequences? How much do these services cost?
- How many people die as a result of alcohol abuse, and what is the economic impact of premature death?
- What impact does alcohol abuse have on individual productivity in the home and workplace?
- How much crime exists because of alcohol abuse, either by definition (e.g., driving under the influence) or physiological effects (e.g., assaults)? What does it cost to protect against these crimes, adjudicate arrests, and punish offenders?
- How much reliance on the social welfare system is caused by alcohol abuse, and at what cost?
- What other impacts are there of alcohol abuse, such as motor vehicle crashes and fire destruction?

COI studies in general and for alcohol abuse in particular are not newly invented, and the general approach to such studies is well established. Studies on alcohol abuse have a near 25-year history, and these in turn built (consciously or otherwise) on 15 years or more of COI studies on various other health problems. There has been a steady evolution of this literature in the United States, certainly along theoretical lines, but, as would be expected with any technology, more development along methodological lines. As the methodology has advanced, there have been greater consistency and comparability across studies (as well as a demand for the same) to the point where the general approach can be considered nearly "standardized" based on the application of "neoclassical" market-oriented economic principles.

All of the studies for alcohol abuse were preceded by COI studies for other types of illnesses and problems, including a study in Great Britain of road crashes,[7] a study in the United States estimating the costs for each of the internationally recognized major classes of illnesses,[8] and a US study on mental illness.[9] Studies prior to these examined various components of what have come to constitute COI studies.

The earliest study focusing on the economic costs of alcohol abuse of which this author is aware was conducted for Australia in 1969–1970.[10] In the United States, the earliest such studies dated from about 1973, including Berry and Boland's[11] study of alcohol abuse and its significantly expanded successor study.[12] There have been a modest number of further studies on the economic costs of alcohol abuse and alcoholism in the United States and other nations since that time. Virtually all of the studies of the illicit abuse of drugs have been in the United States. The most recent and comprehensive substance abuse COI studies have been in Australia,[13] the United States,[4] and Canada.[14]

The alcohol abuse COI studies performed since 1970 have had the explicit objective of demonstrating that a nontrivial amount of expenditures on health (and morbidity and mortality) are due to alcohol abuse, either directly or indirectly. It should be noted that the study by Fein[9] did identify and estimate certain "mental health" costs that were attributed to alcoholism (and drug addiction), and it acknowledged certain other nonmedical costs (e.g., criminal justice system) that were not estimated owing to time limitations.

The central concept in market economics is "opportunity cost," and the studies reviewed employ this basic concept of cost. Opportunity cost is the market value of resources that are redirected away from uses to which they would have been put otherwise.

The opportunity cost concept in health studies has been refined over numerous studies performed since the 1950s. The general approach to this cost methodology in the United States was virtually codified by a task force of the US Public Health Service (PHS) chaired by Dorothy Rice (see refs. 1 and 2 for the guidelines report and a second article that elaborates on the guidelines). The task force was convened in 1978–1979 for the purpose of developing guidelines for COI studies performed or funded by the US PHS. The guidelines were intended to reduce methodological differences between COI studies performed for different illnesses or even for studies of the same illnesses performed by different research teams. It is important to note that the guidelines did not explicitly contemplate or address the conceptual or methodological challenges posed by constructing COI estimates for alcohol abuse. The principles are general in nature, however, and certainly have been found to be applicable to the alcohol abuse COI studies performed since that time.

Table I. Core/Noncore and Direct–Indirect Costs

	Direct (goods and services for treatment)	Indirect (lost productivity)
Core (health)	Cost of treating the illness and its comorbid conditions (e.g., specialty treatment, hospital expenditures)	Lost productivity from deaths and other illness-related factors, including institutionalized populations (e.g., expected lower earnings among diagnosable substance abusers)
Noncore (nonhealth)	Other nonhealth goods and services related to the illness (e.g., crime, social welfare, motor vehicle crashes)	Lost productivity resulting from nonhealth-related sequelae (e.g., crime and motor vehicle crashes)

The primary cost categories in COI studies are "direct" and "indirect" costs (Table I). The direct costs for an illness are represented by the value of tangible goods and services actually delivered to address consequences of that illness. Indirect costs are represented by the value of personal productive services that are not performed owing to the consequences of the illness. A further distinction is usually made in COI studies between costs primarily within the health system or domain ("core" costs) and costs outside of the health system ("noncore" costs).

The US PHS COI guidelines did not actually set standards of practice or break new theoretical or methodological ground. It is probably more accurate to state that the guidelines recognized and described the mainstream of COI practice (as it developed internationally), noted its strengths and weaknesses, and acknowledged the orthodoxy of this approach. Substance abuse COI studies developed in the United States since the guidelines have all been generally based on its approach. There has not been a fundamental challenge to the general approach, although there have certainly been variations and proposed improvements in the methodologies used in prior studies.

3. The Framework for Cost-of-Illness Studies

The construction of COI estimates for substance abuse can be enormously challenging and complex; however, the framework for the study is relatively clear and easy to understand. The design and performance of these studies need to be built around a set of objectives and standards that have scientific validity and can be communicated to the concerned scientific community, policymakers, the media, and the general population. This can be characterized as a three-step process:

- Identify the tangible consequences associated with substance abuse

- Document causality between substance abuse and its consequences, and quantify frequency
- Assign economic values

The initial step in designing a substance abuse COI study is to identify the tangible negative consequences believed to result from alcohol abuse. Identification and definition of these consequences provides a framework for the analysis. The consequences of concern should be tangible and subject to measurement both in their incidence and in the level of resource use associated with their occurrence. A general set of categories of consequences of substance abuse is presented in Table II. Each of the items is actually a category composed of further subsets of consequences, some of which can be quite extensive. For example, the potential health comorbidities of alcoholism and alcohol abuse (i.e., health problems that can be caused by substance abuse or other factors) are quite extensive.

Estimating the role of substance abuse as a causal factor for various adverse consequences is a central issue in any study estimating the COI for substance abuse. First, the analyst must identify the plausible consequences of alcohol abuse. Second, the extent to which alcohol abuse may have caused the specific consequences needs to be quantified. Evidence must be assembled that justifies estimates of how much of the problem is caused by substance abuse.

For some consequences of alcohol abuse, causality is definitional or established by an external source. For example, there are alcohol-specific diagnoses that are attached to health treatment (e.g., alcohol psychosis, alcohol poisoning, alcohol dependence and abuse). Data compiled by International Classification of Diseases and Related Health Problems, ninth revision codes allow certain health services and some deaths to be definitionally attributed to alcohol abuse. In some instances, administrative determinations (usually based on clinical assessments) may be made about the role of alcohol (or drugs). This is the case for some disability programs (Social Security Disability Insurance [SSDI] and Supplemental Security Income [SSI]) in the United States. Also, criminal justice statistics usually have "defined" offenses related to alcohol and drugs (e.g., liquor law violations, driving while intoxicated).

The more challenging situation is when substance abuse is one of multiple potential causes of particular consequences, such as liver disease, certain cancers/neoplasms, motor vehicle crashes, crime of various types, and employment problems. The objective is to develop an estimate of the proportion of the multicause consequence that can be attributed to alcohol abuse. This often requires sophisticated statistical analyses of the sort that are often in the scientific literature. The most important issue is to distinguish between association and causality.

The final step in the COI study is to assign values to the consequences and the associated flows of resources. For example, if half of the episodes of a medical condition are caused by alcohol abuse, then half of the annual expenditure for the treatment of that condition could be allocated to alcohol abuse. The most appropriate measures for this purpose are prices that represent the

Table II. Consequences/Costs Assessed in Cost of Illness Analysis

	Direct (goods and services for treatment)	Indirect (lost productivity)	Generally nonquantifiable costs
Core (health)	• Specialty drug/alcohol treatment and prevention • Support for treatment, including training, research, and insurance administration • Comorbid health treatment provided in hospitals, by outpatient doctors, in nursing homes, with pharmaceuticals; or the continuum of services for certain special disease categories like liver disease, fetal alcohol syndrome, trauma, neoplasms, etc. • Insurance administration for comorbid health problems	• Reduced or lost earnings while impaired or unemployed • Lost earnings due to premature death or to institutionalization	• Pain and suffering • Bereavement • Psychosocial development among substance abusers and their children • Familial health
Noncore (nonhealth)	• Criminal justice system expenses including protection, adjudication, corrections • Victim expenses • Crime-related property destruction • Administration of income transfer programs • Value of substances illicitly consumed • Motor vehicle crashes • Fire destruction	• Lost earnings while crime victims cannot work • Lost earnings while criminals are incarcerated • Lost legitimate earnings, including lost tax dollars, due to "careers of crime"	• Reduced product quality • Secondary market effects • Productivity consequences for family members • Productivity consequences for coworkers and firms that are not reflected in the earnings of alcohol abusers

cost of purchasing, producing, or replacing the resource flow that has been measured.

Direct costs, that is, expenditures for health and nonhealth goods and services, are generally straightforward to value, particularly where resources and services are exchanged in a market. Where resources are in the public sector, social accounting systems usually keep track of the cost of classes of services or resources, although price or cost data for specific units of services often are not available [e.g., the cost of arresting a driver for driving under the influence (DUI)].

Indirect costs, representing lost or missed work and impaired work productivity resulting from alcohol abuse, are usually valued using average wage rates. Lost productivity arises from premature mortality (death at an age prior to an actuarially expected age). A number of studies have found that persons with severe alcohol problems have lower earnings, wage rates, and employment on average than persons of similar sociodemographic backgrounds (e.g., refs. 15 and 16). Note that indirect costs represent lost *potential* productivity, which means work is never done and productivity never delivered because of the impact of alcohol abuse on the amount of productive activity and the productivity of that activity. This also includes the value of household productive services. Average wage rates should be adjusted for several additional factors, including expected level of employment and the value of "fringe" benefits and taxes that may never appear in a paycheck. Also, rates should be adjusted for both age and gender.

4. Findings

This chapter reports the findings and conclusions from the most recent comprehensive study of the economic costs of alcohol (as well as drug) abuse in the United States.[3] Details about the methodology, sources of data, and other references are presented in that report, which can be requested from the National Clearinghouse on Alcohol and Drug Information or the National Institute on Alcohol Abuse and Alcoholism. The summary results are presented in Table III. Findings are briefly discussed below.

4.1. Health Care Expenditures

Total alcohol-related health care expenditures in 1992 were $18.8 billion. Specialized services related to the treatment and prevention of alcohol problems were $5.6 billion. This included specialized detoxification and rehabilitation services ($4 billion for about 1.8 million persons and nearly 3.5 million episodes of specialized care), as well as prevention ($1.1 billion), training ($73 million), and research expenditures ($184 million). Treatment for health problems attributed to alcohol problems (e.g., liver cirrhosis and trauma) were $13.2 billion.

These comorbidity costs are significantly greater than estimates from the Rice *et al.*[4] study, primarily because the earlier study did not utilize epidemiological data about the causal involvement of alcohol problems in comorbid illness other than fetal alcohol syndrome (although Rice *et al.*[4] did use such data in estimating mortality costs). This methodological expansion has added costs for about 500,000 hospital discharges (with 4 million days of care) at

Table III. Estimated Economic Cost of Alcohol Abuse in the United States, 1992[a]

Core	
Direct	
Alcohol abuse services	$5,573
Comorbid health problems	$13,247
Indirect (lost earnings)	
Premature death	$31,327
Due to illness	$67,696
Institutionalized populations	$1,513
Total	$133,498
Noncore	
Direct	
Crime	$6,312
Social Welfare Administration	$683
Motor Vehicle Crashes	$13,619
Fire Destruction	$1,590
Indirect (lost earnings)	
Victims of Crime	$1,012
Incarceration	$5,449
Total	$28,748
Total	$162,246

[a]Millions of dollars.

about $3.3 billion. Data on alcohol-related comorbidities have been summarized in reports such as Stinson *et al.*[17] and *Alcohol and Health.*[6]

4.2. *Premature Mortality*

A total of about 107,400 premature deaths are attributed to alcohol problems for 1992. The estimated cost was $31.3 billion, representing the presented discounted value of expected lifetime earnings (discounted at 6%). The average loss per death was about $300,000. Deaths were bimodally distributed over age groups, among individuals aged 20 to 40 years of age (e.g., motor vehicle crashes, other causes of traumatic death) and among the elderly (from chronic abuse of alcohol due to, e.g., liver disease, neoplasms). There are only modest differences from Rice *et al.*[4]

4.3. *Impaired Productivity*

An estimated $67.7 billion in lost potential productivity was attributed to alcohol abuse in 1992. This accrued in the form of work not performed, including household tasks, and primarily are measured in terms of lost earnings and household productivity. These costs were primarily borne by alcohol abusers and those with whom they lived. This study has not attempted to estimate the burden of alcohol problems on worksites or employers, nor should the estimates in this study be interpreted in this manner.

Among the working age population, there were an estimated 24.5 million persons with a lifetime history of alcohol problems [using the *Diagnostic and Statistical Manual of Mental Disorders* (DSM-IV) standards as applied to the National Longitudinal Alcohol Epidemiologic Survey (NLAES)[5]. The analysis found that negative impacts are detectable among about 13.6 million of the adult population, among males age 18 to 64 years (and statistically significant), while generally negligible and/or not statistically significant among females. Lifetime instead of current year diagnoses are used because alcohol problems can interrupt a career and adversely impact earning over extended periods of time. Individuals with alcohol problems had income roughly 6% lower than persons without alcohol problems, holding other characteristics constant.

4.4. *Motor Vehicle Crashes*

Total costs attributed to alcohol-related motor vehicle crashes were $19.8 billion. This included $11.1 billion from premature mortality (counted/included above), and $13.6 billion from automobile and other property destruction. The costs for health care treatment for injuries are included.

4.5. *Crime*

Costs of crime attributed to alcohol abuse were estimated at $19.8 billion (Table IV). In addition to alcohol-defined crimes (e.g., DUI and liquor law violations), alcohol abuse was causally implicated in about 25 to 30% of violent crimes (with rates differing for different types of crimes). In contrast, rates of about 5% or less were used for the attribution of alcohol to income-generating crime.

Expenditures within the criminal justice system totaled $6.2 billion for alcohol. Costs to victims were $8.0 billion. Most of the estimated victim losses were for lost lifetime earnings of homicide victims, but this estimate also includes medical expenses, lost work, and damaged/destroyed property. A substantial loss of potential productivity to the economy was associated with incarceration of inmates for and alcohol-related offenses (140,000 person years at a loss of potential productivity of $5.4 billion).

4.6. *Social Welfare*

This study estimates that 2.2% of social welfare beneficiaries received benefits *because of* an alcohol-related impairment. These impairments resulted in transfers of $6.1 billion in 1992, with administrative and other direct service expenses of $683 million for those with alcohol problems. While administrative and direct service costs are included in the costs to society, the value of income transfers are not totaled in the "cost to society," because they simply shift or transfer resources from one part of society (a loss to tax payers) to another part of society (a gain to transfer payment recipients). While as many

Table IV. Total Cost of Alcohol Abuse Specific and Related Crime[a]

Type of cost	Cost
Criminal justice system	
Police protection	$1,547
Legal and adjudication	$491
State and federal correction	$1,790
Local correction	$2,326
Total criminal justice system	$6,154
Federal alcoholic beverage control	$62
Public expenditures	$6,216
Private legal defense	$68
Economic costs to victims	
Medical expenses for victims of violent crimes	$400
Property damage	$28
Total, direct costs	$6,712
Homicide (in premature mortality)	$6,589
Victims of crime	$1,012
Incarceration	$5,449
Crime careers	—
Total, indirect costs	$13,050
Total	$19,762

[a]Millions of dollars.

as 15% of government transfer recipients may engage in "heavy drinking,"[19–21] it is estimated that only 4 to 8% may meet clinical DSM-IV criteria for abuse or dependence; it is not clear that for most of these individuals their use of alcohol constituted the primary reason that they did not or could not gain employment.

5. Comparison with Rice *et al.*[4]

The estimated $148 billion costs of alcohol abuse from this study are about 42% greater than the $104 billion population and inflation adjusted total values from Rice *et al.*[4] Figure 1 and Table V compare the total values as well as the respective major components of the costs. Estimates from Rice *et al.*[4] have been adjusted to 1992 based on population growth (about 1% per year) plus inflation (medical CPI for health care expenditures, the Consumer Price Index (CPI) for other direct costs, and the employment compensation index for all indirect costs). The major similarities and differences for the major cost categories are discussed.

5.1. Alcohol Services

The primary difference is that hospital costs were a much larger proportion of alcohol costs in the estimates for 1985. There were more alcohol-

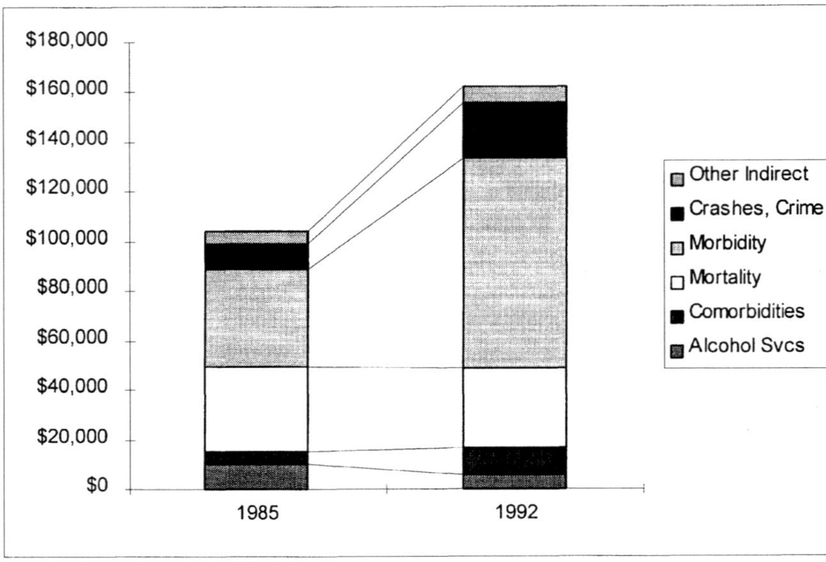

Figure 1. Changes in cost of alcohol abuse between present study and Rice *et al.*[4] The Rice *et al.*[4] estimates for 1985 are adjusted for increases in population and relevant prices.

specific hospital episodes in 1985 (about 500,000 vs. 300,000 in 1992). Moreover, the estimates for 1985 used a much higher cost per hospital day than has been employed in this report. The Rice *et al.*[4] study used the average cost per hospital day for all diagnoses and all types of hospitals (over $800 per day in 1992), while this study has used rates specific to treatment of drug and alcohol patients in hospital specialty treatment units of about $300 per day (based on analysis of a survey of specialized substance abuse treatment providers by

Table V. Changes in Inflation- and Population-Adjusted Costs of Alcohol Abuse between Present Study and Rice *et al.*[4a]

	1985	1992
Specialty substance abuse services	$10,172	$5,573
Comorbid health problems	$4,935	$13,247
Lost earnings—premature death	$34,573	$31,327
Lost earnings—illness	$39,482	$69,209
Crashes and crime	$10,307	$22,204
Other indirect	$4,564	$6,461
Total	$104,033	$148,021

[a]Amounts are millions of 1992 dollars. Rice *et al.*[4] estimates for 1985 adjusted for increases in population and relevant prices.

Harwood *et al.*[22]). Both studies relied on data from specialty treatment providers to develop estimates of services in specialized providers.

5.2. *Treatment of Comorbidities*

This is one of the two major substantive areas of difference between this report and Rice *et al.*[4] and accordingly this study has significantly higher cost estimates in these categories: $13.2 billion versus $4.9 billion. The different approaches of the two studies have been briefly discussed. The primary difference is that this study has drawn on the epidemiological literature (e.g., Stinson *et al.*[17] to identify particular health problems (e.g., liver disease, trauma) and rates of causal linkage to alcohol problems. Rice *et al.*[4] did not use this literature or approach, except in their analysis of premature mortality, where it was the primary approach. Instead, the Rice study analyzed the impact on hospital length of stay from having a nonprimary diagnosis of alcohol or drug abuse or mental illness. The current study has adopted the contribution of calculating the increment in hospital length of stay, but has also incorporated data that make attribution to alcohol abuse of the proportion of hospital stays for selected disorders.

5.3. *Premature Mortality*

The current study has used the same methodology as the previous study, as well as for most of the prior studies. The modest differences in the estimates are accounted for by new epidemiological data for attribution of several disorder to alcohol problems. These changes in mortality attribution were drawn from research developed for the National Institute on Alcohol Abuse and Alcoholism (NIAAA).[17] The current study uses a higher proportion of suicides (28% vs. 13%, which added almost 5000 deaths to the total), a modestly lower attribution factor for motor vehicle deaths (42% vs. 51%), and has also added a small fraction of deaths (7%) associated with cerebrovascular disease (which added about 9000 deaths). Note that this study does not make adjustments for potential benefits to cardiovascular health that may result from moderate consumption of alcoholic beverages.[6]

5.4. *Morbidity—Impaired Productivity*

This is the major difference in terms of impact on cost estimates with the prior study. The current study analyzed a new data set, the NLAES,[5] which yielded roughly comparable prevalence rates. Second, the current study has selected the "indicator" model to measure the impact of alcohol disorders versus the "timing" model. Rice *et al.*[4] developed both sets of estimates, but selected the latter approach, which yields substantially lower impact estimates (as was documented in their report). The indicator model is simpler and less restrictive, and the timing model represents an attempt to model the process with a more restrictive parameterization. Most studies also use an indicator model to analyze the relation of alcohol problems with productivity, earnings, and employment (refs. 15 and 16).

5.5. *Crashes and Criminal Justice Costs*

Very similar methodologies have been used to estimate crime-related costs, although modest changes have been made to the attribution factors, primarily owing to incorporation of more current data. Increases in crime-related costs beyond inflation are attributable to growth between 1985 and 1992 in the overall incarcerated population by about 80%,[23] and in alcohol-related incarcerations specifically by over 60%, from 84,000 in Rice *et al.*[4] to 139,000 in the current report.

Motor vehicle crash costs attributed to alcohol have also increased significantly. This is because new data are available about the causal involvement of alcohol in nonfatal crashes that indicate higher rates of involvement of alcohol than for earlier studies.[24] The causal rates used in the current study for nonfatal alcohol-related crashes are two to three times greater than values used in the prior alcohol studies. The rates used in Rice *et al.*[4] had been used in estimates developed since Berry *et al.*[12]

5.6. *Other Indirect Costs*

These costs are for loss of employment by the incarcerated population. Methodology did not change; therefore, the change is exclusively because of the fact that the corrections system incarcerated over 60% more inmates for alcohol-related offenses in 1992 than in 1985.

6. Comparison with Prior Studies

The estimates from this study are generally comparable to those produced from the prior major studies on the economic impacts of alcohol abuse. While there have been literally hundreds of differences from study to study, and that is true in comparing this study with Rice *et al.*,[4] it is fair to say that relatively consistent methodological approaches have been applied to most of these studies. This is true in terms of the nature of impacts, which have been included in the estimates, and how values have been estimated.

Figure 2 compares the results of the current study with Rice *et al.*[4] and with the prior estimates, making adjustments for inflation and population growth over the 17 years that these estimates cover. Comparisons are made with Rice *et al.*,[4] Berry *et al.*,[12] Cruze *et al.*,[25] and Harwood *et al.*[26] The current estimate for alcohol of $148 billion is about equal to the average of the four prior major studies, although 42% greater than those from Rice *et al.*[4]

The moderated differences in adjusted alcohol cost estimates over the five studies is based on the fact that relatively similar methodological ap-

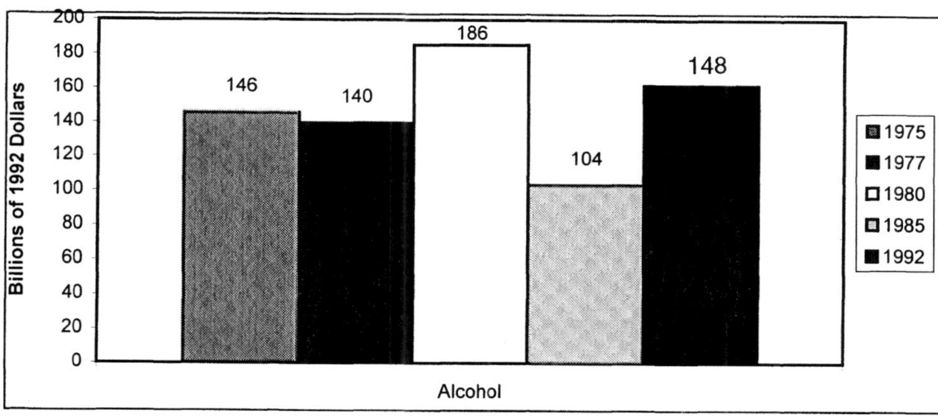

Figure 2. Comparison of estimates from the major cost of illness studies for alcohol abuse adjusted for inflation and population growth. Data for 1975 from Berry *et al.*[12]; 1977 from Cruze *et al.*[25]; 1980 from Harwood *et al.*[26]; 1985 from Rice *et al.*[4]; 1992 from Harwood *et al.*[3] Price and population data are from the *Statistical Abstract of the* United States, 1993, US Department of Commerce.

proaches have been applied to these studies. While each successive study has incorporated the newest data and findings about the nature, extent, and impact of alcohol problems, generally these have not constituted fundamental changes in these estimates. Probably the most fundamentally different estimate was Rice *et al.*,[4] which yielded significantly lower estimates for health expenditures (comorbidities) and reduced productivity than the other studies. This study has given intensive attention to those topics and documents the nature of the differences and the rationale and data that support the findings in this study.

7. Who Bears the Costs of Alcohol Abuse?

One of the conceptual issues raised with COI studies is whether the cost to society should include the cost of impacts such as health problems or losses of earnings experienced by abusers/consumers of alcohol.[27] This study has attempted to estimate who bears the economic burden of substance abuse: users themselves or other members/institutions of society.

For alcohol, losses fall primarily on abusers (including their household members): approximately \$66.8 billion (45%) versus \$81.2 billion for nonabusers (Table VI). Alcohol abusers may bear less of the cost than this, as they shift impacts to household members.

The largest share of the costs that are shifted are borne by government, which ultimately means taxpayers and those who would have received benefits of additional government spending; 38.5% of total alcohol costs fall on government. Private health and life insurance bear 10.2% of alcohol abuse

Table VI. Where the Burden of Alcohol Problems Fall[a]

	Cost
Abusers and households	$66.8
Government	$57.2
Private insurance	$15.1
Victim losses	$8.9
Total	$148.0

[a]Billions of dollars.

costs, while nonabusers directly bear 6.0% of alcohol costs. Of course, all of the costs borne by government and private insurance are ultimately transferred to tax payers and insurance policy holders, who are predominantly nonabusers.

The costs–impacts of alcohol abuse are spread throughout society (to nonusers) through several mechanisms:

- Impacts on nonusers (crime, motor vehicle crashes)
- Government control efforts (prevention, treatment, crime control)
- Insurance and social systems (insurance and tax systems)

First, there is evidence that abuse of alcohol is a material causal factor in crime, as well as transportation accidents that affect nonabusers. Largely because of these impacts on nonusers, society expends substantial resources attempting to control the consequences of alcohol abuse through the criminal justice system and public health efforts. Also, the impacts of alcohol that might appear to fall on the abusers themselves are often shifted to nonusers: the cost of health problems are transferred through private and public health insurance, and lost earnings result in reduced tax revenues and may also be offset through social insurance/welfare programs (unemployment and disability insurance, income supplements).

The fact that alcohol abuse imposes major impacts on the nonabusing public probably is strongly related to how government regulates access to alcohol in our society. If most of the consequences of alcohol abuse fell on and were borne by those who used alcohol, it seems likely that the nature of concern and government involvement with regulation of alcohol could be qualitatively different. One can examine the approach of government toward smoking over the past 30 years for insights into this issue. The primary public health emphasis was on prevention and education (and a minimal level of treatment) until research suggested that passive exposure to smoke might pose a threat to the health of nonsmokers. Since that time much public and private effort has been directed to reducing the exposure of nonsmokers to smoke in order to reduce potential risks.

Thus, the nature and burden (or incidence) of costs can be of interest for policy purposes. While this information does suggest types of impacts and types of policies that may be of interest, it does not yield conclusions about the effectiveness of particular policy initiatives or the relative effectiveness of alternative approaches.

The following sections present the approach taken to estimate how the economic costs of alcohol abuse have been distributed across several major sectors of society: abusers (and their households); federal, state, and local governments; private insurance; and nonabusing victims. The results of the analyses for alcohol abuse are presented in Table VII.

7.1. *The Burden on Work Sites*

Strong note should be given to the fact that no estimates have been developed specifically for work sites. However, costs related to losses in productivity–costs are attributable to worksites.

This study, like those before it (e.g., Rice *et al.*[4]), has estimated work site productivity impacts in terms of lost earnings of alcohol abusers. There are data sets that have been analyzed and yielded plausible estimates about this dimension of alcohol impacts. However, there are few studies (and no rigorous studies) that estimate the other costs to a work site of alcohol abuse among the work force. The analyses of lost earnings in fact indicate that work sites shift at least some of the productivity differential of alcohol-impaired workers to the workers themselves in the form of lower compensation. To the

Table VII. Who Bears the Economic Costs of Alcohol Abuse (millions of dollars)

	Total cost	Abuser and household	Government (total)	Private insurance	Victims of abusers
Health-related costs					
Alcohol treatment—community	$ 3,609	413	2,323	873	
Alcohol treatment—Federal	$ 437		437		
Alcohol prevention	$ 1,088		1,088		
Alcohol research, training	$ 257		257		
Alcohol treatment insurance administration	$ 182		132	50	
Treatment of comorbidity	$ 12,611	2,338	5,347	4,666	260
Comorbidity insurance administration	$ 641		340	296	
Mortality—lifetime earnings	$ 31,327	14,584	9,584	1,278	5,880
Morbidity—lost earnings	$ 69,209	44,243	24,966		
Other related costs					
Crime—CJS and property	$ 6,312	68	6,216		28
Social welfare administration	$ 683		683		
Motor vehicle crashes	$ 13,619	1,149	4,390	6,552	1,531
Fire destruction	$ 1,590			1,431	159
Victims of crime	$ 1,012				1,012
Incarceration—inmate lost earnings	$ 5,449	4,032	1,417		
Total	$148,021	66,828	57,181	15,146	8,870

extent that alcohol-impaired workers perform below the levels implied by their wages/salaries, these costs are borne by the work sites in the form of higher costs. Such costs must then be absorbed by a company by a combination of decreased profits, increased product/service prices, or reduced overall compensation for the workers. There are insufficient data to develop such estimates.

Still, impaired employees' lower earnings are partially shifted to other segments of society at and through the work site, since employers generally withhold income and other social insurance taxes and make contributions toward health insurance and social insurance on behalf of employees. Thus, work sites (and workers earnings) provide a convenient site for making calculations of some of these impacts. Much of the government as well as health insurance share is collected (or failed to be collected, in the instance of lower earnings) through employers.

7.2. The Burden on Households—Families

While the primary finding of this section is that alcohol abusers appear to bear the largest share of the economic impact on society, it should be recalled that this share of the burden also can be shifted. Losses of earnings attributable to alcohol problems impact everyone in a household (children, spouses, and others). Whether earnings are reduced through lower wage rates or reduced days of work, this loss would directly impact the well-being of any additional household members, particularly those who do not work or do not have an independent source of income. Recent surveys of alcohol problems have found that divorced and separated individuals have materially elevated rates of heavy drinking,[6] although it is theoretically possible that family difficulties may induce stress that may cause substance-abusing behavior. When abuse of alcohol causes households and families to break up, this may remove nonabusers from the immediate vicinity of abusers, but may also result in even greater economic hardships.

7.3. Health Care Expenditures

Overall, about 80% of personal health care expenditures are paid through private or public insurance in the United States. It is estimated that almost 90% of health care services for community-based treatment (this excludes prison- and jail-based services to inmates) of alcohol abuse are paid through insurance or direct government financing of services.[22] In addition, the federal government operates treatment services for veterans, dependents of the Department of Defense, and Native Americans. All alcohol abuse prevention and training services have been allocated to government funding, of which it appears that about 85% is from federal sources and 15% is from state and local sources.[28,29] Virtually all alcohol abuse research is federally supported. These values primarily represent budgets for NIAAA.[30]

The costs of treating comorbid disorders attributed to alcohol abuse have been allocated across sources of payment in proportion to national patterns for all personal health services.[31] The costs of administering health insurance systems have been allocated in proportion to estimated payments by sources, as indicated above.

7.4. *Mortality—Lifetime Earnings*

Most of this loss falls on the household members of the alcohol abusers. While life insurance offsets some of the loss of expected lifetime earnings, it is a small fraction. No estimates have been made of the number of households that receive social insurance because of the death of a member. Private life insurance made death benefit disbursements of $26 billion in 1992,[32] or about $13,000 per death in the United States. It is assumed that private life insurance paid out this amount on average for each of the 107,400 alcohol-related deaths in 1992. This number may be low because many of the decedents for alcohol-related causes tend to be in the prime of their working lives and may carry more insurance. However, it is also possible that relatively fewer alcohol abusers may have life insurance because of their relative youth, lifestyles, and problems in their work careers.

7.5. *Morbidity—Lost Earnings*

While lost earnings are generally thought to fall on the alcohol abuser themselves, it would appear that only about 66% of such losses fall directly on the household of the alcohol abusers, respectively. Out of the estimated losses in potential productivity (earnings plus nonmarket activities) from alcohol abuse ($69 billion) governments are estimated to bear almost 25% of such losses through lost employment-related and excise tax payments. This loss only applies to losses of potential market productivity, which is about 85% of total potential productivity (the other 15% is from household productivity; this proportion is about 8% for males and 33% for females). The redistribution–allocation of lost earnings to government is based on shares of 1992 net national product (NNP) of $5.367 trillion. The NNP includes production based in the United States and excludes the import- and export-related components of gross domestic and national product. The federal government received $936 billion (17.44% of NNP) and state and local government received $706 billion (13.15%) from taxes, social insurance fund payments, and excise taxes.[32]

The cost to government is further increased because of the value of social welfare transfer payments that are attributable to impairment or disability from alcohol abuse. While the value of transfer payments do not count in total costs to society (transfers represent almost equal gains to one part of society and losses to another part of society), it does shift part of the burden on alcohol abusers and their families to the rest of society. This was about 2 to 3% (depending on the particular type of social welfare program) of beneficiaries–payments of the national social welfare system and was an estimated $5.6 billion.

7.6. *Crime-Related Costs*

The national criminal justice system spent $74 billion in 1990,[23] or almost $84 billion in 1992 after adjusting for inflation and real growth. This study has attributed $6.2 billion to alcohol abuse, or almost 8% of total national expenditures. Expenditures have been allocated across federal, state, and local governments, based on the most recent Survey of Criminal Justice Expenditures and Personnel.[23] For example, about 90% of prison inmates are in state institutions and 10% in federal prisons. All jail inmates are in local institutions. Federal expenditures on alcohol control (the Bureau of Alcohol, Tobacco and Firearms) are obtained from the federal budget.[30]

7.7. *Social Welfare Administration*

The value of transfer payments (almost $6 billion) has already been included under morbidity (Section 7.5) as a government offset to personal lost earnings. The expense of administering the system, as well as delivering direct services (such as family and child welfare services), is reported in this item. Alcohol-related expenses were estimated at $683 million, respectively, or about 2 to 3% of total system administration expenses (depending on the type of social welfare program). About 80% of social welfare services and transfer payments are from federal funds[32]; thus, 80% of administration costs is allocated to the federal government and 20% to state and local governments.

7.8. *Motor Vehicle Crashes and Fire Destruction*

Estimated losses attributable to alcohol problems of $13.6 billion includes vehicle and roadway damage, legal and court costs, and insurance administration. The allocation of alcohol-related motor vehicle health care costs and mortality (lost lifetime earnings) have been included in estimates under prior sections. All roadway damage ($3.8 billion) was assigned to state and local governments, which are primarily responsible for the upkeep on highways. Insurance administration ($3.1 billion) was assigned directly to private insurance. It was assumed that 90% of vehicle damage (estimated at $3.8 billion) was paid by private insurance and 10% was borne by victims of DUIs. Most states have laws requiring automobile liability insurance, although it is common for policies to not cover collision or to have high deductibles. Automobile insurance premiums (including liability) were $104.5 billion in 1992,[32] several times greater than estimated vehicle damage, suggesting that it is justified to assume that most of this cost was borne by private insurance. It was assumed that of the $2.9 billion in legal–court costs that 20% were state and local costs for court expenses, and that alcohol abusers and victims of alcohol-related crashes had equal levels of expenses (about $1.15 billion each). For the burden of fire damage ($1.6 billion), it is assumed that 90% of the alcohol-related fire damage was paid by private insurance and that 10% was borne by nonabusing victims of such incidents. Fire insurance premiums were $7.1 billion in 1992, just about equal to the value of structural fire losses,[32] which suggests that insurance does pay for most fire losses.

7.9. *Victims of Crime*

Crime losses of $1 billion for alcohol are assumed to have been borne by crime victims in the form of lost earnings. It is conceivable that some if not much of the earnings losses were borne by insurance mechanisms such as sick leave or disability insurance, but for purposes of these calculations it is assumed that victims bore all of these costs. Another cost borne by victims of alcohol-related property crime is the lost cash and property valued at $427 million due to alcohol-related property crime. This value likewise accrues to the benefit of those engaging in crime and serves to offset lost legitimate income. Insurance might offset some of these losses as well. Such losses are again a transfer, albeit involuntary, from one segment of society to another. Thus, the value is not included directly in the calculation of the total economic costs to society, but does figure in the calculations of who bears what part of the total burden.

7.10. *Incarceration and Crime Career Losses—Lost Legitimate Earnings*

There is a substantial loss of potential productivity to the economy from incarceration of alcohol abusers ($5.4 billion, respectively). Almost 140,000 inmates were incarcerated in 1992 because of alcohol-defined and related crimes. While this $5.4 billion in lost potential productivity (almost $39,000 per inmate year) initially constitutes a loss to the inmate, the burden is shifted somewhat as noted in Section 7.5 because of losses in government tax and insurance trust revenues. This loss of potential tax revenue—government spends 30% of NNP (17% federal and 13% state and local), equal to almost $12,000 per inmate year—compounds the cost of keeping inmates incarcerated (about $20,000 per year). It is also likely that members of alcohol abusers' households may require or receive social welfare payments because a potential income earner is incarcerated. However, these costs have not been estimated. Alcohol abusers stole an estimated $427 million, respectively, in cash and property through personal crimes in 1992, and this was borne by victims. No estimates are available for commercial theft losses.

7.11. Summary

The economic costs of alcohol problems are distributed across all of society. While significant of costs arguably fall primarily on the abusers, more than half of all of the costs are shifted to other institutions and members of society. Even the costs that may be most likely to fall on the alcohol abusers themselves may be shifted at least partially to members of their households such as children and spouses. It has not been possible to estimate the losses that fall on employers in this study, as prior studies have also been unable to develop such estimates.

Much of the economic burden of alcohol problems falls on the population that does not abuse these substances. Government bears $57.2 billion (38.6%), compared to $15.1 billion for private insurance, $8.9 billion for victim losses, and $66.8 for alcohol abusers and members of their households.

Costs are imposed on society (nonabusers) in the first instance through alcohol-related crimes and trauma (e.g., motor vehicle crashes), and secondly through government services such as criminal justice and highway safety; they are often spread across society as a whole through social insurance mechanisms such as private and public health insurance, life insurance, pensions, and social welfare insurance.

8. Updated Estimates for 1995

Total costs of alcohol abuse are estimated to have increased 12.5% between 1992 and 1995 (Table VIII). Alcohol abuse costs are an estimated $166.5 billion for 1995. The update estimates incorporate adjustments for population growth (about 1% per year) and price changes (different rates for consumer and medical prices, and for wage increases); however, no adjustment is made for potential changes in the incidence and prevalence of alcohol problems over this period.

Table VIII. Updated Cost Estimates: 1992 Estimates and Inflation- and Population-Adjusted Costs of Substance Abuse for 1995[a]

	1992	1995
Specialty substance abuse services	$5,573	$6,660
Comorbid health problems	$13,247	$15,830
Lost earnings—premature death	$31,327	$34,921
Lost earnings—illness	$69,209	$77,150
Crashes and crime	$22,204	$24,752
Other indirect (incarceration)	$6,461	$7,231
Total	$148,021	$166,543

[a]Millions of current year dollars. Adjustments for population growth and wage and price inflation, respectively.

References

1. Hodgson TA, Meiners MR: *Guidelines for Cost-of-Illness Studies in the Public Health Service.* Bethesda, MD, Public Health Service Task Force on Cost-of-Illness Studies, 1979.
2. Hodgson TA, Meiners MR: Cost-of-illness methodology: A guide to current practices and procedures. *Milbank Q* 60(3):429–462, 1982.
3. Harwood H, Fountain D, Livermore G, *et al: Economic Costs of Alcohol and Drug Abuse in the United States: 1992.* Report to the National Institute on Drug Abuse and the National Institute on Alcohol Abuse and Alcoholism. Fairfax, VA, The Lewin Group, 1998.
4. Rice DP, Kelman S, Miller LS, *et al: The Economic Costs of Alcohol and Drug Abuse and Mental Illness: 1985.* DHHS Publication No. (ADM) 90-1964. Washington, DC, US Department of Health and Human Services, 1990.
5. Grant B, Harford T, Dawson D, *et al:* Prevalence of DSM-IV alcohol abuse and dependence. *Alcohol Health Res World* 18(3):243–248, 1994.
6. National Institute on Alcohol Abuse and Alcoholism: *Eighth Special Report to the US Congress on Alcohol and Health.* 1993.
7. Reynolds D: The cost of road accidents. *J R Stat Soc* 119, 1956.
8. Rice DP: *Estimating the Cost of Illness.* Health Economics Series, No. 6. DHEW Publication No. (PHS)947-6. Rockville, MD, US Department of Health, Education and Welfare, 1966.
9. Fein R: *Economics of Mental Illness.* New York, Basic Books, 1958.
10. Pritchard HM: Economic costs of abuse of and dependency on alcohol in Australia, in Kiloh LG, Bell DS (eds): *Proceedings of the 29th International Congress on Alcoholism and Drug Dependence, February 1970.* Sydney, Australia, Butterworths, 1971.
11. Berry R, Boland J: *The Economic Costs of Alcohol Abuse—1972.* Brookline, MA, Policy Analysis, Inc. 1973.
12. Berry R, Boland J, Smart C, *et al: The Economic Costs of Alcohol Abuse—1975.* Brookline, MA, Policy Analysis, Inc., 1977.
13. Collins DJ, Lapsley HM: *Estimating the Economic Costs of Drug Abuse in Australia.* National Campaign Against Drug Abuse, Monograph Series No. 15. Canberra, Australian Government Printing Service, 1991.
14. Single E, Robson L, Xie X, *et al: The Costs of Substance Abuse in Canada.* Toronto, The Canadian Centre on Substance Abuse, University of Toronto, 1996.
15. Mullahy J, Sindelar J: Gender differences in labor market effects of alcoholism. *Am Econ Rev* 81(2):161–165, 1991.
16. Mullahy J, Sindelar J: Alcoholism, work, and income over the life cycle. *J Labor Econ* 11(3):494–520, 1993.
17. Stinson FS, Dufour MC, Steffens RA, *et al:* Alcohol-related mortality in the United States, 1979–1989. *Alcohol Health Res World* 17(3):251–260, 1993.
18. Eaton W, Kessler L: *Epidemiologic Field Methods in Psychiatry: The NIMH Epidemiologic Catchment Area Program.* Orlando, FL, Academic Press, 1985.
19. Grant B, Dawson D: Alcohol and drug use, abuse and dependence among welfare recipients. *Am J Public Health* 86(10):1450–1454, 1996.
20. US Department of Health and Human Services, Office of the Assistant Secretary for Planning and Evaluation, Public Health Service, National Institutes of Health, National Institute on Drug Abuse: *Patterns of Substance Use and Program Participation.* Washington, DC, National Institute on Drug Abuse, 1994.
21. Weisner C, Schmidt L: Alcohol and drug problems among diverse health and social service populations. *Am J Public Health* 83(6):824–829, 1993.
22. Harwood H, Thomson M, Nesmith T: *Healthcare Reform and Substance Abuse Treatment: The Cost of Financing under Alternative Approaches.* Fairfax, VA, Lewin-VHI, 1994.
23. US Department of Justice: *Sourcebook of Criminal Justice Statistics—1993.* Washington, DC, Bureau of Justice Statistics, 1994.

24. Blincoe L, Faigin B: *Economic Costs of Motor Vehicle Crashes—1990.* Washington, DC, National Highway Transportation Safety Administration, 1992.
25. Cruze AM, Harwood HJ, Kristiansen PC, *et al: Economic Costs to Society of Alcohol and Drug Abuse and Mental Illness, 1977.* Research Triangle Park, NC, Research Triangle Institute, 1981.
26. Harwood HJ, Napolitano DM, Christensen PL, *et al: Economic Costs to Society of Alcohol and Drug Abuse and Mental Illness: 1980.* Report to Alcohol, Drug Abuse, and Mental Health Administration. Research Triangle Park, NC, Research Triangle Institute, 1984.
27. Heien DM, Pittman DJ: The economic cost of alcohol abuse: An assessment of current methods and estimates. *J Stud Alcohol* 50:567–579, 1989.
28. National Association of State Alcohol and Drug Abuse Directors: *State Resources and Services Related to Alcohol and Other Drug Problems for Fiscal year 1992.* Washington, DC, Author, 1994.
29. Office of National Drug Control Policy: *National Drug Control Strategy: Budget Summary.* Washington, DC, Government Printing Office, 1995.
30. Office of Management and Budget: *Budget of the United States Government: 1994.* Washington, DC, Government Printing Office, 1993.
31. National Center for Health Statistics: *Health United States 1994.* DHHS Publication No. (PHS) 95-1232. Washington, DC, US Department of Health and Human Services, 1995.
32. US Department of Commerce: *Statistical Abstract of the United States—1995.* Washington, DC, Bureau of the Census, 1995.

12

The Effects of Price on the Consequences of Alcohol Use and Abuse

Frank J. Chaloupka, Michael Grossman, and Henry Saffer

Abstract. Economists have examined the impact of alcohol prices on various outcomes related to alcohol consumption, including nonfatal and fatal motor vehicle accidents, other accidents, liver cirrhosis, and other alcohol-related mortality, crime, and education attainment. Price, in the context of this research, includes not only the monetary price of alcoholic beverages, but also a wide variety of other "costs" of drinking and heavy drinking, including the time spent obtaining alcoholic beverages and the legal costs associated with drinking and related behavior. This research clearly demonstrates that increases in the monetary prices of alcoholic beverages, which could be achieved by increasing taxes on alcohol, can significantly reduce many of the problems associated with alcohol use and abuse. In addition, control policies that raise other "costs" of drinking, including reduced availability of alcoholic beverages, higher legal drinking ages, and others, are also effective in reducing the consequences of alcohol use and abuse.

1. Introduction

In this chapter, we summarize the research by economists that examines the impact of the price of alcoholic beverages on a variety of outcomes related to

Frank J. Chaloupka • Department of Economics, University of Illinois at Chicago, Chicago, Illinois 60607; and Health Economics Program, National Bureau of Economic Research, New York, New York 10017-5405. **Michael Grossman** • Department of Economics, City University of New York Graduate School, New York, New York 10036; and Health Economics Program, National Bureau of Economic Research, New York, New York 10017-5405. **Henry Saffer** • Department of Economics, Kean University, Union, New Jersey 07083; and Health Economics Program, National Bureau of Economic Research, New York, New York 10017-5405.

Recent Developments in Alcoholism, Volume 14: The Consequences of Alcoholism, edited by Galanter. Plenum Press, New York, 1998.

alcohol consumption, including nonfatal motor vehicle accidents, other potentially alcohol-related accidents, liver cirrhosis mortality, crime, and educational attainment. Since the early 1980s, a growing number of economists have been researching the impact of price on alcohol consumption and its consequences. This research uses a wide variety of aggregate and individual data and generally concludes that increases in the price of alcoholic beverages, by reducing drinking, heavy drinking, and related behavior, are effective in reducing the consequences of alcohol use and abuse. These findings are clearly relevant for policymakers, given that there are a number of aspects of price that are policy manipulable.

Price, in the context of economic research on problems related to alcohol use and misuse, includes not only the monetary price of alcoholic beverages, but also a wide variety of other "costs" of drinking and heavy drinking. The other costs of drinking and related behavior that are commonly included in this research are the time costs of obtaining alcoholic beverages as well as the expected legal costs associated with drinking and related behavior.

Federal, state, and local government policies have raised many aspects of the "full price" of alcoholic beverages in the antidrinking campaign of the past 20 years. Until recently, higher monetary prices for alcoholic beverages, which could be achieved by increased taxation, have generally been ignored in the antidrinking campaign. In January 1991, federal excise taxes on beer and wine were raised for the first time since November 1951, while the tax on distilled spirits was raised for only the second time during that period. As a result of Title XI of the Omnibus Budget Reconciliation Act of 1990, the federal beer excise tax was doubled from 16 cents per six-pack to 32 cents, while the tax on wine was raised nearly sevenfold, from just over 3 cents per 750-ml bottle to about 21 cents. This act also increased the distilled spirits tax by $1.00 per proof gallon, raising the tax from $2.00 per fifth of 80-proof alcohol to $2.16. While there is some evidence that Congress may have been persuaded by the health promotion aspects of higher alcoholic beverage taxes,[1] these increases were well below those recommended by numerous public health organizations. They also fell far short of the 25-cent tax per ounce of pure alcohol in any beverage that was initially proposed by the Bush Administration (the rates resulting from the 1991 tax increase are approximately 10 cents, 7 cents, and 21 cents for beer, wine, and distilled spirits, respectively).

Like the federal government, state and local governments have raised taxes on alcohol modestly and infrequently, almost always with the intent of increasing revenues rather than discouraging alcohol use and abuse. Due in part to the stability of these taxes, the real prices for alcoholic beverages (i.e., their prices after accounting for the effects of inflation) have declined significantly over time. For example, between 1975 and 1990, the real price of distilled spirits fell by 32%, the real price of wine fell by 28%, and the real price of beer fell by 20%.

The 1991 increases in the federal alcoholic beverage excise taxes fell far short of those needed to offset the effects of inflation since 1951. For example, the distilled spirits tax would have needed to have been more than four times larger than what was enacted ($8.80 per fifth of 80 proof liquor) to have the same real value as it had in 1951. Similarly, more than a fivefold increase in the beer tax, to 84 cents per six-pack, would have been needed. The increase in the wine tax, however, was large enough to offset the effects of inflation since 1951. If alcohol abuse is affected by price, as economists have argued,[2,3] then allowing the real value of alcoholic beverage taxes and consequently prices to decline will exacerbate the problems associated with alcohol use and abuse.

In contrast to their relative inactivity with respect to raising alcoholic beverage taxes, the federal, state, and local governments have engaged in an active campaign over the past two decades to reduce heavy drinking and its consequences. Much of this campaign has focused on youths and young adults, given the disproportionate incidence of alcohol-related problems in this population. The most important element of the antidrinking campaign with respect to adolescent alcohol abuse has been the upward trend in state minimum legal ages for the purchase and consumption of alcoholic beverages. The Twenty-sixth Amendment, which lowered the voting age from 21 to 18 years in 1972, led 29 states to reduce their legal drinking ages in the period from 1970 to 1975. This downward trend was reversed, however, when Minnesota raised its drinking age from 18 to 19 years in 1976. This was followed by increases in 27 other states prior to the passage of the Federal Uniform Drinking Age Act of 1984 (Public Law 98-363). This act accelerated the upward trend by withholding federal highway funds from states that failed to raise drinking ages on all alcoholic beverages to 21 years by October 1, 1986. By 1987, all states had complied, although grandfather clauses in some states kept the effective age below 21 years until 1990. Increases in the legal drinking age are expected to significantly raise the full price of alcoholic beverages to youth by reducing availability and increasing the expected legal costs of drinking.

Other policies in the antidrinking campaign have targeted all segments of the population and focus on problems related to alcohol use and abuse. For example, the Federal Alcohol Traffic Safety Act of 1983 (Public Law 97-364), provided financial incentives for states to adopt and enforce more stringent policies related to drinking and driving. These measures include easing the standards required for arresting and convicting drunk drivers, more severe and certain penalties for conviction of drunk driving, and the increased allocation of resources for the apprehending drunk drivers. In the several years after this Act, hundreds of new state and local laws related to drinking and driving were adopted.[4,5] Moreover, this trend shows no signs of abating, with numerous new and stronger laws being enacted throughout the 1990s. In addition to the laws targeting all drinking drivers, several states have recently adopted laws targeting underage drinking drivers by making it per se illegal to drive with either blood alcohol concentrations well below those used for adults or, in some states, any measurable amount of alcohol (the so-called "zero tolerance" laws).

These new laws were designed to both punish drunk drivers and to deter others from drinking and driving. The assumption of rational behavior provides a foundation for the deterrence effect. While driving when drunk may not be a rational decision, the joint decision to drink and then drive can be thought of as a rational process. In his economic theory of crime, recent Nobel laureate Gary S. Becker[6] shows that the number of offenses committed by an individual is inversely related to the cost of each offense. In the context of drunk driving, the laws increasing the probabilities of arrest and conviction for drunken driving, as well as those raising the penalties upon conviction, raise the cost of drinking and driving.

Another key element in the antidrinking campaign is Public Law 100-690, which, since November 1989, has required that all alcoholic beverages sold in the United States must carry a warning label informing drinkers of such dangers as drunk driving, drinking during pregnancy, and other (unspecified) health problems. The warning label can raise the full price of alcoholic beverages by raising the perceived health costs of drinking.

In addition to reducing the availability of alcohol to youth, many states and localities have adopted other policies that limit availability for all drinkers. These include regulations that limit the places and/or times where alcoholic beverages can be sold, as well as dram shop laws (either statutes or case laws), which hold servers liable for the harmful actions of their patrons who drink to excess. In many states, there are special provisions in the dram shop laws that relate to serving underage drinkers. By raising the full price of drinking and excessive drinking, these limits on availability can reduce the consequences of alcohol use and abuse. Other policies that are becoming increasingly prevalent, including restricting or banning "happy hours," training and/or licensing servers, penalizing parents who allow underage drinking parties in their homes, can also raise various components of the full price of drinking and consequently reduce the consequences of alcohol use and abuse.

2. Theoretical and Analytical Framework

Perhaps the most fundamental principle of economics is that of the downward sloping demand curve that states that as the price of any good rises, the consumption of that good falls. Noneconomists, as well as some economists, have argued that the consumption of a potentially addictive good, such as alcohol, might be an exception to this rule. However, numerous econometric studies,[2] including those that explicitly model the addictive aspects of consumption,[3,7,8] confirm that this principle does apply to the demand for alcoholic beverages.

However, the impact of price on outcomes related to alcohol use and abuse in part depends on the effect of price on different patterns of drinking, which may differ with respect to the frequency and/or quantity of alcohol consumption. For example, it may be that the heaviest drinkers and/or binge drinkers are relatively insensitive to price,[9,10] implying that while price increases may reduce overall alcohol consumption, they would have little impact on outcomes related to excessive or abusive consumption. Alternatively, recent theoretical economic models of addictive behavior[3,11,12] predict that addicted consumers will be more price responsive in the long run than their nonaddicted counterparts.

The empirical model used in many of the economic analyses of the effects of price on outcomes related to alcohol use and abuse can be derived from a theoretical model consisting of two equations. The first is termed a "production function," which describes how alcohol consumption (A) and various other inputs ($\mathbf{X}$) are related to a particular output (y):

$$y = f(A, \mathbf{X}) \tag{1}$$

In the context of this chapter, the outputs include motor vehicle or other accidents, deaths from liver cirrhosis, crime related to alcohol use and abuse, and educational attainment. The vector $\mathbf{X}$ contains other factors related to the outcome; for example, when modeling motor vehicle accidents, this vector includes variables that measure traffic density, roadway conditions, vehicle quality, and other motor vehicle safety measures.

The second equation is the demand for alcohol:

$$A = g(p, \mathbf{Z}) \tag{2}$$

where p reflects the full price of drinking and the vector $\mathbf{Z}$ captures other determinants of demand, including income, the prices of complements to or substitutes for alcohol, and other determinants of tastes. Again, the full price includes not only the monetary price of alcoholic beverages, but also other costs associated with drinking in the context being examined. For example, when examining drinking and driving, A reflects the demand for alcohol shortly before or while driving, while the full price of alcohol in this context includes the monetary price, measures of alcohol availability, the probabilities of apprehension and conviction for drunken driving, and the penalties associated with apprehension and conviction.

Substituting the alcohol demand equation (2) into the production function (1) produces a reduced form equation in which the effects of price and other factors on outcomes related to alcohol consumption can be estimated:

$$y = f(p, \mathbf{X}, \mathbf{Z}) \tag{3}$$

This equation can either be estimated using data on individuals or it can be aggregated across individuals.

3. Review of Empirical Studies

3.1. Drinking, Driving, and Motor Vehicle Accidents

There have been a large number of econometric studies estimating the effects of the full price of alcohol on drinking and driving in the United States.[5,13–34] Nearly all of these studies use alternative measures of aggregate motor vehicle accident fatality rates as the measure of drinking and driving, given the evidence that alcohol plays a significant role in many of these fatal accidents.[35] Most of these studies employ state level data, although some employ county level data[29–31] and still others use other aggregate measures.[23] A relatively small number of studies use self-reported, individual level data on drinking and driving and/or involvement in nonfatal traffic accidents.[20,21,24,26,34]

The motor vehicle accident fatality measures used in these studies are generally constructed from the National Highway Traffic Safety Administration's (NHTSA) Fatal Accident Reporting System (FARS) and are expressed as rates (i.e., deaths per person in the relevant population). Some, however, use alternative measures such as deaths per mile of roadway or deaths per mile traveled. Many of these studies include measures of fatality rates defined for all age groups, while a large number also include a variety of age-specific fatality rates, including several focused on teenagers and young adults (generally ages 15 through 17 years, 18 through 20 years, and 21 through 25 years). Similarly, a wide variety of motor vehicle accident fatality rates are defined based on anticipated alcohol involvement. For example, in addition to total motor vehicle accident fatality rates, several researchers use measures based on the time of day, given that alcohol is much more likely to be involved in nighttime fatal accidents than in daytime accidents.[36] Similarly, several measures are based on the role of the individual killed in the accident (driver, passenger, pedestrian/other) as well as the number of vehicles involved in the accident. Finally, Chaloupka *et al.*[18] use the information on blood alcohol concentration (BAC) of dead drivers to construct measures of alcohol-involved driver fatality rates based on a BAC of 0.05%, the level used by most states to define alcohol involvement.

3.1.1. Alcoholic Beverage Taxes and Prices. The most commonly used measure for the monetary price of alcoholic beverages in these studies is the excise tax on beer. This choice is made for a variety of reasons, most notably because beer is the most popular alcoholic beverage in the United States and because meaningful data on wine and distilled spirits taxes are only available for states that license the sale of all alcoholic beverages. In addition, some have argued (Ruhm,[19] for example) that the tax is a more relevant measure for policymakers as well as that the tax can be considered exogenous, while the price may depend on the interaction of the supply and demand for alcoholic beverages.

Finally, a few studies, most notably those using individual level data, have employed actual alcoholic beverage price data (either for beer or for a composite alcoholic beverage based on a weighted average of the prices of beer, wine, and distilled spirits).

Nearly every study that includes a measure of the price of alcoholic beverages concludes that higher prices lead to significant reductions in drinking and driving. This is true not only for self-reported measures of drinking and driving, but for both nonfatal and fatal accidents related to drinking and driving. For example, Kenkel[20] estimates that a 10% increase in price would reduce the probability of drinking and driving by approximately 7.4% for males and 8.1% for females. Moreover, he predicts even larger reductions in drinking and driving by those ages 21 years and under, with the 10% price increase expected to reduce drinking and driving by 12.6% and 21.1% for young males and young females, respectively.

Kenkel's estimates from the individual level data are consistent with the predicted effects of alcoholic beverage price increases in the aggregate data. For example, a 10% increase in price is predicted to reduce overall motor vehicle accident fatalities by between 5 and 10%.[5,13,18,19] Measures of fatality rates that reflect greater levels of alcohol involvement (i.e., single vehicle nighttime driver rates, BAC-based estimates of alcohol involved fatality rates) are found to be more responsive to changes in alcoholic beverage prices than overall measures of fatality rates, as expected. Similarly, price is found to have a greater impact on motor vehicle accident fatalities for younger persons, which was expected given the research that finds that youth drinking and heavy drinking is more responsive to price than adult drinking (i.e., Kenkel[20]) and that younger individuals have less experience with both driving and drinking. The estimates from studies that employ youth motor vehicle accident fatality rates predict that a 10% increase in alcoholic beverage prices would reduce youth fatalities by between 7 to 17%.[14,15,18,19]

3.1.2. Alcohol Availability. Several measures of alcohol availability, an additional component of the full price of alcoholic beverages, are employed in the various econometric studies of drinking and driving. Studies of youth and young adult drinking and driving, as well as many of those that look at other age groups, include a measure of the minimum legal drinking age for alcoholic beverages. Higher minimum legal drinking ages are expected to increase the amount of time a youth spends obtaining alcohol, whether it results from spending additional time and money to obtain fake identification or from spending time finding a store that does not demand proof of age.

Virtually every study that examines the impact of drinking ages on youth drinking and driving concludes that higher minimum legal drinking ages significantly reduce self-reported drinking and driving as well as fatal accidents related to drinking and driving.[14–16,18–20,27,34]

Kenkel,[20] for example, predicts that a nationally uniform legal drinking age of 21 years for all alcoholic beverages—an increase of about 2 years in the average legal drinking age for his sample—would have reduced self-reported drinking and driving among young males by 14% and among young females by 21% in 1985. Similarly, Chaloupka *et al.*[18] predict that had a uniform drinking age of 21 years been in effect for the years 1982 through 1988, motor vehicle accident fatalities among 18- to 20-year-olds would have been reduced by just over 3% per year. In contrast, they predict that a uniform age of 18 years would have raised fatalities in this group by nearly 10% per year.

Another commonly used measure of availability captures localities that prohibit the sale of alcoholic beverages ("dry areas") or other limits on alcoholic beverage sales (i.e., restrictions on sales for on-premise consumption). Some have argued that these types of restrictions encourage more driving and increase the likelihood of drinking and driving[32,33] (the same argument can be made for higher drinking ages leading to more underage drinking and driving by youth living in high drinking age states but who live near low drinking age states). However, most have argued that these types of limits on availability significantly increase the time and travel costs associated with obtaining alcohol, which should reduce consumption and related outcomes.

Several of the studies using state aggregates have included a variable measuring the fraction of the state population that resides in dry areas[14,15,18] in an effort to examine the impact of availability on motor vehicle accidents. Others have used an indicator for dry counties in studies employing county level data for a single state over time.[29,30] These studies produce consistently strong evidence that restricting the availability of alcoholic beverages leads to significant reductions in motor vehicle accident fatality rates.

Jewell and Brown,[29] in their study using data on 254 Texas counties, present some interesting estimates of the responsiveness of various accident rates to changes in time and travel costs associated with obtaining alcoholic beverages. They estimate that a 10% increase in the time and travel costs leads to a 4.5% reduction in the probability of a fatal accident and a 5.6% reduction in the probability of a fatal or nonfatal accident. These estimates are consistent with the range estimated for the effects of the money price of alcoholic beverages on fatal accidents.

Several recent studies have included indicators for states with dram shop laws as an additional measure of availability.[18,19,23] Dram shop laws are expected to reduce availability, since these laws hold the person or establishment that served the alcohol liable for the damages caused by intoxicated patrons. In general, these studies find that dram shop laws significantly reduce the probability of a fatal motor vehicle accident, supporting the hypothesis that these laws are effective in reducing the availability of alcohol. In general, the dram shop laws are found to have less of an impact on drinking and driving by youth.[18,19] Chaloupka *et al.*[18] argue that this is to be expected, given that underage drinkers are likely to have difficulty being served in the on-premise drinking establishments where the dram shop laws are expected to have their greatest impact.

3.1.3. Laws Related to Drinking and Driving. Several recent studies have attempted to analyze a wide variety of state legislation and other activities related to drinking and driving.[5,16–21,24–26,28] The expected legal costs of drinking and driving (a component of the full price of alcohol) will rise with increases in the expected probabilities of apprehension and conviction as well as with an increase in the penalties imposed upon conviction. The use of sobriety checkpoints, increased police activity, open container laws, and laws allowing the prearrest use of a preliminary breath test to establish probable cause for a driving under the influence (DUI) arrest are likely to raise the probability of detection and apprehension of drunk drivers. Similarly, per se illegal laws, which make it an offense to operate a motor vehicle with a BAC level above some specified level (generally 0.10%), and no plea bargaining laws are likely to significantly increase the probability of conviction for DUI. Finally, administrative per se laws and mandatory minimum penalties can raise the penalties upon either arrest or conviction for DUI.

In general, there is little, if any, consensus produced in the numerous studies of the impact of DUI laws on motor vehicle accident fatalities related to drinking and driving. For example, estimating fixed effects models with state level data from 1975 through 1986, Evans, Neville, and Graham[6] conclude that none of their individual measures (including preliminary breath tests, sobriety checkpoints, no plea bargaining provisions, mandatory jail sentences, illegal per se laws, open container laws, and administrative license sanctions) significantly reduces drinking and driving. They do, however, suggest that there may be synergistic effects of multiple laws designed to increase the probability of detection and arrest (i.e., sobriety checkpoints and preliminary breath tests).

In contrast, Chaloupka *et al.*,[18] using annual state aggregates from 1982 through 1988 and a more comprehensive set of laws related to DUI, conclude that several of these laws do act as deterrents to drinking and driving. For example, while existing administrative license laws with relatively weak penalties were found to have little impact, they find that a relatively severe mandatory administrative license suspension of 1 year would lead to significant reductions in fatal accidents related to drinking and driving. They make similar conclusions with respect to mandatory minimum fines and license sanctions upon conviction for DUI, although these have less of an impact than the administrative actions. Finally, they find that preliminary breath test laws and no plea bargaining provisions also deter drunk driving, while other laws—open container laws and mandatory jail sentence and community service—did not.

In the most recent comprehensive evaluation of the impact of drunk driving laws on fatality rates, Ruhm[19] attempts to examine the stability of the estimated effects of these laws across a variety of model specifications. He suggests that one reason for the differences in estimates among earlier studies is that they include different sets of explanatory variables (not only for the drunk driving laws but for a variety of other factors likely to be related to drinking and driving) and that the omission of potentially key variables in each may bias the estimates for the included variables. To at least partially address this problem, Ruhm estimates fixed effects models, which include a relatively comprehensive set of explanatory variables. In addition, he examines a variety of different model specifications to determine how the omission of some variables affects the estimates for the included variables. He does find sharp differences for the estimates obtained from alternative models specifications, with the estimated impact of some policies falling by as much as 70% when more complete specifications are estimated. Among the various drunk driving laws he examines, only the administrative per se laws are found to consistently deter drinking and driving.

3.1.4. Other Issues. In an interesting paper, Sloan and Githens[24] merge automobile insurance data with self-reported individual level data on drinking and drinking and driving to examine the impact of state-mandated automobile insurance premium surcharges on the probability of drinking and driving. These surcharges could be viewed as an additional legal cost of drinking and driving and therefore as an additional component of the full price of alcoholic beverages. They conclude that these surcharges do significantly reduce drunk driving, estimating that a $1000 surcharge for the first DUI offense would reduce the probability of drinking and driving by 50% among those who drink.

3.2. Health

3.2.1. Liver Cirrhosis Mortality. One commonly used measure of long-term heavy alcohol consumption is the liver cirrhosis mortality rate. Cook and Tauchen[37] were the first to use this indicator to explore the possibility that heavy drinking is responsive to price. Using annual state-level measures of per capita distilled spirits consumption and liver cirrhosis mortality rates for states that license the private sale of alcoholic beverages over the period from 1962 through 1977, Cook and Tauchen[37] examine the impact of increases in distilled spirits excise taxes. They conclude that the state excise tax rate on distilled spirits has a negative and statistically significant effect on both consumption and cirrhosis mortality rates. Moreover, they estimate that a $1 increase in the distilled spirits tax would reduce per capita consumption by 6.2% and that cirrhosis deaths would fall by approximately the same amount (between 5.4 and 10.8%). Cook and Tauchen[37] conclude that "liquor consumption, including consumption of heavy drinkers, is quite responsive to price" (p. 387). This finding contradicted the then-conventional wisdom that addictive alcohol consumption was not responsive to price.

More recently, Chaloupka *et al.*[7] apply an economic model of addictive behavior[3,11,12] to similar outcomes using state level data for all states of the United States and the District of Columbia from 1961 through 1984. The theoretical and empirical model employed in this research explicitly accounts for the tolerance, reinforcement, and withdrawal that distinguish the consumption of an addictive substance from the consumption of a nonaddictive substance. Specifically, unlike nonaddictive models, the intertemporal linkages in the demand for addictive substances are captured by making current consumption decisions dependent on past choices. In addition, this research treats addicts as rational in the sense that they take account, at least partially, of the future consequences of their addictive consumption decisions. This is in contrast to myopic models of addiction that assume that addicts completely ignore the future implications of their addictive consumption. Perhaps the most important implication of this model is that the long-term effect of price on addictive consumption will be larger than the short-term effect.

Three outcomes related to alcohol consumption are examined: per capita distilled spirits consumption, per capita total alcohol consumption, and the age-adjusted liver cirrhosis mortality rate for the population age 30 and older (as a measure of addictive alcohol consumption). The measure of price employed in this research is an index based on the prices of the three leading brands of distilled spirits during the time period covered by the data.

Chaloupka and co-workers'[7] estimate indicates that per capita distilled spirits consumption and total alcohol consumption are not characterized by addictive behavior. This is not surprising, given that there are many light, moderate, and infrequent drinkers who are not addicted to alcohol. Nevertheless, aggregate alcohol demand was found to be quite responsive to price. In addition, the estimates do indicate that long-term heavy alcohol consumption, as reflected by the liver cirrhosis mortality rate, is an addictive behavior. These estimates imply a permanent 10% increase in the price of alcoholic beverages would lead to a long-term reduction of 8.3 to 12.8% in addictive consumption.

3.2.2. Other Health Consequences of Alcohol Use and Abuse. Sloan *et al.*[25] examine the impact of the full price of alcoholic beverages on a variety of state level death rates related to alcohol use and abuse for the period from 1982 through 1988. The death rates were constructed from the vital statistics data on mortality for the 48 contiguous states of the United States, and capture deaths in six categories: (1) diseases where alcohol is the primary cause, as identified by the decedent's physician (including liver cirrhosis); (2) motor vehicle traffic accidents; (3) homicides; (4) suicides; (5) diseases for which alcohol is considered an important contributory cause (includes various cancers); and (6) other accidental deaths frequently related to alcohol use and abuse (including drowning, accidental falls, fires, and others).

Sloan *et al.*[25] constructed state level measures of alcoholic beverage prices from the American Chamber of Commerce Researchers Association quarterly price reports, which were adjusted to reflect changes in the relative prices of alcohol consumed at home compared to out of home during the time period covered by the sample. Various mandatory penalties for DUI conviction, dram shop laws, and alternative measures of police activity were included in the analyses as additional components of the full price of alcoholic beverages.

Sloan *et al.*[25] conclude that the monetary price of alcoholic beverages reduces some mortality rates but does not reduce deaths where alcohol is the primary cause. This is somewhat surprising, given that this measure largely consists of deaths from liver cirrhosis, which others have found to be negatively related to price.[7,37] They do estimate a negative and statistically significant effect of the money price on suicides and on deaths where alcohol is a contributing cause, but they do not find that higher prices would reduce other accidents related to alcohol use. In addition, they find that alcohol availability, as reflected by dram shop laws, does have a significant effect on many of the death rates they estimate, including deaths where alcohol is the primary cause, suicides, and deaths from drowning, falls, and other accidents.

In a similar examination of the impact of alcoholic beverage prices on accidents, Ohsfeldt and Morrisey[38] examine the impact of beer taxes on state level measures of workplace accidents. Using data for the period from 1975 through 1985, they predict that a 25-cent increase in the beer tax in 1992 would have reduced work-loss days from nonfatal work-related injuries by 4.6 million, thereby reducing lost productivity by $491 million. However, they found no effect of availability, as measured by the proportion of the state population in dry areas, on nonfatal workplace accidents.

3.3. *Crime*

Chaloupka and Saffer[39] and Cook and Moore[40] examined the impact of the full price of alcoholic beverages on various crime rates constructed from the Federal Bureau of Investigation's Uniform Crime Reports. Similarly, Sloan *et al.*,[25] as described above, use data from the vital statistics to examine the impact of full price on homicide death rates.

Chaloupka and Saffer[39] use annual state level crime rates for the 50 states of the United States and the District of Columbia, for the period from 1975 through 1990, in their analysis of the impact of alcohol control policies on crime. Ten alternative measures of crime are employed, including: total crime, violent crime, property crime, homicide, rape, assault, robbery, burglary, larceny, and motor vehicle theft. Using the beer tax as their measure of the monetary price of alcoholic beverages, they conclude that increases in price would lead to statistically significant reductions in nearly every crime rate; the only crime they find apparently unresponsive to price is assault. Their estimates suggest, for example, that doubling the federal excise tax on beer during the period covered by their data would have reduced total crime rates by approximately 1.3%, homicides and rapes by 3%, robberies by 4.7%, burglaries and larceny by 1.3%, and motor vehicle thefts by 3%.

Somewhat surprisingly, given that a disproportionate share of crime is committed by youths and young adults, Chaloupka and Saffer[39] find no evidence that higher minimum legal drinking ages reduce crime. However, they do find strong evidence that there is a positive relationship between increased availability of alcoholic beverages and all measures of crime.

Similarly, Cook and Moore[40] use the state level data from the Uniform

Crime Reports for the period from 1979 through 1987 to examine the impact of per capita alcohol consumption on violent crime rates. Using fixed effects models in which the only independent variable other than state and year indicators was the measure of alcohol consumption, they find that there is a significant relationship between consumption and assault, rape, and burglary, but do not find a significant effect of consumption on homicide. Given the literature that finds an inverse relationship between drinking and alcoholic beverage prices, they then estimate the effects of beer taxes on the various crime rates. They conclude that higher beer taxes would significantly reduce rapes and robberies, predicting that a 10% increase in the tax would lead to 1.3% and 0.9% reductions in the number of rapes and robberies, respectively.

Finally, Sloan *et al.*,[25] using the data described above, find evidence that higher alcoholic beverage prices as well as reduced availability of alcohol significantly reduce homicides.

3.4. Educational Attainment

Two recent studies use data from the National Longitudinal Survey of Youth (NLSY) to examine the impact of alcohol use and heavy use, as well as the full price of alcoholic beverages, on educational attainment.

Yamada *et al.*[41] use the NLSY data to examine the impact of alcohol and marijuana use by high school seniors in 1982 on the probability of high school graduation. They find strong evidence that increases in the frequency of drinking and/or marijuana use, as well as increases in the consumption of wine and distilled spirits, significantly reduce the probability of high school graduation. In addition, using the beer tax as their measure of price, Yamada *et al.* find that drinking by high school seniors is significantly reduced by higher alcoholic beverage prices. Using these estimates, they predict that a 10% increase in the beer tax would raise the probability of high school graduation by approximately 3%. Similarly, they conclude that higher minimum legal drinking ages would also raise the probability of high school graduation.

Cook and Moore[42] use the data for the two youngest cohorts in the NLSY (those aged 14 and 15 when the survey began) as well as a subsample of these data on youth who were high school seniors in 1982 to consider the impact of drinking during high school on post-high school educational attainment. They estimate a structural model consisting of an equation for drinking that includes the beer tax and minimum legal drinking age as measures of the full price of alcoholic beverages, as well as an equation for educational attainment that includes alcohol consumption during high school. In addition, they estimate reduced form models that directly estimate the effects of beer taxes and drinking ages on educational attainment.

Cook and Moore[42] find that frequent drinking during high school significantly reduces post-high school education, with high school seniors who are frequent drinkers going on to complete 2.3 fewer years of college than their less frequent drinking counterparts. In addition, they find strong evidence that higher beer taxes and legal drinking ages are effective in reducing the frequency of drinking by high school seniors. The estimates from their reduced form model provide even clearer evidence that increases in the full price of alcoholic beverages raise educational attainment. Based on these estimates, Cook and Moore[42] predict that, in 1982, raising the beer tax from 10 cents a case to $1 a case would increase the probability of attending and graduating from a 4-year college or university by 6.3%. Similarly, they predict that raising the minimum legal drinking age from 18 years to 21 years would raise the probability of college graduation by 4.2%.

4. Conclusions

This chapter summarized the economic research that examines the impact of the full price of alcoholic beverages on several outcomes related to alcohol use and abuse, including drinking and driving and motor vehicle accidents, health consequences of alcohol consumption, other accidents related to drinking, crime, and educational attainment. This research clearly demonstrates that increases in the monetary prices of alcoholic beverages, which could be achieved by increasing federal, state, and local alcohol taxes, can significantly reduce many of the problems associated with alcohol abuse, as well as improve educational attainment. However, alcoholic beverage prices, in large part because of the infrequent and relatively small changes in federal and state taxes, have been allowed to decline relative to the prices of other goods and services. Given the evidence discussed above, falling prices will lead to increases in many of the problems associated with alcohol use and abuse.

Other policies can be used to offset the impact of declining real prices on the consequences of alcohol use and abuse. For example, the research described in this chapter generally finds a strong positive relationship between the increased availability of alcoholic beverages and the consequences of alcohol use and abuse. Thus, efforts to reduce the availability of alcoholic beverages, including higher minimum legal drinking ages and the widespread adoption of dram shop laws, have been found to be effective in reducing motor vehicle and other accident fatalities related to drinking, crime, and other consequences of alcohol abuse.

References

1. Cook PJ, Moore MJ: Taxation of alcoholic beverages, in Hilton ME, Bloss G (eds): *Economics and the Prevention of Alcohol-Related Problems.* Washington, DC, US Government Printing Office, pp 33–58, 1993.

2. Leung SF, Phelps CE: My kingdom for a drink. . . . ? A review of estimates of the price sensitivity of alcoholic beverages, in Hilton ME, Bloss G (eds): *Economics and the Prevention of Alcohol-Related Problems*. Washington, DC, US Government Printing Office, pp 1–31, 1993.
3. Grossman M: The economic analysis of addictive behavior, in Hilton ME, Bloss G (eds): *Economics and the Prevention of Alcohol-Related Problems*. Washington, DC, US Government Printing Office, pp 91–123, 1993.
4. Ross HL: Deterring drunken driving: An analysis of current efforts. *Alcohol Health Res World* 14:58–62, 1990.
5. Evans WN, Neville D, Graham JD: General deterrence of drunk driving: Evaluation of recent American policies. *Risk Anal* 11:279–289, 1991.
6. Becker GS: Crime and punishment: An economic approach. *J Polit Econ* 76:169–217, 1968.
7. Chaloupka FJ, Grossman M, Becker GS, Murphy KM: Alcohol addiction: An econometric analysis. Presented at the annual meeting of the Allied Social Science Associations, Anaheim, CA, December 1992.
8. Grossman M, Chaloupka FJ, Sirtalan I: An empirical analysis of alcohol addiction: Results from the Monitoring the Future panels. National Bureau of Economic Research Working Paper Number 5200. Cambridge, MA, National Bureau of Economic Research, 1995.
9. Manning WG, Blumberg L, Moulton LH: The demand for alcohol: The differential response to price. *J Health Econ* 14:123–148, 1995.
10. Chaloupka FJ, Wechsler H: Binge drinking in college: The impact of price, availability, and alcohol control policies. *Contemp Econ Policy* 14:112–124, 1996.
11. Becker GS, Murphy KM: A theory of rational addiction. *J Polit Econ* 96:675–700, 1988.
12. Becker GS, Grossman M, Murphy KM: Rational addiction and the effect of price on consumption. *Am Econ Rev* 81:237–241, 1991.
13. Cook PJ: The effect of liquor taxes on drinking, cirrhosis, and auto fatalities, in Moore M, Gerstein D (eds): *Alcohol and Public Policy: Beyond the Shadow of Prohibition*. Washington, DC, National Academy of Sciences, 1981, pp 255–285.
14. Saffer H, Grossman M: Drinking age laws and highway mortality rates: Cause and effect. *Econ Inquiry* 25:403–417, 1987.
15. Saffer H, Grossman M: Beer taxes, the legal drinking age, and youth motor vehicle fatalities. *J Legal Stud* 16:351–374, 1987.
16. Saffer H, Chaloupka FJ: Breath testing and highway fatality rates. *Appl Econ* 21:901–912, 1989.
17. Zador PL, Lund AK, Fields M, Weinberg K: Fatal crash involvement and laws against alcohol-impaired driving. *J Public Health Policy* 10:467–485, 1989
18. Chaloupka FJ, Saffer H, Grossman M: Alcohol control policies and motor vehicle fatalities. *J Legal Stud* 22:161–186, 1993.
19. Ruhm CJ: Alcohol policies and highway vehicle fatalities. *J Health Econ* 15:435–454, 1996.
20. Kenkel DS: Drinking, driving and deterrence: The effectiveness and social costs of alternative policies. *J Law Econ* 36:877–913, 1993.
21. Mullahy J, Sindelar JL: Do drinkers know when to say when? An empirical analysis of drunk driving. *Econ Inquiry* 32:383–394, 1994.
22. Saffer H: Alcohol advertising and motor vehicle fatalities. *Rev Econ Stat* 79(3):431–442, 1997.
23. Sloan FA, Reilly BA, Schenzler CM: Tort liability versus other approaches for deterring careless driving. *Int. Rev Law Econ* 14:53–71, 1994.
24. Sloan FA, Githens PB: Drinking, driving and the price of automobile insurance. *J Risk Insurance* 61:33–58, 1994.
25. Sloan FA, Reilly BA, Schenzler C: Effects of prices, civil and criminal sanctions, and law enforcement on alcohol-related mortality. *J Stud Alcohol* 55:454–465, 1994.
26. Sloan FA, Reilly BA, Schenzler CM: The effects of tort liability and insurance on heavy drinking and drinking and driving. *J Law Econ* 38:49–78, 1995.
27. O'Malley PM, Wagenaar AC: Effects of minimum drinking age laws on alcohol use, related behaviors, and traffic crash involvement among American youth: 1976–1987. *J Stud Alcohol* 52:478–491, 1991.

28. Wilkinson JT: Reducing drunken driving: Which policies are most effective. *South Econ J* 54:322–334, 1987.
29. Jewell RT, Brown RW: Alcohol availability and alcohol-related motor vehicle accidents. *Appl Econ* 27:759–765, 1995.
30. Winn RG, Giacopassi D: Effects of county-level alcohol prohibition on motor vehicle accidents. *Soc Sci Q* 74:783–792, 1993.
31. Blose JO, Holder HD: Liquor-by-the drink and alcohol-related traffic crashes: A natural experiment using time series analysis. *J Stud Alcohol* 48:52–60, 1987.
32. Colon I: County-level prohibition and alcohol-related fatal motor vehicle accidents. *J Safety Res* 14:101–104, 1983.
33. Colon I, Cutter HSG: The relationship of beer consumption and state alcohol and motor vehicle policies to fatal accidents. *J Safety Res* 14:83–89, 1983.
34. Chaloupka FJ, Laixuthai A: Do youths substitute alcohol and marijuana? Some econometric evidence. *Eastern Econ J* 23:253–276, 1997.
35. Zobeck TS, Stinson FS, Grant BF, Bertolucci D: *Trends in Alcohol-Related Traffic Crashes, United States, 1979–1991*. Surveillance Report 26. Washington, DC, National Institute on Alcohol Abuse and Alcoholism, 1993.
36. National Highway Traffic Safety Administration: *Fatal Accident Reporting System, 1984*. Washington, DC, US Department of Transportation, 1986.
37. Cook PJ, Tauchen G: The effect of liquor taxes on heavy drinking. *Bell J Econ* 12:379–390, 1982.
38. Ohsfeldt RL, Morrisey MA: Beer taxes, workers' compensation and industrial injury. *Rev Econ Stat* 79(1):155–160, 1997.
39. Chaloupka FJ, Saffer H: Alcohol, illegal drugs, public policy and crime. Presented at the annual meeting of the Western Economic Association, San Francisco, CA, July 1992.
40. Cook PJ, Moore MJ: Economic perspectives on reducing alcohol-related violence, in Martin SE (ed): *Alcohol and Interpersonal Violence: Fostering Multidisciplinary Perspectives*. Washington, DC, US Government Printing Office, 1993, pp 193–212.
41. Yamada T, Kendix M, Yamada T: The impact of alcohol consumption and marijuana use on high school graduation. *Health Econ* 5:77–92, 1996.
42. Cook PJ, Moore MJ: Drinking and schooling. *J Health Econ* 12:411–430, 1993.

13

Drinking, Problem Drinking, and Productivity

John Mullahy and Jody L. Sindelar

Abstract. This chapter surveys and critiques the recent economic literature dealing with the relationships between labor market productivity and alcohol use and misuse. The focus here is twofold. First is to present and discuss the relevant conceptual issues that must be appreciated in assessing such relationships. Second is to summarize and assess the empirical findings that have been offered in the literature.

1. Introduction

This chapter summarizes what is known about the impact of alcohol on labor market productivity. More specifically, it reviews the literature in the economics field that assesses the impact of alcohol consumption and/or problem drinking on labor market productivity. It has been estimated that about two thirds of the "economic costs" of alcohol use and misuse may be due to reductions in labor productivity, broadly speaking.[1] An examination of the role of drinking and problem drinking as determinants of labor market outcomes is thus of considerable relevance. Various measures of productivity—wages, earnings, income, employment—will be considered. The distinction between alcohol consumption per se and problem drinking as determining productivity will be of particular concern. We use the term *problem drinking* to refer to a category including abusive or dependent drinking and alcoholism.

John Mullahy • Department of Preventive Medicine, Bradley Memorial, University of Wisconsin, Madison, Wisconsin 53706. **Jody L. Sindelar** • Department of Epidemiology and Public Health, Yale University School of Medicine, New Haven, Connecticut 06520.

Recent Developments in Alcoholism, Volume 14: The Consequences of Alcoholism, edited by Galanter. Plenum Press, New York, 1998.

This discussion is selective in two respects. First, the research surveyed is drawn primarily from the economics literature and the focus is on productivity impacts of alcohol. Second, the discussion is confined for the most part to relatively recent research. For a review of earlier literature see ref. 1 and Chapter 11, this volume.

Finally, more information on the topics discussed in this chapter is available in several useful surveys: Cook[2] provides a general overview of economic aspects of alcohol-related problems; Mullahy[3] assesses the economic aspects of labor market productivity and drinking; and Sindelar[4] reviews differences by gender in the impact of alcoholism on productivity.

2. Alcohol Use and Labor Market Outcomes

2.1. *Wages, Earnings, Income, and the Use and Abuse of Alcoholic Beverages*

2.1.1. Conceptual and Methodological Issues. Labor market productivity or labor market success can be measured variously by using measures of wages, earnings, income, labor supply, and employment. Alcohol consumption or problem drinking also can be measured in many ways. Thus, in making comparisons across studies, differences in measures used must be considered. Although there are variations in measures used, most economists take a similar perspective in statistical formulations. In most cases, productivity is treated (at least implicitly) as if it were causally determined by alcohol use or misuse. Such "structural relationships" are at least implicit in statistical formulations in which the productivity measure is treated as the outcome variable and the relevant alcohol measure is included among the explanatory covariates. However, the possibility that alcohol consumption or problem drinking is correlated with unobserved determinants of labor market outcomes must be addressed statistically in order to appropriately interpret causality, with causality intended in the standard statistical counterfactual sense.[5]

The issue of causation in the economics literature runs from alcohol use or problem drinking to labor market outcomes: Does problem drinking of some degree of severity cause unemployment, and if so, what is the magnitude of this relationship? Does alcohol consumption at a particular level cause lower (or, as has been speculated by some, higher) wages, and if so, what is the magnitude of this relationship?

The main problem in attempting to ascribe a causal interpretation to such relationships is an empirical, not a logical, one. Questions of causality like those raised in the previous paragraph are logically meaningful (at least in a statistical sense). However, in general it would be expected that alcohol use or problem drinking will be correlated with factors that determine productivity but that are unobserved by empirical analysts.

Another important conceptual issue to consider involves the definition of the labor market outcome to be analyzed. Specifically, it must be borne in mind that outcomes, like earnings, weekly wages, and income, are the product of two distinct (yet related) economic processes. The first is what economists refer to as the *wage rate,* or the amount an individual receives for each unit of time worked (e.g., hourly wage). The second component involves the outcomes of whether or not the individual works at all, and if so, the amount of labor the individual actually supplies to the labor market (referred to as *labor supply*). Earnings as generally defined are the product of the wage rate and the amount of labor supplied (e.g. a wage rate of $20/hr times 2000 hours worked per year implies earnings of $40,000).

At the conceptual level, the important consideration is that alcohol use and/or problem drinking may have distinctly different implications for each of these components of earnings or income. Some empirical studies have focused on samples consisting only of working individuals.[2,6–9] As one impact of alcoholism may be to reduce employment, it is important to remember that inferences drawn from workers only are conditional on the fact that individuals are already working. Some results[10–12] suggest that there are important relationships as well between alcohol use/misuse and employment propensity and labor supply. The fundamental message is that in order to obtain an accurate view of the entire picture of such productivity relationships both components must be addressed.

One final methodological issue arises when income is used as a measure of labor market productivity. Transfer payments and income earned or generated by other household members can be a part of measured income. However, this can create problems of interpretation. All else being equal, higher levels of transfer payments should represent lower productivity, since eligibility for and receipt of public transfer payments often coincide with subpar productivity. However, to the extent that measures of individual or household income include transfers received by the individual or household, then precisely the "wrong" signal is being sent by reference to such aggregated income data. Analogous, albeit somewhat more complex, arguments apply when analyzing household income measures. All else being equal, it is recognized that household incomes may increase when the alcohol problems of one spouse triggers increased labor supply of other spouse.

2.1.2. Recent Empirical Research. Owing to their theoretical linkages to worker productivity, wages, earnings, and income have proved to be the labor market outcomes most studied by economists interested in alcohol's economic costs. As mentioned above, when comparing across studies, it is important to recognize differences in conceptualization and measurement of alcohol and income. Some of the literature has focused primarily on the effects of various measures of problem drinking, whereas other studies have used various measures of alcohol consumption in their research. For example, whereas one study may focus on all levels of alcohol consumption, another may employ measures of chronic alcohol dependence. Considerable care should be exercised in making general inferences about "alcohol and earnings" in such cases where the underlying measurements may be vastly different.

In one of the earliest attempts to relate alcohol problems in the household to economic success, Berry and Boland[13] use data from the 1969 Berkeley Social Research Group Survey to relate household incomes to alcohol problems. For this study, alcohol problems are measured as whether or not an alcohol-abusing male resides in the household. Berry and Boland find overall that households in which no alcohol-abusing male resides have 22.5% higher mean incomes and 24.3% higher median incomes than households where alcohol-abusing males reside.

An early and well-known study of the economic costs of alcohol-related problems is Harwood *et al.*[14] [commonly known as the Research Triangle Institute (RTI) study]. This study uses data from the 1979 National Survey of Attitudes and Interests in Drinking Practices and Problems (National Alcohol Survey) and assesses relationships between household income from all sources and various measures of drinking (quantity/frequency) and problem drinking. The key result from the Harwood *et al.*[14] regression analyses is that problem drinking is associated with a 21% reduction in household income from all sources. The results suggest that consumption is beneficial (in terms of household income) over low levels of consumption but harmful beyond about 2.0–2.6 ounces per day.

Heien and Pittman[15] have offered a critique of the Harwood *et al.*[14] results (see also ref. 16). They use the 1979 National Alcohol Survey data on household incomes and various measures of the quantity and frequency of alcohol consumption and of problem drinking. In a raw comparison, Heien and Pittman find that households in which no problem drinker resides have incomes 13.6% lower than households that include at least one problem drinker. In a regression setting, they find no statistically significant relationships between household incomes and either the quantity/frequency measures or the problem drinking measures.

A recent study by Rice *et al.*,[17] whose main objective is to update and revise the Harwood/RTI economic cost estimates, contains some results that are useful for the purposes at hand. As a component of their economic cost computations, Rice *et al.* estimate a set of relationships between income and disorders including alcoholism. The authors use multiple-site data from the Epidemiological Catchment Area (ECA) surveys in conjunction with the *Diagnostic and Statistical Manual of Mental Disorders*, 3rd edition (DSM-III)[18] diagnosis of ever having alcohol abuse or dependence. The income measure used in this study is personal income. Rice *et al.*'s key finding is that lifetime alcohol dependence or alcohol abuse is negatively related to personal income for males and females. They estimate a range from a low of about 0.8% for individuals aged 18 to 24 and a high of 18.7% for those 55 to 64.

Berger and Leigh[6] use data from the 1972–1973 Quality of Employment Survey (QES) to assess the relationships between alcohol consumption and wages. For this analysis, drinkers are defined as individuals reporting drinking alcoholic beverages at least one or two times per week. The key sample selection criteria are that the individual had to be at least 18 years old and working for pay at least 20 hr per week. Even their most conservative approach to estimating wage differentials suggests sizable wage advantages for drinkers over nondrinkers, with the differentials particularly large for females (8% for males, 21% for females).

In his comprehensive survey of the social costs of drinking, Cook[2] attempts to replicate the Berger and Leigh results using the QES sample described above. Cook's results basically confirm the Berger and Leigh findings. While Cook's statistical analysis is more direct than the Berger and Leigh selection-correction methodology, essentially the same message emerges: At least over some range of moderate drinking, workers' earnings increase with alcohol consumption. The key relationship Cook estimates is a positive relationship between alcohol consumption and earnings up to the level of one drink per day. This amount, unless concentrated on a few drinking occasions, would typically not constitute problem drinking behavior. No statistically significant positive or negative association is found beyond this level of consumption.

In a series of recent papers, Mullahy and Sindelar utilize data on males from the ECA survey's New Haven site to analyze a variety of relationships between alcoholism and labor market success. Mullahy and Sindelar[11] summarize the key results from this work insofar as income is concerned (see also Ref. 32). The income measure used by Mullahy and Sindelar is the individual's income brought in from all sources. Mullahy and Sindelar consider several measures of alcoholism problems. Their key results are based on the DSM-III measure of ever having met criteria for alcohol dependence and/or alcohol abuse. Focusing on the "prime working age" population (ages 30–59), Mullahy and Sindelar's main finding is that alcoholism has a negative and statistically significant relationship with individual income. The size and the significance of the relationships, however, depends crucially on what other covariates are controlled. Their empirical analyses produced estimates of between 17 to 31% reductions in income due to alcoholism.

Miller and Kelman[19] also use the ECA data to assess the impact of productivity losses from not only alcoholism, but also mental health and drug abuse. They examine men and women separately. They focus on time dimensions of each of these disorders, using the data in the ECA on first symptoms of a disorder for those who ultimately exhibit the disorder. They estimate a variety of functional forms and select a few as their "best" estimates. They conclude that both men and women suffer productivity losses from alcohol abuse/dependence. However, they conclude that the negative impact for men is more closely related to current disorder, while for women the impact is more closely related to the length of time that they have exhibited symptoms. Specifically, they conclude that alcohol abuse/dependence reduces income for men ranging from 1% for those 18 to 24 years old to a high of 9.8% reduction for those 55 to 64 years old. Young women, like young men, suffer a 1% reduction in income; but for older women, the impact is larger than it is for men.

Bryant *et al.*[20] use data from the National Longitudinal Survey of Youth (NLSY) to determine whether alcohol use affects labor market incomes. The analysis is confined to young, white males, this (presumably) being the subsample for which the statistical results would be most reliable and robust. Several statistical models (in many respects analogous to those employed by Berger and Leigh[6]) are employed to obtain the result of primary interest: wage rates and labor earnings of drinkers are greater than wage rates and labor earnings of nondrinkers (on the order of 25 cents/hr for the wage differential, on the order of $500/year for the labor earnings differential).

Like Bryant *et al.*,[20] Kenkel and Ribar[10] have employed data from the NLSY to characterize empirically a broad set of structural economic relationships involving alcohol consumption and young adults' socioeconomic success. Some of their results are more appropriately summarized below. Their results on earnings are of primary interest at this juncture. Kenkel and Ribar present a comprehensive set of estimates of these relationships, which correspond to a rich set of alternative statistical assumptions, methodologies, and alternative definitions of drinking and problem drinking.

While it is not appropriate to offer a simple, single summary statement about Kenkel and Ribar[10] results, a general message is that problem drinking is often associated with reduced earnings for males and is sometimes associated with lower earnings for females. In perhaps the most interesting and statistically sophisticated set of specifications estimated by Kenkel and Ribar, the magnitudes of some of these estimated effects are considerable, on the order of 25% in some instances. However, Kenkel and Ribar estimate a number of specifications and the estimated impact can include a small positive effect. Note that the finding for males stands in contrast with the conclusion of Bryant *et al.*[20]

Taken together, French and Zarkin[21] and Zarkin *et al.*[9] show how results can be fragile and that two similar studies can have conflicting results. In the first paper in this set, French and Zarkin[21] collected data at four large work sites and used this sample to address the question of whether moderate alcohol consumption is related to wages. Using bounded-influence regression methods to mitigate the problems of outlying observations in their sample, French and Zarkin analyzed the relationship between weekly wages and a set of drinking behavior measures. The main finding in this study is that abstainers have lower wages than drinkers and heavy drinkers have lower wages than moderate drinkers. The peak of the alcohol–wage relationship is in the range of 1.5–2.5 drinks per day.

Zarkin *et al.*[9] attempt to replicate the French and Zarkin[21] paper, using a different data source: the 1991 and 1992 National Household Surveys on Drug Abuse. Also, in contrast to the first study, this study analyzes men and women separately and uses drinking categories instead of a continuous variable for alcohol consumption. They analyze prime-aged workers. In this study, they fail to find evidence of the inverted U-shape found in the previous paper. Instead they find a wage premium related to consumption. For men, the wage premium is relatively consistent over the alcohol categories and is in the range of about 7%. Although a wage premium for women is observed, it is not significant.

Heien[22] also explores the hypothesis of a ∩-shape relationship between alcohol use and earnings. Further, he hypothesizes that two categories of nondrinkers should be distinguished: lifetime abstainers and ex-drinkers. Using the 1979 and 1984 National Household Surveys on Alcohol Use, he finds evidence that moderate drinkers earn more than nondrinkers and heavy drinkers.

2.2. *Alcohol Use and Abuse, Labor Supply, and Employment*

2.2.1. Conceptual and Methodological Issues. In analyzing employment, economists differentiate three states relating to labor supply and labor force participation. The first is *employment;* that is, the individual is either working (or on vacation or some other type of temporary leave from a place of employment). The second is *unemployment;* that is, actively seeking work yet not having secured labor market employment. The last category is referred to as *out of the labor force;* that is, not working and not actively seeking a job.

Finally, it should be noted that work loss or absenteeism is, in an important sense, one manifestation of labor supply behavior. The decision to miss work on what would otherwise be a scheduled work day is in essence a decision to not supply labor to the market on that day. To the extent that drinking and/or drinking problems are found to be determinants of work loss, it is thus reasonable to interpret such relationships within this broader context of labor supply and employment issues.

2.2.2. Recent Empirical Research. Mullahy and Sindelar[11] have found for the New Haven ECA sample of males that ever having met the DSM-III criteria for alcohol dependence or abuse is negatively and significantly related to full-time work propensity (78% for nonalcoholics vs. 72% for alcoholics). The relatively small differences between alcoholics and nonalcoholics when pooled over all age groups mask striking differences seen for specific age groups. For males 30–44 and 45–59, the differences between the full-time work propensities of alcoholics and nonalcoholics are significant (88% vs. 73% in the younger group; 86% vs. 68% in the older group). These significant negative effects of alcoholism carry over to a regression setting where age, race, and other covariates are controlled.

Using the NLSY sample, Kenkel and Ribar[10] employ a variety of estimation strategies to examine the number of hours worked by young males and females. In their benchmark models, Kenkel and Ribar find only small labor supply effects of heavy drinking—negative and statistically significant for males, and positive and statistically insignificant for females. Alcohol abuse has small positive but statistically insignificant relationships with labor supply for both males and females. Using alternative statistical methods, however, Kenkel and Ribar find considerably larger negative, though statistically insignificant, effects of their problem drinking measures on hours worked for males, and considerably larger positive and statistically significant effects of the problem drinking measures on hours of females' labor supply.

Mullahy and Sindelar[12] further analyze the result that they and others (e.g., ref. 10) have found, indicating a perhaps positive impact of alcoholism on women's participation in the labor market; this is in sharp contrast to the negative impact found for men in studies using the same data and methods. Using the 1988 Alcohol Survey of the National Health Interview Survey, they find that the positive association between labor market participation and alcoholism holds for white women only. Further, they find somewhat surprisingly that for white women, alcoholism is associated with higher educational attainment, a smaller family size, and a lower probability of being married. These in turn are associated with a higher labor force participation rate, thus partly explaining the puzzle of contrasting impacts by gender. Nonwhite women, however, appear to have impacts of alcoholism more like those of men; that is, reducing employment. For both white and nonwhite women, and for men, alcoholism is associated with increased unemployment. This study also explores the impact of lifetime abstention from alcohol consumption on employment and human capital accumulation. Several curious heretofore unexplained results are found, including that abstention is associated with lower employment, unemployment, and education for both white and nonwhite women.

Also analyzing youths, Zarkin *et al.*[9] use the 1991 National Health Interview Survey for their initial estimates and use the data from the same survey, but from 1992, to check the robustness of their results. They examine not only the consumption of alcohol, but also use of cigarettes and other drugs and their impact on young men's hours worked. Much of the focus is on the impact of drugs, not alcohol. However, with regard to alcohol, they find that consumption of alcohol in the past month is significantly associated with increased hours worked relative to nondrinkers in all categories except one of the lower categories (8 to 23 drinks). Another significant finding is that individuals who never in their lifetime drank had significantly lower hours of work than drinkers.

A rather distinct issue concerning wages, income, and welfare is considered in Mullahy and Sindelar.[23] In this study, the authors argue that an important shortcoming of standard productivity-based welfare arguments is that such analyses fail to account for real-world *ex ante* uncertainty in wage and income outcomes. Uncertainty with regard to future income is a negative to many individuals, holding all else constant. Thus, if drinking problems increase the uncertainty, then simply using *ex post* productivity will generally result in underestimates of the welfare losses associated with problem drinking. Using the ECA sample described above, Mullahy and Sindelar[23] provide empirical support for the hypothesis that problem drinking is associated with increases in the variance of income.

The recent study by Ruhm[24] provides an altogether different perspective on relationships involving employment and unemployment and alcohol-related problems. Specifically—and in addition to the hypotheses he addresses concerning tax effects discussed earlier—Ruhm considers the hypothesis that both total alcohol consumption as well as the motor vehicle fatality rate might be causally affected by unemployment conditions. Employing a variety of statistical approaches to the problem and using a pooled time-series, cross-section state level sample, Ruhm finds no evidence that drinking or drunk driving rates increase during economic downturns (i.e., periods with relatively high unemployment rates). His conclusion is based in part on the finding that alcohol use is positively related to disposable income (i.e., alcoholic beverages are "normal goods") and that disposable incomes tend to decline during periods of relatively high unemployment.

There has been little economic analysis of the relationships between work loss or absenteeism and alcohol use. Two exceptions are Manning *et al.*[25] and French and Zarkin.[7] Manning *et al.* utilize data from the Rand Health Insurance Experiment and from the 1983 National Health Interview Survey to test a set of hypotheses regarding work loss and alcohol use. The Manning *et al.* results from their analysis of the Health Insurance Experiment data indicate that former drinkers have 38% more work loss compared to abstainers and infrequent current drinkers. However, these researchers found no statistically significant relationships for current drinkers between the monthly volume of reported alcohol consumption and the amount of work loss. The National Health data yield somewhat different conclusions. Like the Health Interview results, the National Health analysis turned up no significant relationships between quantity consumed by drinkers and work loss; however, the significant former drinker results found in the Health Interview analysis are not replicated in the National Health analysis.

French and Zarkin[7] use the data on four large manufacturing work sites from the 1995 French and Zarkin paper.[21] While they focus primarily on the impact of mental health on absenteeism, they examine alcohol use as a covariate. Using an overall index of quantity and frequency of consumption, they find that alcohol consumption is associated with significantly greater absenteeism, whether measured as a dummy variable or as the number of days lost out of the last 30 days. Three measure of drunkenness were used as covariates in addition to the overall index: drunk infrequently, occasionally, or frequently. None of these were significant when the dependent variable was the binary indicator on absenteeism. However, both the "occasionally" and the "often" indicators were significant and negative in regressions of the number of days absent.

It should be emphasized that the caveats earlier about the conditional interpretation of wage/earnings studies apply with equal force in analyses of absenteeism or work loss. Put simply, individuals cannot lose time from work unless they are already employed.

2.3. *Alcohol Use and Human Capital*

2.3.1. Conceptual and Methodological Issues. Mullahy and Sindelar[11,27] have argued that the effects on labor market success of alcohol consumption and/or problem drinking may not be fully captured in the standard statistical analyses. To the extent that other productive determinants (i.e., "human capital") of labor market outcomes are themselves determined by problem drinking, then some of the effects of problem drinking on labor market outcomes are indirectly channeled through these other covariates; that is, there may be both direct as well as indirect effects of problem drinking on labor market success. For example, early onset of alcoholism may reduce educational attainment. Thus, estimates of earnings regressions that use education as an explanatory variable may underestimate the true impact of alcoholism on earnings; that is, the total impact of alcoholism would incorporate the lower educational attainment. Economists consider schooling attainment, work experience, health status, and family structure as important component of human capital.

2.3.2. Recent Empirical Research. Relatively little is known empirically about how youth drinking affects the level of schooling attainment and its quality. Mullahy and Sindelar[27–29] present some results suggesting that onset of alcoholism's symptoms during youth is associated with reduced schooling attainment; specifically, first onset of alcoholism's symptoms before age 19 is found to be related to an 11% reduction in schooling attainment, controlling for other covariates, but only an 8% raw difference. It should be stressed that the direction of causality between alcoholism symptoms and schooling cannot be ascertained with confidence in this study.

Cook and Moore[30] have also utilized data from the NLSY to determine empirically whether youthful drinking behavior affect educational outcomes, and, based on the logic spelled out above, thus ultimately result in productivity reductions during the prime working years. The particular outcome measure analyzed by Cook and Moore is the highest year of completed schooling, which is related to a set of variables measuring the individual's alcohol use and abuse behavior while in high school. Cook and Moore use statistical methods designed to mitigate problems of reverse causation (i.e., does the propensity to be a youthful alcohol abuser result in reduced schooling attainment, does the propensity to have reduced schooling attainment result in alcohol abuse, or both).

Cook and Moore's central finding is that the measures of high school drinking behavior (number of drinks per week, frequency of drinking, and frequency of being drunk) are each found to be negative and statistically significant determinants of the highest year of schooling completed. In quantitative terms, their estimates suggest that frequent drinking while a high school senior results in completion of 2.3 fewer years of college when compared with otherwise similar individuals who are not frequent drinkers.

For their NLSY sample of young adults, Kenkel and Ribar[10] have examined how the probability of being married may be related to problem drinking. Across the various statistical specifications and measures of problem drinking they employ, Kenkel and Ribar estimate almost universally negative and statistically significant relationships between marriage probability and problem drinking for both males and females. These general results even tend to stand up (though are statistically somewhat weaker) when Kenkel and Ribar attempt to control for possible reverse causation (i.e., marital status influencing drinking behavior rather than drinking behavior causally influencing marital status).

Kenkel and Wang[31] examine the impact of alcoholism on occupational choice, another possible pathway of indirect effects. The broad concept is that alcoholism may cause an individual to prefer some nonwage attributes of a job. This may lead to a preference for one occupation over another, because of, for example, the availability of health insurance. Empirical findings for men suggest that nonwage attributes are associated with alcoholism. For example, male alcoholics are more likely to be injured on the job, are less likely to receive some types of fringe benefits, and tend to work for smaller firms. They estimate that about 20% of the productivity lost estimated is due to nonwage attributes. Alcoholics are more likely to be in blue-collar jobs, but alcoholics in white-collar jobs are estimated to earn 15% less than their nonalcoholic peers.

The basic message emerging from the limited empirical evidence available to date on this topic both within economics and outside (see ref. 32) is highly suggestive: Indirect effects of drinking and problem drinking may be as important as the direct effects. Thus, an important line of research would be to obtain more detailed and reliable information on the magnitude and type of indirect effects. Indirect effects could include the quality and quantity of schooling attainment, the formation of households, the choice of spouse and friends, the level and quality of labor market experience, and other key components of human capital is of considerable importance.

3. Summary

This chapter analyzes and reviews of some of the main research on the economic aspects of drinking and problem drinking, also referred to as alcohol use and abuse. The findings are intriguing, if not always consistent across studies. Some of the inconsistency relates to differences in specific questions addressed, and some relates to data sources, sample selection, measures of alcohol, and measures of labor market productivity. Recent methodological advances (e.g., theories of addiction and econometric advances) have permitted and will continue to permit more ambitious empirical efforts in these areas of inquiry. There is a need for more detailed and specific measures of both labor market productivity and alcohol use, situation of use, misuse, and dependence. With the methodological advances and the promise of new data sources, the literature may soon be able to provide a better and more unified understanding of how alcohol use and abuse is associated with labor market productivity.

References

1. US National Institute on Alcohol Abuse and Alcoholism: *Eighth Special Report to the US Congress on Alcohol and Health.* NIH Publication No. 94-3699, Washington, DC, National Institutes of Health. 1993.
2. Cook PJ: The social costs of drinking, in *Expert Meeting on Negative Social Consequences of Alcohol Use.* Oslo, Norway, Norwegian Ministry of Health and Social Affairs, 1991.
3. Mullahy J: Alcohol and the labor market, in Hilton ME, Bloss G (eds): *Economics and the Prevention of Alcohol-Related Problems.* Rockville, MD, NIAAA Research Monograph No. 25, NIH Publication No. 93-3513, 1993, pp 141–174.
4. Sindelar JL: The effect of alcoholism on women's labor market outcomes, in Howard JM, Martin SE, Mail PD, *et al.* (eds): *Alcohol and Women: Issues for Prevention Research.* Rockville, MD, NIH, NIAAA Research Monograph No. 32, 1996, pp 291–314.
5. Mullahy J, Manning WG: Statistical issues in cost-effectiveness analyses, in Sloan F (ed): *Valuing Health Care: Costs, Benefits, and Effectiveness of Pharmaceuticals and Other Medical Technologies.* Cambridge, England, Cambridge University Press, 1995, pp 144–184.
6. Berger MC, Leigh JP: The effect of alcohol use on wages. *App Econ* 20:1343–1351, 1988.
7. French MT, Zarkin GA: Mental health, absenteeism, and earnings at a large manufacturing worksite. Mimeo, Research Park, NC, Research Triangle Institute (undated).
8. Zarkin GA, French MT, Mroz T, Bray JW: Alcohol use and wages: New results from the national household survey on drug abuse. Mimeo, Research Park, NC, Research Triangle Institute, 1996.
9. Zarkin GA, French MT, Mroz T, Bray JW: The relationship between drug abuse and labor supply for young men. Mimeo, Research Park, NC, Research Triangle Institute, 1996.
10. Kenkel DS, Ribar DC: Alcohol consumption and young adults' socioeconomic status. *Brookings Papers on Economic Activity: Microeconomics* 1:119–161, 1994.
11. Mullahy J, Sindelar JL: Alcoholism, work, and income. *J Labor Econ* 11:494–520, 1993.
12. Mullahy J, Sindelar JL: Employment, unemployment, and problem drinking. *J Health Econ* 15:409–435, 1996.
13. Berry R, Boland J: *The Economic Costs of Alcohol Abuse.* New York, Free Press, 1977.
14. Harwood HJ, Napolitano DM, Kristiansen PL, Collins JJ: *Economic Costs to Society of Alcohol and Drug Abuse and Mental Illness: 1980.* Research Park, NC, Research Triangle Institute, 1984.
15. Heien DM, Pittman DJ: The economic costs of alcohol abuse: An assessment of current methods and estimates. *Stud Alcohol* 50:567–579, 1989.
16. Heien DM, Pittman DJ: The external costs of alcohol abuse. *J Stud Alcohol* 54:302–307, 1993.
17. Rice DP, Kelman S, Miller LS, Dunmeyer S: *The Economic Costs of Alcohol and Drug Abuse and Mental Illness: 1985.* Washington, DC, PHS/ADAMHA DHHS Publication No. (ADM) 90-1694, 1990.
18. American Psychiatric Association: *Diagnostic and Statistical Manual of Mental Disorders, Third Edition.* Washington, DC, Author, 1980.
19. Miller LS, Kelman S: Estimates of the loss of individual productivity from alcohol and drug abuse from mental illness, in Frank R, Manning W (eds): *Economics and Mental Health.* Baltimore, Johns Hopkins Press, 1992, pp 91–129.

20. Bryant RR, Samaranayake VA, Wilhite A: The influence of current and past alcohol use on earnings: Three approaches to estimation. *J Appl Behav Sci* 29:9–31, 1993.
21. French MT, Zarkin GA: Is moderate alcohol use related to wages? Evidence from four worksites. *J Health Econ* 14:319–344, 1995.
22. Heien DM: Do drinkers earn less? *South Econ J* 63:60–68, 1996.
23. Mullahy J, Sindelar JL: Health, income, and risk aversion: Assessing some welfare costs of alcoholism and poor health. *J Human Resources* 30:439–460, 1995.
24. Ruhm CJ: Economic conditions and alcohol problems. *J Health Econ* 14:583–603, 1995.
25. Manning WG, Keeler EB, Newhouse JP, *et al: The Costs of Poor Health Habits.* Cambridge, MA, Harvard University Press, 1991.
26. Mullahy J, Sindelar JL: Gender differences in labor market effects of alcoholism. *Am Econ Rev* 81:161–165, 1991.
27. Mullahy J, Sindelar JL: Life cycle effects of alcoholism on education, earnings, and occupation. *Inquiry* 26:272–282, 1989.
28. Mullahy J, Sindelar JL: Direct and indirect effects of alcoholism on human capital. *Milbank Q* 72:359–375, 1994.
29. Mullahy J, Sindelar JL: Women and work: Tipplers and teetotlers. *J Health Econ* 6:533–537, 1997.
30. Cook PJ, Moore MJ: Drinking and schooling. *J Health Econ* 12:411–429, 1993.
31. Kenkel DS, Wang P: Are alcoholics in bad jobs? Mimeo, Ithaca, NY, Cornell University, 1996.
32. Miller-Tutzauer C, Leonard KE, Windle M: Marriage and alcohol use: A longitudinal study of "maturing out." *Stud Alcohol* 52:434–440, 1991.

14

The Cost Offsets of Alcoholism Treatment

Harold D. Holder

Abstract. While the effectiveness of alcoholism treatment is an important concern in alcohol research, the cost of such treatment and its benefits are also important research matters. There is substantial research that examines the possible benefits of alcoholism treatment in reducing the cost of all medical care, including the cost of alcoholism treatment itself. This is referred to as cost offsets. This chapter reviews the research evidence of alcoholism treatment cost offset, that is, the ability of alcoholism treatment to reduce the cost of medical care of persons participating in such treatment. The chapter gives an overview summary of the cost offset findings for alcoholism treatment and concludes with an identification of future research needs and opportunities, especially surrounding the popular increase in the use of managed care.

1. Introduction

Evaluation of alcoholism treatment has most often focused on the effectiveness of any intervention to reduce dependency. Effect analysis focuses on patient outcomes, usually changes in drinking behavior. In the past 20 years, the treatment of alcoholism has been subjected to a number of controlled clinical evaluations of effectiveness. See Hester and Miller[1] and Miller and Hester[2] for summaries of treatment effectiveness research for alcoholism. While there have been a number of treatment effectiveness studies, few have considered the actual cost of treatment. Such a simultaneous consideration is important, since cost as well as the effects of treatment must also be considered for a more complete assessment.

Harold D. Holder • Prevention Research Center, Berkeley, California 94704.

Recent Developments in Alcoholism, Volume 14: The Consequences of Alcoholism, edited by Galanter. Plenum Press, New York, 1998.

2. Economic Aspects of Alcoholism Treatment

A consideration of the economic or cost aspects of alcoholism treatment involves three general domains of concern:

1. *Cost:* The actual cost to deliver alcoholism treatment itself, usually influenced by the treatment modality or approach used to achieve recovery or rehabilitation, as well as the physical setting in which the treatment occurs, for example, inpatient, residential facility, outpatient, halfway house, and so forth.
2. *Cost/Effectiveness:* The relationship of the cost of treatment to the effects achieved, on the average, for patients.
3. *Cost/Benefits:* The relationship of the cost of treatment to the benefits achieved as a result of treatment. Benefits are most often expressed in economic terms, such as changes in income, reduced social services and associated costs, reduced expenditures for other services for alcoholics or their families, and increased economic productivity resulting from a longer life or reduced impairment.

One cost–benefit consideration that has been given considerable attention over the past 15 years has been the cost offset of alcoholism treatment. This typically refers to the reduction in health care utilization and associated costs that can be attributed to alcoholism treatment and whether there are sufficient savings in health care cost reduction to offset the cost of the alcoholism treatment itself. The most basic criterion would be that some of the cost of alcoholism treatment would be accounted for (or "offset," if you will) in reduced other health care costs, and the highest criterion would be that there was a net overall reduction in total health care costs including the costs of alcoholism treatment itself.

Cost offset studies have particular appeal as a part of the cost–benefit consideration for alcoholism treatment in that: (1) these analyses involve actual health care costs and not imputed costs, such as expected years of productive labor or expected personal income, and (2) health care costs are a particularly central economic issue in the United States.

This chapter will first review some of the recent research on cost–effects analyses of alcoholism treatment and then provide a longer review and discussion of cost/offset research.

2.1. *Cost–Effects Studies*

Effectiveness has been defined in various ways through a large number of clinical studies. Examples include abstinence, relapse, or readmission for treatment; changes in drinking levels; improved social or interpersonal relationships; and employment and/or work absences. In practice, number days of abstinence is probably the most popular criterion. Holder *et al.*[3] completed a first approximation of a cost and effect analysis for alcoholism. In their analysis, they combined average unit cost per treatment modality (based on the least expensive appropriate type of facility in which the treatment modality could be delivered) and a weighted number of positive controlled effectiveness studies (using whatever criterion of effectiveness each study employed). They concluded that increased alcoholism treatment cost was not positively related to treatment effectiveness and that lower-cost treatment could have significant effect on reducing drinking.

Finney and Monahan[4] replicated the treatment effects evaluation of Holder *et al.*,[3] with some differences in the conclusions about expected cost effectiveness of specific treatment modalities; but they also concluded that lower-cost treatment modalities are good investments.

Walsh *et al.*,[5] in a recent study, randomly assigned 227 workers who were identified as abusing alcohol to one of three treatment alternatives: (1) compulsory inpatient treatment, (2) compulsory attendance at Alcoholics Anonymous (AA), and (3) a choice of options. All three groups improved. Alcohol-abusing workers who used inpatient treatment did better than those who used AA or who were given free choice on subsequent drinking and drug use. Since AA and choice groups required additional inpatient treatment more often than the initial hospital group, the estimated costs for inpatient treatment for these two groups were found to be only 10% less than for the initial inpatient only group.

2.2. *Cost Offset Research*

As noted previously, the cost offsets of alcoholism treatment is to determine if other health care costs are reduced when treatment is begun. This determination examines how much of other costs are saved because of the investment in alcoholism treatment. In other words, is there cost reduction or "offset" associated with treatment. Since alcoholics are known to consume medical care at a much higher rate than their age and gender cohorts,[3,6] then savings in medical costs is an economic benefit resulting from alcoholism treatment. We are concerned with cost savings or offset yielded, that is, the dollar savings in medical costs per dollar spent on treatment.

There have been a number of cost offset studies over the past 20 years. Jones and Vischi[7] and Saxe *et al.*[8] provided the first reviews of such studies. They concluded there was initial evidence that alcoholism treatment can reduce the costs of other types of health care. A subsequent review by Holder[9] reached a similar conclusion. Holder *et al.*[10] have provided a more recent summary of this research.

This chapter will summarize some of the salient research of the past 20 years concerning cost–benefits of alcoholism treatment.

2.3. *Early Cost Offset Research*

Early studies in the 1970s sought evidence of positive cost offsets (or savings) associated with the treatment for alcoholism. In one of the earliest controlled studies, Edwards *et al.*[11] compared 48 inpatients with 46 advice-only (minimum treatment) control patients and found that the costs for the inpatient treatment were greater than for the control group.

In a study from January 1, 1972 through June 30, 1975 (2 years before first referral and 2 years after initial treatment), Forsythe *et al.*[12] compared 191 treated alcoholics with 191 matched nonalcoholic controls in a California health maintenance organization (HMO) and found that costs increased after treatment for both groups.

In one of the first longitudinal studies, Holder and Hallan[13] conducted a 6-year study (from 1974 to 1979) to determine whether the treatment of alcoholism as a primary diagnosis results in a reduction of total health care cost and/or utilization for the alcoholic and other nonalcoholic family members. All health care costs and utilization were tracked for a group of 90 families (representing 245 individuals) enrolled with Blue Cross/Blue Shield through the health benefits division of the California public employees retirement system. At least one member in each family received treatment under a specific diagnosis of alcoholism during the period July 1, 1974 to December 1, 1975. All health care utilization and costs were obtained for a 12-month period before initial treatment for alcoholism and up to July 1, 1979. A matched group of 83 comparison families (291 persons) with no alcoholic members was selected to reflect comparable family composition, age, and sex. The results indicated that overall health care utilization and costs for both alcoholic individuals and their nonalcoholic family members dropped after alcoholism treatment began and ultimately reached a level similar to the matched comparison group. These findings held for both inpatient and outpatient care.

Holder and Hallan[13] concluded from this 6-year (1974–1979) study that:

- Contrary to insurance carriers' expectations of greater utilization of alcoholism treatment as a result of insurance coverage, the utilization rate of alcoholism treatment following the advent of specific coverage of primary diagnosis of alcoholism was only 0.5 of 1% of the entire enrolled population.
- Over time, inpatient alcoholism treatments decreased while the use of outpatient alcoholism care increased.
- For each $1 spent on alcoholism treatment, there was at least 42 cents in projected savings to insurance carriers and prepaid plans from reduced general health care costs for the alcoholic to offset alcoholism treatment costs.

Two experimental studies produced evidence of decreasing costs following alcoholism treatment. Hayami and Freeborn[14] found small decreases in costs for medical office visits, emergency room visits, and hospital admissions, but only during the second 6-month posttreatment period. Medical costs increased during the first posttreatment period. Although this study supports the hypothesis that in the long run costs of alcohol treatment are offset by reduced health care costs, it has been criticized as lacking internal validity because it used no untreated control group and the sample size was relatively small. The study by McLellan *et al.*[15] of 460 veterans also produced evidence of posttreatment cost decreases, but it too lacked an untreated control group.

Four naturalistic studies examined health care records and found evidence of posttreatment health care cost decreases.[16–19] As with most naturalistic studies, none included untreated alcoholic control groups or employed a standardized clinical treatment.

Holder and Blose[20] examined the effect of alcoholism treatment services on overall health care utilization and costs for health insurance enrollees under the Federal Employees Health Benefit Program (FEHBP) with Aetna Insurance Company. Four-year average per capita monthly medical care costs for families with an alcoholic member were $209.60 or almost 100% higher than comparable costs ($106.54) for families with no apparent alcoholic members. Most of this difference resulted from higher monthly inpatient costs.

From 12 to 36 months before alcoholics began alcoholism treatment, their medical care costs gradually increased. During the year before treatment began, however, total medical care costs rose much faster. The average monthly medical care cost rose to $452 in the 6-month period before alcoholism treatment and to $1370 in the final month. After treatment began, total medical care costs dropped fairly rapidly for about 12 months. This drop continued, though more slowly, during the next 2 years. Total health care costs averaged $294 per month during the 6 months following treatment initiation, but only $190 per month by the third posttreatment initiation year.

Holder and Blose[20] also examined patterns of health care cost by gender and age. The pattern of overall medical care costs was almost identical for both men and women. Alcoholics of different ages, however, showed distinct medical care cost patterns. Three age groups were used: less than 45 years, 45 to 64 years, and 65 years and older. The middle-age group was most like the modal age of groups typically represented in previous studies of treated alcoholics. Although alcoholics in each age group followed the general pattern of the total group, there was a clear association between age and the extent of the drop in medical care costs following the start of alcoholism treatment. By 36 months after the start of treatment, the average monthly total costs of those younger than 45 years (N = 440) had dropped to a level comparable with that experienced 36 months prior to treatment.

The health care costs of the middle group (N = 823) also dropped significantly following the start of alcoholism treatment, although they did not reach levels as low as those existing several years prior to treatment. The oldest group (N = 434), which consisted primarily of retirees, experienced the highest overall medical care costs and showed the least convergence with the levels that existed prior to initiation of alcoholism treatment.

Holder and Blose[21] in a later replication analyzed data from treated alcoholics (both employees and dependents) who were health insurance enrollees of a large midwestern manufacturing firm. A total of 3729 alcoholics were identified (3068 of whom received treatment and 661 of whom did not) who had filed insurance claims from 1974 to 1987. Untreated alcoholics were those identified by primary or secondary diagnoses of a physical health problem clearly related to chronic drinking, but for whom there was no evidence of participation in an organized alcoholism treatment program with the goal of recovery.

Time-series analyses found that following treatment initiation, the total health care costs of treated alcoholics—including the cost of alcoholism treatment—declined by 23 to 55% from their highest pretreatment levels. Costs for identified but untreated alcoholics rose following identification. In a second design, analysis of variance was used to control for group differences including pretreatment health status and age. This analysis indicated that the posttreatment costs of treated alcoholics were 24% lower than comparable costs for untreated alcoholics.

Blose and Holder[22] found no treatment-related differences in overall health care cost between men and women. Significant differences were found by age: On the average, individuals in the 30 and under and the 31–50 age groups experienced declines in health care costs following initiation of treatment, whereas those over 50 experienced increasing costs.

The studies, which might be considered efficacy studies, demonstrate the clear potential of alcoholism treatment to assist by contributing to reductions in medical or health care cost. The results contribute to the policy question of whether providing alcoholism treatment is more cost beneficial than not providing such care. The results across studies are generally consistent in finding actual offset or potential for offset via a reduction in medical care utilization, especially fewer hospital days. In other words, these offset studies demonstrated the potential that part of the cost of alcoholism treatment is returned via lower health care costs.

3. Factors Affecting Cost of Alcoholism Treatment

The cost of medical care other than alcoholism treatment is a major factor in determining the potential for reductions in such costs following treatment initiation. This is especially true for the major source of medical care costs: inpatient treatment. Longitudinal analyses of cost components demonstrate that it is inpatient treatment that is most affected by alcoholism treatment. In some cases, outpatient treatment is actually increased in response to aftercare health care utilization, but at a substantially lower cost than inpatient.

Goodman *et al.*[23] examined several factors that predict long-term alcoholism treatment costs. They found that the probability of long-term treatment depends on whether the diagnosis used in initiating treatment is for alcohol abuse or alcohol dependence. The short-term treatment costs are higher when the treatment is for abuse rather than dependence. Patients with a dependence diagnosis are much more likely to receive subsequent treatment in an inpatient setting than those with abuse diagnoses. In addition, if there is a comorbidity for drug abuse, the probability for subsequent alcoholism treatment is substantially increased. The interaction with mental health and drug comorbidity was demonstrated by Goodman *et al.*[24] in that inpatient treatment is much more likely to be the location of treatment, and thus increase the treatment costs by $500 to $1500 for the first 6-month period following initial alcoholism treatment. If the alcoholism condition can be treated on an outpatient basis, then the total cost of such treatment is obviously lower and the potential for a cost offset net effect is substantially increased.

The hospital with its medical supervision is a much more costly site for alcoholism treatment than a nonmedically supervised residential facility, which is itself more costly than outpatient treatment. A part of total cost is the cost of alcoholism treatment itself, including the initial detoxification, if required, for the patient. Hayashida *et al.*[25] investigated comparable costs of detoxification occurring in an inpatient versus an outpatient setting for mild-to-moderate alcohol withdrawal syndrome. They randomly assigned 164 Veterans Administration patients to one of the two detoxification settings. The mean duration of treatment was shorter for outpatient than inpatient treatment, though more of the inpatients completed detoxification than the outpatients. Both groups had fewer alcohol problems after a 6-month follow-up; there were no significant differences between the groups themselves. The detoxification costs for inpatients were up to ten times those of the detoxification for outpatients ($3319–$3665 versus $175–$388).

Longabaugh *et al.*[26] compared the posttreatment costs of 60 extended inpatients with 114 partial hospital treatment patients (patients who remain in the hospital only during the day) and found the partial hospital group to have lower costs, largely as the result of the lower cost of the partial hospital treatment costs. The posttreatment follow-up period was probably too short for substantial health improvements to emerge and thereby reduce average health care costs. These early studies, while not definitive in themselves, provided evidence that the location of treatment affected the total costs and that there were not always obvious differences in effectiveness by site of treatment.

4. Generalizability

How generalizable are the findings of health care cost reduction associated with alcoholism treatment? This requires a determination that these results can be generalized across patient populations as well as an examination of differences in cost offset by the specific treatment modality utilized.

The research of Booth and colleagues[27–30] and Magruder-Habib *et al.*[31] have analyzed changes in medical care utilization before and after alcoholism treatment for Veterans Administration (VA) patients. These studies found that VA patients are lower socioeconomic persons with more disability than patients in other medical care situations. They also found that following the completion of inpatient alcoholism treatment (in the VA), there was an increased use of inpatient and outpatient services compared to other forms of alcohol-involved inpatient care and increased mental health hospitalizations with alcohol dependence as a secondary diagnosis. Booth *et al.*[32] did find that a substantial number of alcoholics receiving alcoholism treatment did experience major decreases or no other inpatient utilization. Booth *et al.*[33] conducted an analysis of the use of outpatient mental health treatment following inpatient alcoholism treatment by over 7000 VA patients. They found that those who completed an extended inpatient treatment stay had higher utilization of outpatient mental health care than those with a brief (usually for detoxification only) hospital stay. These studies of the VA population did find that this population did not achieve the overall cost offsets found in studies using employed populations (see ref. 10). Booth *et al.*[34] concluded in a study of VA patients that supportive interventions and networks reduced readmission by alcoholics, thus increasing the potential for lower utilization and associated costs.

Comparable populations to the VA are those enrolled under Medicare. There was an opportunity to study this population as part of a federal demonstration by the Heath Care Financing Administration and the National Institute on Alcohol Abuse and Alcoholism to study the costs of alcoholism treatment in freestanding residential alcoholism treatment facilities compared with hospital treated patients. Lo and Woodward[35] examined whether Medicare patients had lower health care utilization following initiation of alcoholism treatment than patients only treated in hospitals. A comparison group was formed of a randomly selected population of Medicare patients who were not treated directly for alcoholism but for the physical health consequences of heavy chronic alcohol use. Lo and Woodward[35] found that patients treated for alcoholism in both freestanding facilities and hospital settings had lower overall health care costs following treatment initiation. However, those treated in freestanding facilities had lower overall costs than those treated in hospital settings, controlling for sex, age, and initial alcohol diagnoses. The comparison group did not have an equivalent reduction in health care costs following treatment initiation.

This replicated earlier findings by Lawrence Johnson and Associates,[36] who examined the health records for alcoholics and a general cohort of Medicaid and Medicare patients across eight quarters (2 years). Although they found differences between groups in the expected direction prior to treatment, the posttreatment costs of alcoholics decreased substantially while those of the general cohort increased.

The other issue of complexity is whether there are differences in cost offset between specific alcoholism treatment modalities. As noted previously, Holder *et al.*[3] and Finney and Monahan[4] have completed early approximations of cost effectiveness of various unique treatment modalities. These studies established the standard of examining cost to deliver treatment and the expected effectiveness of treatment across controlled clinical trials. Treatment costs are in all cases derived from clinical judgments of the "minimum necessary" professional staff and treatment events necessary to effectively deliver each treatment modality. The unit costs are not derived from actual empirical data and the effectiveness of modalities are expressed in terms of the outcome criteria of the clinical trial (usually abstinence) but not in terms of changes in medical care utilization and costs. In other words, these early approximations do not assist us in the cost offset deliberations.

The differential effectiveness of treatment modalities has been addressed by several clinical trials as noted above. Project MATCH is a most recent effort to determine if there are patient attributes that are better matched with treatment modalities.[37] Project MATCH, a large clinical trial involving nine research sites, found modest differences in effectiveness across three treatment modalities while all three were effective in reducing drinking outcomes. A study involving two of the MATCH clinical sites to determine if there are differential treatment modality cost offset effects is under way.

5. Summary of Research Findings

This chapter has described the research findings from a number of cost offset studies of alcoholism treatment. In broad terms, the overall findings of this research can be summarized as follows:

1. Untreated alcoholics use health care and incur costs at a rate about twice that of their age and gender cohorts.
2. Prior (usually about 6 month's pretreatment) to alcoholism treatment initiation, there usually is a substantial and rapid rise in health care utilization (most often inpatient care) and associated costs.
3. Once treatment begins, total health care utilization and costs begin to drop (even allowing for expected regression to the mean), reaching a level that is lower than pretreatment initiation costs after a 2- to 4-year period.
4. There are no apparent gender differences in these trends for alcoholics. The pre- and posttreatment patterns of alcoholic females and males are virtually identical.
5. There are age differences that support the value of early intervention. Younger treated alcoholics have pretreatment total cost levels that are lower than pretreatment levels for older alcoholics (say 55 years and older), and other alcoholics have a much poorer prognosis. The older treated alcoholic is unlikely to experience lower health care costs following treatment initiation than before treatment.
6. Part of the increase in health care costs is a function of maturation. The difference between patients and their age and/or gender cohorts is relatively constant during the period prior to treatment. Once treatment begins, there is a clear tendency for cost trends to reverse direc-

tion and go down. Convergence with the expected age–gender baseline is quite possible over time.

The results of research provide consistent support for the cost effectiveness of alcohol treatment. That is, we find support if we define cost effectiveness in terms of treatment's ability to offset its own cost by reducing future health expenses.

6. Future Cost Offset Research Needs and Opportunities

The 1990s have brought a major reexamination and realignment of health care services in the United States.[38] Such realignment was apparently motivated by demands for cost control by insurance carriers, the federal and state governments, employers who pay for insurance or are self-insured, labor unions, and consumers. The issue of the cost of alcoholism treatment (along with mental health and drug abuse treatment) is a significant aspect of these health policy discussions.

Important cost questions include: What is the cost of alcoholism treatment (in total and by specific treatment modality)? Can such treatment reduce other health care utilization (or at least transform utilization to less costly alternatives)? What are the cost reductions that could be expected?[39] The managed care organization as a broker of health care for enrolled clients is clearly motivated to seek ways to reduce overall costs while providing an acceptable level of care. Thus, both the issue of units (or total costs) for treating alcoholism and the issue of potential savings are of concern.[40] See Coyle *et al.*[41] for an example of an effort to document unit and total costs for alcohol and drug abuse services.

The issue of cost of alcoholism treatment as a defined approach to recovery from alcohol dependency is hardly a simple one. Such costs are typically known through the billing of inpatient, residential, or outpatient treatment providers to their patients or the patient's insurance program. Such costs are typically defined in terms of time, for example, a hospital day or outpatient visit. In all cases, these units of charge represent averages across all patients and the types of facilities, professional staff, and other services included in average. Thus, for a unit rehabilitation day costs, a variety of services may be included in per day cost, depending on the facility. The specific therapeutic approach (or approaches) is not reflected specifically by the unit cost. In most cases, the cost of the facility that is the site of care drives the total average unit costs.

As Booth and Zhang[42] have noted, most prior studies have been based upon patient populations in clinical research or fee-for-service settings. There is a need now for replication of these studies in managed care environments. These future studies should be guided by considering the interactive effects of the physical location of treatment, the specific modality or modalities of treat-

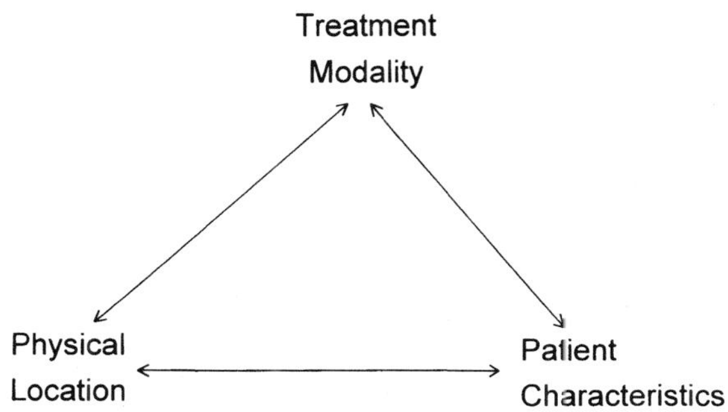

Figure 1. Mutual interaction of three basic elements in cost offset research.

ment delivered, and the patient characteristics. This mutual interaction is illustrated in Fig. 1. Each of the elements and interactions is described below:

1. *Physical location of treatment* usually refers to the facility or institution or setting in which treatment occurs. As has been noted, inpatient care (both in a general medical/surgical hospital as well as a specialized psychiatric facility) is likely to be the most expensive location for treatment.
2. *Treatment modality* refers to the therapeutic approach or means utilized to achieve the clinical objectives. Treatment can involve one type of treatment or multiple treatment modalities and can be educational, psychotherapeutic, supportive, and pharmacological in nature. Some treatment modalities may be delivered only in a specific setting, such as aversion therapy, or by a medical professional such as pharmacotherapy. Thus, as Holder *et al.*[3] demonstrated, there are minimum necessary locations or professional personnel required for most modalities. Therefore, there is a location and treatment modality interaction that affects cost of treatment.
3. *Patient characteristics* include such factors as the sociodemographics of the patient, especially their age, their drinking history and level of dependency, and level of physical health. One aspect of a consideration of this factor is the matching hypothesis that there are certain modalities that are better suited therapeutically to persons of specific characteristics. This was a basis for Project MATCH.[37] In addition, persons who already have disabled physical health may require treatment in an inpatient facility in order to receive concurrent medical treatment for their health. Since level of social support (family, friends, and coworkers) can influence treatment effectiveness, there is a possible interaction with treatment modality.

The above is not intended to be a definitive discussion of possible research interactions. Rather, the figure and the discussion illustrates the level of complexities that future cost offset research should address.

In summary, the efficacy of alcoholism treatment to yield reductions in other health care costs has been demonstrated by prior research. Now the research challenge is to determine if and in what ways these findings can be generalized to other patient populations, to specific treatment modalities, and to the physical location of the treatment. This is especially true in the situation where managed care is rapidly becoming the dominant form of health care organization.

ACKNOWLEDGMENT. Research and preparation of this chapter were supported in part by the National Institute on Alcohol Abuse and Alcoholism Research Center grant AA06282 to the Prevention Research Center, Pacific Institute for Research and Evaluation.

References

1. Hester RK, Miller WR (eds): *Handbook of Alcoholism Treatment Approaches: Effective Alternatives.* Elmsford, NY, Pergamon Press, 1989.
2. Miller WR, Hester RK: Matching problem drinkers with optimal treatment, in Miller WR, Heather N (eds): *Treating Addictive Behaviors: Processes of Change.* New York, Plenum Press, 1986, pp 175–203.
3. Holder HD, Longabaugh R, Miller WR, *et al:* The cost of effectiveness of treatment for alcohol problems: A first approximation. *J Stud Alcohol* 52(6):517–540, 1991.
4. Finney JW, Monahan SC: The cost effectiveness of treatment for alcoholism: A second approximation. *J Stud Alcohol* 57(3):229–243, 1996.
5. Walsh DC, Hingson R, Merrigan DM, *et al:* A randomized trial of treatment options for alcohol-abusing workers. *N Engl J Med* 325:775–782, 1991.
6. Putnam SL: Alcoholism, morbidity and care-seeking: The inpatient and ambulatory service utilization and associated illness experience of alcoholics and matched controls in a health maintenance organization. *Med Care* 10(1):97–121, 1982.
7. Jones KR, Vischi JR: Impact of alcohol drug abuse and mental health treatment on medical care utilization: A review of the research literature. *Med Care* 17:1–82, 1979.
8. Saxe L, Dougherty D, Esty K, *et al: The Effectiveness and Costs of Alcoholism Treatment.* Report prepared under contract to the Office of Technology Assessment, Washington, DC, Congress of the United States, 1983.
9. Holder HD: Alcoholism treatment and potential health care cost saving. *Med Care* 25:52–70, 1987.
10. Holder HD, Lennox RD, Blose JO: The economic benefits of alcoholism treatment: A summary of twenty years of research. *J Employee Assist Res* 1(1):63–82, 1992.
11. Edwards G, Orford J, Egert S, *et al:* Alcoholism: A controlled trial of treatment and advice. *J Stud Alcohol* 38:1004–1031, 1977.
12. Forsythe AB, Griffiths B, Reiff S: Comparison of utilization of medical services by alcoholics and nonalcoholics. *Am J Public Health* 72:600–602, 1982.
13. Holder HD, Hallan JB: Impact of alcoholism treatment on total health care costs: A six-year study. *Adv Alcohol Subst Abuse* 6(1):1–15, 1986.
14. Hayami DE, Freeborn DK: Effect of coverages on the use of an HMO alcoholism treatment program, outcome and medical care utilization. *Am J Public Health* 71:1133–1144, 1981.
15. McLellan AT, Luborsky L, O'Brien L, Woody AE, Druley KA: Is treatment for substance abuse effective? *JAMA* 247:1423–1428, 1982.
16. Gregory D, Jones RK, Rundell OH, Stanitis T, Stanhope P: Feasibility of an alcoholism health insurance benefit, in Gallanter M (ed): *Currents in Alcoholism: Recent Advances in Research and Treatment,* vol VIII. New York, Grune and Stratton, 1981, pp 195–202.

17. Becker FW, Sanders BK: The Illinois Medicare/Medicaid alcoholism services demonstration; Medicaid cost trends and utilization patterns—managerial report. Springfield, IL, Center for Policy Studies and Program Evaluation, Sagamon State University. Report prepared under contract with the Illinois Department of Alcohol and Substance Abuse, September 21, 1984.
18. Sanders BK, Becker FW: Average medical expenditures reimbursed by Medicaid for services provided to clients in the Illinois alcoholism services demonstration, SFY's 1982–85. Springfield, IL, Center for Policy Studies and Program Evaluation, Sagamon State University, 1985.
19. Plotnick DE, Adams KM, Hunter HR, *et al: Alcoholism Treatment Programs within Prepaid Group Practice HMOs: A Final Report* (Contract No. ADM 281 80 004). Rockville, MD: National Institute on Alcohol Abuse and Alcoholism, 1982.
20. Holder HD, Blose JO: Alcoholism treatment and total health care utilization and costs: A four-year longitudinal analysis of federal employees. *JAMA* 256(11):1456–1460, 1986.
21. Holder HD, Blose JO: The reduction of health care costs associated with alcoholism treatment: A 14-year longitudinal study. *J Stud Alcohol* 53:293–302, 1992.
22. Blose JO, Holder HD: The utilization of medical care by treated alcoholics: Longitudinal patterns by age, gender, and type of care. *J Subst Abuse* 3:13–27, 1991.
23. Goodman AC, Nishiura E, Hankin J, *et al:* Long-term alcoholism treatment costs. *Med Care Res Rev* 53:441–464, 1996.
24. Goodman AC, Holder HD, Nishiura E, *et al:* Analysis of short-term alcoholism treatment cost functions. *Med Care* 30(9):795–809, 1992.
25. Hayashida M, Alterman AI, McLellan AT, *et al:* Comparative effectiveness and costs of inpatient and outpatient detoxification of patients with mild-to-moderate alcohol withdrawal syndrome. *N Engl J Med* 320(6):358–365, 1989.
26. Longabaugh R, McCrady B, Fink E, *et al:* Cost effectiveness of alcoholism treatment in partial vs. inpatient settings: Six-month outcomes. *J Stud Alcohol* 44:1049–1071, 1983.
27. Booth BM, Yates WR, Petty F, *et al:* Longitudinal characteristics of hospital use before and after alcoholism treatment. *Am J Drug Alcohol Abuse* 16:161–170, 1990.
28. Booth BM, Yates WR, Petty F, *et al:* Patient factors predicting early alcohol-related readmissions for alcoholics: Role of alcoholism severity and psychiatric co-morbidity. *J Stud Alcohol* 52:37–43, 1991.
29. Booth BM, Blow FC, Cook CAL, *et al:* Age and ethnicity among hospitalized alcoholics: A narrative study. *Alcohol Clin Exp Res* 16:1029–1034, 1992.
30. Booth BM, Cook CAL, Blow FC, *et al:* Utilization of outpatient mental health services after inpatient alcoholism treatment. *J Mental Health Admin* 19:21–30, 1992.
31. Magruder-Habib K, Luckey JW, Mikow V, *et al:* Effects of alcoholism treatment on health services utilization patterns: Final report—IIR #82-026. Washington, DC, Department of Veterans Affairs, 1985.
32. Booth BM, Blow FC, Cook CAL, Bunn JY, Fortney JC: Relationship between inpatient alcoholism treatment and longitudinal changes in health care utilization. *J Stud Alcohol.* 58(6):625–637, 1997.
33. Booth BM, Cook CAL, Blow FC, Bunn YJ: Utilization of outpatient mental health services after inpatient alcoholism treatment. *J Mental Health Admin* 19(1):21–30, 1992.
34. Booth BM, Russell DW, Soucek S, Laughlin, PR: Social support and outcome of alcoholism treatment: An exploratory analysis. *Am J Drug Alcohol Abuse* 18(1):87–101, 1992.
35. Lo A, Woodward A: An evaluation of freestanding alcoholism treatment for Medicare recipients. *Addiction* 88:53–68, 1993.
36. Lawrence Johnson and Associates, Inc: HCFA alcoholism services demonstration briefing handouts of slide presentations. Report prepared for Health Care Financing Administration and the National Institute on Alcohol Abuse and Alcoholism. Washington, DC, Lawrence Johnson and Associates, Inc. 1985.
37. Project MATCH Research Group: Matching alcoholism treatments to client heterogeneity: Project MATCH posttreatment drinking outcomes. *J Stud Alcohol* 58(1):7–29, 1997.

38. Kenkel PJ: Provider-based managed-care programs continue growth trend. *Mod Health Care* 23(19):26–28, 30, 32, 1993.
39. Adams RP, Grimes RM: Alcohol and chemical dependency treatment: A study of cost and outcomes. *Health Care Innovations* 5(1):32–36, 1995.
40. French M, Dunlap L, Galinis D, Rachal JV, Zarkin, JA: Health care reforms and managed care for substance abuse services: Findings from eleven case studies. *J Public Health Policy.* 17(2):181–203, 1996.
41. Coyle D, Godfrey C, Hardman G, *et al:* Costing substance misuse services. YARTIC Occasional Paper 5. Centre for Health Economics, University of York, Leeds Addiction Unit, York, England, 1994.
42. Booth BM, Zhang M: Cost-effectiveness of alcohol services. Prepared for the Subcommittee on Health Services Research, National Institute on Alcohol Abuse and Alcoholism (unpublished manuscript), 1995.

IV

An International Perspective of the Biobehavioral Consequences of Alcoholism

Alfonso Paredes, Section Editor

Overview

Alfonso Paredes

Section IV presents perspectives on the biological and behavioral consequences of alcoholism derived from research conducted in four different sociocultural and geographic settings. This work is not necessarily representative of the research in these countries. The investigations are presented to illustrate some interesting issues raised by investigators from four countries: Finland, Mexico, Japan, and Spain. The importance of these topics transcends the locale where the research was conducted. The following summaries of the topics in Section IV are presented as preludes to these important contributions.

Like many other countries, Mexico experiences alcohol and drug abuse problems. Drug use problems are less prominent than in the United States, however. Whereas 34% of the general population in the United States report having used drugs of abuse at some point in their life, in Mexico only 4% have used such substances.[1] On the other hand alcohol problems are common. Chapter 15, Medina-Mora, Carreño, and de la Fuente, reviews the experience in Mexico with the Alcohol Use Disorders Identification Test (AUDIT). This work derives from the collaborative activities of the Mexican Institute of Psychiatry and the International Labor Office/World Health Organization. This agency has been interested in developing model programs for alcohol prevention in the workplace. According to the investigators, the characteristics of alcohol problems have local features. Daily consumption of alcohol is not normative in Mexico, but when the person engages in drinking, the individual commonly consumes alcohol to the point of intoxication. Among males, the most frequent pattern of drinking is low frequency with high quantities per drinking occasion. Heavy drinking is a prominent feature of festive occasions

Alfonso Paredes • Laboratory for the Study of the Addictions, West Los Angeles VA Medical Center, Los Angeles, California 90073.

Recent Developments in Alcoholism, Volume 14: The Consequences of Alcoholism, edited by Galanter. Plenum Press, New York, 1998.

that may occur infrequently. Incidentally, the proportion of abstainers is high in Mexico: 46% of the urban population between 18 and 65 years of age. The pattern of drinking mentioned brings with it specific problems. Twenty-two percent of the trauma victims evaluated in emergency rooms showed positive breathalizer alcohol readings. Only 6% of these individuals were consistent daily heavy drinkers. Paradoxically, harmful drinking consequences such as trauma are more prevalent among nondependent drinkers. Health authorities have adopted aggressive preventive approaches, placing less emphasis on the identification and treatment of alcohol dependence. More attention is given to the behavior of occasional heavy drinkers.

Investigators have given a prominent place to the AUDIT as a research tool. This instrument has been ranked fourth among the self-report screening measures more commonly used to identify hazardous drinkers; that is, drinkers whose pattern of drinking poses a high risk of future damage to physical or mental health. Harmful drinkers, also identified by the instrument, would be persons whose pattern of alcohol use is already resulting in problems. The technique therefore shifts the focus from alcoholism as a clinical entity to a public health perspective aimed at the earlier detection of a broad range of alcohol-related problems, only one of which is alcohol dependence.[2] Data on the validation of this instrument are presented in the chapter. With the assistance of this tool, categories of drinkers were identified depending on the level of risk. The Mexican team has used this instrument to evaluate needs among special populations and as the basis for intervention programs. For example, the AUDIT was used to identify patients with alcohol-related problems in work settings, primary care environments, and emergency rooms. Interestingly, as many as 44% of workers were considered hazardous drinkers, 16% harmful, and 3% alcohol dependent. As mentioned throughout, the interest of the investigators has not been just with those individual likely to become dependent on the substance, but also with those for whom drinking represents a risk for accident and/or psychosocial problems.

In Chapter 16, Campillo, Romero, Saldívar, and Ramos are part of the team of Mexican researchers participating in the WHO collaborative project mentioned. This group has been particularly interested in studying the prevalence of hazardous and harmful drinking in a clinical population of persons receiving primary health care from outpatient clinics in two major general hospitals. Patients who clearly met diagnosis of alcohol dependence were excluded from the investigation. The group included drinkers who consumed approximately 29 standard drinks a week for males and 19 drinks females. Identification of hazardous drinkers among these men and women would help to define at-risk groups suitable for testing intervention procedures designed to lower the risk of alcohol-related problems. The investigators rated behavior using instruments, most of them with psychometric characteristics reported in the literature. The dimensions explored included symptoms of alcohol dependence, physical trauma experience, family history of alcoholism, situations that placed the individual at risk for drinking and adverse social consequences.

The findings suggest that the group as a whole experienced significant social, legal, medical, and occupational problems. These individuals required considerable health care, were less productive in their jobs, and had difficulties at work. Among the unmarried, strained interpersonal relationships and angry behavior were often reported. Their families were the first to express concern about their drinking. Health providers were less likely to raise questions about drinking. Circumstances that placed patients at risk of drinking included festive social occasions, weekends, or vacations. Socializing with friends in bars or parties were common situations that placed these persons at risk. A high prevalence of alcohol-related problems were reported among family members, particularly the father. Among members of this group of people who had not been identified as alcohol dependent, drinking was not without consequences. Hazardous drinking was not easy to identify, given that a large proportion of the group reported considerable alcohol-related problems. Given the findings of this research, the validity of the concept of hazardous drinking could not be fully supported. The line between harmful and hazardous was not easy to draw.

The drinking of alcoholic beverages is to a great extent a cultural phenomenon influenced by the social matrix in which this behavior occurs. It is therefore interesting to view this behavior from this vantage point. In Chapter 17, Tiina Arppe, a researcher from the Academy of Finland currently doing investigations in Paris, presents an insightful perspective of alcohol-drinking behavior attributed to the French existentialists during and after World War II. Arppe indicates that periods of economic boom are characterized by increased social interaction. Drinking during these times is "not only normal" but almost a duty. The situation is more complex, however. She uses as an illustration the behavior attributed to Sartre and his followers during the period mentioned. She also examines the significance of the image of the lifestyle given by the intellectuals themselves and by daily papers of the time. The French existentialists had gained considerable public visibility because of their literary and philosophical work, as well as the perception of their behavior presented by the media. The existentialists were criticized severely and in a moralizing way in the daily papers for their extravagant way of life. Jean-Paul Sartre and Simone de Beauvoir, "a teacher's son" and "a girl brought up in the best tradition of French nobility," were seen as determined to corrupt a great part of French youth by means of their "obscure philosophy and filthy lifestyle." Collective drinking is an activity that creates and maintains a feeling of togetherness. It may also become an endeavor of a secret fraternity for groups who perform their ritual behavior away form the world's gaze. Hotel life, contingent love affairs, the love of certain excesses, drinking, and the use of stimulants were attributed to the group. Their behavior was seen as a form of rebellion within the refined French culture. In the terminology of the author, feasting and the temporary transgression of the rules of everyday life, and the promotion of excess and extravagance acquire a "sacred nature." Their leader becomes "a sanctified accursed." The sacred therefore appears almost entirely in a negative way through the challenge of prohibitions. A great deal of effort is made during the feast to act in a way completely different from ordinary times. Excess is part of a "rite" with "sacred power." The chaos created helps nature and communities to renew themselves. Turning everything upside down seems to prove the possibility of a return to the creative epoch of chaos, after which the universe needs to be made again. To be created again is the function of the feast in the community; it actualizes their relationships and gains new strength. Jean-Paul Sartre's position as the leading intellectual figure of the time was partly propelled by his ambiguous reputation. His reputation and visibility also "sanctifies" him. The behavior of the group creates a transgressive myth of rebellion that contributed to the visibility mention and perhaps to emulation by the many.

The concurrent use of cocaine and alcohol is common, as survey data indicate. Furthermore, studies with clinical populations suggest that more than one half of those individuals diagnosed with cocaine dependence also meet criteria for the alcohol dependence.[3,4] Interactions between the two drugs at behavioral and pharmacological levels are likely to occur. In Chapter 18, a research team from Barcelona, Spain including Camí, Farré, Gonzáles, Segura, and de la Torre examine these interactions and share some of their expertise and research experience in this area. According to the investigators, combinations of these drugs induce certain behavioral changes and increase toxicity. Cocaine and alcohol accentuate the risks of medical and legal complications. The administration of alcohol in cocaine abusers increases the magnitude and duration of the euphoric effects of cocaine and reduce some of the dysphoric withdrawal symptoms. A study on drug preference is reported in which alcohol pretreatment significantly increased the choice of cocaine over placebo in nondependent cocaine users. The combination of both drugs enhanced euphoric and cardiovascular effects. Interactions occur at the pharmacodynamic and pharmacokinetic levels. Plasma levels of cocaine are higher when alcohol and cocaine are administered concurrently, and cocaine clearance is reduced significantly. Metabolic inhibition of the metabolism of cocaine in the presence of alcohol is therefore present. These changes involve alterations of cocaine kinetics and metabolism and the biosynthesis of newly active metabolites such as cocaethylene. This compound has a pharmacological profile similar to that of cocaine. Cocaethylene has less pronounced subjective effects. Equimolar doses of cocaine and cocaethylene produce similar subjective and cardiovascular effects, but cocaethylene appears to be eliminated more slowly than cocaine.

Hepatitis C virus (HCV) was first recognized as an independent disorder in 1974. The virus responsible for this infection was identified in 1988. The virus belongs to the family of flaviruses and pestiviruses.[6] A clinically important feature of the infection is its tendency to become chronic and to lead to disorders such as cirrhosis of the liver and hepatocellular carcinoma. Fifty to eighty percent of the patients infected with the virus will develop chronic hepatitis, and in 20 to 30% the disorder will progress to cirrhosis.[7] This, called by some the silent epidemic, is of considerable public health importance. The disease has been of increasing interest to physicians working with addictive disorders. According to some studies, the seroprevalence of HCV antibody is as high as 94% among heroin users.[8] The infection is common in alcoholics: 36 to 39% of alcoholics with cirrhosis of the liver are positive for the HVC antibody. Fifty-six to seventy-six percent of the alcoholics with hepatocellular carcinoma are positive for the antibody.[9] It is therefore useful to review aspects of this infection. With this purpose in mind, in Chapter 19, Yoshihara, Noda, and Kamada review the interrelationships between alcohol intake and liver cirrhosis. According to the authors, alcohol intake may exaggerate the severity of the liver disease and promote carcinogenesis in patients with chronic hepatitis. Alcohol is likely to be an important modulator in the progression of chronic viral hepatitis. Heavy drinkers exhibit significantly higher levels of serum HCV-RNA than nondrinkers. Increasing mutation of the HCV genome might be related directly or via immune response to the production of acetaldehyde, a metabolite of alcohol; genetoxin, which is induced by alcohol and activated by cytochrome P450 IIE1; and free radicals produced by ethanol metabolism. This activity may promote an increase in the occurrence of carcinoma in alcoholic patients with hepatitis C. HCV may not be oncogenic by itself but may act as a cofactor by inducing necroinflammation, regeneration, and possibly malignant transformation to hepatocellular carcinoma. Abstinence therefore may contribute to the prevention of hepatocarcinogenesis and have favorable effects in the clinical course of HCV.

References

1. Bordon A: Ignoran que consumen drogas [They ignore their own consumption of drugs]. *Reforma* 4(1193):2A 1997, March 15.
2. Allen JP, Litten RZ, Ferig JB, Babor T, A review of research on the Alcohol Use Disorders Identification Test, AUDIT. *Alcohol Clin Exp Res* 21:613–619, 1997.
3. Higgins ST, Budney, AJ, Bickel, WK, *et al:* Alcohol dependence and simultaneous cocaine and alcohol use in cocaine dependent patients. *J Addict Dis* 13:177–189, 1994.
4. Kahlsa H, Paredes A, Anglin MD: The role of alcohol in cocaine dependence, in Galanter M (ed): *Recent Developments in Alcoholism*, vol 10.
5. Prince AM, Brotman B, Grafdy GF: Long-incubation posttransfusion hepatitis without serological evidence of exposure to hepatitis B virus. *Lancet* 2:241–246, 1974.
6. Choo Q-L, Kuo G, Weiner AJ: Isolation of a cDNA clone derived from a blood-borne non-A, non-B viral hepatitis genome. *Science* 244:359–362, 1989.
7. Alter MJ, Margolis H, Krawczynski K, *et al:* The natural history of community-acquired hepatitis C in the United States. *N Engl J Med* 327:1899–1905, 1992.
8. Tennant F, Moll D: Seroprevalence of hepatitis A, B, C, and D markers and liver function abnormalities in intravenous drug addicts. *J Addict Dis* 14:35–49, 1995.
9. Noda K, Yoshihara K, Suzuki K, *et al:* Progression of type C chronic hepatitis to liver cirrhosis and hepatocellular carcinoma—Its relationship to alcohol drinking and the age of transfusion. *Alcohol Clin Exp Res* 29:95A–100A, 1996.

15

Experience with the Alcohol Use Disorders Identification Test (AUDIT) in Mexico

Elena Medina-Mora, Silvia Carreño, and Juan Ramon De la Fuente

Abstract. This chapter describes the development of the Alcohol Use Disorders Identification Test (AUDIT) among various Mexican populations, the evaluations that followed the World Health Organization international research project from where this screening instrument was derived, its use in nonclinical settings, modifications introduced in its wording, the development of a short version, and validity and reliability tests. It also describes rates of hazardous, harmful, and dependent drinkers and biobehavioral consequences of abuse among various Mexican populations. Data drawn from different samples showed adequate levels of specificity and sensitivity. Findings from general population samples confirmed previous observations in general practice: That the AUDIT could capture not only regular consumption at hazardous levels, but also episodic heavy drinking. Data from an International Labor Office/World Health Organization project on model programs for alcohol prevention in the workplace showed that it was possible to derive a short version, easily used for intervention programs, that differentiated categories of drinkers at various risk levels. Rates of problem drinkers in clinical samples varied between 28 and 43% for males and 3.6 and 4.8% among females. Hazardous drinking varied between 0.7 and 15.5% among males and females in general populations and reached 44% in a sample of male workers; in clinical settings, harmful drinking ranged from 7 to 16% among males and dependence from 3 to 10%.

Elena Medina-Mora and Silvia Carreño • Instituto Mexicano de Psiquiatria, Calzada, CP 14370 México, DF. **Juan Ramon De la Fuente** • Secretary of Health, Lieja 7, México DF 06693.

Recent Developments in Alcoholism, Volume 14: The Consequences of Alcoholism, edited by Galanter. Plenum Press, New York, 1998.

1. Introduction

Problems that derive from the abuse of alcoholic beverages represent a main burden to the public health of many societies, and Mexico is not an exception. In this country, hepatic cirrhosis is one of the ten leading causes of death;[1] 1.3 of each ten adult males living in urban areas are dependent on alcohol,[2] and a high burden is derived from events of acute intoxication that also result in a high rate of violence and accidents.

The prevalence of problem drinking in nonpsychiatric clinical settings is also high. De la Fuente,[3] using a modified version of the Self-Administered Alcoholism Test (SAAST)[4]—the Cuestionario Administrado de Alcoholismo (CUAAL)—found a rate of 30% and 5% of excessive intake among the male and female, respectively, inpatient and outpatient populations of a third-level hospital. A multicenter study among male outpatients detected 22% of problem drinkers, and in 17% there was a suggestion of dependence.[5] The rates of hazardous and harmful use in two general hospitals in Mexico was estimated by Campillo[6] in 14% among male and 1% in female outpatients using the World Health Organization (WHO) questionnaire on health and lifestyles.[7] Other studies have also documented the low level of identification of these populations at risk in the general practice,[8] suggesting the need of simple screening instrument.

The purpose of this chapter is to describe the development and use of a screening instrument, the Alcohol Use Disorders Identification Test (AUDIT) in Mexico. It describes its development and the evaluations that followed the WHO international research project where this instrument was developed, its use in nonclinical settings, modifications introduced in its wording, the development of a short version, and its validity and reliability tests. It also discusses its utility when used in nonclinical populations to consider the specific way alcohol is consumed in the country. It also describes survey results of the biobehavioral consequences of alcohol abuse among various populations.

2. Alcohol Use Disorders Identification Test

2.1. *Background Information: Patterns of Alcohol Consumption and Related Problems among the Mexican Population*

In Mexico per capita consumption of alcohol (5 liters in 1994)* is lower than that observed in the United States or Spain. Notwithstanding, alcohol consumption is not evenly distributed among the population; data from a national survey on addictions[2] showed that 25% of the heaviest drinkers consume 78% of the available alcohol.

Daily consumption of alcohol is not a common practice in Mexico, but consumption to the point of intoxication if frequent. There is a high propor-

* Estimated for the population 15 years of age and over, through legal production.[32]

tion of abstainers*: 46% of the urban population between 18 and 65 years of age of the country (63% among females and 27% among males); only 31% and 5% of males and females, respectively, of the population drink once a week or more often. More than half (59%) of the females and one fifth (20%) of the males who drink alcohol do so less than once a month. Among males the most frequent pattern of drinking is of low frequency (at least once a month, less than once a week) with high quantities (five of more drinks per sitting at least once a year) per drinking occasion (66% of the drinkers).

Cross-cultural comparisons, through household surveys conducted among adult populations in selected regions of Mexico and Spain, have shown how patterns of frequent use (once a week or more often) with low quantities (one or two drinks per sitting) are almost nonexistent in Mexico (3% as compared to 46% in Spain), while infrequent use (once a month/less than once a week) with high quantities (five or more drinks per sitting at least once a year), the most frequent pattern in Mexico (24%), is practically not observed in the country of comparison[9,10] (1%).

This pattern of drinking is linked to a high proportion of alcohol-related problems. Data from emergency rooms show that alcohol-related injuries are most linked to acute intoxication than with chronic ingestion; 22% of the traumatic events evaluated in a representative sample of emergency rooms showed positive alcohol readings through a breath analyzer, but only 6% were heavy drinkers.[11] A similar study conducted by Cherpitel,[12] in a county in California, showed the following distribution: 11% of the cases of traumatic injuries entering emergency rooms had positive alcohol levels (around half of what was observed in Mexico), but the proportion of all admissions due to this type of event (being heavy drinkers) was more than three times higher (21%).

According to a national survey on addiction,[2] negative consequences of drinking are more prevalent among nondependent drinkers; for instance, only 18% of persons reporting being involved in a car accident or having work problems because of alcohol intake were dependent on alcohol. These data reflect the "prevention paradox"; that is, even though heavy drinkers or alcoholics may be at higher risk for injury or death than other members of the population, they constitute a small segment of the population. The largest proportion of problems occur among nondependent drinkers, thus supporting the shift in the focus of intervention programs toward the prevention of alcohol-related problems, independently of whether or not they occur to alcohol-dependent persons.

Surveys undertaken in the general population consistently have found an unusually high report of problems, not necessarily explained through frequency of alcohol intake. The WHO international project on early detection of harmful alcohol consumption, from which the AUDIT was developed, detected a "disproportionate experience of dependence and problems in rela-

* Persons that reported not having taken any alcohol in the 12 months previous to the survey.

tion to intake" among general practice patients in Mexico compared to the data obtained from five other countries participating in the study.[13]

Similar findings have been derived from general population surveys that also have shown that it is common for persons who drink less than once a month to report having consumed alcohol first thing in the morning, or to feel guilt due to their use, or to feel the need to reduce their consumption.[14,15] Underlying these self-reports of Mexican respondents might be a sense of social desirability; however, they also are a result of cultural practices, where drinking during festivities that might happen once a year occurs for several days, from morning to night,[16] when the above-mentioned problems might occur without being a result of chronic use.

Furthermore, the experience gained from the WHO project on community responses to alcohol-related problems[17] has suggested that the high rate of problems reported in Mexico might be more linked to events of acute intoxication than to chronic use. In fact, other general population surveys have shown how total alcohol intake in the month previous to the interview explained only 11% of the variance of problems, whereas 81% of drinkers with problems consumed high quantities per occasion.[18]

This evidence suggest that the burden of alcohol in this country is linked both with chronic use and frequent events of acute intoxication that increase the risk for accidents or other psychosocial problems; also, it is more related with being intoxicated in situations where people are not supposed to be. Consequently, an ideal instrument should be able to detect both types of problem drinkers.

2.2. The Development and Validation of the AUDIT in Mexico

The AUDIT was developed in 1982 by an international group of researchers and conveyed by the WHO[13,19] to be an instrument able to identify persons with early alcohol-related problems. The screening instrument is a ten-item questionnaire, which contains three questions on the amount and frequency of drinking (global frequency of alcohol intake, number of drinks on a typical day, and frequency of ingesting six or more drinks on one occasion), three questions on alcohol dependence, and four on problems caused by alcohol, including adverse psychological reactions, selected on the basis of their ability to distinguish light drinkers from those with harmful drinking. A score of 8 or more qualified for a positive case; high scores on the first three items indicate "hazardous alcohol use" and high scores on the problem items suggest "harmful alcohol use"; the same procedure may be followed to indicate possible "alcohol dependence." In certain medical settings and for group of patients that might be uncooperative, it might be accompanied by a second clinical screening procedure that consists of two questions about traumatic injury and five items on clinical evaluation and a blood test—the serum γ-glutamate transpeptidase (GGT). Results of Mexican patients studied as part of the WHO international project showed the AUDIT to be a highly sensitive (80%) and specific (89%) screening instrument, with mean positive and negative predictive values of 60% and 90% respectively.[5]

In order to allow the use of the AUDIT by lay interviewers and in nonclinical settings, a new test of the wording was conducted. A total of 45 interviews were conducted with persons with different drinking patterns: 15 heavy drinkers, 15 moderate drinkers, and 15 light drinkers, of low school status (1–6 years of school completed). All subjects, through a face-to-face interview, were asked to complete the AUDIT and then to report what they understood by each item. The main results suggested the need of changing the wording of one item where the word used to translate "injured" included not only the concept of physical damage but also a sense of emotional harm ("hurt"), thus resulting in an overreporting of this problem among the lighter drinkers; therefore, the item was reworded.

Factorial structure of the AUDIT when used in nonclinical samples was analyzed in a sample of 2050 male workers as part of an international labor organization (ILO)/WHO initiative that tested a model of intervention among this group. Of the sample, 21.5% had finished elementary school and only 6.3% had studied at a university. Approximately half of the workers lived in rural areas. The average age was 28, ranging between 16 and 61 years of age; 19.9% were younger than 21 years of age.[20]

Through a factor analysis with varimax rotation, using the statistical package for the social sciences (SPSS) for Windows, it was possible to derive two factors, one containing items one to three that evaluate frequency and quantity of alcohol intake and one containing items that evaluate problems. The only exemption was item ten: "Has a friend, relative, doctor or other health worker been concerned about your drinking or suggested you cut down?" which had high loading (above 0.40) in both factors; alpha coefficients were 0.88 and 0.81 for frequency/quantity and problem factors, respectively. The complete AUDIT was found to have an internal reliability coefficient of 0.87, indicating an adequate consistency in the responses of the workers. The removal of item ten (others being concerned) did not improve the total alpha coefficient (Table I).

Reliability scores are similar to the ones reported by Barry and Fleming[21] among a rural primary care sample in the United States. Similarly to what these authors report, item nine, which evaluates injuries due to drinking, although more frequently reported among the Mexican sample showed in both samples the lowest item to total correlation. The removal of this item had practically no effect in the alpha coefficient (0.81) (Table II).

2.2.1. Interclass Reliability of Conceptual Domains. Several sections of the questionnaire were devised as scales: three questions of drinking behavior (frequency and quantity of alcohol intake), four questions indicating psychosocial problems (guilt, injuries, others concerned), and three indicators of dependence. The drinking behavior scale had the highest intrascale reliability, with values for Chronbach's alpha among workers of 0.87. Chron-

Table I. Factor Analysis of the AUDIT Symptoms

Items	Factor 1: Alcohol-related problems[b]	Factor 2: Pattern of alcohol intake
1. How often do you drink?	0.21	**0.86**
2. How many drinks on a typical day?	0.18	**0.84**
3. Six or more drinks on one occasion?	0.31	**0.84**
4. Unable to stop drinking?	**0.68**	0.28
5. Failed to do what was expected?	**0.73**	0.11
6. Needed a first drink in the morning?	**0.60**	0.29
7. Felt guilt or remorse?	**0.65**	0.36
8. Unable to remember?	**0.74**	0.16
9. You or someone else injured?	**0.48**	0.15
10. Friend, relative, doctor or other, concerned/suggested you cut down?	**0.41**	**0.51**

[a]Rotated factor matrix (varimax rotation).
[b]Boldface indicates factor where items loaded with values above .40.

Table II. Estimates of AUDIT Item-to-Total Correlations[a]

Items	Item mean (standard deviation)	Item to total correlation	Alpha if item deleted
1. How often do you have a drink containing alcohol?	0.80 (0.80)	0.70	0.80
2. How many drinks containing alcohol do you have on a typical day when you are drinking?	1.08 (1.26)	0.64	0.81
3. How often do you have six or more drinks on one occasion?	0.70 (0.88)	0.74	0.79
4. How often during the last year have you found that you were unable to stop drinking once you started?	0.21 (0.56)	0.56	0.82
5. How often during the last year have you failed to do what was normally expected of you because of drinking?	0.11 (0.38)	0.48	0.83
6. How often during the last year have you needed a first drink in the morning to get yourself going after a heavy drinking session?	0.15 (0.46)	0.52	0.82
7. How often during the last year have you felt guilt or remorse after drinking?	0.27 (0.63)	0.61	0.81
8. How often during the last year have you been unable to remember what happened to the night before because of drinking?	0.15 (0.45)	0.52	0.82
9. Have you or someone else been injured as the result of your drinking?	0.18 (0.71)	0.37	0.83
10. Has a friend, relative, doctor or other health worker been concerned about your drinking or suggested you cut down?	0.67 (1.34)	0.56	0.83

[a]This analysis included the total sample of abstainers and drinkers. Reliability coefficients: alpha = 0.8377; standardized item alpha = 0.8660.

Table III. AUDIT's Reliability Scores

Scales	Items	Chronbach's alpha	Correlation between frequency/quantity and problem scales
Frequency/quantity	1–3	0.87	
Psychosocial	7–10	0.69	0.57
Dependence	4–6	0.69	0.52
Total problem scale	4–10	0.81	0.61
Total scale	1–10	0.87	

bach's alpha coefficients for the adverse psychosocial problems and dependence scales were similar: 0.69. When the seven questions of problems were considered together as a scale, the alpha coefficient reaches 0.81 (Table III).

2.2.2. Interrelationship among Conceptual Domains. The interrelationship of alcohol-specific domains and those measuring problems were examined by correlation analysis. The correlation between questions measuring frequency/quantity of alcohol intake and psychosocial problems was 0.57, and with the dependence scale, 0.52. The correlation between the two problem scales was higher, reaching 0.61.

When the questions of frequency and quantity were analyzed separately, it was evident that the former indicator was more related with problems; between two and three more drinkers of high quantities (five or more drinks per sitting) experienced the psychosocial or dependence problems compared to drinkers that limit the amount consumed, independently of the frequency of intake (Table IV).

2.3. *The Development of Brief Version*

The ILO/WHO project recommended the development of a brief version, using only the three first questions, to facilitate its use among workers in

Table IV. Relation between Quantity of Alcohol Intake and Problems

	Low quantities per sitting	High quantities per sitting
1. Unable to stop drinking?	4%	8%
2. Failed to do what was expected?	0%	2%
3. Needed a first drink in the morning?	2%	3%
4. Felt guilt or remorse?	4%	7%
5. Unable to remember?	1%	3%
6. You/someone else injured?	13%	49%
7. Friend, relative, doctor or other, concerned/suggested cut down?	22%	34%

order to make an initial assessment of their way of drinking and to follow the advice according to their level of risk, including those with low levels of formal education. Using the data from one of the companies, where all workers came from rural areas, the answers to these three questions* were compared with the full AUDIT. Through Roc curves, a cutoff point of three quarters was selected; adequate levels of sensitivity and specificity† (92% and 82%, respectively) with this cutoff point for the brief version were observed; probable dependence was determined with a cutoff point of seven eighths, as all positive cases in the full version scored 8 or more in the first three questions.

As for this analysis, the three first questions were included in both sets of the data that compared (brief vs. full versions); further analyses were conducted comparing only the brief version versus the dependence scores, versus the seven questions on problems and problems without dependence.

The comparison between the brief version and the presence of high scores (three quarters) in the three dependence symptoms showed that 100% of the workers with positive scores in the three symptoms also had a score of 8 or more in the brief version; only 4% of the workers without dependence obtained this score. On the other hand, none of the respondents who scored between 0 and 3 in the brief version had a dependence symptom. Consistency with social problems was tested by dividing the population in three groups: drinkers at a low risk level (scores 0 to 3 in the brief version), excessive drinkers without dependence, and excessive drinkers with dependence symptoms. Self-report of alcohol-related injury varied between 2, 13, and 40%, respectively; concern on behalf of others was reported by 9, 43, and 73%, respectively; frequency of drunkenness during festivities ranged from 7 to 44% and to 85%; problems at work were reported by 8, 13, and 46%, respectively; and quasi-accidents due to alcohol by 7, 9, and 45%, respectively, suggesting an adequate differentiation of drinkers according to risk levels.

3. Prevalence of Drinking at Various Risk Levels

The AUDIT has been used successfully in general population surveys,[22] in studies at the work place,[20,23] in emergency rooms,[24] in the general practice, at third-level services in the Mexican Institute of Social Security,[25,26] and in general hospitals[27] (Table V).

Data from a general population survey in a marginal population of a city located in central Mexico show a similar rate of problem drinkers evaluated

* The total score resulted from adding the individual responses to the three questions; it ranged from 0 to 12.

† These estimations were made by comparing the score in the short version versus the score in the full instrument.

Table V. Rates of Hazardous, Harmful, Dependent, and Problem Drinkers in Various Mexican Populations

Study	Population	Gender	Hazard-ous	Harmful	Depen-dence	Problem drinkers
Díaz *et al.*[22]	Household survey of general population	Males	15.5%	6.0%	9.7%	
		Females	0.7%		0.25%	
Medina-Mora *et al.*[23]	Workers	Males	44%	16%	3%	
Guevara *et al.*[27]	General hospitals	Males				43%
		Females				3.6%
Peña-Corona[26]	General practice	Males				28%
		Females				4.8%
Borges[24]	Emergency rooms (persons that reported drinking in the last 12 months)	Males				35%
		Females				7%

through the AUDIT and the Composite International Diagnostic Interview 1.0 (CIDI). Díaz[22] conducted a study in the general population of the capital city of a central state in Mexico, and the sample design was of multiple stages, with blocks, houses, and individuals being units of selection at the different stages. One person per household was interviewed, and data were weighted according to the probability of selection. The sample was also stratified by social level with an oversample of high-risk areas, defined by low levels of income and services, as well as by high levels of delinquency. A total sample of 608 individuals was obtained. The study reported rates of 15.5% hazardous drinkers, 6.8% of harmful drinkers, and 9.7% of dependents among males, and of 0.7, 0, and 0.25%, respectively, among females. Using the CIDI 1.0 among this same population, the rate of abuse–dependence was estimated in 14.1% and 0.25% among males and females, respectively.

Guevara-Arnal[27] used the AUDIT in nine general hospitals in a sample of adult patients (18–59 years of age) and found 3.6% positive cases among females and 43% among males. Medina-Mora[20] used the AUDIT in a sample of 2050 workers who answered a questionnaire through a face-to-face interview, in which the rate of nonresponse was 9.8%. In both cases, all male workers from the chosen plants were selected. Anonymity was ensured, the name of the worker was not written in the questionnaire, and no records were made available that could match the worker with the answers provided in the questionnaire. Approximately one third of the workers (35%) were drinking at a low-risk level, 44% qualified as hazardous drinkers, 16% as harmful drinkers, and 3% as dependents. Workers with dependence had experienced between one and three more problems than harmful drinkers at work caused by their alcohol intake. No differences were observed between low-risk and hazardous drinking; between 8 and 11% of the low-risk drinkers had interpersonal problems due to alcohol compared to 11 and 42% of harmful drinkers and 26 and 64% of workers with dependence; rates of absenteeism varied from 7% among low-risk drinkers to 41% among dependent drinkers and accidents between 5 and 10%, respectively.

Hazardous and low-risk drinkers were less likely than harmful drinkers or those where there was evidence of dependence to present the studied problems; however, because of the fact that they represent a higher proportion of the population, more than 60% of problems at the work place related to alcohol intake occurred in this group, reflecting the previously mentioned prevention paradox (Table VI).

4. Other Developments

The AUDIT has been used in Mexico both as a research tool and to evaluate needs among special populations as a basis for intervention programs. For example, it was used to identify patients with alcohol-related problems at the general practice from the Mexican Institute of Social Security, and it was applied to a total sample of 41,121 patients in the whole country; 4.8% of the females and 28% of the males were drinking at various risk levels. Later, the same group of researchers used the AUDIT to detect drinkers at risk from a total sample of 204 patients in six outpatient third-level services; these results were used as a basis for the addictions program implemented in that institution.[25,26]

Borges[24] used the AUDIT in an emergency room study in a representative sample of persons who attended the emergency rooms available in a city located near the capital. A total of 871 persons (52% males and 48% females), attending because of accidents or violence (56%) or medical emergencies (44%), submitted to a breath test and participated in a face-to-face interview using a standardized questionnaire. Eight percent of the cases were positive in the breath analysis (13% of the accidents and 4% of the medical emergen-

Table VI. Relation between Type of Drinker and Problems

	Low risk (n = 434)	Hazardous (n = 543)	Harmful (n = 198)	Dependence[a] (n = 41)
Friends criticized	11%	12%	42%	64%*
Alcohol/complicated relations	9%	8%	11%	26%*
Supervisor commented	8%	10%	22%	41%*
Problems at work	10%	10%	22%	46%*
Quasi-accidents	7%	7%	12%	45%*
Absenteeism	9%	11%	20%	41%*
Accidents	5%	4%	3%	10%
Percentage from total sample (N = 1244)	35%	44%	16%	3%

[a]$*p \geq .001$.

Table VII. Relation between Emergency Room Entrances and AUDIT Scores

	Negative AUDIT	Positive AUDIT
Injuries	67%	33%
Burns/near drowning	73%	27%
Alcohol/drug intoxication/abstinence	54%	46%
Heart condition/shortness of breath	65%	34%
Liver/stomach condition	62%	18%
Other medical conditions	71%	29%

cies); 35% of the males and only 7% of the females who reported any drinking in the year previous to the interview had a positive score in the AUDIT (score 8 or more); this occurred in 32% of the accidents, it rose to 50% when the accident included violence, and it appeared in 44% of the medical emergencies. Positive scores were more prevalent in cases attending because of intoxication with substances (46%); for various types of injuries (33%), burns, or drownings (27%); heart conditions or shortness of breath (34%); than in those attending for liver or stomach conditions (18%) (Table VII).

Finally, the AUDIT also has been used successfully to identify cases and noncases in several studies, for example, to distinguish alcoholic and nonalcoholic cirrhotics, for a determination of the prevalence of *Helicobacter pylori* and its relationship to the etiology of cirrhosis and liver function,[28,29] to investigate the contribution of structural differences in genes in the predisposition to develop alcohol-induced liver damage,[30] and to establish the role of the menstrual cycle in ethanol pharmacokinetics associated with changes in body composition.[31]

5. Discussion, Conclusions, and Recommendations

Because of the specific alcohol consumption patterns observed in Mexico, an ideal screening instrument should include not only problems derived from chronic use but also those related to acute intoxication. It should be able to identify persons not only at risk for becoming problem drinkers or alcoholics but also persons who might not be at special risk of developing dependence but whose way of drinking represents a risk for accidents or other psychosocial problems more related with events of intoxication. Results from the above-mentioned studies show that the AUDIT can successfully capture both problems.

The data from general population surveys have confirmed the observations drawn from the WHO international project from which the AUDIT was derived[13] that "the samples of Mexico and Zambia included a high proportion of total abstainers, and a large group of individuals who drank relatively infrequently, but when they did so, drank large quantities and often experienced problems." By including questions on overall frequency of drinking, amount consumed on special occasions, and frequency of excessive drinking, the AUDIT is able to capture not only regular consumption but also episodic heavy drinking.

This feature represents an advantage when compared to instruments that either include only problems derived from drinking or that inquire about number of days of alcohol intake in the last week, which are not useful for our context. As seen before, this pattern of inquiry would only include about one third of the males (30%) and 5% of the females in the general population. By controlling for the overall frequency and quantity, it allows one to rule out those cases of single episodes of heavy drinking that occur during special festivities that can take place as infrequently as once a year.

The AUDIT, developed from studies conducted in multicultural settings with different levels of alcohol intake, does not share the cross-cultural problems of other screening and diagnostic instruments used in the United States or Western Europe, where patterns of drinking and problems differ considerably. The research protocols that have included the AUDIT as a screening instrument have also shown that it is a useful instrument to identify drinkers with different levels of intake and degree of related problems, thus being a valuable tool for case–control studies.

Data from the ILO/WHO project on model programs for alcohol prevention in the work place also showed that through the AUDIT it was possible to derive a short version, easily used for intervention programs, that differentiated three categories of drinkers: those not at special risk, those that were drinking at a high-risk level either because of high quantities of intake or the presence of problems, and persons with symptoms that suggested dependence. Using this instrument, it is possible to study the likeness of heavy drinkers or persons with alcohol dependence to present problems and the proportion of problems that are the responsibility of hazardous drinkers; it is also a very useful tool for prevention programs. Nonetheless, the data now available do not fully support the validity of the category of hazardous drinker; consequently, it is important to conduct further research to address this issue.

References

1. Secretaría de Salud: *México, Estadísticas de Salud* [Health statistics], Ministry of Health, Mexico City, 1996.
2. Medina-Mora ME, Tapia R, Villatoro J, *et al:* Problems of alcohol use in Mexican urban population: Results from a National Survey. Paper presented at Signatuna, Sweden, 17th Annual Alcohol Epidemiology Symposium, 1991.
3. De la Fuente JR, Gutiérrez RLM, Rivero MF, *et al:* Detección precoz del alcoholismo en una población hospitalaria [Early detection of alcoholism in a hospital population]. *Rev Invest Clín* 34:1–6, 1982.
4. Swenson WM, Morse RM: The use of a self-administered alcoholism screening test (SSAST) in a medical center. *Clin Pro* 50:204, 1975.

5. De la Fuente JR, Kersenobich D: El alcoholismo como problema médico [Alcoholism as a medical problem]. *Rev* la Facultad Med 35:47–51, 1992.
6. Campillo C, Díaz R, Romero M, Padilla P: El médico general frente al bebedor problema [The general doctor and the problem drinker]. *Salud Men* 11:4–11, 1988.
7. Saunders JB, Aasland OG, Babor TF, *et al: WHO Collaborative Project on Identification and Treatment of Persons with Harmful Alcohol Consumption.* Geneva, World Health Organization, 1987.
8. Campillo C, Padilla P, Díaz R, *et al:* La frecuencia de los problemas relacionados con el alcohol en la práctica médica general [Frequency of alcohol-related problems in the general practice]. Memorias de la III Reunión de Investigación y Enseñanza, México City, Instituto Mexicano de Psiquiatría, 1986, pp 181–187.
9. Caetano R, Medina-Mora ME: Acculturation and drinking among people of Mexican descent in México and the United States. *J Stud Alcohol* 49:462–471, 1988.
10. Martines RM, Martin ML, Calve A: Alcohol consumption prevalence in the autonomous region of Madrid. NIDA Monograph Series, 85, 1988.
11. Rosovsky H, García G, López JL, *et al:* El papel del consumo de alcohol en las urgencias médicas y traumáticas [Role of alcohol use in injuries and medical emergencies]. IV Reunión de Investigación. Mexico City, Instituto Mexicano de Psiquiatría, 1988, pp 261–267.
12. Cherpitel Ch: Epidemiology of alcohol related trauma. *Alcohol Health Res World* 16:191–196, 1992.
13. Saunders JB, Aasland OG, Amunsen A, *et al:* Alcohol consumption and related problems among primary health care patients: WHO collaborative project on early detection of persons with harmful alcohol consumption. *Int J Addict* 88:349–362, 1993.
14. Calderón G, Campillo C, Suarez C: *Respuestas de la Comunidad ante los Problemas Relacionados con el Alcohol* [Community responses to alcohol-related problems]. México, Organización Mundial de la Salud, Mexico City, Instituto Mexicano de Psiquiatría, 1981.
15. Medina-Mora ME, Rascón ML, Otero BR, Gutierrez E: Patrones de consumo de alcohol en México [Alcohol drinking patterns in Mexico], in J. Gilbert (ed): *Alcohol Consumption among Mexicans and Mexican Americans: Binational Perspective.* Los Angeles, CA, 1988, pp 27–52.
16. Natera G: El consumo de alcohol en zonas rurales de México [Alcohol use in rural areas]. *Salud Mental* 10:59–66, 1987.
17. Roizen R, Brace S, Cameron T, *et al: Drinking Behavior in Cross-Cultural Perspective: Some Preliminary Findings from the World Health Organization Project, Community Responses to Alcohol Related Problems* (Alcohol Research Group, eds.). Berkeley, CA, 1980.
18. Medina-Mora ME: Diferencias por género en las practicas de consumo de alcohol [Gender differences in alcohol drinking practices]. México, DF, Tesis para optar por el grado de doctor en psicología social, Universidad Nacional Autónoma de México, 1993.
19. Babor T, De la Fuente JR, Saunders JB, Grant M: *The Alcohol Use Disorders Identification Test: Guidelines for Use in Primary Health.* WHO/MNH/DAT/89.4, Geneva, World Health Organization, 1989.
20. Medina-Mora ME, Ortiz A, Carreño S, *et al:* Model program for the prevention of abuse of alcohol and other drugs by workers and their families. International Labor Office, United Nations Drug Control Program. México, World Health Organization, Secretaría de Salud, Consejo Nacional contra las Adicciones, Instituto Mexicano de Psiquiatría, unpublished report AD/GLO/92/586, 1996.
21. Barry K, Fleming M: The Alcohol Use Disorders Identification Test (AUDIT) and the SMAST-13: Predictive validity in a rule primary care sample. *Alcohol Alcohol* 28:33–42, 1993.
22. Díaz R, Osornio A, Díaz A, *et al: La Salud Mental en el Municipio de Querétaro: Estudio Epidemiológico de la Población Marginada* [Mental health in the municipality of Querétaro: Epidemiological study of population living in poor areas]. Queretaro, México, Sociedad de Salud Mental del Estado de Querétaro, 1994.
23. WHO/ILO: Model program of abuse prevention in the industry. International Labor Office, United Nations Drug Control Program. Mexico, World Health Organization, Secretaria de

Salud, Consejo Nacional contra las Adicciones, Instituto Mexicano de Psiquiatría, unpublished report AD/GLO/92/586, 1994.
24. Borges G: The detection of alcohol-related problems at emergency rooms (ongoing project). Pachuca, Hidalgo, México, Mexican Institute on Psychiatry, 1997.
25. Peña-Corona MP: Resultados de la encuesta AUDIT en trabajadores del IMSS [Results of the AUDIT study among IMSS workers]. Paper presented at the "Alcohol Consumption: New Medical Perspectives," Seminar, Mexico City, August 1996.
26. Peña-Corona MP: Consumo de alcohol en pacientes del IMSS [Alcohol consumption in patients from the Mexican Institution Social Security]. Paper prepared for the National Council against Addictions meeting, Mexico City, October 1996.
27. Guevara-Arnal L, Zapata L, Kaplan M, *et al:* Excessive alcohol intake among Mexican patients. *J Addict* 2:170–176, 1995.
28. De la Fuente JR, Kersenobich D: Detección oportuna del paciente alcohólico y sus alteraciones hepáticas. *Salud Mental* 10:76–80, 1987.
29. Schmulson M, De León G, Kershenovich A, *et al: Helicobacter pylori* infection among partients with alcoholic and nonalcoholic cirrhosis. Submitted for publication.
30. Taba SS, Cruz C, Green-Renner D, et al: Association between type I procollagen genes with alcoholic liver cirrhosis. Submitted for publication.
31. Kershenobich D: Effect of menstrual cycle in ethanol pharmacokinetcs. Submitted for publication, 1997.
32. Rosovsky H: Data bases of alcohol statistics. Mexico City, Center of Information on Alcohol, Mexican Institute on Psychiatry, 1996.

16

Problems Associated with Hazardous and Harmful Alcohol Consumption in Mexico

Carlos Campillo, Martha Romero, Gabriela Saldivar, and Luciana Ramos

Abstract. This chapter presents research findings from a collaborative project between Mexican investigators from the Mexican Institute of Psychiatry and the World Health Organization on the identification and treatment of harmful and hazardous drinking. A sample of 189 individuals who met criteria for hazardous drinking was selected for the study after screening 2319 outpatients attending clinics in two general hospitals in Mexico City. We present here the characteristics of this sample along dimensions that include alcohol related problems, history of trauma, alcohol dependence scores and family history of alcoholism. We rated, utilizing structures interviews, situations that place these individuals at risk of drinking. The possibility of constructing a typology of harmful and hazardous drinking was also explored. The significance of the findings of this investigation for health care clinicians is discussed.

1. Introduction

Alcohol research in the last decade has shown a growing awareness of the potential for adverse consequences associated with what used to be referred as social or moderate drinking. Programs designed to identify and treat drinkers at risk for developing alcohol-related problems have received considerably less attention than those dealing with the treatment of alcohol dependence and chronic alcoholism.[1] Worldwide, there are now a number of innovative projects of research that focus on secondary prevention efforts for a special

Carlos Campillo, Martha Romero, Gabriela Saldivar, and Luciana Ramos • Instituto Mexicano de Psiquiatría, Tlalpan, 14370 México, DF.

Recent Developments in Alcoholism, Volume 14: The Consequences of Alcoholism, edited by Galanter. Plenum Press, New York, 1998.

group that may be called hazardous and harmful drinkers. The characteristics of this group may vary in different cultural contexts.

According to Kranzler *et al.*,[2] the term *hazardous drinking* refers to a level of alcohol consumption or pattern of drinking that, should they persist, are likely to result in harm to the drinker. In contrast, harmful drinking is defined as alcohol use that has resulted in adverse mental or physical effects for the individual. The aim of the terminology is to provide clinicians and researchers with guidelines for the identification of individuals at risk who may not meet the criteria for alcohol dependence.

A variety of screening procedures have been created to facilitate the early identification of this population. Among the most important efforts were the development of instruments such as the Michigan Alcoholism Screening Test (MAST),[3] the CAGE,[4] the T-ACE,[5] and the Alcohol Use Disorders Identification Test (AUDIT) by the World Health Organization (WHO).[6]

Following the development of the screening instruments, the question that arose was how to design intervention approaches that were capable of modifying drinking patterns and related behaviors as well as changing attitudes of nondependent drinkers. From a growing international literature dealing with what have been variously described as early intervention and secondary prevention programs emerged a WHO project on identification and management of alcohol-related problems.[7] In Mexico, we experienced a growing concern regarding the public health consequences of hazardous alcohol consumption. The need for more effective measures in primary health care therefore became evident.[8–10] Mexico participated in the task as a WHO collaborative center. The principal aim of the project was to evaluate brief intervention procedures directed at heavy drinkers who are not seriously dependent on alcohol. For instance, we intended to determine whether simple advice or brief counseling, delivered within the context of a single consultation in a medical setting, would result in a significant reduction in the patient's drinking over a 6-month period. To the extent that the quantity and frequency of drinking can be reduced in hazardous drinkers, it was expected that the likelihood of alcohol-related problems would be reduced within the time frame mentioned. Hypotheses along this line have been validated and analyzed elsewhere.[11] The aim of the present chapter is to describe the characteristics of the harmful and heavy drinkers who took part in the study, to see if a typology of this category of drinkers would emerge considering their related problems, and to show that in spite of the fact that they have some characteristics in common (like their drinking habits), they form an heterogeneous group.

2. Methods and Procedures

2.1. Study Site, Screening, and Recruitment

2.1.1. Inclusion Criteria. The study was carried out by the Mexican Institute of Psychiatry, in Mexico City, at a clinic, which was one of the units belonging to the network of facilities from the Mexican Institute of Social Security, and in the general hospital "Dr. Manuel Gea Gonzalez." Patients for the project were recruited from outpatient clinics, either from the clinical record files or from patients in the waiting room. Recruitment was conducted in two steps. First, the Health and Lifestyle (Screening) Questionnaire was administered. This instrument was employed to: (1) provide a brief explanation to prospective subjects; (2) identify subjects who met minimal eligibility criteria; and (3) screen out subjects who were ineligible either because they drank too much or too little.

If the individual was eligible, a standard explanation was employed to inform the patient that the health adviser wished to: (1) conduct a 20-min interview using a general health survey developed by researchers at the WHO (the WHO Composite Interview); (2) *possibly* give them some health information and brief advice based on the interview results; (3) have them fill out a brief self-report questionnaire; and (4) have them return for a follow-up health survey in about 6 months. No information was provided about the specific purpose of the study.

Patients were then randomly assigned to three possible groups: a control group, a simple advice group, and a brief counseling group. Patients from the control group were thanked for their participation in the study and were asked to return for a follow-up interview in approximately 6 months.

Patients assigned to the other two conditions received either simple advice or brief counseling directed toward changing their drinking habits and were asked to return in 6 months for a follow-up interview. At that time, a revised version of the WHO Composite Interview was administered in addition to several self-report questionnaires such as the Inventory of Drinking Situations, Moos Depression Scale, Self-Confidence Questionnaire, Family History of Alcoholism, and California Personality Inventory (CPI) scale of sociopathy among others.

Only 196 individuals were interviewed at follow up. Four of the patients died and data from 14 files were excluded from most of the analyses because of missing information. Table 1 summarizes the inclusion criteria.

2.1.2. Exclusion Criteria. The exclusion criteria were designed to exclude drinkers who were inappropriate for the intervention. Exclusion criteria included: prior treatment for alcoholism, drug abuse, liver disease, or mental disorder; being warned by a physician or other health professional to refrain completely from drinking alcohol; past or recent history of morning drinking on a relatively frequent basis; and recent alcohol consumption. Also excluded were individuals who drank less than the levels recommended in the inclusion criteria or extremely high amounts per day (150 g or more), pregnancy, lack of social–residential stability, and patients who were less than 18 years of age and older than 70 years of age.

2.2. *Sample*

A total of 2319 patients were screened, 1748 at the clinic and 571 at the hospital. Of these groups a total of 244 patients met the inclusion criteria, 84%

Table I. Inclusion Criteria[a]

	Males	Females
Regular[b]		
A. Average quantity per week	350 g/week (29 standard drinks)[c]	225 g/week (19 standard drinks)
B. Frequency of intoxication	100 g on one occasion two times per month or more	65 or more g on one occasion, two times per month or more
Reduced[d]		
C. Average quantity per week if perceives problem	300 g/week (25 standard drinks)	200 g/week (17 standard drinks)
D. Frequency of intoxication if perceives problems or desires to cut down	100 g on one occasion once per month	65 g on one occasion once per month

[a]Adapted from Babor and Grant.[7]
[b]Either A or B qualified for patient inclusion.
[c]US standard drink was estimated to contain 12 g of absolute alcohol. This may differ in other countries.
[d]If patient perceived a problem or had tried to cut down in past 3 years, the inclusion criteria were somewhat lower.

from the clinic and 16% from the hospital. Only seven women met selection criteria. As mentioned, 196 male patients were included in the final study sample; the rest were excluded either because they met a criteria for alcohol dependence or drank at levels below inclusion criteria. For the final analysis all woman were excluded.

Before conducting the analysis, patients were assigned to the three study conditions and were compared on demographic characteristics and drinking behavior at intake. Age, socioeconomic status, average daily consumption, intensity of drinking, and days of abstinence are shown in Table II.

Table II. Demographic Characteristics of Male Hazardous and Harmful Drinkers Recruited in Mexico[a]

Mean years of age	32.84
Mean years of education	8.46
Mean occupational prestige[b]	39.65
Single	30.1%
Married	66.8%
Separated/divorced	3.0%

[a]N = 196.
[b]To measure occupational status across the samples, the Standard International Occupational Prestige Scale was used as a determinant of socioeconomic status. Range, 0–100. The scale provides prestige ratings for over 100 occupations.

3. Results

3.1. *Adverse Social Consequences*

The social problems associated with harmful or hazardous drinking may be result of single episodes of drinking or because of persistent alcohol abuse. These consequences impact not only the drinker but also the drinker's family, friends, and associates and others with whom the drinker may come into contact. Moreover, the cost to society of adverse outcomes of alcohol use is high.[12] Individuals with alcohol-related problems require more general health care and may be less productive at their jobs.

In this study the resulting adverse social consequences were striking. Family members were the first to be highly concern by the drinking habits of their relatives. This group of Mexican drinkers revealed a characteristic pattern of alcohol consumption: high quantities on special occasions, weekends, or vacations. In the case of drinkers who consumed alcoholic beverages once a week, 32.6% of the spouses expressed concern with this frequency of drinking. (Figs. 1 and 2). For those patients who were not married, the problems were more likely to be reflected in strained interpersonal relationships, broken relationships, and expressed anger (Fig. 3). Job problems reached almost 40% (Fig. 4); 3.9% of the subjects had lost their job within the last 6 months and 7.9% were disciplined for their alcohol-related behavior; 30% had had problems with legal authorities (Fig. 5). Only 30.3% had been in contact with a health worker who expressed concern for their drinking habits (Fig. 6).

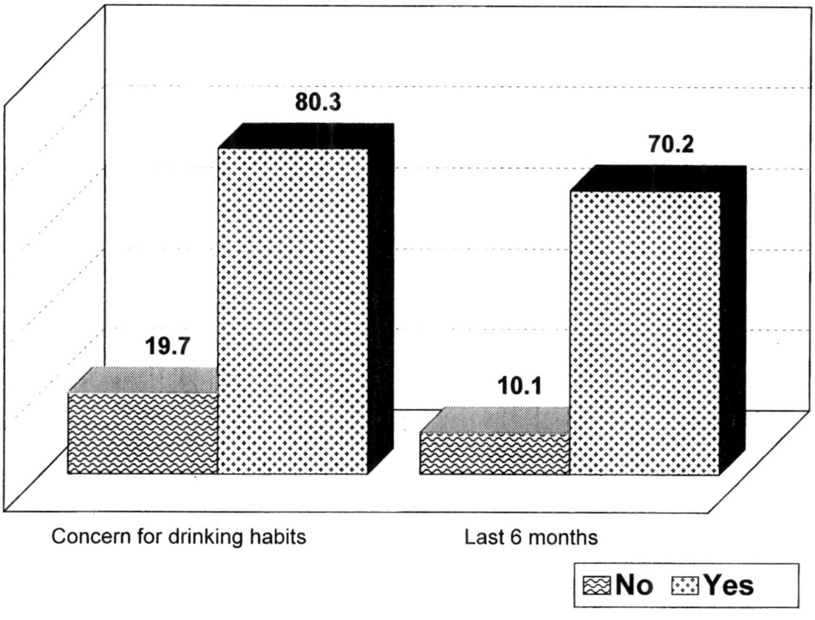

Figure 1. Family concern ($N = 178$). Percentages obtained from the total sample.

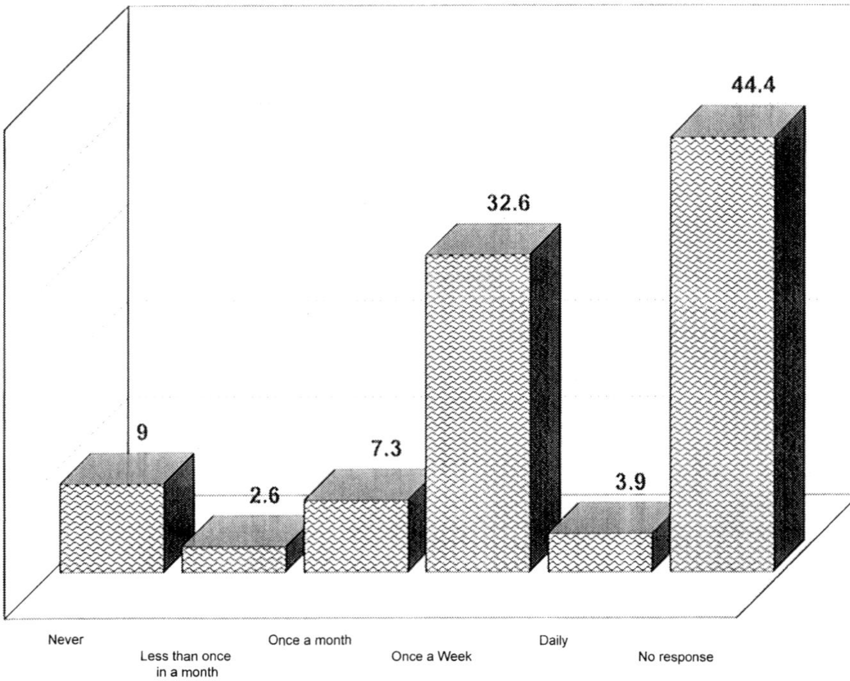

Figure 2. Spouse concern (N = 178). Percentages obtained from the total sample.

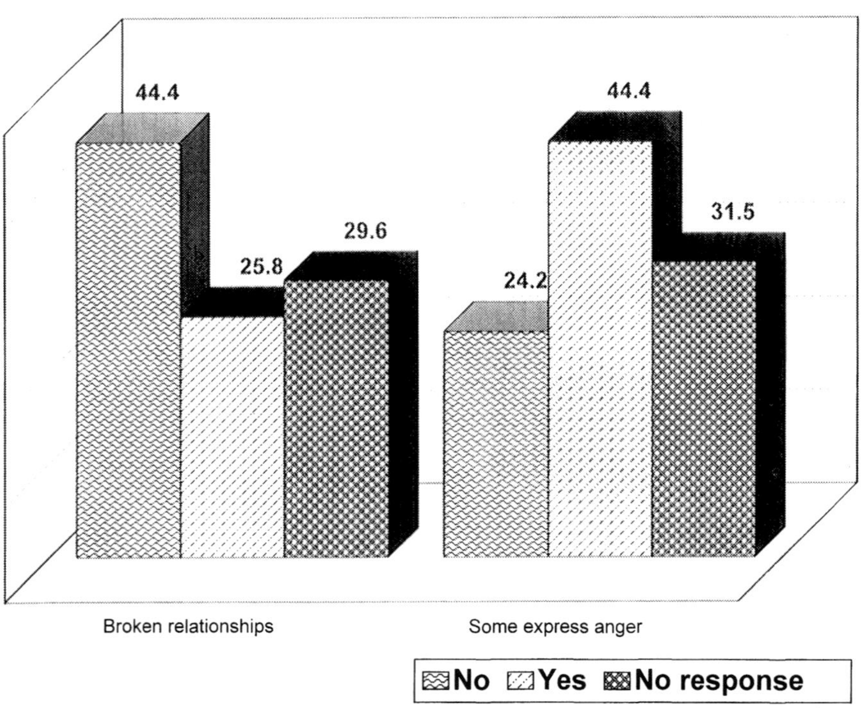

Figure 3. Strained interpersonal relationships (N = 178). Percentages obtained of the total sample.

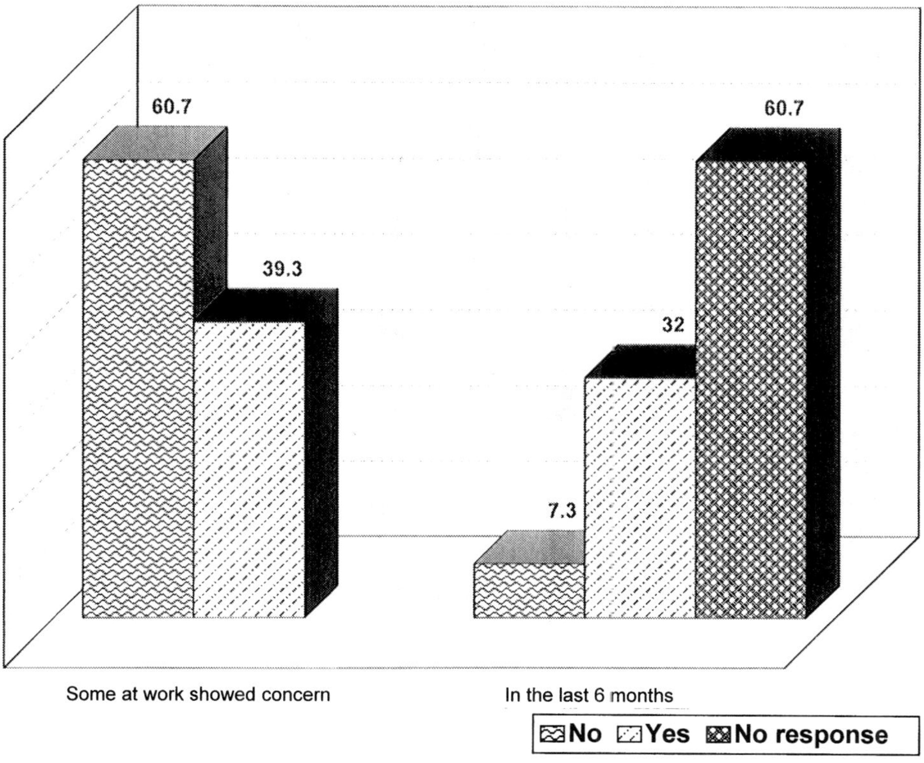

Figure 4. Job problems (N = 178). Sample percentages.

In order to give a comprehensive view of alcohol consumption patterns and alcohol-related problems below we describe the areas covered in our investigation.[7]

3.1.1. Average Daily Alcohol Consumption. This measure estimates the average amount of alcohol ingested per day (in centiliters of absolute alcohol) during the past 6 months. It is computed by dividing the total amount of alcohol reported during a typical month by 30. When interpreting results, it may be useful to remember that one standard drink contains approximately 1.5 cl of absolute alcohol.

3.1.2. Typical Intensity of Alcohol Consumption. This measure estimates the amount of alcohol typically ingested on those days when the respondent actually drank. The total amount of alcohol reported during a typical month is divided by the actual number of drinking days.

3.1.3. Days Drinking. This measure is the patient's estimate of the number of days that alcoholic beverages were ingested during a typical month within the 6-month reference period.

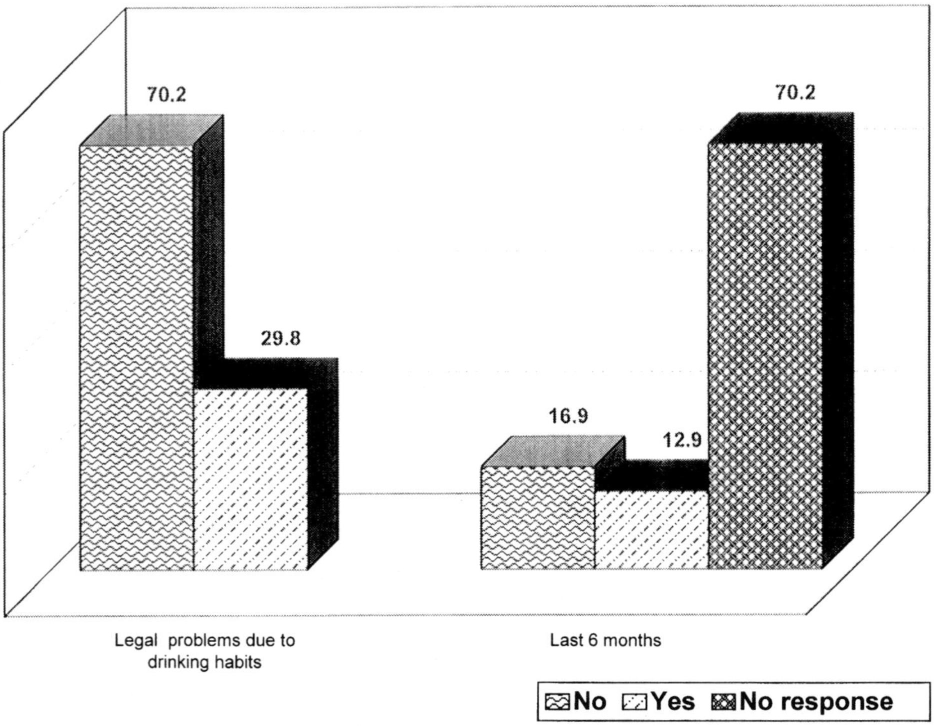

Figure 5. Problems with legal authorities (N = 178). Total sample percentages.

3.1.4. Dependence Score. Six questions were included in the interview to estimate the frequency of dependence symptoms. The items asked about skipping meals while drinking, being unable to stop once drinking began, gulping drinks, staying drunk for several days at a time, attempts to reduce drinking and experiencing morning shakes. Each item was rated on a five point scale in terms of its frequency of occurrence (0 = never to 4 = daily) during the previous 6 months. The patients total score could range between 0 to 24.

3.1.5. Problem Score. This measure estimates the number of alcohol-related social, legal, medical, and employment problems experienced by the patient during the previous 6-month period. It is computed by adding positive responses to questions about family concern, strained interpersonal relationships, anger expressed by others, job difficulties, problems with legal authorities, and concern expressed by a health worker. The range of possible scores varies between 0 and 7.

3.1.6. Concern Score. This is an estimate of the frequency with which persons in the patient's family and immediate social network expressed concern

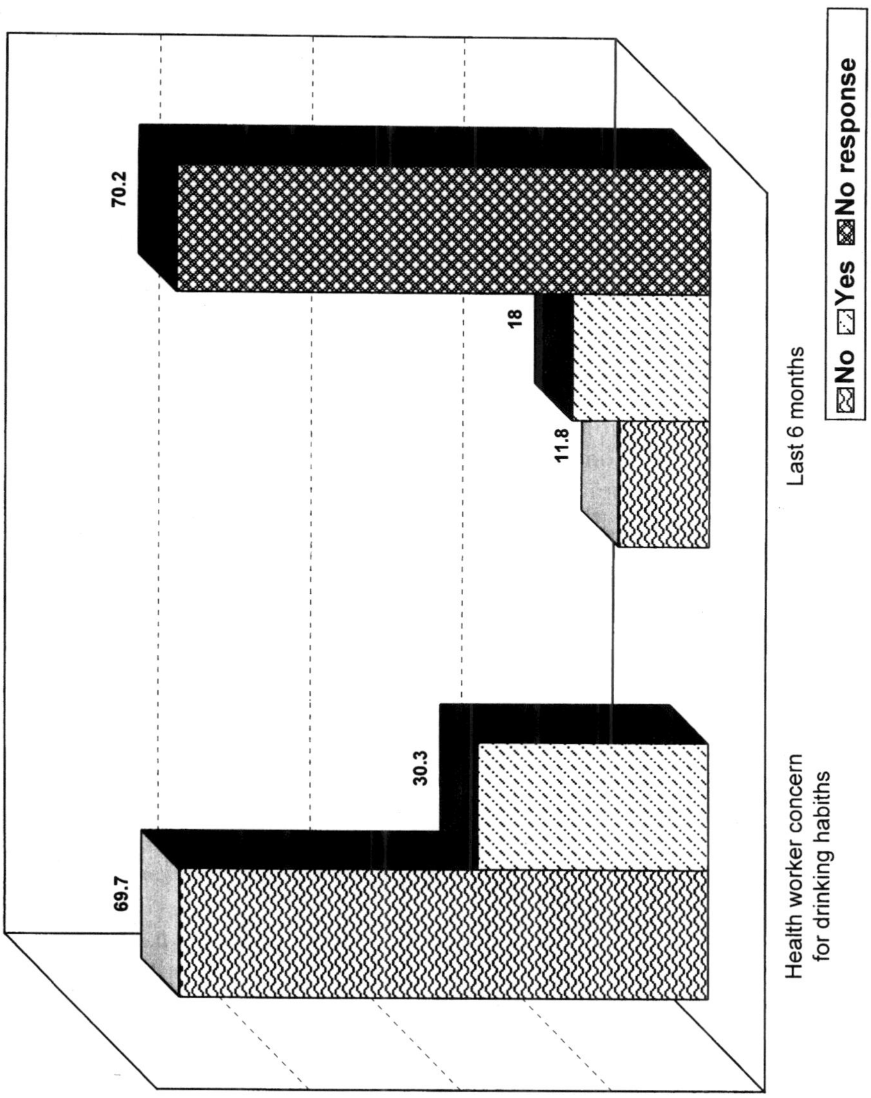

Figure 6. Health problems ($N = 178$). Total sample percentages.

Table III. Measures of Alcohol Consumption and Alcohol-Related Problems[a]

Average daily consumption	4.90[b]
Intensity of drinking	14.53[b]
Days of drinking	10.78
Dependence score	5.06
Concern score	1.96
Problem score	1.51

[a]From Babor and Grant.
[b]In centiliters of absolute alcohol. One standard drink contains 1.5 cl absolute alcohol or 12 g of absolute alcohol.

about the patient's drinking during the past 6 months. Six categories of social relationships (spouse, parents, children, living companion, other family member, friend) were rated on a five-point scale (0 = never to 4 = daily) in terms of the frequency they expressed their concern to the patient. The main findings along the measures of alcohol consumption and alcohol-related problems are summarized in Table III.

3.2. Familial History of Alcohol Consumption

Family studies have consistently revealed a two- to fourfold increased risk for severe alcohol-related life problems in close relatives of alcoholics. The

Table IV. Positive Familial History

	Father		Mother		Brothers and sisters	
	n	%	n	%	n	%
Never lived with	9	8.6	5	4.8		
Less than a year	1	1.0	0			
Between 1 and 5 years	11	10.5	6	5.7		
More than 5 years	84	80.0	94	89.5		
Mental problems	26	24.8	33	31.4	23	21.9
Suicide	2	1.9	0		2	2.0
Alcohol problems	76	72.4	4	3.8	66	62.9
Legal problems	14	13.3	1	1.0	22	21.0
Alcohol-related problems	(N = 76)		(N = 4)		(N = 66)[a]	
Legal problems	25	23.5	0		31	29.5
Health problems	44	41.9	2	1.9	34	32.4
Marital problems	55	52.4	2	1.9	52	49.5
Work problems	23	21.9	2	1.9	33	31.4
Treatment	11	10.5	1	1.0	11	10.5
Social problems	25	23.8	0		37	56.1

[a]Total sample, 105.
[b]Of the brother or sister with the worst problem.

effects of parental alcohol abuse may involve both genetic and experiential factors; a genetic factor would increase the likelihood of alcohol-related problems. Another factor, perhaps experiential, such as living with an alcoholic parent, may increase the likelihood of depressive symptoms.[13] Consistent with the possibility of genetic influences, the risk for severe life problems related to alcoholism appears to increase with an increasing number of alcoholic relatives, the closeness of the genetic relationship to these family members, and perhaps with the severity of their disorder. While more controversial, there also are data to indicate that relatives of primary or uncomplicated alcoholics do not have higher risks for schizophrenia, manic–depressive disease, heroin dependence, or most of the major anxiety disorders.[14]

All patients from the sample answered at follow-up a number of questions regarding the frequency of alcohol problems in the family. The main results are shown in Table IV. Positive history of alcohol problems was more frequent in the father (72.4%), followed by brothers and sisters (62.9%), and finally the mother (3.8%). Significant differences also were found concerning psychological problems. It is necessary to note that the column on siblings indicates either the brother or sister as having the highest frequency of alcohol problems. If each one who was positive was counted, the proportion of alcohol-related problems would be higher.

3.3. *Trauma Scale*

Research to measure and understand alcohol's role in accidents and trauma is essential for planning prevention programs and obtaining baselines for evaluation. Research has suggested that the severity of trauma is greater among intoxicated victims; also, heavy alcohol consumption is frequently related to criminal behavior.[12,15]

As another indicator for harmful drinking, a modified version of the Trauma Scale developed by Skinner *et al.*[16] was used in order to see how well this scale would work with this specific population, which is different from those alcoholics with demonstrated alcohol dependence. As is shown in Table V, the best indicator was to have had a history of fractured bones. No significant differences were found between patients with positive familial history and those without it. The frequency of bone fractures was similar to that found in Mexican studies in emergency room services[15] where 27.7% of the male injuries cases had positive blood alcohol levels.

3.4. *Drinking Situations*

Harmful and hazardous drinkers may differ in the involvement in psychosocial situations that place them at high risk for alcohol consumption. In order to obtain an estimate, the Inventory of Drinking situations (IDS) was administered.[17,18] This instrument was designed by Annis in 1982 to obtain a specific measure of the high-risk psychosocial situations in which a patient

Table V. Trauma History and Positive Familial History[a]

	Total sample (n = 178)		HF+ (n = 105)		HF− (n = 73)	
After 18 years	n	%	n	%	n	%
Accidents	35	19.7	21	20	14	19.2
Head injuries	40	22.5	22	21	18	24.7
Bone fractures	53	29.8	36	34.3	17	23.3

[a]HF+, positive history of bone fractures; HF−, negative history of bone fractures.

may have a relapse to alcohol consumption. The inventory is based on a microanalysis of the situations that, with some frequency, precipitated excessive alcohol consumption within the previous 6 months.[19] From the prevention research point of view, the IDS is a useful instrument to identify situations that place individuals at risk for alcohol consumption in a given population. The instrument is useful to study treatment success and relapse.

Prior to statistical analysis of the inventory responses, all the 42 items were reviewed in order to assure that each question was answered. Twenty-five subjects were excluded of the sample because of missing responses. Therefore, only 166 subjects out of the original sample were used in the analysis.

Descriptive statistics on the percentages of each item response were obtained. These responses were then grouped in two categories: never–seldom and frequently–always. This analysis was done without including the demographic variables. The following items elicited the highest response rates in the categories of frequently and almost always:

I was more likely to drink:

(7) When I went with our friends and they stopped at a bar for a drink (23.5%)
(16) When I went out with friends and wanted to increase my enjoyment (27.1%)
(23) When I was at a party and other people were drinking (3.3%)
(28) When I wanted to celebrate with a friend (18.1%)
(31) When something good happened and I felt like celebrating (19.9%)
(36) When I was enjoying myself at a party and wanted to feel even better (28.3%)
(41) When I was relaxed with a good friend and wanted to have a good time (18.1%)

As a next step, a variance analysis (ANOVA), which included the different age groups, was done in order to see which items reached statistical significance. Only the eight items that are shown in Table VI were statistically

Table VI. Analysis of Variance (ANOVA) of the IDS Items by Age

	Means by age					Statistics		
IDS items	<26	26–35	36–45	46–55	>55	*F*	*P*	Subscale
4. When I had trouble sleeping	1.10	1.23	1.06	1.00	1.50	2.7075	<0.03	2
7. When I went out with friends and they went to a bar for some drinks	2.28	1.93	2.06	1.66	2.12	2.0837	<0.08	7
18. When I do get along with people	1.20	1.15	1.03	1.20	1.50	2.4042	<0.05	3
24. When I felt pressured by the demands of my boss or supervisor to finish a job	1.16	1.17	1.09	1.20	1.75	3.3105	<0.01	3
32. When I thought that one drink wouldn't hurt me	1.55	1.74	1.45	1.53	2.25	2.3643	<0.05	8
33. When I was confused about what I had to do	1.18	1.23	1.12	1.33	2.00	5.9718	<0.0002	1
35. When I did not get along with the people I work with	1.30	1.23	1.16	1.13	1.75	2.4169	<0.05	3
41. When I am with a good friend and we want to have a good time	1.83	1.90	2.35	1.66	22.25	3.6159	<0.0075	2

significant. Three of the eight items pertain to the subscale of social problems at work.

In order to analyze the items in relation to the test subscales, a problem index was obtained. Then we proceeded to obtain the global sample profile (Fig. 7), which revealed the areas of major risk for excessive consumption. The bar length of each category illustrates the magnitude of the problems the respondents experienced in given situations. As the figure shows, the largest percentage of problems fall under the category of "positive social situations." With an ANOVA by age groups, it was found that subscale three (social problems at work) was statistically significant ($p < 0.03$).

3.5. *Typologies*

Although typologies in the alcoholism field are at least 100 years old, more recently clinicians and researchers have proposed several typologies of substance-abusing individuals using empiric rules, clinical wisdom, and theories about the etiology of substance abuse. Subgroups have been proposed on the basis of psychological, biological, and social characteristics of the individual.[20,21]

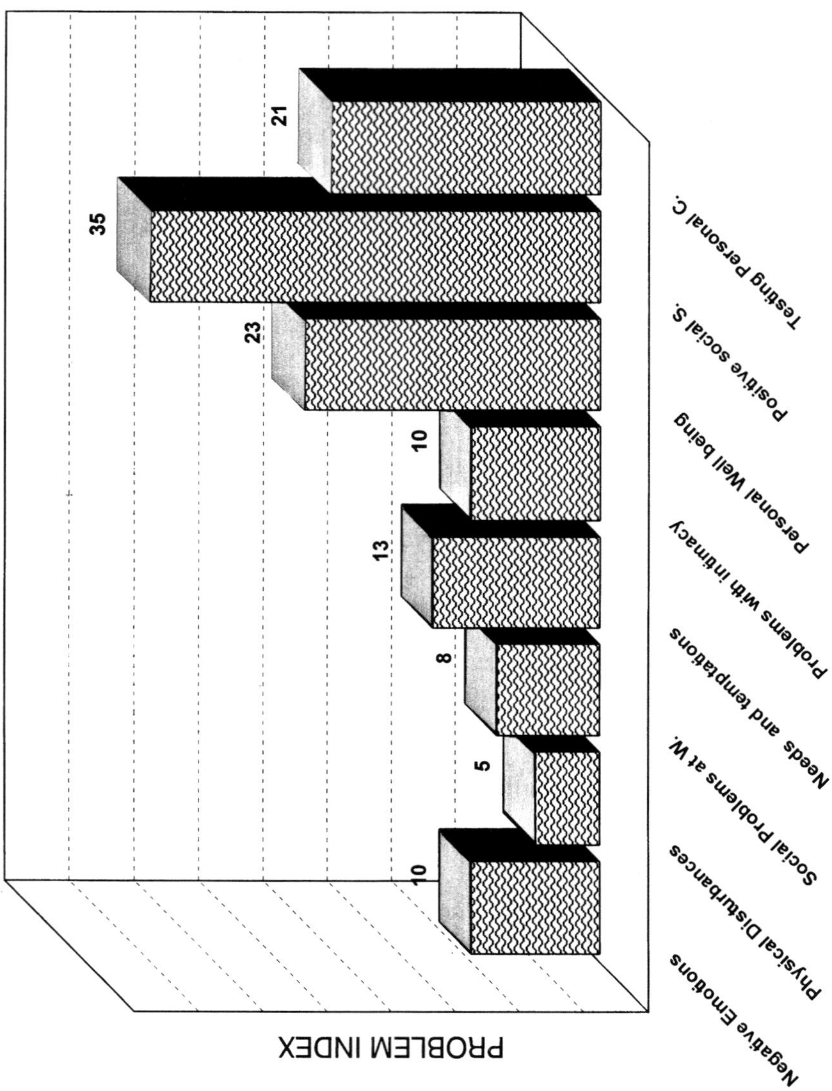

Figure 7. Drinking situations ($N = 166$). Percentages obtained of the total sample.

Table VII. Group Comparison: Patients' Alcohol Dependence Score and Familial History[a]

Variable	Number of cases	Mean	SD	SE of mean
ALCDEP				
Group 1	20	8.8500	1.66	.372
Group 2	25	3.5200	1.475	.295

[a]*T*-test = 11.38 (df 43, $P = 0.00$)

The results obtained with the variables mentioned above led us to consider the construction of groups with different characteristics. Two procedures were employed to obtain separate typologies. First a *K*-means empirical clustering technique[22] was used to identify homogeneous subtypes based on the following variables: familial history, accidents, injuries, bone fractures, concern of the family, problems at work, legal problems, health problems, and alcohol dependence. Once the clusters had been formed, a *t*-test was used to check the significance of the differences in the groups. Two major groups were differentiated: one with positive paternal family history of alcohol consumption (group 1) and another that joins maternal and sibling positive history of alcohol (group 2). Alcohol dependence was the main variable that separated the clusters. Results are shown in Table VII.

4. Discussion

The 1993 world development report found that alcohol-related diseases affect 5 to 10% of the world's population each year, and accounted for approximately 2% of the global burden of disease in 1990.[23] In spite of its importance, the literature has pointed out that in many countries the relationship between hazardous drinking and harmful consequences of drinking are not fully recognized by the medical profession. This is regrettable given that primary care physicians are in a key position to make early diagnoses of alcohol use disorders. Some of them misdiagnose, while others underdiagnose because of stereotypes regarding alcohol problems or inadequate training in this area. There is still a tendency to think about alcohol-related problems only in terms of heavy dependence or alcoholism. An approach designed to influence hazardous drinking patterns will have to define its target group clearly.[7]

As our results indicate, a large number of medical and social problems are typically present in harmful and hazardous drinkers. It is essential to take these different types of drinkers and the different medical and social problems into account, both to obtain a proper diagnosis of the alcohol problems and to make appropriate clinical decisions. It is also important to point out that in this sample only men were included. The screening instrument was found not to be as useful for women. Consequently, further research will have to be done in order to determine the problems associated with hazardous or harmful patterns of consumption in women. Woman may respond differently than men, thus requiring gender-specific intervention strategies.

References

1. Babor T, Korner P, Wilber C, *et al:* Screening and early intervention strategies for harmful drinkers: Initial lessons from the Amethyst Project. *Australian Drug Alcohol Rev* 6:325–339, 1987.
2. Kranzler H, Babor T, Lauerman R: Problems associated with average alcohol consumption and frequency of intoxication in a medical population. *Alcohol Clin Exp Res* 14:119–126, 1990.
3. Selzer ML, Vinokur A, van Rooijen L: A self-administered Short Michigan Alcoholism Screening Test (SMAST). *J Stud Alcohol* 36:117–126, 1975.
4. Clark WD: Alcoholism: Blocks to diagnosis and treatment. *Am J Med* 71:275–285, 1981.
5. Sokol RJ, Martier SS, Ager JW, *et al:* The T-ACE questions: Practical prenatal detection of risk-drinking. *Am J Obstet Gynecol* 160:863–879, 1989.
6. Babor T, De la Fuente JR, Saunders J, *et al:* AUDIT: *The Alcohol Use Disorders Identification Test: Guidelines for Use in Primary Health Care.* Geneva, World Health Organization, 1992.
7. Babor T, Grant M: *Project on Identification and Management of Alcohol-related Problems. Report on Phase II: A Randomized Clinical Trial of Brief Interventions in Primary Health Care.* Geneva, Programme on Substance Abuse, World Health Organization, 1992.
8. Medina-Mora ME, Ortiz A, Natera G, Carreño S, Tiburcio M: Model program for the prevention of the abuse of alcohol and other drugs by workers and their families. ILO/UNPIDC, WHO Report, Mexico 1996.
9. Orford J, Natera G, Casco M, Nava A, Ollinger E: Estrategias que utiliza la familia en México frente al uso de alcohol y otras drogas [Strategies that Mexican families use to cope with alcohol and drugs]. Secretaria de Salud, CONADIC, Instituto Mexicano de Psiquiatría, Mexico City, 1993.
10. Natera G, Orford J: Manual destinado a los orientadores de prevención de alcohol y otras drogas para su intervención y apoyo a las familias que se enfrentan a problemas de consumo excesivo de sustancias en sus hogares [Manual for counselors for the prevention and intervention of alcohol and drugs: support of families that have excessive substance consumption]. Secretaria de Salud, CONADIC, Instituto Mexicano de Psiquiatría, Mexico, 1995.
11. Campillo SC, Diaz R, Romero M, *et al:* Mexico City, Mexico, in Babor T, Grant M (eds): *Project on Identification and Management of Alcohol-Related problems. Report on Phase II: A Randomized Clinical Trial of Brief Interventions in Primary Health Care.* 1992, pp 129–142.
12. National Institute of Alcohol Abuse and Alcoholism: *Alcohol and Health.* US Department of Health and Human Services, 1990.
13. Parker D, Harford T: Alcohol-related problems, marital disruption and depressive symptoms among adult children of alcohol abusers in the United States. *J Stud Alcohol* 49:306–313, 1988.
14. Shuckit M: Advances in understanding the vulnerability to alcoholism, in O'Brien CP, Jaffe JH (eds): *Addictive States.* New York, Raven Press, 1992, pp 93–108.
15. Rosovsky H, Casanova L, Gutiérrez L, *et al:* Los accidentes y la violencia en México: El consumo de alcohol como factor de riesgo [Accidents and violence in Mexico: Alcohol consumption as a risk factor]. *ANALES* 5:61–64, 1994.
16. Skinner HA, Holt S, Schuller R, *et al:* Identification of alcohol abuse: Trauma and laboratory indicators, in *Early Identification of Alcohol Abuse.* Rockville, MD, NIAAA Research Monograph 17, 1985, pp 285–301.
17. Romero M, Campillo C, Cerrud J: The use of the inventory of drinking situations in Mexican population. *New Trend Exp Clin Psychol* 10:165–171, 1994.

18. Annis HM, Graham M, Davis CH: *Inventory of Drinking Situations (IDS) User's Guide.* Toronto, Canada Addiction Research Foundation, 1987.
19. Peachey JE, Annis HM: New strategies for using alcohol sensitizing drugs, in Naranjo CA, Selleres EM (eds): *Research Advances in New Psychopharmacological Treatment for Alcoholism.* New York, Elsevier Science Publishers, 1985.
20. Babor T, Hofmann M, DelBoca F, *et al:* Types of alcoholics. I. Evidence for an empirically derived typology based on indicators of vulnerability and severity. *Arch Gen Psychiatry* 49:599–608, 1992.
21. Bohn M, Meyer R: Typologies of addictions in Galanter M, Kleber H (eds): *Textbook of Substance Abuse Treatment.* Washington, DC, The American Psychiatric Press, 1994, pp 11–24.
22. Norusis MJ: *SPSS/PC + Professional Statistics.* Version 5.0. Chicago, SPPS, Inc, 1992.
23. Desjarlais R, Eisenberg L, Good B, Kleinman A: *World Mental Health: Problems and Priorities in Low-Income Countries.* New York, Oxford University Press 1995, pp 382.

17

Sanctification of "the Accursed"

Drinking Habits of the French Existentialists in the 1940s (A Case Study)

Tiina Arppe

Abstract. The chapter deals with the drinking habits of the French existentialists during and after World War II (roughly from 1943 to 1948). It attempts to show that the phenomenon cannot be understood separately from their lifestyle as a whole, which in this case (as I claim) is primarily manifested through a certain (mythical) structure of meanings related to the category of the sacred. Jean-Paul Sartre's position as the leading intellectual figure of the time is also to be seen as a result of his ambiguous reputation as a "prophet" and a "criminal" in the yellow press. What is involved is a single mythical structure, where "decadent" life is precisely one aspect of sanctification. On the other hand, Sartre's "bohemian lifestyle" and his desire to break bourgeois habits can be seen as a variant of the bourgeois myth of the artistic lifestyle created in the 19th century. From this angle, existentialism can in a certain sense be considered the last hybrid expression of the "transgressive" myth of rebellion which this sort of lifestyle had crystallized.

1. Introduction

> A month later, the first Gallimard cocktail party was given; Astruc went to sleep behind a sofa; when he woke up the room was empty; he tried to feel his way out, stumbled into the dining room, where the Gallimard family had just gathered for dinner, and stuck both his hands in the soup tureen.[1(p74)]

> To celebrate my return I gave a party in the *cave* into which the Lorientais [the group Claude Luter had formed] had moved in the Rue de la Mon-

Tiina Arppe • Department of Sociology, The University of Helsinki, 00200 Helsinki, Finland.

Recent Developments in Alcoholism, Volume 14: The Consequences of Alcoholism, edited by Galanter. Plenum Press, New York, 1998.

> tagne-Sainte-Geneviève. Vian, who was tending bar for me, immediately began to serve the most merciless concoctions; many of the guests sank into a stupor; Giacometti went off to sleep. I was careful and kept going till dawn; I forgot my purse when I left, and went back with Sartre in the afternoon to get it. "And the eye?" the concierge asked us. "Don't you want the eye?" A friend of Vian's, known as the Major, had put his glass eye on the piano and left it there.[1(p143)]

The above extracts are from *La Force des Choses*, memoirs by Simone de Beauvoir, and they describe the way of life of French intelligentsia in Paris after World War II. What is described in particular is the circle of friends of de Beauvoir and Jean-Paul Sartre, which consisted mainly of people from the upper middle class who were engaged in art or literature. Judging from these people's own descriptions and from biographies written about them, it would seem that Parisian intelligentsia drank not only often but in great quantities during the years after World War II: drinking oneself senseless until finally passing out was clearly not unheard of among the people here discussed. How do we explain this way of drinking and how exceptional was it in fact?

The most obvious explanation is the period of prosperity and economic growth that followed World War II: Alcohol, among many other things, was again available. In addition to the explanation emphasizing economic factors, we may refer to the "spiritual climate" of periods of crisis or boom: The increased social interaction typical of such times makes drinking not only normal but almost a moral duty.[2]

It is obvious that contextual factors as well as factors related to the nature of the times have their role in the phenomenon. Yet there are considerations that make it difficult to accept an interpretation based solely on these factors. To begin with, the intellectuals did not start drinking heavily only after World War II, but while it was still going on. According to the Beauvoir, some members of the "Sartre family" drank rather heavily as early as in the 1930s.[3(pp184,260–270)] Second, it should be noted that the general atmosphere during the period under study was not perhaps quite so tolerant or positive toward drinking as might be assumed: The existentialists were criticized severely and in a moralizing way in the daily papers for their extravagant ways of life. "A teacher's son" and "a girl brought up in the best tradition of French nobility" were seen as determined to corrupt a great part of French youth by means of their obscure philosophy and filthy lifestyle characterized by corruption, dirt, lechery, atheism, and immorality. *Samedi-Soir* and *France Dimanche* particularly excelled in criticizing Sartre and his immediate circle of friends: "Shady hotels, nauseating drunkenness, abortion, dreary nights, stuffy love: in the novels of Sartre and de Beauvoir we can see the image of what is most crooked in the human existence."[4] My aim is to examine precisely *the image* of lifestyle given by the intellectuals themselves and by a few daily papers of the time (an integral part of this image being, as we shall see, the use of alcohol). The time period under study is roughly from 1943 to 1948 (the choice is mainly based on the exceptional number of descriptions of drinking that exists from this period). My thesis is that the drinking of French intellectuals during the above-mentioned period cannot be understood apart from a certain lifestyle as a whole, which in this case (as I claim) is primarily manifested through a certain (mythical) structure of meanings. My main aim, therefore, is not to find out how much or how often French intellectuals "really" drank, but to look at the ways in which their drinking has been described and to draft a possible structure of meanings based on these descriptions.

2. Feast and Transgression

> It required great care and severe self-restraint to amass the provisions and bottles with which we stacked the buffet; then, suddenly, we found ourselves eating and drinking all we could put away. . . . It was, primarily, drink which aided our break with the daily humdrum round: when it came to alcohol, we never held back, and none of us had any objections to getting drunk. Some even regarded it as a duty. Leiris, among others, set about the task enthusiastically and made a most admirable job of it. I can see him now, bumping down the staircase at Taverny on his bottom. . . . Each of us turned himself, more or less deliberately, into some sort of clown for the others' benefit, and there was no shortage of special attractions. . . . Dora Marr used to mime a bullfighting act; Sartre conducted an orchestra from the bottom of a cupboard; Limbour carved up a ham as though he were a cannibal; Queneau and Bataille fought a duel with bottles instead of swords; Camus and Lemarchand played military marches on saucepan lids [. . .].[3(pp662–663)]

The above description of a fiesta probably arranged in March–April 1944 (the exact date is not given in the sources) combines several of the features attached to the feast by Roger Caillois, the French anthropologist, in his studies on primitive communities.[5] Caillois studies the feast as a kind of simulacrum of the creation, where life in the community reaches not only its religious but also its economic climax (the recycling of riches, the distribution of accumulated stocks, and sacrifice). The sacred nature of the feast becomes manifest in the momentary transgression of the rules of everyday life and the promotion of excess and extravagance.

Caillois links the feast particularly to the sacred, its structures and functions in primitive communities (he says that he aimed with his theory at presenting a kind of "syntax" of the sacred). According to him, the sacred appears almost entirely in a negative way—through prohibitions—on the level of everyday life. The prohibitions maintain the profane life built by means of work and make sure that it endures. However, the universe must at times be created again, or made young again, which is the function of the feast. In fact, the feast appears as a recreation of the early years of the universe. "Urzeit" represents the time when nothing had stabilized and when the entire universe was plastic, in flux, inexhaustible. On the other hand, it is also the era of exuberant and turbulent creations, an undifferentiated and dark chaos. By dipping again in this ever-actual eternity, the world has a chance of becoming young again and of finding again the superabundance of life and power, which makes it possible for man to defy time. Therefore, the feast always takes place in mythical time and space. It is a means by which the members of the community actualize their relationships and get new strength. On the other hand, the excess and the sacrificial atmosphere of the feast bring the sense of death to the act of recreating the communal link—death, which is a necessary condition of creation.[5(pp130–131)]

Since the feast is an actualization of creative chaos, everybody is required to act against the rules. The opposite nature of the feast and everyday life is also emphasized by the period of fasting or silence that precedes the feast. The fast and silence are contrasted by the excesses that are integral to the feast: collective excitement, gestures and cries, rash impulses, intensive emotions, excessive eating and drinking, wasteful spending of riches, even downright destruction. According to Caillois, the excesses are not only a by-product of the ceremony, a "kind of mechanical outcome of the excessive excitement created by the ceremony" as, for example, Durkheim would have had it.[6(pp547–548)] On the contrary, they are necessary for the ceremony to succeed. Excess is part of the sacred power of the rites; it helps nature and communities to renew themselves, which is the aim of the feast. That is why a great deal of effort is made during the feast to act in a way completely different from ordinary times. Turning everything upside down seems an obvious proof of a return to the creative epoch of chaos. Although the breach of rules always remains a sacrilege, in primitive communities such sacrileges are considered equally sacred and ritualistic as the prohibitions that they transgress. Schematically put, the sacred related to prohibitions organizes and maintains the creation attained by means of the sacred related to the transgression of the rules.[5]

We can find a kind of "archischeme" of the feast in the passage from Simone de Beavoir's memories quoted at the beginning of this chapter. First, there is a period of fasting and quiet life, accumulating stocks and obeying rules (hard work and strict self-denial, wartime restrictions); after this, the everyday order is turned upside down all at once (breaking loose from everyday routine). Now begins a period of eating and drinking to one's heart's content, making a fool of oneself either consciously or unintentionally (collective excitement, gestures: swordplays with bottles or playing military marches with pots and pans), engaging in impulsive activities (bumping down the stairs on one's bottom). Second, drinking and feasting are highly collective activities that create and maintain the feeling of togetherness. De Beauvoir emphasizes the fact that the participants were happy just to be together as friends,; there was a kind of mutual understanding or "being accomplices in a crime" that was further strengthened by the circumstances:

"We were isolated from our fellows by an impassable circle of silence and darkness. No one could pass either into or out of the ring [refers to the curfew]; we might have been living in the Ark. We became a sort of secret fraternity, performing its rites away from the world's common gaze.[3(p662)]

Third, even though the intellectuals' parties cannot be considered a simulacrum of the timeless early moment of the universe or of creative chaos, they may, paradoxically, be seen as a kind of memorial ceremony of future creation. Hitler had not yet been defeated nor Paris liberated, but an anticipation of these historical events, the euphoria created by a new (and better) world opening up in the middle of the chaos, saturated the atmosphere of the parties. De Beauvoir herself offers such an interpretation: As the events were yet to become real (the "mythical" dawn of the new world), "magic tricks" were required to celebrate them (cf. sympathetic magic):

[. . .] How was one to celebrate events that had not yet happened? There exist certain magical conductors that abolish both temporal and spatial distances: the emotions. We worked up a vast atmosphere of collective emotionalism that fulfilled all our longings in a trice: in the fever that it kindled victory became tangible reality.[3(p662)]

Although the drinking habits of the Parisian intelligentsia may in reality have been no more than a "profane" way of having fun during a time of crisis, we may yet say that the picture that de Beauvoir gives of it is, in spite of everything, sacred. It would be interesting to study why de Beauvoir chose to emphasize the sacral aspects of feasting, considering that her and Jean-Paul Sartre's entire philosophy is at odds with such a conception (with their emphasis on the individual's freedom of choice and the contingency of existence, projects aiming toward the future, a linear conception of time, and so on; it must also be of some significance that this is the only point in de Beauvoir's memories where she seeks to analyze the drinking habits of her intimates by taking an entire theory as its background).

In *Saint Genet—Comédien et Martyr*, Sartre[7] emphasizes the cyclical nature of the time related to a feast, which, according to him, is a distinctive feature of a sacred period of time. He also compares the writer he analyzes, Jean Genet, to a sacrificial animal, which, as it is taken to the place of sacrifice "tries to borrow from the crowd which is to survive it, a dazzling memory of itself *in order to memorise its future death*.[7(p307)] In other words, Genet lives his own life as a kind of myth, the eternal return of a certain archetypal event (the moment of his metaphorical "death," which occurred during his childhood). In his analyses of the sacred, Sartre refers, among others, to Mircea Eliade, according to whom the taking into possession of reality in archaic ontology takes place solely by means of repetition or participation.[8(p63)] There is actually nothing new in the world, because everything is a repetition of the same fundamental archetypes; by actualizing the mythical moment when the archetypal (creative) gesture first became revealed, repetition keeps the world continually in the moment of the dawn of origin (in the continually present eternity). It goes without saying that a philosopher who is committed to a utopian progress (universal liberation achieved by means of socialism) can only see mythical sacredness of this kind as illusory:

> I, like many others, think that we should cut short the convulsions of a world that is dying, to assist in the birth of a community of production and to try, together with the workers and militants, to lay the table with new values. This is why Saintliness, with its sophisms, its rhetoric and its morose delight is repugnant to me; it has but one use today: to allow men of bad faith to reason incorrectly.[7(p230)]

It might, therefore, be more appropriate to talk about "utopia" (understood as a progressive orientation toward the future) in connection with Sartre and de Beauvoir, rather than of "myth" (the eternal return of the same); it is, however, interesting that the expectation of future utopia is analyzed (at least retrospectively) by means of categories related to the sacred and even in the cyclic time characteristic of the myth (as a memorial ceremony of a future event). De Beauvoir also emphasizes two features of the feast, which she connects with the specific conditions of wartime life: the feast is a celebration of the present moment and it always carries an undercurrent of death:

> When the days pass smoothly and happily, there is no stimulus towards a fête. But if hope is rekindled in the very midst of despair, if you regain your hold upon the world and the times—then the magic moment catches fire, and you can plunge into it and be consumed with it: *that* is a fête. . . . beneath the lively wine-flown raptures there is always a faint taste of death, but for one resplendent moment death is reduced to nothingness.[3(p661)]

From this point of view, the unusual conditions of wartime life provide an essential incentive for "the fervent adulation of the present moment," a kind of timeless timeliness, which drives a radical wedge between the past and the future and at the same time makes the feast a euphoric anticipation of the renewal of the world and a new creation. Considering that the intellectuals have always perceived themselves as some kind of heralds of a new age, this attitude is not particularly surprising. On the other hand, the feasts of the intellectuals reproduced in a smaller and more "innocent" scale the violation of everyday rules, which were broken in a much more fatal way by war on the level of society as a whole.

If we present the two basic axes that articulate the relationship between the sacred and the profane (the feast and everyday life) in Caillois's theory of the feast, and which also occupy an important position in the descriptions by de Beauvoir, in a cross tabular form, we get Table I. The dimension that is outlined on the order–disorder axis could be called "transgressive"; here, the sacred, by means of the momentary transgression of the prohibitions constituting everyday life, may manifest itself in the form of a feast, for example, or waste and sacrifice (in a sense, the prohibitions themselves are sacred: they

Table I. Field 1: Caillois's Theory of the Feast

	(Prohibitions) Order	(Transgression) Disorder
Communality	1. "Normal," conventional life in a community	2. State of war; "continuous revolution"; euphoria of creative chaos or feast; a secret society of accomplices
Individuality	3. "Alienated" bourgeois living in atomistic individuality; the saint, the priest	4. Anarchy of marginal individuals; "the accursed sacred"

are the level on which the sacred manifests itself in everyday life). On the communality–individuality axis, however, the archaic sacred is fundamentally constituted as a communal factor creating, renewing, and maintaining togetherness ("the saint" actually only steps into the picture with the personal relationship with God manifest in the Christian religion).

If we study the texts of Sartre and de Beauvoir in the light of the field described above, we might say that the intellectuals who, together with "workers and militants," committed themselves to a new communal order after the war are particularly attracted by the dimension of transgression, which opens through disorder (fields 2 and 4 in Table I) and is opposed to the "normality" they despised. While de Beauvoir emphasizes the secret society of accomplices and the rites of transgression that the feasting intelligentsia represents, Sartre is obviously fascinated by the anarchistic efforts of marginal individuals, a kind of "sacred evil" (the surrealists, Jean Genet, Charles Baudelaire). On the other hand, it should be noted that his interest also points toward members of some "secret society" that exists on the margins of society (the surrealists as a rebellious group of avant garde, Genet as a member of the community of criminals and thiefs, Baudelaire as a member of a kind of parasitic society of "dead authors").

Although Sartre, who is "engaged," only brings up the parasitic heroes of disorder and the sacred evil in order to illustrate their self-deception, we may also ask why it should be so important for the Sartre after the engagement to reveal the self-deception manifested by the romantic glorification of the sacred and the evil (field 4). For the "young" Sartre of the 1920s and 1930s, the prototypes of self-deception were represented by the alienated bourgeois (with double morality) and the society they stood for (e.g., fields 1 and 3). An obvious and rather attractive answer would be that Sartre himself seemed to live in a state of similar self-deception before the end of World War II and before adopting the doctrine of engagement. This becomes evident in Sartre's own, but particularly in de Beauvoir's, opinions on the status of the writer and artist in society and on writing as a profession or lifework.

> He kept his sympathy for those thaumaturge-like characters who, shut off form the City with its logic and mathematics, wandered alone in the

> wilderness and only trusted the evidence of their own eyes as a guide towards knowledge. Thus it was only to the artist, the writer, or the philosopher—those whom he termed the "solitaries"—that he granted the privilege of grasping living reality.[3(pp52–53)]

The writer or artist is by nature an outsider in the society surrounding him or her. He or she bears the mark of a rebel ("continuous revolution"), because he or she loves his or her own (anarchistic) freedom and loneliness. This again makes him or her independent and equips him or her with superior clear-sightedness compared with the bourgeoisie struggling in the jungle of its roles and hypocritical conventions. The artists form the free, powerless, clear-sighted and miserable pariah class of society who get their sanctification from the very fact of their marginality, from being rejected or abandoned. The same romantic myth is also revealed in the way writing was perceived: de Beauvoir, for example, emphasizes the free choice of the individual, on the one hand (choosing for oneself, understanding that writing is a profession that has to be learned), but on the other hand, she sees writing as a mystical calling (an impersonal "voice" that forces the writer to do it), the result of "fate" rolling dice for the writer or choosing him or her out.[3(pp215,420)]

The idea of a writer as guided by a calling, an anarchist and outcast of society, a bearer of the "cure" (stigma) can already be seen in the "art for art's sake" movement of the 19th century (the social conditions for the birth of this movement have been analyzed by Anna Boschetti and Jerrold Seigel, among others).[9,10] In this tradition, the rejection of the values of the existing ("normal", bourgeois) society occupies an important position, which also becomes apparent in the writings of the existentialists (in spite of Sartre's criticism of the "art for art's sake" school[11)] (p 77). A free, anarchistic spirit is fascinated by all the groups of outcasts rejected by society or whom the society tries to exclude from its midst.

On the level of lifestyle, some commentators have seen Sartre's "bohemian" lifestyle as a thoroughly thought-out compromise between the obligatory extravagance of genius and the requirements of productivity (notable, Anna Boschetti suggests this kind of interpretation). Hotel life, contingent love affairs, and the love of certain excesses (drinking, use of stimulants) are from this angle "seamlessly linked with a certain organisation of holiday and work periods, which is completely finalised by the conditions of productivity."[9(p172)] This would therefore represent (according to the Bourdieu model) a kind of strategy to build a habitus with the purpose of achieving a dominant position in the field of intellectual power. We may study, however, the phenomenon by taking the lifestyle factors more seriously or by giving them a status that is less dependent on the structures of production or individual power struggles. Then the question is not so much of the struggle of individuals in the field of symbolic power, or of the material conditions of this struggle, or of the conditions related to the individuals' *symbolic capital* in it, as it is of the mythical structures of signification inherent in culture, which influence the conscious subjects in spite of their explicit–implicit goals and efforts and which, above all, influence the picture that the subjects build of themselves and the picture that public life builds of the subjects. A closer study of lifestyle in fact brings into the picture a third distinction of the sacred (the ambivalence of the sacred), which plays its role even in the myth of the "accursed" writer: it is a question of the opposite nature of the pure and the impure, which I will analyze in the following section.

3. Sanctification of the Accursed

While the drinking habits of the studied group of intellectuals before and during the war can be regarded as a phenomenon related to the feelings of togetherness shared by a small circle of friends, "decadent life" after the war was incarnated in two basic "phenomena," that is, in the person of Jean-Paul Sartre and in the movement labeled "existentialism." In the autumn of 1945, Sartre became very famous in a very short time; he became the symbol of existentialism. That was the time when the first volumes of the series, *Chemins de la Liberté* were published, the first issues of the paper founded by Sartre, *Les Temps Modernes,* came out, and he gave a tremendously successful lecture, "L'Existentialisme Est-Il un Humanisme?" in a small club in Paris. Sartre was of course quite well known even before this (particularly for his *Nausée* and *L'Être et le Néant*), but his fame was mostly limited to critics and experts in a narrow field. In 1945, however, Sartre became a phenomenon by becoming a highly public figure, who was made even more interesting by the fact that certain concepts that can be called philosophical in a very narrow and technical sense suddenly became the property of the general public (as Annie Cohen-Solal, for example, points out[12]).

The social conditions of Sartre's success and the effects of his celebrity have already been studied fairly conclusively[9] and I will not get into them here. My purpose is to study the *image* of the intelligentsia given by the intellectuals themselves and by the public life of the time, particularly as related to existentialism as a kind of total lifestyle. As Boschetti, for example, notes, because of Sartre's celebrity, everything about him became a public figure posed in front of everyone's eyes:

> His deeds outshine one another, colouring themselves by the anti-conformist lifestyle. . . . Behind his novels, as behind his plays, philosophical essays and critiques one can already see a great figure, a corruptor of youth or a moral guide, whom it is impossible to ignore.[9(p80)]

Judging from the intellectuals' own descriptions, drinking and feasting were relatively common among them during the years following World War I. On the other hand, we also should bear in mind that, as Sartre's reputation grew, his doings and those of his closest entourage were looked at under a magnifying glass in the daily newspapers. Thanks to the articles and brief news in *Samedi-Soir* and *France Dimanche,* Sartre quickly became a virtual prophet of decadent life and loose morals.

> In the early hours of the dawn, the philosopher is pleased to find clothes scattered here and there, saucers full of ash overturned haphasardly, sheets of paper scribbled full of text turning up everywhere, including in the bed.[13]

Celebrity also forced Sartre and de Beauvoir to change their lifestyles to a certain extent: they went out less and started to avoid "Le Flore," "Les Deux Magots," and "Lipp"—the cafés they had frequented earlier. As Sartre has later remarked, for him celebrity meant hatred above anything else.[14(p754)] Simone de Beauvoir sees the mudslinging as a direct result of Sartre's extremely democratic principles:

> All these eccentricities would have been forgiven if only Sartre had taken shelter behind his role as a writer. . . . But public opinion was shocked. Ignorant of the real seriousness of a writer's work, the public only forgives him his privileges if he appears to them as the Other, flattering their taste for myths and idols and disarming envy. . . . Then, determined to identify him as the Other while noticing that he was just like them, people began to denounce him as a barefaced hoaxer. . . . Insofar as he was unable to conform to bourgeois behaviour, his very simplicity became a weapon that could be used against him. The fact is that there was something suspect about it; it implied democratic convictions too extreme for the élite not to feel its superiorities were being challenged.[1(pp54–55)]

From this angle, Sartre, who had as good as risen to the position of a prophet exactly because of his lifestyle, appears to be a kind of champion of extreme democracy. Yet the dimension of lifestyle may in this case be studied from an entirely different perspective as well. In the light of the theory of the sacred, it may be seen as the "dark" pole of the saint–criminal pair, which is equally sacred as the position of the prophet or saint (as Hubert and Mauss[15] have shown, in primitive societies, the violation of religious laws or contact with unclean things cause impurity, which in a certain way corresponds to sanctification: the criminal just as the sinner is a sacred being).

On a more general level, the opposing pair of saint–criminal can be linked with the ambivalence of the sacred, which Robertson Smith, Emile Durkheim, and Georges Bataille, among others, have analyzed.[6,16] The relationship between the sacred and the profane is fundamentally organized on the basis of the prohibition concerning the sacred. In fact, however, the prohibition is directed toward two seemingly mutually exclusive realities: what is sacred and what is impure. The ambivalence results from the fact that sacred things are beneficial and desirable on one hand and dangerous on the other (if let loose they can spread uncontrollably and cause immeasurable destruction). The same duality is also revealed in the reactions caused by the sacred: it is the object of fear, terror, and repulsion and at the same time it manifests itself as something that arouses respect and appeal. From the point of view of profane life, however, both poles are equally sacred. They represent a poorly controllable, contagious, and dangerous power, which should be warded off in everyday life with the help of prohibitions.

In Sartre's case, therefore, we might say that the earlier marginal position of the lonely, "accursed" hero was changed into the status of prophet–criminal when he became the object of public sanctification–defamation. What is involved is a single (mythical) structure, where "decadent" life reveals itself as one aspect of sanctification. By way of contradicting Simone de Beauvoir, we might claim that Sartre, because of his lifestyle exactly, takes the position of the Other (the "accursed" Other). He does not cause offense because his figure is perceived by people as similar to theirs ("he was no different from the others"), and they consequently feel cheated, but because the mythology of celebrities emphasizing amorality makes Sartre an ambiguous bearer of the feelings of repulsion and appeal experienced by the general public. Purity and impurity are both essential parts of his "otherness."

In fact, we might claim that although Sartre, in the later half of the 1940s, wanted to identify with the pariah class of society par excellence, that is, the proletariat, he actually ended up in the structural position of an "exceptional individual" (prophet–criminal), but not at all necessarily against his own will. Simone de Beauvoir describes Sartre's embarrassment concerning his celebrity in her memoirs. According to her, fame came as a shock to the writer of the old school, who had considered loneliness to be the price of genius paid, for example, by Baudelaire, Stendhal, and Kafka; it was almost a sign of mediocrity to him.[1(p52)] Yet in a way Sartre was saved from his abhorred "mediocrity" by rejection: he neither enjoyed the trust of the bourgeoisie nor a contact with the masses. "He did not mind his isolation, because it tickled his sense of adventure. His essay oozes absolute despair and yet is radiant with joy."[1(p146)] In a series of interviews given to David Rousset in 1948, Sartre himself speaks about the positive effects of hatred: "To feel hated; an element of culture."[1(p164)] Large-scale idolatry would become embarrassing without the element of the sanctifying curse that opens the way to "great and free loneliness, choosing oneself in anxiety."[17]

According to Sartre, Flaubert is one of those who are unable to take this dreary choice of the lonely hero to its bitter end. Instead, he strives to compensate for the absolute freedom (which potentially leads to madness) created by a symbolic disengagement from one's social class by means of finding a mythical community (of marginals or parasites) that one can identify with. In Flaubert's case, this community consisted of dead writers. As sanctification by society has been rejected (by the writer himself, because he has disengaged himself from the bourgeoisie which would have been able to provide it), it is searched for in a kind of imaginary "community of the sacred." What Sartre fails to notice is that he ends up turning his own "curse" (rejection by the bourgeoisie and proletariat, defamation by the press) into a similar sign of elective choice. Although there is no God, the condemnation coming from the others is absolute: "The hatred of the others reveals to me my objectivity."[1(p164)] The rejection of the community becomes for Sartre a sign of his prophetlike status (his heroic loneliness) and the most secure guarantee of his sanctification. The myth of the scapegoat or martyr is, however, strongly communal by nature (for example, the Christian myth of the self-sacrifying God, whose "blood" and "body" is the foundation of the Christian community, the communion of the faithful). It is the ambivalent structure of the sacred–sanctification that makes it possible for an "exceptional individual" to appear as both "master" and "criminal" (the epithets attached to Sartre by *Samedi-Soir*, November 17, 1945).

From a historical or "contents-based" point of view, the same mythical structure can be localized in the bohemian subculture of artists and writers at the end of the 19th century and in the concept of "the accursed writer" often associated with the writings of Baudelaire and Rimbaud. As far as the artists are concerned, bohemian lifestyle largely meant the identification of art with a particular way of life: the identification of art with experience, sensation, and emotion and the search for authentic and free subjectivity by means of art heightened the role of the artistic lifestyle (for example, in the romantic "art for art's sake" movement of the 1830s). On the other hand, bohemian lifestyle was also a crystallization of the fundamental conflict of values of bourgeois society: the demand for personal freedom and immediate gratification (giving up social rigidity, "pamperping oneself") on the one hand and the preservation of independence achieved and maintained through hard work (putting off immediate gratification, the idealization of poverty, ascetism) on the other. Seigel, [10(p58)] for example, claims that bohemian lifestyle was a highly visual dramatization of the ambivalence that characterized the relationship of many members of the new bourgeois class with their own identity and fate. "Bohemia" was necessary for the early bourgeois class of the 19th century as a kind of contrast, which helped it define itself.

As Seigel[10] has shown, at the end of the 19th century, bohemian lifestyle was particularly localized in the artists' cafes ("les cabarets") that had sprung up in the Montmartre area. These were public places for having fun, where the artists gathered to attract and entertain a clientele, which mainly consisted of the new bourgeois middle class. From the beginning, the cabarets were a means of advertising themselves for the poets and artists who joined them. They made "Bohemia" also into a social theatre, a form of public life. As the new middle class started to reform the worlds of consumption, politics, and culture, the importance of publicity was emphasized in more and more fields of life. The cafes of Montmartre represented a new Bohemia directed at the bourgeoisie, a place where they could leave behind the increasingly organized and regulated life of a big city, if only for one night. They were places where the bourgeoisie could look for liberation from conventional social barriers and participate in the game of breaking taboos and conventions.

From this angle of history and contents we therefore might say that Sartre's bohemian lifestyle and his desire to break bourgeois habits were not so much an expression of his extremely democratic principles but of the bourgeois myth of the artistic lifestyle created in the 19th century to make the bohemian the bourgeois' "other," his opposite, which was attractive in an ambivalent way. Like Sartre, the "accursed writers" of the 19th century aroused horror and disgust as well as fascination in the general public. As Seigel[10(p10)] points out, Bohemia was certainly not located outside bourgeois life: in fact, it was an expression of a conflict that arose from the core of that life itself. Bohemia sprang up where the borders of bourgeois life were obscure and uncertain and where the margins of the society were constantly put to test. And although the bohemian lifestyle rebellion as a wider social phenomenon started to evaporate even before World War I, in a certain sense existentialism can be considered the last hybrid expression of the "transgressive" myth of rebellion that it had crystallized (I shall get back to this in the end of the chapter).

4. "Existentialism" as a Phenomenon—Lifestyle and Publicity

The ambivalent structure of the sacred becomes particularly obvious when we study another phenomenon taken up by the contemporary daily press and associated right from the start with the name of Sartre, that is, "existentialism" and its bearers "the existentialists". Although the flamboyant night life of the Saint-Germain-des Près was associated with Sartre's person, he himself had little to do with it. Most of the young people who frequented Le Tabou and Club Saint-Germain (two much-talked about jazz clubs) were existentialists only in name (according to Ory and Sirinelli,[18(p148)] for example, the "village of the existentialists" was largely an invention of *Samedi-Soir* and *France Dimanche*). The following contemporary descriptions may serve as examples:

> *The existentialists:* never has a term grown more remote from what it is supposed to express. To do nothing but drink in small caves is to be an existentialist. It is as if there were relativists in New York who danced in caves and people believed that Einstein was there dancing among them.[18(pp148–149)]

> The public takes the bait. An elegant lady lets slip a four-letter word. In mock horror, she exclaims, "Oh, my God! I've turned into an existentialist!" An effeminate young man walks by. Comments are heard, "Look! An existentialist!" An agricultural labourer, who is an avid reader and regular visitor at the municipal library, commits murder. It is an existentialist crime.[19]

If we take a closer look at the articles that appeared in the daily papers, it seems that the term "existentialism" denoted a certain bundle of specific connotations, where lifestyle and its assumed impurity were essential dimensions. The two daily papers chosen for the study are *France Dimanche* and *Samedi-Soir* (which could be classified as belonging to the so-called "yellow press"), because they may have had the strongest role in the birth of the legend of both Sartre and existentialism. For *Samedi-Soir*, the years 1945–1947 have been studied and for *France Dimanche*, the years (1946–1947 (it was only founded in 1946). There are altogether 35 articles and news items touching on

Sartre and existentialism during this time period, five of which may be considered feature articles. The general tone of the texts, with the exception of a few openly disapproving ones, is mocking and sarcastic, sometimes also humoristic. The most disapproving articles are about the literary production of the existentialists and the twisted or perverse foreign influence it showed; this is particularly so in *Samedi-Soir,* whose cultural line here might be considered clearly conservative, even if it also quotes the rather venomous letter of complaint signed by the neighbours of Le Tabou concerning its nightlife. It is clear, that the papers had their own economic interest at stake, but so, in certain cases, had the existentialists (Anne-Marie Cazalis, the owner of Le Tabou, actually participated in writing an openly sensational article about her place in *Samedi-Soir*). If the publicity given to Sartre and the existentialists is compared with the offense caused by the surrealists in the press, we have to say in all honesty that the press in fact treated Sartre more softly than Simone de Beauvoir and he allowed to be known. (There was often fascination and even admiration in the mockery, and Sartre's success as a writer and playwright abroad, for example, was frequently pointed out.)

If we examine the articles published in *Samedi-Soir* and *France Dimanche* during the period under study, we may, in the light of an analysis based on a very rough listing of nouns and adjectives, outline a few categories that may give new interest to the phenomenon. The categories picked out from the materials are dress and looks, environment, the general characteristics of the existentialists, the writings and their world, and existentialism as a philosophy and phenomenon. On the basis of this preliminary categorization, "existentialism" and "the existentialists" appear more or less as follows (the terms in quotations are the ones used by the papers).

First, the existentialists dress either outright badly (they wear "stained pajamas" or "frayed clothes"—Sartre wears an "old and stained jacket" with "shiny sleeves," his trousers have pockets that "hang down to the knees" and they are "yellow between the legs") or at least in an unconventional or extravagant way (existentialist painters wear "Portuguese shirts decorated with many-coloured checks"; more generally, male existentialists wear "bright socks with stripes in many colours"). Otherwise, what catches the eye in the way they look is their untidy hair: they are "long-haired," the men have "matted hair hanging down the forehead," some "haven't combed their hair in a year." The intellectuals are also described as "bare-legged," and the women, it seems, are forbidden to wear "make-up." Some of them sport "dark glasses" in order to cover the "bruises they have received when hit" (Anne-Marie Cazalis, the owner of Le Tabou).

This badly dressed, untidy, and bizarre tribe lives in "dark," "unwholesome," and "smoky" "caves" (jazz clubs, particularly Le Tabou), "as in limbo" or "in damp hotels." Its members write their first books "on the benches of some provincial lycée," which they leave to settle in "hotels," "cafes," "restaurants," "clubs," "bars," and "local bistros." Their domain is also the "toilets" and "telephone booths" of the restaurants (which they daub with graffiti). There the members of the new "animalistic" literary school are picked up by patrolmen and taken to "the zoo" (i.e., locked up in jail). The chief of the tribe, Jean-Paul Sartre, lodges in a room at the Lousiana Hotel full of "dusty furniture," "pieces of clothing scattered everywhere," "sheets of paper scribbled over in illegible scrawl," and "saucers overflowing with cigarette ash, some turned upside down here and there." All in all, the room resembles "hell." On the other hand, the chieftain also moves on less primitive scenes as befits his rank ("magazines," "theatres," "restaurant galas"). Yet, all in all, "he and his likes" are only happy living on "a dunghill."

One of the key characteristics of the existentialists seems to be their age: they are young. In addition, these "little student girls," "little starlets," other flibbertigibbets and "silly young men" are usually less than intelligent: Their "affected intelligence" is not even enough to allow them to control their "animal drives." This bunch, which is "saturated in alcohol," "gaudy," and "no good," forms the "indefatigable crowd" of the Cafe Flore, for example, with "an eye for alcohol" and an inclination to move "in the night" or "in the small hours." They are "so-called intellectuals" who dance a "wild" "jitterburg" or "swing" with "sturdy black men" in restaurants, but who also sit in the corner of bars "listless" and "staring with glazed eyes at their glasses filled with tepid water." The majority of this "noisy," "idle," and "fanatic" crowd are "poor," "from good families" and "disowned by their fathers." (There are so many professional categories that I shall not get into them here.) They are always "drowning in debt" and are therefore "pursued by their creditors"; in order to escape their plight, they "sell books," "play the roles of servants" in Sartre's plays, "bury an old aunt who has forgotten to disinherit them," and "lunch on credit." The leader of these "young hopes," Jean-Paul Sartre, seems to be a man of many interests: He is "the pope," "a lycée teacher," "a philosopher," "a writer," "the leader of a literary school," "a government official," "a lecturer," "a master," and "a criminal." Compared with "crowd of worshippers" that surrounds him all of the time, he is "rich" and "clever." In the eyes of his previous teacher colleagues, he appears "pedantic" and "unsociable"; his students again remember him as "sharp," "original," and "confusing." Generally, he is the "most famous and active" of all Parisian writers, yet on the other hand also "a snob," "insignificant," "wretched," and downright "depraved."

The texts and writings of the "existentialists" (most of whom are "writers" and "actors") are full of "cliches" and their "raving obscenities" are "almost humorous." They are characterized by "romanticism soaked in whisky," "passion," and "anxiety." As writers, most existentialists are too young: They write their first books "on the benches of provincial lycées" and describe mostly "their own experiences and sufferings" in them. That they are young is also evident in that "some of them have had no time to study ortography." That is why the "younger generation" no longer expresses itself in "works" but "communiqués" and "graffitis" with "inexistence," "graves," and "suicide" as their motives. Where before the war, "literature was written"; it is now "drunk, danced, vomited, sketched, imitated, and roared; it is an engaged and re-engaged literature reached by a short-cut." In addition, Sartre's and de Beauvoir's novels and plays are particularly characterized by "violence," "nauseous realism," "perverse habits," and "hellishness." The picture of life given in them is "twisted": "crippled hotels, repulsive drunkenness, dreary nights, stale love affairs." The "influence of American novels" ("promiscuity," "incest," "sensual pleasures," "nights drowned in whisky and rape") becomes "false" when transferred to French soil.

As a phenomenon, existentialism is closely linked with "the generation" that is "young" and "new." It is "a literary revolution," "a fashion," "a school," "a philosophy," "the triumph of publicity," and "a mission." As a philosophy, it is "obscure," "abstract," and "of German origin." What is more, one of the key figures in its background, Martin Heidegger, is "a Nazi."

On the basis of the last categorization, existentialism would appear to mean at least a religion (a sect with "a pope" as its leader and "a mission" to carry out), a philosophical discipline, a lifestyle or fashion, and a literary school. In all these fields it appears impure, disorganized, primitive, and Other (with pure, organized, civilized and the Same as their opposite pairs). As a religion, it could be studied on the axis organized–disorganized: It clearly resembles a sect, with a prophet of its own, separated from the organized churches. As a philosophy, it is characterized by being Other or alien as opposed to the solid identity of traditional French philosophy (it is "obscure" and, particularly, "of German origin"). As a lifestyle, existentialism is associated with a marked impurity, which becomes obvious through certain external signs or "stigmas" (dirty and ragged clothes, untidy hair, unhealthy and gloomy living environment), but also through deviant behavior (uncontrolled instincts, nightlife, heavy drinking, wild orgies with "black people" [Others]). As a literary school, it is primitive compared with the best (most civilized) traditions of French literature ("courtesy," "elegance," "sophisticated emotions," "linguistic harmony").

If we study the picture of the phenomenon given in *France Dimanche* and *Samedi-Soir* by means of two opposing pairs related to the sacred, namely purity–impurity and order–disorder, we get the following field, which describes both a particular structure and the attitude assumed when faced with it (Table II). In the table, the pure–impure axis is related to the inherent ambivalence of the sacred (and to the attitude assumed when faced with it); the order–disorder axis regulates the relationship between prohibitions and transgressions, a certain structure (whose both poles, however, are considered equally sacred). On the basis of the field outlined in Table II, we might say that the primary feeling experienced toward bourgeois (and in this case, specifically French) society or organized daily life is respect. The same goes for French literature in its traditional form. The proletariat, again, is in a sense part of the organized society (revolutionary efforts are channeled into an established and organized form, such as trade unions); but because of its impurity and a kind of "beastliness," it also evokes a vague repulsion. Sim-

Table II. Field 2: Pure–Impure Sacred

	Pure	Impure
Prohibition (Order)	1. Bourgeois (French) society; traditional art and literature	2. Proletariat; foreign influence in literature
Transgression (Disorder)	3. Individual holy, charismatic leaders ("pope," "master," "leader of discipline")	4. Existentialists, anarchists ("criminal")

ilarly, American literature, which describes its own (obviously disorganized) cultural environment in a "natural" and "authentic" way, becomes "twisted" and "false" when transferred to French (organized) culture. Individual holy and charismatic leaders are, on the one hand, clearly outside the organized forms of society (in this case, the church or political parties), but, on the other, arouse a kind of respect because of their symbolic purity (charisma, genius, personal grace). The groups settled in the last field, for their part, are both outside social order and impure and repulsive in a symbolic sense.

Therefore, what we get as a result is a space of significations and values structured through the category of the sacred, which in this case could be called "conservative" or "conventional." The position that most clearly is a bearer of deviance is the one where disorder is combined with impurity (of lifestyle) (field 4). Impurity that appears inside some kind of order (field 2), however, is tolerated with certain reservations (even if this order is in some way "Other" than the one identified with). The same is true for disorder that is "purified" by personal genius, for example (field 3). What is interesting in this connection is that Sartre simultaneously occupies two of the positions in the transgressive dimension: He is both a charismatic and respected "master" (prophet) basking in the sunshine of a kind of personal grace and a hated and defamed "criminal" (an anarchist living on a "dunghill," an existentialist), who is yet sacred because of the rejection he undergoes. In any case, he has been shut out of both positions of order constituted by means of prohibitions—bourgeois society and the proletariat.

The world of values of the yellow press is, in this analysis, a kind of diametric opposite of the intellectuals' own world of values: Where the press praises organized (French) bourgeois society and abhors anarchism, the intelligentsia for its part admires the creative anarchy of exceptional individuals (and American cultural products) and despises the bourgeois order. In both cases, transgression is understood in the same way (as breaking the norms of bourgeois society). But while the press condemns it, the intellectuals set it up as a kind of absolute value. The underlying structure remains essentially the same, only with the poles of the hierarchy turned upside down.

Therefore, the forms of rebellion demonstrated by the intelligentsia engaged to a Marxist revolutionary theory still seem rather "romantic" on the level of lifestyle. And even though Sartre turns to the revolutionary (heroic) proletariat after World War II, there is never a question of identification: The prophet no more than the criminal can identify himself with ordinary people, because both in a sense exist in the margins of established order (one on the basis of his purity, the other on the basis of his impurity) and thereby mark its borders. A ritually unregulated contact with either one or the other would threaten the symbolic categories of established order, causing a dangerous confusion of these categories. With the birth of mass media, we could claim that this ritual mediating task has been transferred to the media: modern "saints" (film stars, sports heroes, rock stars; and in the Paris of the 1940s, even writers and philosophers) and well-known criminals are "mediatized" so that some contact with the "masses" becomes possible.

5. The End of the "Transgression Cult"

It is, in fact, quite curious that there is such an abundance of descriptions of drinking in the material studied, and also that the question was discussed with considerable frequency even in the contemporary daily press. That drinking should be a form of rebellion in French culture, where alcohol has always been drunk rather freely, seems strange also because the golden years of this type of avant-garde rebellion were already far behind in the past in the 1940s. If we think that the intellectuals have always considered themselves to be the heralds of new times in one way or the other, we may well ask what was the kind of modernity that could be articulated by means of drinking alcohol in the 1940s? What was it regarded as opposing?

One possible answer or interpretation might be found in the fact that the drinks that were consumed were mostly of foreign and specifically (as is interesting) of American origin (for example, in de Beauvoir's *The Mandarins*, a two-volume prose work describing the life of the French intelligentsia after World War II, where the most-often-mentioned single drink by far is whisky). It is somewhat paradoxical that the consumption habits of the intelligentsia, who preached a Marxist class theory in their meetings, communiqués, and magazines, were so clearly attracted by American products (and this was not true only of alcohol but also of literature, films, music, etc). Jean Cau, who worked as a secretary to Sartre in the 1940s and 1950s, has pointed out the same thing—in rather cutting remarks.

> To sign the "Stockholm appeal," condemn the actions of the General Ridgway in Korea and proclaim the innocence of Julius and Ethel Rosenberg while at the same time never ceasing to drink whisky, smoke Lucky Strikes and devour the books by James Hadley Chase seemed to me but a way of covering up vices . . . [20(p30)]

The interest shown by Sartre and de Beauvoir in the products of American culture in fact dated back to the time long before World War II (as Sartre tells us in his satirical "autobiography," in his case, this interest went back to his childhood[21]). It was in the 1930s that they already went to see Hollywood films, listened to blues, jazz, and Negro spirituals, and devoured the works of Hemingway, Dos Passos, Faulkner, and Hammet, among others. Simone de Beauvoir herself has pointed out the ambivalence inherent in the attitudes of the couple: On the one hand, they felt attracted by the United States, whose administration they condemned, and on the other hand, the Soviet Union, whose experiment of communism they admired, left them cold in all other respects.[1(p162)]

> At the age of twenty, in about the year 1925, we heard about skyscrapers. To us, they were symbols of the fabulous wealth of America. We were amazed to see them in the movies. They were the architecture of the future, just as the cinema was the art form of the future and jazz the music of the future.[22(pp122–123)]

In a certain sense we might say that the romantic myth or marginalism and rebellion characteristic of the French intelligentsia ever since the 19th century, where bohemian lifestyle and even drinking had an important role, reaches not only its culmination but also its point of extinction in existentialism. The Americanization of the habits of consumption and the slow extinction of the "cult of transgression" are, in fact, essentially related with each other: When a bohemian rebellion (which in the 1940s was above all articulated in existentialism) becomes fashionable as it becomes highly publicized by the mass media, that is, when the intelligentsia is no longer able to distinguish itself as a subculture or marginal culture of its own by means of "different" ways of life, the limit to be overstepped is more and more transferred from everyday bourgeois conventions (the ritual dimension) to the level of the ideology of the entire bourgeois society (the mythical dimension). Transgression can only exist as a momentary breaking of the rules of everyday life; when it becomes a fashion, that is, the rule, it disappears (following Jean Baudrillard,[23] we might speak about the "implosion" of transgression). From this point of view, preaching Marxist theory on the strength of whisky, Lucky Strikes, and James Hadley Chase is no longer paradoxical in the least, as transgression based on lifestyle began to lose its importance among the intelligentsia of the 1940s.

The ambivalence related to the ritualization of the way-of-life rebellion is also apparent in the existentialists'—and particularly Sartre's—use of intoxicants. In a later interview, Sartre justified his drinking and use of amphetamine, for example, by saying that amphetamine helped him to think and write at a pace about three times as fast as his normal rhythm.[14(p149)] When the interviewer pointed out that Sartre also ruined his health by his too excessive use of intoxicants, Sartre said that it was more important for him to write something significant and meaningful for himself ("Critique of Dialectical Reason") than to be in good health (health, so to speak, is there to be ruined). Therefore, the use of intoxicants is justified from a very utilitarian point of view and simultaneously in a mythical and heroic mode ("who cares about health, I have sacrificed myself for my work").

Sartre's attitude is a combination of the ideology of productivity promoted by market economy and the old romantic vision of the writer or artist as a kind of martyr of his own works. It is notable, however, that it does not show any of the ambivalence between hedonism and ascetism that Seigel, for instance, considers typical of 19th-century Bohemia (and, more generally, of the morality of contemporary bourgeois society).[10(p55)] It seems that hedonism and overindulgence were not important to Sartre, who does not emphasize the dimension of pleasure related to consumption, for example. The fundamental conflict of Sartre's modernism may be positioned rather between the Marxist ethos of productivity and the romantic ethos of uselessness, between production and pure waste as an end in itself. On the one hand, he takes a strategically critical attitude toward pure, unproductive waste: The cult of pure consumption is not sufficient as an instrument in questioning the bourgeois ideology of usefulness (total criticism, because of its totality, can never really destroy anything). Consequently, it is inadequate and useless as a means of criticism (of course, we could add ironically, because waste once reduced to a means would no longer be pure).

On the other hand, Sartre prides himself with the meaninglessness, demotivation, and uselessness of literature, but only as far as these attributes are combined in an appeal to the reader's freedom, "a categorical imperative" that demands the reader to overcome his present (alienated) state and to reach out for something better. The sacrifice of the writer, his celebration or "gift," is in this sense never without self-interest: What still looms in the background is the protestant ethics of utility and redemption, where waste is always submitted to the purposes of production (regardless that the final objective of Sartrean dialectics is the universal and concrete liberation of the entire mankind). Despite the bohemian lifestyle linked with it, Sartre's modernism therefore appears as highly ascetic, even Christian.

The paradox of Sartre, or of the modern intellectual, can also be claimed to reflect the conflict characterizing modern society itself, which is not, however, located between hedonism and ascetism, but rather between production and unproductive waste (pleasure is permissible as long as it remains within the limits of moderation). In the system of maximal investment and recycling, it is waste in its different forms (as opposed to rational consumption participating in the reproduction of the system) that turns against (established) reason and also becomes something vaguely sinful (morally reproachable). Characteristically, "modern" Sartre finds the sacred distasteful exactly as a remnant of archaic wasteful societies.[7(pp226–227)] In the context of modernity, it is reduced to the last reflection of the agony of the already disappearing artistocracy, with the sole function of enabling the people living in self-deception (the conservatists) to reason incorrectly. The sacred is defined as the sphere of unproductive waste (as George Bataille, a writer and philosopher contemporary of Sartre, pertinently remarked). This is what makes it impossible to integrate with the "modern" discourse of usefulness, even for Sartre, who wrestled with this "archaic remnant" in book after book (Baudelaire, Genet, Mallarmé, Flaubert).

From the point of view of modern society, therefore, it may well appear that the sacred and the mythical dimensions of signification related to it are nothing but an archaic residuum, whose status in our times is at best marginal. This is true, however, only if the sacred is conceived of as something strictly related to religion (Christianity, in particular) and religious institutions. If, however, it is studied as a broader structure of significations parsing culture or as a system of classification, it can be used to analyze different phenomena of modern culture. From this angle, Sartre and existentialism represent an example of the possibility to use certain attributes that essentially articulate the dimension of meaning of the sacred in a study—in the context of modernity—of the image constructed of the artist–intellectual as far as both their self-images and public images are concerned.

ACKNOWLEDGEMENT. This chapter is an abridged version of a larger study published in 1996 by the Social Research Institute of Alcohol Studies in Finland, "The Feasting Intelligentsia and the Sanctification of 'The Accursed'" (Research Report No. 190).

References

1. Beauvoir S. de: *La Force des Choses.* Paris, Gallimard, 1963.
2. Koski-Jännes: Pullon henki ja kirjailija (The spirit of the bottle and the writer). *Nuori Voima* 5–6, 1983.
3. Beauvoir S. de: *La Force de L'Âge.* Paris, Gallimard, 1960.
4. *Samedi-Soir* November 3, 1945. ("En découvrant l'Amérique les romanciers français n'enrichissent pas notre littérature.")
5. Caillois R: *L' Homme et le Sacré.* Paris, Gallimard, 1950.
6. Durkheim É: *Les Formes Élémentaires de la Vie Religieuse.* Paris, 1990.
7. Sartre J-P: *Saint Genet—Comédien et Martyr.* Paris, Gallimard, 1952.
8. Eliade M: *Le Mythe de l'Éternel Retour.* Paris, Gallimard, 1949.
9. Boschetti A: *Sartre et "Les Temps Moderns."* Paris, Minuit, 1985.
10. Seigel J: *Bohemian Paris—Culture, Politics, and the Boundaries of Bourgeois Life, 1830–1930.* New York, Viking Harmondsworth, 1986.
11. Sartre J-P: Qu'est-ce que la littérature? in Sartre J-P: *Situations II.* Paris, Gallimard, 1948, p 77.
12. Cohen-Solal A: *Sartre 1905–1980.* Paris, Gallimard, 1985.
13. *Samedi-Soir* November 17, 1945. ("Jean-Paul Sartre et Simone de Beauvoir existentialistes professent le dépassement des ustensiles.")
14. Sartre J-P: Autoportriat de soixante-dix ans (propos recueillis par Michel Contat), in Sartre J-P: *Situations X.* Paris, Gallimard, 1976, p 154.
15. Hubert H, Mauss M: Essai sur la nature et la fonction du sacrifice, in Mauss M: *Oeuvres I.* Paris, Minuit, 1968. p 258.
16. Bataille G: Attraction et répulsion II—la Structure sociale, in Hollier D (ed): *Le Collège de Sociologie.* Paris, Gallimard, 1979.
17. Sartre J-P: *Baudelaire.* Paris, Gallimard, 1947.

18. Ory P, Sirinelli J-F: *Les Intellectuels en France, de L'Affaire Dreyfus à nos Jours*. Paris, A. Colin, 1992.
19. Hanoteau G: *L'Âge d'Or de Saint-Germain-des-Près*. Paris, 1965.
20. Cau J: *L'Ivresse des Intellectuels—Pastis, Whisky et Marxisme*. Paris, Plon, 1992.
21. Sartre J-P: *Les Mots*. Paris, Gallimard, 1964.
22. Sartre J-P: New York—ville coloniale, in Sartre J-P: *Situations III*. Paris, Gallimard, 1949.
23. Baudrillard J: Quand Bataille attaquait le principe métaphysique de L'économie. *Quinzaine Litt* 233, 1976.

18

Cocaine Metabolism in Humans after Use of Alcohol

Clinical and Research Implications

Jordi Cami, Magi Farré, Maria Luisa González, Jordi Segura, and Rafael de la Torre

Abstract. The simultaneous administration of cocaine and alcohol implies a pharmacological interaction at pharmacodynamic and pharmacokinetic levels. The latter involves an alteration of cocaine kinetics and metabolism, as well as the biosynthesis of newly active metabolites, such as cocaethylene. Cocaethylene is metabolized along the same pathways as cocaine. Its detection in biological samples indicates the combined consumption of cocaine and alcohol. From epidemiological and toxicological data, it has been suggested that the combination of alcohol and cocaine produces an increased toxicity in addition to behavioral changes. There has been some debate regarding the contribution of cocaethylene to this rise of toxicity. Its pharmacological and toxicological profile is very similar to cocaine. During the interaction of both substances, the rise in cocaine plasma concentrations can explain many of cardiovascular and behavioral effects observed. The contribution of cocaethylene to the interaction is probably minor; its effects are likely additive to those of cocaine. Perhaps its longer elimination half-life can help in understanding long-lasting effects of the alcohol–cocaine combination.

Jordi Cami • Institut Municipal d'Investigació Médica and Universitat Pompeu Fabra, Barcelona, Spain. **Magi Farré** • Universitat Pompeu Fabra and Universitat Autónoma de Barcelona, Barcelona, Spain. **Maria Luisa González, Jordi Segura, and Rafael de la Torre** • Institute Municipal d'Investigació and Universitat Autónoma de Barcelona, Barcelona, Spain.

Recent Developments in Alcoholism, Volume 14: The Consequences of Alcoholism, edited by Galanter. Plenum Press, New York, 1998.

1. Cocaine and Alcohol Consumption: Epidemiological and Toxicological Data

1.1. *Epidemiological Data*

The simultaneous use of cocaine and alcohol is very common. In the 1985 national survey on drug abuse done in the United States, prevalence rates for the simultaneous use of alcohol and cocaine (defined as the use of both drugs at the same time or within 2 hr) were 2.4% for the past month and 4.7% for the past year. Population estimates associated with these figures might suggest that 4.5 million Americans are using this drug combination each month.[1]

Recent data seem to indicate that a large proportion (64%) of patients who reported simultaneous cocaine and alcohol use most of the time (more than 50%) when using cocaine met criteria for alcohol dependence.[2] In a sample of 212 problem drinkers who participated in an alcohol treatment program, the prevalence of polydrug use was investigated, particularly the use of alcohol and other drugs in combination or on the same day. The majority of subjects (61%) reported simultaneous polydrug use. The most frequent alcohol–drug combination was alcohol with cocaine (60% of subjects reporting polydrug use) followed by alcohol with marijuana (51%) and alcohol and sedatives (31%).[3]

It appears that important differences could be found between cocaine-dependent subjects and subjects who fulfill criteria for both cocaine and alcohol dependence. Cocaine–alcohol-dependent persons had higher depression and global severity scores and were more likely to experience paranoid psychosis with cocaine use and to abuse of additional substances. The combination-dependent subjects attended fewer therapeutic sessions. These features suggest that these patients could require a more intensive treatment.[4] It has been described that simultaneous use of alcohol and cocaine contributed to a high prevalence of violent behavior. Patients using both substances had a higher likelihood of associated current homicidal behavior than cocaine-only and alcohol-only abusers.[5]

Cocaine abusers reported that the administration of alcohol produced an increase both in magnitude and duration of some of the euphoric effects of cocaine, and additionally a reduction of some of the unpleasant symptoms associated with the warning of cocaine effects ("crash").[6] In an interesting study on drug preference, it has been demonstrated that alcohol pretreatment significantly increased choice of cocaine versus placebo in nondependent cocaine users. Ratings of pleasurable-related effects and cardiac output were higher in those subjects who chose cocaine and were pretreated with ethanol as compared with those who selected cocaine but did not receive alcohol.[7]

1.2. *Toxicological Data*

The use of cocaine has been related to the appearance of social problems, mainly related to violent behaviors, including homicides, suicides, and accidents. The use of cocaine and alcohol seems to increase the risks of medical and legal complications.

In forensic studies, cocaine and ethanol are frequently identified in biological samples from fatally injured drivers.[8,9] and in homicide victims.[10] In a sample of driver fatalities, it was found that almost one of four drivers had used cocaine within 48 hr of death. Fifty-six percent of all drivers killed in fatal traffic accidents had cocaine metabolites, alcohol, or both detected at autopsy. In 10% of all fatalities, cocaine metabolites and alcohol were found.[8]

In a study designed to assess the presence of different drugs of abuse in 2824 homicide victims, cocaine or benzoylecgonine were found in 31.3% of victims, cocaine–benzoylecgonine without other drugs in 13.4%, cocaine–benzoylecgonine with ethanol in 10.6%, cocaine–benzoylecgonine with opiates in 7.3%, alcohol alone in 21.1% and opiates alone in 2%.[10]

A group of 325 cocaine abusers seen in an emergency room was divided into those who screened positive for benzoylecgonine ($n = 190$) and those positive for benzoylecgonine and alcohol ($n = 135$). Patients positive for both drugs were more frequently involved in violent trauma and presented higher heart rate and blood pressure levels on admission than cocaine-only-positive patients. Two subjects with myocardial infarction were positive for both drugs, but the incidence of rhabdomyolysis was lower in this group of patients.[11]

Cocaethylene, as a marker of simultaneous cocaine and ethanol use,[12] was detected in 25% of patients examined in a hospital emergency room who had positive urines for benzoylecgonine in a urinary screening for drugs of abuse.[13] In a sample of 416 trauma patients, urine was tested for the presence of benzoylecgonine. A total of 158 (38%) subjects tested positive for this metabolite. In 114 of these patients, a blood sample was obtained in order to determine cocaine, cocaethylene, and ethanol. Cocaethylene was detected in blood samples in 60% of tested patients, with a mean concentration of 41 ng/ml (range 3 to 213 ng/ml). All patients tested positive for cocaine, with a mean concentration of 92.9 ng/ml (range 3.8 to 699.9 ng/ml), but only 56% were positive for ethanol. The results suggest that cocaethylene could be present in more than half of the subjects who tested positive for cocaine (more precisely, benzoylecgonine present in urine samples).[14]

2. Cocaine and Alcohol Interactions in Humans

2.1. *Pharmacological Effects of the Cocaine and Alcohol Combination*

The effects of the combination of cocaine and ethanol in healthy volunteers have been assessed in a number of studies, all of which included the evaluation of subjective and physiological effects; several studies presented data on the pharmacokinetics of cocaine and its metabolites, including cocaethylene.[6,15–18]

Summarizing the results of these studies, it seems that the administration of cocaine in subjects who had consumed social-like doses of ethanol produced an enhancement or an antagonism of some of the characteristic effects of each drug. The combination of both drugs induced a significant increase in euphoriclike effects ("high," "good effects," "liking") and caused a clinically significant increase in the cardiovascular effects of cocaine with a very important rise of heart rate and blood pressure. Cocaine also antagonized in part some of the deleterious effects of alcohol, producing lower ratings of drunk feelings and an amelioration of some psychomotor performance tasks altered by alcohol. Subjects performed better under the drug combination condition than under the use of alcohol alone but significantly worse than under placebo or cocaine alone.[17,19] At the neuroendocrine level, the drug combination induced an increase in cortisol levels[19] that was greater than that observed after cocaine administration. Cocaine alone seems to decrease serum prolactin levels,[20] which is in contrast with that reported for ethanol. However, the administration of cocaine did not change the increase in prolactin induced by the administration of alcohol.[19]

2.2. *Pharmacokinetics of the Cocaine–Alcohol Interaction*

In several clinical trials in healthy volunteers, where different doses of alcohol and cocaine were coadministered, similar pharmacokinetic results have been observed.[6,16,18,19]

Plasma levels of cocaine in the drug combination condition were higher than in the cocaine-only condition, and cocaine plasma clearance was reduced by one half. No differences were found in the elimination half-life values.

Plasma levels of benzoylecgonine were significantly higher in the cocaine condition than in the drug combination condition. No differences were found between conditions in the elimination half-life and in any of the pharmacokinetic parameters derived from ecgonine methyl ester plasma concentrations. Plasma levels of norcocaine in the drug combination were higher than in the cocaine condition.[6,19]

The metabolites cocaethylene and norcocaethylene were present only in the condition receiving the drug combination. When the area under the curve (AUC) of cocaine and cocaethylene were compared at 0 and 8 hr, plasma levels of cocaethylene accounted for about one fifth of those calculated for cocaine. No significant differences were observed in the alcohol pharmacokinetics.[6,19]

In summary, cocaine plasma concentration are higher in the combination conditions. However, benzoylecgonine plasma concentrations are lower in the same condition. Combining these observations with the absence of differences in cocaine elimination half-life and reduction by half of its plasma clearance, there is strong support for the hypothesis of a metabolic inhibition in the metabolism of cocaine in the presence of alcohol. Cocaine is metabolized to benzoylecgonine by spontaneous hydrolysis in plasma and by the action of a hepatic nonspecific carboxylesterase.[21,22] In the presence of ethanol, this enzyme is responsible for the *trans*esterification of cocaine, forming

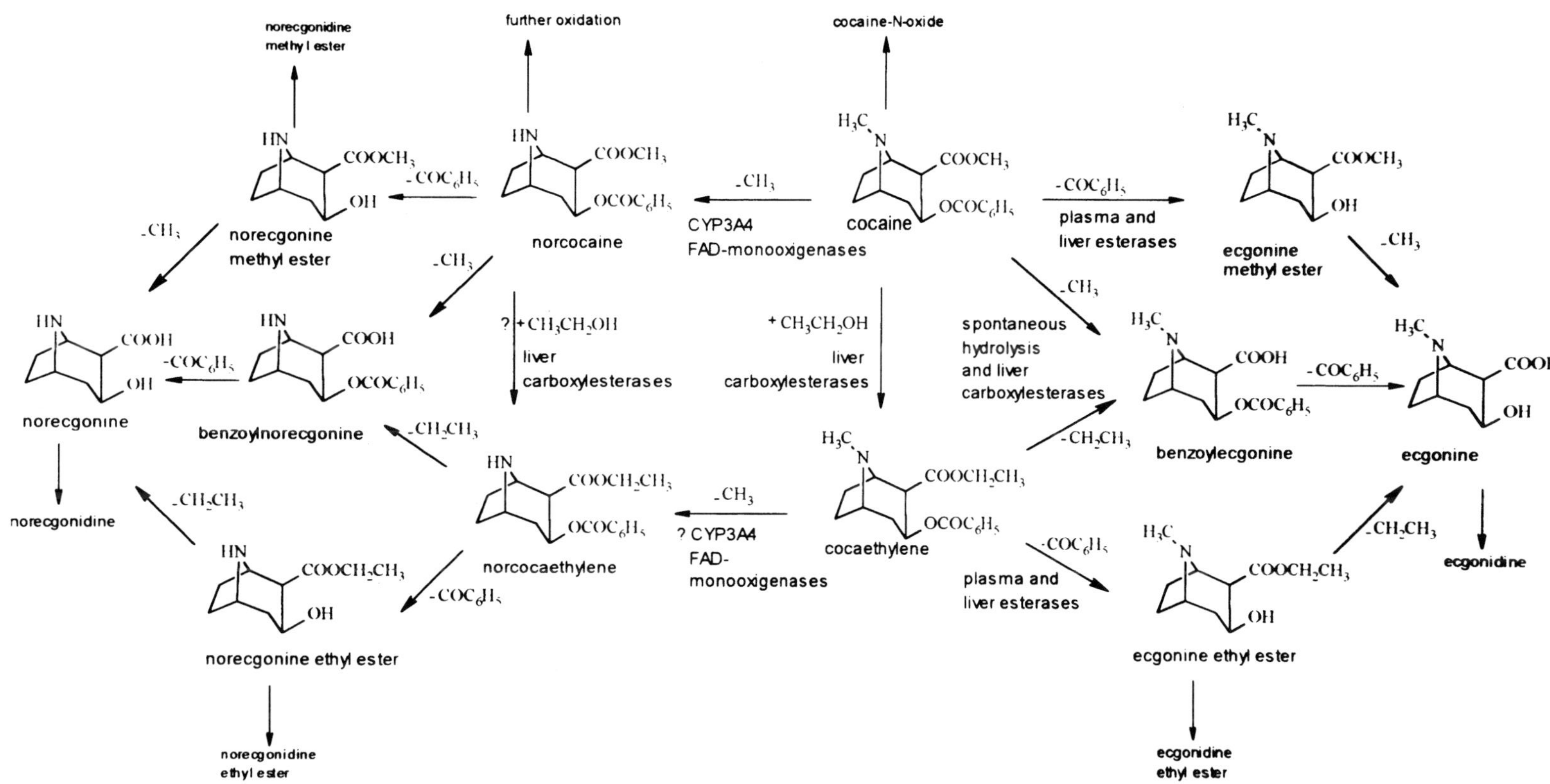

Figure 1. Cocaine and cocaethylene metabolic pathways.

the active metabolite cocaethylene.[23,24] Some of the pharmacokinetic findings could be explained by a competitive mechanism between both substrates, since the same enzyme regulates both metabolic pathways. Cocaine and cocaethylene metabolic reactions are summarized in Fig. 1. The order of drug administration could be a crucial factor in this interaction. In one study, no differences in cocaine plasma concentrations were observed when alcohol was administered 30 min after cocaine snorting.[25]

3. Cocaethylene

Cocaethylene (benzoylethylcocaine) is a pharmacologically active metabolite of cocaine initially found in cases of cocaine and ethanol intoxication.[12,26] It has been identified in plasma and urine of healthy volunteers,[6,27] as well as in postmortem samples from trauma victims.[28–30] Cocaethylene has been found in urine, blood, and tissues of subjects who consumed cocaine and alcohol simultaneously. Recent reports have documented the presence of high levels of cocaethylene in blood samples of patients who had recently ingested cocaine and ethanol. In some cases, concentrations of cocaethylene were higher than those of cocaine. In a series of 41 patients, the ratio of cocaethylene–cocaine concentrations in plasma showed a mean value of 1.3, ranging from 0.1 to 4.7.[30]

3.1. *Basic Pharmacology*

Cocaethylene has a pharmacological profile similar to that of cocaine.[29,31–33] It displays equal affinity for the dopamine transporter as cocaine. It also blocks dopamine uptake at the presynaptic level, increasing concentrations of dopamine in the synaptic cleft. Apparently, cocaethylene is a more selective indirect dopamine agonist, as it is a lesser inhibitor of serotonine uptake than cocaine. In animal models, cocaethylene increases locomotor activity and it is self-administered by nonhuman primates.

3.2. *Pharmacological Effects of Cocaethylene in Humans*

There are three published studies where cocaethylene was administered by different routes (intravenous or intranasal) to evaluate its pharmacological effects in comparison with those of cocaine.

In a pilot study[34] that included three male recreational users of cocaine, cocaethylene was administered at doses of 0.025, 0.05, 0.1, 0.15, 0.20, and 0.25 mg/kg by the intravenous route (as a bolus during 1 min). After that, the same subjects were given an intravenous injection of cocaine (0.25 mg/kg). In the case of cocaethylene, no effects on subjective or cardiovascular parameters were reported for doses below 0.15 mg/kg. The subjective effects, described as increases in the feelings of arousal, pleasure, and increased energy, rated more intensely in a dose-dependent manner. These feelings were stronger at 0.25 mg/kg dose. Also, a dose–response effect was observed on heart rate (30% increase from baseline at the highest dose), but minimal changes were observed on blood pressure. In comparison to cocaine, cocaethylene produced tachycardic effects of similar magnitude, and subjects judged the effects of cocaethylene as more pleasant but less intense than those produced by cocaine.

In a single-blind, cross-over study,[35] six male recreational users of cocaine were given intravenous injections of cocaine (0.25 mg/kg as a cocaine base) and cocaethylene (0.25 mg/kg as a cocaethylene base). Several variables were collected over a period of time including subjective effects ("high"), cardiovascular parameters (heart rate, blood pressure), and blood samples to measure cocaine and cocaethylene. The results showed that cocaethylene was less potent than cocaine, producing changes of lower magnitude in "high" feelings (65%) and heart rate (43%) as compared with cocaine.

In a third study,[36] eight male cocaine abusers (mean dose 3.6 g/week) who were not seeking treatment participated in four experimental sessions. One of the following drugs by intranasal route was given in each session: cocaethylene (0.48 or 0.95 mg/kg), cocaine (0.92 mg/kg), or placebo (lactose, 1 mg/kg). Different variables were measured at baseline and after drug administration. These included different self-rated visual analogue scales ("high," "pleasant", etc) and physiological measures (heart rate, blood pressure). Blood samples were obtained to determine the concentrations of cocaine and cocaethylene. Cocaethylene 0.95 mg/kg and cocaine produced similar effects on "high" rating, but peaks were observed some minutes later in the cocaethylene condition (15 vs. 30 min). Subjects were unable to distinguish between both conditions. With regard to cardiovascular parameters, similar effects on heart rate and blood pressure were recorded, but after cocaethylene administration these effects peaked later. The effects induced by the lowest cocaethylene dose were significantly lower than those induced by cocaine and the highest cocaethylene dose. As a summary, equimolar doses of cocaine and cocaethylene produced similar subjective and cardiovascular effects.

3.3. *Pharmacokinetics of Cocaethylene*

Most of the pharmacokinetic parameters of cocaethylene derive either from two experiments[35,36] in humans, where this substance was administered by the intranasal and the intravenous route at different dose levels, or from studies of cocaine alcohol interaction.[6,19] While studies that administer pure cocaethylene are more suitable for the estimation of pharmacokinetic parameters, it is closer to the real situation to evaluate it in the context of the concomitant consumption of alcohol and cocaine. In experimental studies in volunteers using social doses of both cocaine and ethanol, the concentrations of cocaethylene were lower than those of cocaine. The ratios of peak concentrations or AUC between both substances, seems to be around 15–25%.[6,19] Table

I summarizes pharmacokinetic parameters of cocaethylene in both situations. Pharmacokinetic parameters of cocaine calculated for each experiment have been included as a "control" group for better comparison with those estimated for cocaethylene. There is good agreement between experiments on pharmacokinetic parameters either for cocaine or cocaethylene. The main differences between both drugs are related to their body clearence. Cocaethylene appears to be eliminated more slowly than cocaine, and thus might be expected to accumulate during a binge, which is consistent with analyses of forensic and clinical samples.[37] Differences observed in plasma half-lifes[38] between cocaine and cocaethylene may be explained because of renal tubular reabsorption of cocaethylene. This observation is most probably related to the higher hydrophobicity of cocaethylene as compared with cocaine.

Norcocaethylene, an *N*-demethylated product of cocaethylene, has also been detected in plasma and urine of subjects given alcohol and cocaine concomitantly. Its estimated elimination half-life is 162 ± 59 min, which is greater than that of norcocaine (110 ± 29 min).[19]

Urinary recoveries (24 and 48 hr) for cocaethylene and norcocaethylene are presented in Table II. Urinary excretion rates are presented in Fig. 2. One interesting finding that deserves further research is that recovery of oxidative products like norcocaine in addition to norcocaethylene in the combination groups is higher (100%) than in the cocaine groups. It is unclear whether this observation is a direct effect of alcohol on liver metabolism or a larger availability of substrate (i.e., cocaine), because of metabolic inhibition, for oxidation. In addition, and based on plasma AUC ratios between cocaethylene and norcocaethylene and urinary recoveries, there is apparently an increase in oxidative metabolism of cocaethylene as compared with cocaine. Table III summarizes cocaine and metabolite urinary concentrations in subjects (n = 48) testing positive for cocaine metabolites by fluorescence polarization immunoassay (FPIA) in a noncontrolled setting. Subjects were not overdose or trauma victims but were a population of heroin addicts (n = 354) consuming cocaine concomitantly. Samples testing positive for cocaine by FPIA were reanalyzed by gas chromatography/mass spectrometry (GC/MS).[39] Among other substances, cocaethylene was detected in a 71% of cocaine-positive tested samples (34 of 48).

3.4. *Cocaethylene and Cocaine Metabolism*

What is known about cocaethylene metabolism is quite close to cocaine (see Fig. 1). In summary, cocaine is extensively metabolized in humans and only a small percentage is excreted unaltered in urine.[22,40,41] Cocaine is rapidly metabolized to ecgonine methyl ester by plasma and liver cholinesterases.[23,42–44] Cocaine is also spontaneously hydrolyzed in plasma to benzoylecgonine[22,44] and also by a recently identified human liver carboxylesterase.[23,24] Both are known as the main metabolites excreted in urine. The percentage of these metabolites found in plasma depends on the

Table I. Cocaethylene Pharmacokinetic Parameters in Humans

Study/drug	Dose	Admin. route	$t_{1/2a}$ (min)	$t_{1/2}$ (min)	t_{max} (min)	C_{max} (ng/ml)	V (liter)	CL (liter/min/kg)
McCance[36]								
Cocaine	0.92 mg/kg	Snorting	17.0	111.0	64.0	144.0		
	0.48 mg/kg	Snorting	10.0	155.0	43.0	128.0		
Cocaethylene	0.95 mg/kg	Snorting	13.0	138.0	41.0	251.0		
Perez-Reyes[35]								
Cocaine	0.25 mg/kg	IV		64.2		170.3	205.0	133.0
Cocaethylene	0.25 mg/kg	IV		100.8		159.6	211.0	86.0
Farré[6]								
Cocaine	100 mg	Snorting		78.0	37.9	343.8	229.0	
Cocaethylene[a] (cocaine/alcohol)	100 mg/1 g/kg	Snorting		99.0	121.0	53.3		
Farré[20]								
Cocaine	100 mg	Snorting	14.7	76.1	41.3	330.5	270.0	
Cocaethylene[a] (cocaine/alcohol)	100 mg/0.8 g/kg	Snorting		113.2	116.0	48.7		

[a]Cocaethylene derived from the interaction of cocaine and alcohol

Table II. Urinary Recoveries of Cocaine and Cocaethylene in Healthy Subjects[a]

	Recovery (μmole)[b]		Recovery (%D)	
Compound	C	C/A	C	C/A
A. Urinary excretion recovery at 24 hr of cocaine and its main metabolites in healthy volunteers ($n = 7$) after the simultaneous use of cocaine intranasal (100 mg) and ethanol (1 g/kg)				
Cocaine	5.6 ± 3.1	11.7 ± 4.3	1.9 ± 1.1	4.0 ± 1.4
Benzoylecgonine	72.3 ± 16.4	59.0 ± 15.6	24.6 ± 5.7	20.1 ± 5.3
Ecgonine methyl ester	66.8 ± 38.9	66.7 ± 25.8	22.7 ± 13.22	22.7 ± 8.8
Cocaethylene	ND	1.9 ± 0.6	ND	0.6 ± 0.2
Norcocaine	0.65 ± 0.26	1.34 ± 0.52	0.22 ± 0.09	0.46 ± 0.18
Total	145.35	140.64	49.42	47.86
B. Urinary excretion recovery at 48 hr of cocaine and its main metabolites ($n = 6$) after simultaneous use of cocaine intranasal (100 mg) and ethanol (0.8 g/kg)				
Cocaine	2.9 ± 0.8	9.4 ± 2.5	0.9 ± 0.2	3.2 ± 0.8
Benzoylecgonine	89.0 ± 17.9	84.0 ± 18.9	30.2 ± 6.1	28.5 ± 6.4
Ecgonine methyl ester	67.0 ± 14.2	73.9 ± 13.4	22.8 ± 4.8	25.1 ± 4.6
Cocaethylene	ND	2.1 ± 0.8	ND	0.7 ± 0.3
Norcocaine	0.19 ± 0.08	0.34 ± 0.13	0.06 ± 0.03	0.12 ± 0.04
Norcocaethylene	ND	0.18 ± 0.08	ND	0.06 ± 0.00
Total	159.09	169.92	53.96	57.68

[a]The results are expressed as μmole (mean ± standard deviation) and the percentage of the dose (D, 294.3 μmole of cocaine base).
[b]C, cocaine group; C/A, combination group; ND, not detected.

administration route. In human studies carried out after intranasal administration of doses of 2 mg/kg^{-1} of cocaine, plasma concentrations of ecgonine methyl ester were about one third of those of benzoylecgonine.[45] When cocaine was smoked or injected, the concentrations of ecgonine methyl ester were lower (about 5% of those of benzoylecgonine).[46,47]

Norcocaine is a *N*-demethylated minor active metabolite of cocaine in humans (between 2 and 6% of the dose)[21] produced by liver isoenzymes of the cytochrome P450 (CYP3A)[48,49] and also through FAD mono-oxygenases, which form first the *N*-oxide of cocaine and then it is *N*-demethylated by the action of the cytochrome P450 to form norcocaine.[50–53] The subsequent oxidation of norcocaine has been associated with hepatotoxicity derived from cocaine consumption in experimental animal models[52,54–56] and also in humans.[57,58]

Cocaethylene is formed by the interaction between cocaine and ethanol. The human liver carboxylesterase recently identified[23,24] is responsible not

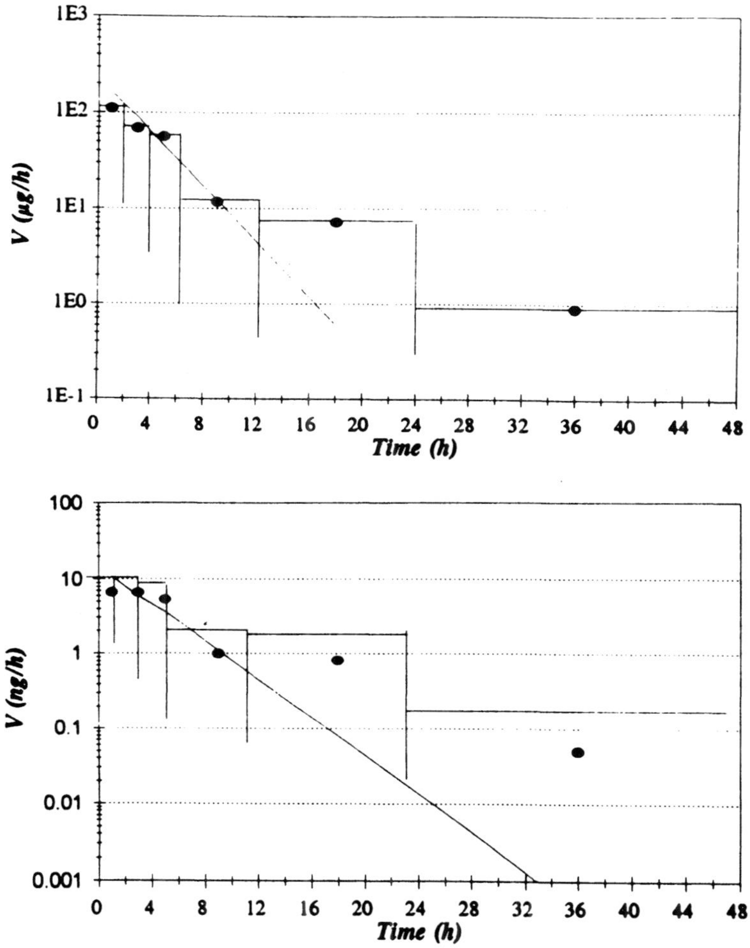

Figure 2. Urinary excretion rates of cocaethylene (upper) and norcocaethylene (lower) in a collection period 0–48 hr after the simulatneous use of cocaine 100 mg and ethanol 0.8 mg/kg.

only for the hydrolysis of cocaine to benzoylecgonine but also of cocaethylene formation by ethyl *trans*esterification of cocaine in the presence of ethanol. It also has been shown that cocaethylene is not formed from benzoylecgonine by *trans*esterification.[23,32] Recently, it has been reported that the enzyme responsible for the esterification of fatty acids in the presence of ethanol can also produce cocaethylene from cocaine.[59] Cocaethylene seems to be metabolized to benzoylecgonine and ecgonine ethyl ester in the same way as cocaine. The corresponding *N*-demethylated metabolite of cocaethylene (equivalent to norcocaine for cocaine), norcocaethylene, is present in plasma and urine of individuals using cocaine and alcohol concurrently.[19,39]

Table III. Urinary Cocaine and Metabolite Concentrations in Heroin Addicts Concomitantly Using Cocaine

Substance	Cocaine	Benzoylecgonine	Ecgonine methylester	Cocaethylene	Norcocaine	Norcocaethylene
Median (μg/mL)	0.098	3.44	0.47	0.15	0.032	0.022
Range	0.009–20.72	0.042–424.71	0.038–112.28	0.007–7.94	0.006–2.6	0.016–0.052
n^a	46	48	33	34	27	3

[a]Refers to the number of urines testing positive for a particular substance. Total number of urines analyzed = 48.

There also are some other minor metabolites of cocaine, such as methyl ecgonidine derivatives, the corresponding ethyl derivatives of which are present in urines of individuals who are concomitant consumers of cocaine and alcohol.[39] Nevertheless, it is still controversial whether these compounds are degradation products from dehydration reactions occurring either in the process of smoking (crack)[60,61] or during the analysis of biological fluids by gas chromatographic techniques,[62] or whether they are real metabolites of cocaine and cocaethylene. Urinary metabolic profiles of cocaine administered alone or concomitantly with alcohol are shown in Fig. 3.

3.5. *Cocaethylene Toxicity*

Cocaethylene toxicity is a controversial issue. The combination of cocaine and ethanol has shown higher toxicity compared with the administration of cocaine and ethanol alone.[63,64] It is unclear what is the contribution of cocaethylene to this general observation. Some reports suggested that cocaethylene was more potent than cocaine in mediating lethality.[65] There are several studies that suggest that it can be more hepatotoxic than cocaine.[65] However, some clinical studies do not seem to support data found in *in vitro* studies and in animal models. For example, hepatotoxicity is not increased in alcoholics with positive urinary cocaine metabolites. Alcoholics abusing cocaine do not have a larger prevalence of severe hepatotoxicity; in those cases where it is observed, it may represent comorbidity.[66] Several clinical studies have described an increase in cocaine oxidative metabolism. In particular, cocaethylene seems to be oxidized to norcocaethylene in a larger proportion to what is observed for cocaine. Its significance in terms of hepatotoxicity is still unknown.[6,19] In addition, animal models seem to support that cocaine-induced liver injury appears to be reversible.[67]

Cocaethylene shows similar immunotoxicity to that associated with cocaine,[68] and especially to *N*-demethylated metabolites (norcocaine and norcocaethylene and their rise during cocaine–alcohol interaction), which are potentiated by ethanol.[69] This observation is not surprising, since cocaine (cocaethylene) immunotoxicity is related to cytochrome P450 activation by cocaine.[70]

Cocaethylene is as cardiotoxic as cocaine, but it is less toxic than cocaine plus ethanol, probably because of the pharmacological interaction; in fact, cocaine at the same doses produced similar effects to cocaethylene.[71] It has been reported to reduce cardiac function in a dose-dependent manner and may be responsible for the delayed but substantial cardiotoxicity that occurs in individuals who use both cocaine and alcohol.[72]

Most probably, the increased toxicity in those individuals who combine cocaine and alcohol compared with that observed for these drugs abused alone is due to increased cocaine plasma concentrations; this is most likely because the metabolic interaction described previously is marginally related to cocaethylene. There also are several other factors that are involved, such as

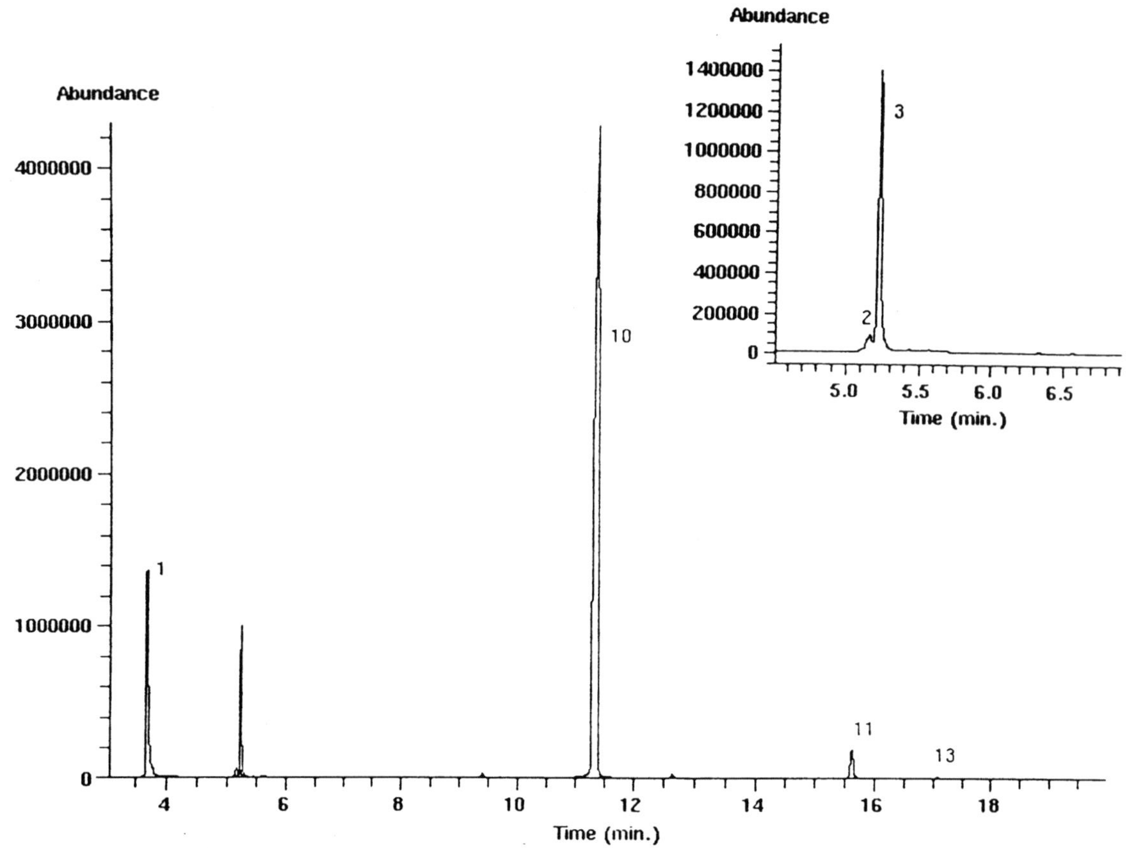

Figure 3. Total ion current profile (SIM acquisition mode) from the GC/MS analysis of a derivatized urine from a healthy volunteer who consumed cocaine (A) alone and (B) cocaine and alcohol. (1) COO-HFIP-ecgonidine; (2) ecgonidine methyl ester; (3) O-PFP-ecgonine methyl ester; (4) ecgonidine ethyl ester; (5) *O*-PFP-ecgonine ethyl ester; (6) *N*-PFP-norecgonidine methyl ester; (7) *N,O-bis*-PFP-nor-

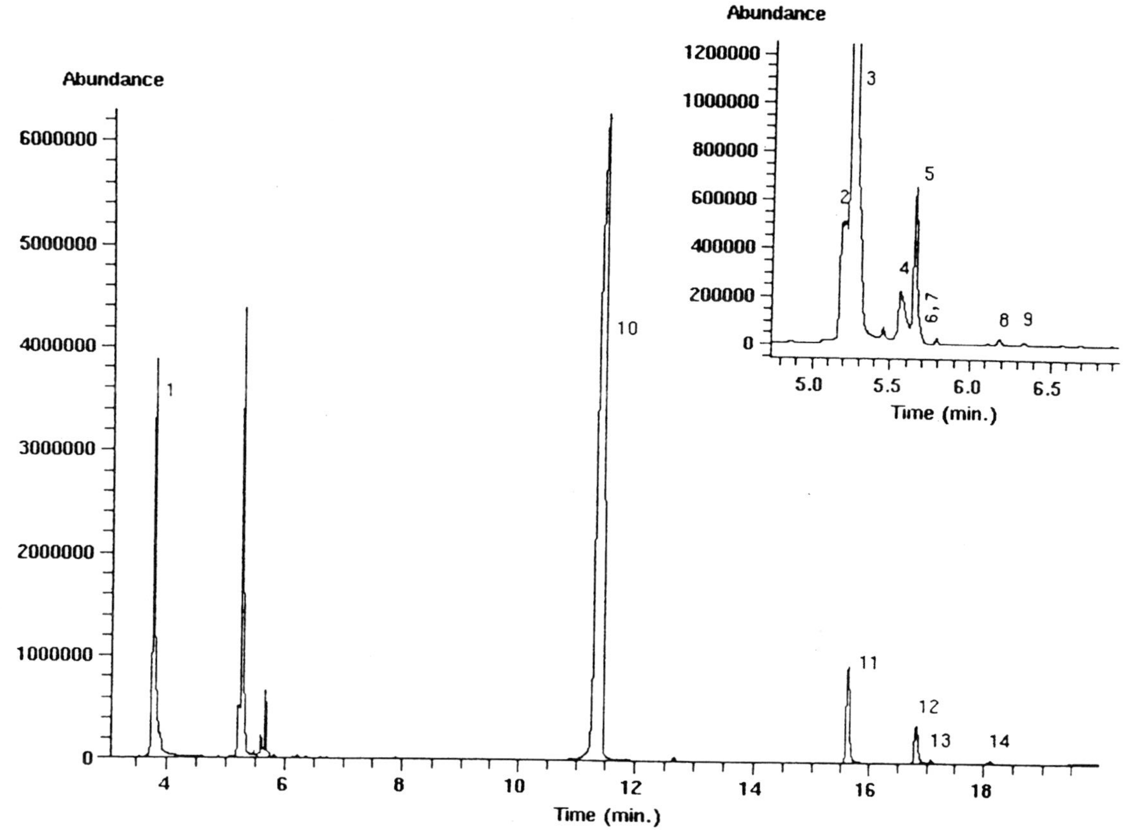

ecgonine methyl ester; (8) *N*-PFP-norecgonidine ethyl ester; (9) *N,O-bis*-PFP-norecgonine ethyl ester; (10) COO-HFIP-benzoylecgonine; (11) cocaine; (12) cocaethylene; (13) *N*-PFP-norcocaine; (14) *N*-PFP-norcocaethylene.

the route of administration, acute versus chronic use, and the order and timing of administration that can modify effects.

In summary, the simultaneous administration of cocaine and alcohol implies both a pharmacological interaction at a pharmacodynamic level and a pharmacokinetic interaction. The latter involves an alteration of cocaine kinetics and metabolism and also the biosynthesis of newly active metabolites, such as cocaethylene. Cocaethylene is metabolized according to the same pathway as cocaine and its detection in biological fluids is indicative of the concomitant consumption of cocaine and alcohol.

ACKNOWLEDGMENTS. This work was supported by grants from 'Fondo de Investigación Sanitaria' (92/0152), CIRIT (GRQ93-9303), and CITRAN Foundation.

References

1. Grant BF, Harford TC: Concurrent and simultaneous use of alcohol with cocaine: Result of a national survey. *Drug Alcohol Depend* 25:97–104, 1990.
2. Higgins ST, Budney AJ, Bickel WK, *et al:* Alcohol dependence and simultaneous cocaine and alcohol use in cocaine-dependent patients. *J Addict Dis* 13:177–189, 1994.
3. Martin CS, Clifford PR, Maisto SA, *et al:* Polydrug use in an inpatient treatment sample of problem drinkers. *Alcohol Clin Exp Res* 20:413–417, 1996.
4. Brady DT, Sonne S, Randall CL *et al:* Features of cocaine dependence with concurrent alcohol abuse. *Drug Alcohol Depend* 39:69–71, 1995.
5. Salloum IM, Daley DC, Cornelius JR, *et al:* Disproportionate lethality in psychiatric patients with concurrent alcohol and cocaine abuse. *Am J Psychiatry* 153:953–955, 1996.
6. Farré M, de la Torre R, Llorente M, *et al:* Alcohol and cocaine interactions in humans. *J Pharmacol Exp Ther* 266:1364–1373, 1993.
7. Higgins ST, Roll JM, Bickel WK: Alcohol pretreatment increases preference for cocaine over monetary reinforcement. *Psychopharmacology* 123:1–8, 1996.
8. Budd RD, Muto JJ, Wong JK: Drugs of abuse found in fatally injured drivers in Los Angeles County. *Drug Alcohol Depend* 23:153–158.
9. Marzuk PM, Tardiff K, Leon AC, *et al:* Prevalence of recent cocaine use among motor vehicles fatalities in New York City. *JAMA* 263:250–256, 1990.
10. Tardiff K, Marzuk PM, Leon AC, *et al:* Cocaine, opiates, and ethanol in homicides in New York City: 1990 and 1991. *J Forensic Sci* 40:387–390, 1995.
11. Vanek VW, Dickey-White H, Signs SA, *et al:* Concurrent use of cocaine and alcohol by patients treated in the emergency department. *Ann Emerg Med* 28:508–514, 1996.
12. Rafla FK, Epstein RL: Identification of cocaine and its metabolites in human urine in the presence of ethyl alcohol. *J Anal Toxicol* 3:59–63, 1979.
13. Wu AHB, Onigbinde TA, Johnson KG, Wimbish GH: Alcohol-specific cocaine metabolites in serum and urine of hospitalized patients. *J Anal Toxicol* 16:132–136, 1992.
14. Brookoff D, Rotondo MF, Shaw LM, *et al:* Cocaethylene levels in patients who test positive for cocaine. *Ann Emerg Med* 27:316–320, 1996.
15. Foltin RW, Fischman ME: Ethanol and cocaine interactions in human: Cardiovascular consequences. *Pharmacol Biochem Behav* 31:877–873, 1989.
16. Perez-Reyes M, Jeffcoat R: Ethanol/cocaine interaction: Cocaine and cocaethylene plasma concentrations and their relationship to subjective and cardiovascular effects. *Life Sci* 51:553–563, 1992.
17. Higgins ST, Rush CR, Bickel WK, *et al:* Acute behavioral and cardiac effects of cocaine and alcohol combinations in humans. *Psychopharmacology* 111:285–294, 1993.

18. McCance-Katz EF, Prince LH, McDougle CJ, *et al:* Concurrent cocaine–ethanol ingestion in humans: Pharmacology, physiology, behavior, and the role of cocaethylene. *Psychopharmacology* 111:39–46, 1993.
19. Farré M, de la Torre R, González ML, *et al:* Cocaine and alcohol interactions in humans: Neuroendocrine effects and cocaethylene metabolism. *J Pharmacol Exp Ther* 283:164–176, 1997.
20. Heesch CM, Negus BH, Bost JH, *et al:* Effects of cocaine on anterior pituitary and gonadal hormones. *J Pharmacol Exp Ther* 278:1195–1200, 1996.
21. Inaba T, Stewart DJ, Kalow W: Metabolism of cocaine in man. *Clin Pharmacol Ther* 23:547–552, 1978.
22. Inaba T: Cocaine: Pharmacokinetics and biotransformation in man. *Can J Physiol Pharmacol* 67:1154–1157, 1989.
23. Dean RA, Christian CD, Sample RHB, Bosron WF: Human liver cocaine esterases: Ethanol-mediated formation of ethylcocaine. *FASEB J* 5:2735–2739, 1991.
24. Brzezinski MR, Abraham TL, Stone CL, *et al:* Purification and characterization of a human liver cocaine carboxylesterase that catalyzes the production of benzoylecgonine and the formation of cocaethylene from alcohol and cocaine. *Biochem Pharmacol* 48:1747–1755, 1994.
25. Perez-Reyes M: The order of drug administration: Its effects on the interaction between cocaine and ethanol. *Life Sci* 55:541–550, 1994.
26. Smith RM: Ethyl esters of arylhydroxy- and arylhydroxymethoxicocaines in the urines of simultaneous cocaine and alcohol users. *J Anal Toxicol* 8:38–42, 1984.
27. De la Torre, R, Farré M, Ortuño J, *et al:* The relevance of urinary cocaethylene as a metabolite of cocaine under the simultaneous administration of alcohol. *J Anal Toxicol* 15:223, 1991.
28. Bailey DN: Serial plasma concentrations of cocaethylene, cocaine and ethanol in trauma victims. *J Anal Toxicol* 17:79–83, 1993.
29. Jatlow P, Elsworth JD, Bradberry CW, *et al:* Cocaethylene: A neuropharmacologically active metabolite associated with concurrent cocaine-alcohol ingestion. *Life Sci* 48:1787–1794, 1991.
30. Bailey D: Comprehensive review of cocaethylene and cocaine concentrations in patients. *J Clin Pathol* 106:701–704, 1996.
31. McCance-Katz EF, Price LH, McDougle CJ *et al:* Concurrent cocaine–ethanol ingestion in humans: Pharmacology, physiology, behavior, and the role of cocaethylene. *Psychopharmacology* 111:39–46, 1993.
32. Hearn WL, Flynn DD, Hime GW: Cocaethylene: A unique cocaine metabolite displays high affinity for the dopamine transporter. *J Neurochem* 56:698–701, 1991.
33. Katz JL, Terry P, Witkin JM: Comparative behavioral pharmacology and toxicology of cocaine and its ethanol-derived metabolite, cocaine ethylester (cocaethylene). *Life Sci* 50:1351–1361, 1992.
34. Perez-Reyes M: Subjective and cardiovascular effects of cocaethylene in humans. *Psychopharmacology* 113:144–147, 1993.
35. Perez-Reyes M, Jeffcoat R, Myers M, *et al:* Comparison in humans of the potency and pharmacokinetics of intravenously injected cocaethylene and cocaine. *Psychopharmacology* 116:428–432, 1994.
36. McCane EF, Price LH, Kosten TR, Jatlow PI: Cocaethylene: Pharmacology, physiology and behavioral effects in humans. *J Pharmacol Exp Ther* 274:215–223, 1995.
37. Bailey DN: Plasma cocaethylene concentrations in patients treated in the emergency room or trauma unit. *Am J Clin Pathol* 99:123–127, 1993.
38. Bailey DN, Bessler JB, Sawrey BA: Cocaine- and cocaethylene–creatinine clearance ratios in humans. *J Anal Toxicol* 21:41–43, 1997.
39. De la Torre R, Ortuño J, Gonzàlez ML, *et al:* Determination of cocaine and its metabolites in human urine by gas chromatography/mass spectrometry after simultaneous use of cocaine and alcohol. *J Pharm Biomed Anal* 13:305–312, 1995.
40. Fish F, Wilson DC: Excretion of cocaine and its metabolites in man. *J Pharm Pharmacol* 21:135S–138S, 1969.

41. Ambre JJ, Fischman M, Ruo TI: Urinary excretion of ecgonine methyl ester, a major metabolite of cocaine in humans. *J Anal Toxicol* 8:23–25, 1984.
42. Jatlow P, Barash PG, Van Dyke C, *et al:* Cocaine and succinylcholine sensitivity: A new caution. *Anesth Analg* 58:235–238, 1979.
43. Stewart DJ, Inaba T, Tang BK, Kalow W: Hydrolysis of cocaine in human plasma cholinesterase. *Life Sci* 20:1557–1564, 1977.
44. Stewart DJ, Inaba T, Lucassen M, Kalow W: Cocaine metabolism: Cocaine and norcocaine hydrolysis by liver and serum esterases. *Clin Pharmacol Ther* 25:464–468, 1979.
45. Brogan III WC, Kemp PM, Bost RO, *et al:* Collection and handling of clinical blood samples to assure the accurate measurement of cocaine concentration. *J Anal Toxicol* 16:152–154, 1992.
46. Isenschmid DS, Fischman MW, Foltin RW, Caplan YH: Concentration of cocaine and metabolites in plasma of humans following intravenous administration and smoking of cocaine. *J Anal Toxicol* 16:311–314, 1992.
47. Cone EJ: Pharmacokinetics and pharmacodynamics of cocaine. *J Anal Toxicol* 19:459–478, 1995.
48. Le Duc B, Sinclair PR, Shuster L, *et al:* Norcocaine and *N*-hydroxynorcocaine formation in human liver microsomes: Role of cytochrome P450 3A4. *Pharmacology* 46:294–300, 1993.
49. Pellinen P, Honkakoski P, Stenbäck F, *et al:* Cocaine *N*-demethylation and the metabolism-related hepatotoxicity can be prevented by cytochrome P450 3A inhibitors. *Eur J Pharmacol* 270:35–43, 1994.
50. Kloss MW, Rosen GM, Rauckman EJ: *N*-Demethylation of cocaine to norcocaine. Evidence for participation by cytochrome P450 and FAD-containing monooxygenase. *Mol Pharmacol* 23:482–485, 1983.
51. Shuster D, Casey E, Welankiwar SS: Metabolism of cocaine and norcocaine to *N*-hydroxynorcocaine. *Biochem Pharmacol* 32:3045–3051, 1983.
52. Kloss M, Rosen G, Rauckman E: Cocaine-mediated hepatotoxicity: A critical review. *Biochem Pharmacol* 33:169–173, 1984.
53. Roberts SM, Harbison RD, James RC: Human microsomal *N*-oxidative metabolism of cocaine. *Drug Metab Dispos* 19:1046–1051, 1991.
54. Thompson ML, Shuster L, Shaw K: Cocaine-induced hepatic necrosis in mice—The role of cocaine metabolism. *Biochem Pharmacol* 28:2389–2395, 1979.
55. Freeman RW, Harbison RD: Hepatic periportal necrosis induced by chronic administration of cocaine. *Biochem Pharmacol* 30:777–783, 1981.
56. Evans MA: Role of protein binding in cocaine-induced hepatic necrosis. *J Pharmacol Exp Ther* 224:73–79, 1983.
57. Perino LLE, Warren GH, Levine JS: Cocaine-induced hepatotoxicity in humans. *Gastroenterology* 93:176–180, 1987.
58. Wanless IR, Dore S, Gopinath N, *et al:* Histopathology of cocaine hepatotoxicity. Report of four patients. *Gastroenterology* 98:497–501, 1990.
59. Heith AM, Morse CR, Tsujita T, *et al:* Fatty acid ethyl ester synthase catalyzes the esterification of ethanol to cocaine. *Biochem Biophys Res Commun* 208:549–554, 1995.
60. Jacob P III, Lewis E, Jones R, Elias-Baker B: A pyrolysis product, anhydroecgonine methyl ester:methylecgonidine, is in the urine of cocaine smokers. *J Anal Toxicol* 14:353–357, 1990.
61. Cone EJ, Hillsgrove MJ, Darwin WD: Simultaneous measurement of cocaine, cocaethylene, their metabolites and "crack" pyrolysis products by gas chromatography-mass spectrometry. *Clin Chem* 40:1299–1305, 1994.
62. Gonzàlez ML, Carnicero M, de la Torre R, *et al:* Influence of the injection technique on the thermal degradation of cocaine and its metabolites in gas chromatography. *J Chromatogr Biomed Appl* 664:317–327, 1995.
63. Ponsoda X, Jover R, Castell JV, Gòmez-Lechón J: Potentiation of cocaine hepatotoxicity in human hepatocytes by ethanol. *Toxic in Vitro* 6:155–158, 1992.
64. Smith AC, Freeman RW, Harbison RD: Ethanol enhancement of cocaine-induced hepatotoxicity. *Biochem Pharmacol* 30:453–458, 1981.

65. Hearn WL, Rose S, Wagner J: Cocaethylene is more potent than cocaine in mediating lethality. *Pharmacol Biochem Behav* 39:531–533, 1991.
66. Worner TM: Hepatotoxicity is not inreased in alcoholics with positive urinary cocaine metabolites. *Drug Alcohol Depend* 35:191–195, 1994.
67. Pellinen P, Stenbäck F, Kojo A, *et al:* Regenerative changes in hepatic morphology and enhanced expression of CYP2B10 and CYP3A during daily administration of cocaine. *Hepatology* 23:515–523, 1996.
68. Chiappelli F, Kung MA, Villanueva P, *et al:* Immunotoxicity of cocaethylene. *Immunopharmacol Immunotoxicol* 17:399–417, 1995.
69. Pirozhkov SV, Watson RR, Chen GJ: Ethanol immunosuppression induced by cocaine. *Alcohol Alcohol Suppl* 2:75–82, 1993.
70. Jeong TC, Jordan SD, Matulka RA, *et al:* Immunosuppression induced by acute exposure to cocaine is dependent on metabolism by cytochrome P-450. *J Pharmacol Exp Ther* 276:1257–1265, 1996.
71. Henning RJ, Wilson LD: Cocaethylene is as cardiotoxic as cocaine but is less toxic than cocaine plus ethanol. *Life Sci* 59:615–627, 1996.
72. Wilson LD, Henning RJ, Sutheimer C, *et al:* Cocaethylene causes dose-dependent reductions in cardiac function in anesthetized dogs. *J Cardiovasc Pharmacol* 26:965–973, 1995.

19

Interrelationship between Alcohol Intake, Hepatitis C, Liver Cirrhosis, and Hepatocellular Carcinoma

Harumasa Yoshihara, Katsuhisa Noda, and Takenobu Kamada

Abstract. The discovery of a cDNA clone of hepatitis C virus (HCV) genome in 1989 has resulted in numerous reports of high rates of the prevalence of HCV antibody in patients with alcoholic liver disease, in particular, alcoholic liver cirrhosis and hepatocellular carcinoma. Thus, the interaction between alcohol intake and HCV infection has become of great importance. In terms of the effect of alcohol on HCV-RNA levels, the data are controversial; in some reports, alcohol increases HCV-RNA levels, and in the other reports it does not. There are several reports suggesting the possibility of an elevated quasi-species of hypervariable region 1 in the HCV genome caused by alcohol drinking. Recent studies have documented that alcohol intake exaggerates the responsiveness of interferon therapy for chronic hepatitis C; however, its mechanism is still obscure. Several studies have suggested the promoting effect of alcohol on the development of hepatocellular carcinoma in type C liver cirrhosis, which has been similarly observed in type B chronic liver disease, whereas its mechanism is limited to speculations.

1. Introduction

The cDNA clone of hepatitis C virus (HCV) genome was discovered in 1989 by Choo *et al*,.[1] who subsequently developed a serological assay for the detection of antibody to a polypeptide of the nonstructural region of the HCV

Harumasa Yoshihara, Katsuhisa Noda, and Takenobu Kamada • Department of Gastroenterology, Osaka Rosai Hospital, Osaka 591-8025, Japan.

Recent Developments in Alcoholism, Volume 14: The Consequences of Alcoholism, edited by Galanter. Plenum Press, New York, 1998.

genome (anti-C100-3).[2] Recently, various new assays for antibodies to the core or the other regions of HCV genome and for HCV-RNA have been established.[3–5] This discovery has resulted in numerous reports of the prevalence of antibody to HCV (anti-HCV) in patients with alcoholic liver disease.[6,7] In particular, high rates of the prevalence of anti-HCV were observed in alcoholic liver cirrhosis and hepatocellular carcinoma (HCC); HCV is therefore assumed to be intimately related with the development of alcoholic liver injury to liver cirrhosis and HCC. It has been reported that alcohol intake exaggerates the liver disease and promotes the carcinogenesis of the liver in patients with chronic hepatitis B.[8–11] These investigations suggest that alcohol is an important factor that modulates the development and prognosis of chronic viral hepatitis; however, little is known about interaction between alcohol intake and chronic hepatitis C.

On the other hand, interferon (IFN) therapy recently has been proved to be effective for chronic hepatitis C,[12] although some patients show a resistance to IFN therapy. Several studies have attempted to clarify the factors determining the efficacy of IFN therapy, but there have been few reports concerning the effect of alcohol intake on the efficacy of IFN therapy in patients with chronic hepatitis C. Therefore, in the current chapter, how alcohol drinking affects the development of chronic liver disease and the responsiveness to IFN therapy in type C chronic hepatitis are reviewed.

2. Effect of Alcohol Intake on Serum HCV-RNA Levels and Sequence Diversity of Hypervariable Region 1 in Patients with Chronic Hepatitis C

The development of type C chronic hepatitis to liver cirrhosis (LC) or HCC in drinkers is assumed to be associated with the factors of ethanol as well as HCV. These effects of alcohol on quality or quantity of HCV and host immunity might be determining factors for the development of liver disease and the responsiveness to the therapy. In particular, HCV is known to exhibit extremely frequent genomic mutation of the hypervariable region 1 (HVR1) in the E2/NS1 region of HCV genome, which is supposed to be most intimately connected with quasi-species of the HCV genome and to act as a target epitope of host immune reaction.[13,14] Recently, it has been reported that nucleotide diversity in HVR1 and/or amino acid quasi-species in NS5A of the HCV genome are intimately related with the responsiveness to IFN therapy[15] and the development of liver disease in patients with chronic hepatitis C.[16] We[17] also studied whether the nucleotide diversity of HVR1 is predictive for the efficacy of IFN therapy employing fluorescence single-strand conformation polymorphism sequence analysis (FSSA). We concluded that the efficacy of IFN therapy showed no relationship with the mutant clones but it showed a significant relationship with the nucleotide diversity. Also, multivariate logistic analysis revealed an intimate relationship of genotype, serum HCV-RNA levels, and nucleotide diversity with the efficacy of IFN therapy, in this order.

As to the effect of alcohol on quantity and quality of HCV, we[18] evaluated the effect of alcohol drinking on HCV-RNA levels and the nucleotide diversity of HVR1. Sixty-three patients were diagnosed histologically as type C chronic active hepatitis. HCV-RNA levels, genotype, and nucleotide diversity of HVR1 were measured by competitive reverse transcription polymerase chain reaction (RT-PCR),[19] RT-PCR,[20,21] and FSSA, respectively. For the FSSA method, serum HCV-RNA was extracted and the sequence of HVR1 was amplified with nested PCR, and PCR products were subjected to autosequencer. The mutant clones (the number of constituent clones of HCV-RNA quasi-species) were measured, and the nucleotide diversity (the number of substitutive nucleotides in HVR1) was also measured. Subjects were divided into three groups: nondrinkers, ethanol intake less than 46 g/day, and ethanol intake more than 46 g/day. HCV-RNA levels in nondrinkers (n = 33), less than 46 g/day (n = 16), and more than 46 g/day (n = 14) were 4.9 ± 1.6, 4.9 + 1.4, and 4.4 ± 1.6 (log, copy/ml), and the mutant clones were 4.5 ± 2.2, 5.8 ± 2.7, and 5.3 ± 2.4, respectively, showing no significant difference; however, the nucleotide diversities were 9.3 ± 6.7, 9.8 ± 3.9, and 11.9 ± 6.6, respectively, resulting in a trend of higher value in the more than 46 g/day group than the less than 46 g/day group. The analysis only in men (n = 44) revealed no difference in HCV-RNA levels among three groups and a trend of higher value of the mutant clones in drinkers than in nondrinkers (4.3 ± 1.9, 5.6 ± 2.8, and 5.3 ± 2.4). However, the nucleotide diversities in nondrinkers, less than 46 g/day, and more than 46 g/day were 7.3 ± 5.0, 9.0 ± 3.4, and 11.9 ± 6.6, resulting in a significant difference between nondrinkers and more than 46 g/day ($P<0.05$) (Table I). In conclusion, these data suggest a possibility that alcohol drinking might increase the nucleotide diversity of HVR1 of HCV genome without affecting the HCV-RNA levels.

Ohnishi *et al.*[22] also reported significantly lower levels of serum HCV-RNA in drinkers than in nondrinkers with type C chronic hepatitis. By contrast, it is supposed that drinkers should show higher serum HCV-RNA levels than nondrinkers because of an increased viral proliferation based on the reduced capacity of cellular immunity[23] or genetic drift to HCV clones

Table I. Relationship between the Nucleotide Diversity of HVR1 and Alcohol Intake in Male Patients with Chronic Hepatitis C

	Mutant clone (PCR-SSCP method)	Nucleotide diversity (direct sequence method)
Nondrinker (n = 16)	4.3 ± 1.9	7.3 ± 5.0
<46 g/day (n = 14)	5.6 ± 2.8	9.0 ± 3.4
≥46 g/day (n = 14)	5.3 ± 2.4	11.9 ± 6.6[a]

[a]$P < 0.05$ vs. nondrinker.

with more rapid viral proliferation. In fact, heavy drinkers have been documented to exhibit significantly higher levels of serum HCV-RNA than nondrinkers,[24] and that HCV-RNA levels in some habitual drinkers decrease after abstinence and again increase when drinking resumes.[25] Thus, the data concerning the effect of alcohol on serum HCV-RNA levels are controversial. This controversy may be attributed to the difference in the amount of alcohol intake or length of abstinent period to sampling of blood in subjects. In order to clarify this problem, the time course of serum HCV-RNA levels during drinking and after abstinence is required in larger numbers of drinkers with type C chronic hepatitis.

In terms of the effect of alcohol drinking on nucleotide diversity of HCV genome, Finkelstein *et al.*[26] reported that quasi-species in the NS5 RNA polymerase region was significantly higher in drinkers than in nondrinkers. We suggested a possibility of an elevated nucleotide diversity of HVR1 by alcohol drinking as described above; however, there have been few reports about the effect of alcohol on the nucleotide diversity of HVR1. The mechanism of an enhanced nucleotide diversity of HVR1 in drinkers possibly could be as follows: ethanol has not been reported to directly produce a mutation of DNA or RNA, so that an increase in mutation of HCV genome might be related directly or via the immune response of the host with a production of acetaldehyde,[27,28] a metabolite of alcohol, genetoxin activated by cytochrome P450IIE1 induced by ethanol,[29–31] and free radicals produced by ethanol metabolism.[32] Such an increase in mutation of HVR1 may be involved in the mechanism of the resistance to IFN therapy and/or promotion of an occurrence of HCC in alcoholic patients with hepatitis C.

3. Effect of Alcohol Intake on the Responsiveness to IFN Therapy in Patients with Chronic Hepatitis C

Interferon has been used in the treatment of chronic hepatitis C since the report by Hoofnagle *et al.*,[12] and its efficacy has been established in normalizing serum alanine aminotransferase (ALT) levels, diminishing serum HCV-RNA, and improving liver histological findings. However, some patients with chronic hepatitis C show a resistance to IFN therapy, and the factors for these nonresponders have been documented so far. A study with multiple logistic regression demonstrated that the total dose of IFN, age, method of IFN administration, liver histology, and gender were the factors that affect the response to IFN therapy.[19] It is generally accepted that a poor response to IFN therapy could be observed in the patients with increased serum levels of HCV-RNA, genotype Ib, histologically advanced stages of liver damage, and old age. In particular, serum HCV-RNA levels and genotype are the most important determining factors for the responsiveness of IFN therapy in patients with chronic hepatitis C.

Although alcohol has been reported to be an important factor that modulates the development and prognosis of chronic viral hepatitis, little is known

Table II. The Efficacy of Interferon Therapy and the Disappearance Rate of HCV-RNA after the Therapy in Patients with Chronic Hepatitis C[a]

	Sustained responder	HCV-RNA disappearance
Nondrinker	8/15(53.3%)	7/12(58.3%)
<70 g/day	6/14(42.9%)	2/10(20.0%)
≥70 g/day	0/10(0%)[b,c]	1/8(12.5%)[d]
Total	14/39(35.9%)	10/30(33.3%)

[a]HCV-RNA was detected 6 months after the cessation of interferon therapy.
[b]$P < 0.01$ vs. nondrinker.
[c]$P < 0.01$ vs. <70 g/day.
[d]$P < 0.05$ vs. nondrinker.
Chi-square test.

about the interaction of alcohol intake and chronic hepatitis C, particularly of alcohol intake and the responsiveness to IFN therapy in type C chronic hepatitis. Hereby, we[33] examined whether alcohol drinking affects the effectiveness of IFN therapy for chronic hepatitis C by comparing the effectiveness in drinkers with that in nondrinkers (Table II). Thirty-nine patients with chronic hepatitis C were divided into three groups on the basis of the amount of alcohol intake before IFN therapy: group 1 ($n = 15$), nondrinkers; group 2 ($n = 14$), less than 70 g/day; and group 3 ($n = 10$), more than 70 g/day of ethanol intake for at least 10 years. The IFN (total dose, 330 ± 206 MU) was administered daily for 2 weeks and thereafter intermittently. Drinkers stayed abstinent for at least 1 month before, during, and after IFN therapy. The sustained responder was defined as the patient who showed normal ALT levels continuously for more than 6 months after the therapy. The liver histology (histological activity index [HAI] score)[34] and serum HCV-RNA[35] were also examined before and after the therapy. There was no significant difference among three groups in the level of ALT before IFN therapy, age, total dose of IFN, and liver histology. The rates of sustained responders in groups 1, 2, and 3 were 53.3%, 42.9%, and 0%, respectively, resulting in a significantly lower rate in heavy drinkers (group 3) than in nondrinkers (group 1) ($P<0.01$) and light drinkers (group 2) ($P<0.01$) and a fall of the ratio in parallel with an elevation of alcohol intake. The serum HCV-RNA turned negative after the therapy in 58.3%, 20.0%, and 12.5% of groups 1, 2, and 3, respectively, leading to a significantly lower rate of disappearance of HCV-RNA in group 3 than in group 1 ($P<0.05$). Nondrinkers showed a significant histological improvement in category 1 of the HAI score after IFN therapy, whereas drinkers did not. Thus, there was no significant difference in age, daily dose, total dose of IFN, duration of IFN therapy, and histological liver findings before IFN therapy between nondrinkers and drinkers with chronic hepatitis C, whereas IFN therapy for chronic hepatitis C was less effective in heavy drinkers than in nondrinkers with regard to normalization of serum ALT levels, disappearance of serum HCV-RNA, and histological improvement of the liver after the therapy.

IFN therapy is more effective for the patients with lower titers of HCV-

RNA and with mild histological changes of the liver, implying that the initial HCV-RNA titer is the most important factor affecting the sustained response to IFN therapy.[19] In terms of how alcohol affects the proliferation of HCV in patients with chronic hepatitis C, Oshita *et al.*[24] reported that the titers of HCV-RNA in serum quantified by means of a competitive RT-PCR assay in subjects drinking more than 69 g/day ethanol showed significantly ($P<0.01$) higher titers than nondrinkers and drinkers of less than 46 g/day ethanol, and that the IFN therapy for chronic hepatitis C was less effective in heavy drinkers than in nondrinkers. Similarly, a recent study demonstrated the promotion of HCV-RNA replication in heavy drinkers with chronic hepatitis C.[25,36] These data suggest the possibility that the serum levels of HCV-RNA are higher in drinkers than in nondrinkers with chronic hepatitis C, which, in turn, may be attributed to a lower effectiveness of IFN therapy in drinkers than in nondrinkers. On the contrary, Matsuo *et al.*[22] studied the relationship, employing multivariate logistic analysis, between alcohol drinking and HCV-RNA levels, liver histology, and responsiveness to IFN therapy in patients with chronic hepatitis C. They concluded that habitual alcohol intake does not affect the liver histology of chronic hepatitis C; however, it is a factor contributing to a progression of alcoholic liver fibrosis, and it reduces the serum levels of HCV-RNA and exaggerates the efficacy of IFN therapy. Recently, our investigation[18] also demonstrated similar levels of serum HCV-RNA in drinkers compared with nondrinkers. Thus, there are a couple of reports indicating the lower effectiveness of IFN therapy in drinkers with HCV; however, the reports are controversial concerning the serum levels of HCV-RNA in drinkers. It will be necessary in the future to examine how the serum level of HCV-RNA changes following abstinence in individual drinkers. Alternatively, the difference in HCV genotype between drinkers and nondrinkers could be one of the causes for the difference in effectiveness of the IFN therapy[37]; that is, a high incidence of genotype K1 in heavy drinkers has been reported; however, we could not find a difference in genotype between drinkers and nondrinkers. During the suppression of the immunologic response to HCV in habitual drinkers,[23,38,39] mutational alteration in the HCV genome could easily occur, and such a diversity of HCV quasi-species population of HVR1 or NS5A region of HCV genome[13,14,18,21,26] might affect the resistance to IFN therapy in drinkers. More work will be required to discern the difference in diversity of the other regions of HCV genome between drinkers and nondrinkers. The difference in immunologic reaction of the host might be also involved in this mechanism, although it is still obscure.

4. Effect of Alcohol Intake on the Progression of Type C Chronic Hepatitis to Liver Cirrhosis and Hepatocellular Carcinoma

Since the development of the C100-3 antibody (a tool for the serological assay of HCV[1,2]), various studies using this method revealed that HCV is the major cause of non-A, non-B hepatitis, and that persistent infection with this virus is intimately related with the occurrence of LC and HCC. In addition, these studies showed that approximately 36 to 39% of alcoholic LC and 56 to 76% of alcoholic HCC were positive for HCV antibody.[9,40] Thus, the association between alcohol intake and hepatitis C is of great importance in the progression of liver disease.

It has been reported that habitual alcohol intake promotes the progression of liver disease from chronic hepatitis B to LC and/or HCC; that is, alcohol is a factor modulating the development and prognosis of chronic hepatitis B. Ohnishi *et al.*[11] demonstrated that the average age for the diagnosis of LC was significantly younger by 10.5 years in hepatitis B surface antigen (HBsAg)-positive patients who drank >23 g/day ethanol than in those who drank <23 g/day ethanol, and that the average age for the diagnosis of HCC was significantly younger by 9 years in HBsAg-positive patients who drank >23 g/day ethanol than in nonalcoholic, HBsAg-positive patients. Austin *et al.*[41] also reported using a case–control study in patients with HBV that daily intake of alcohol beverages increased dose dependently the risk for developing HCC. However, it still is not clear whether habitual alcohol intake facilitates the progression of type C hepatitis to LC or HCC. Similar studies in patients with HCV have not been possible because of the lack of a specific diagnostic test for HCV. Takase *et al.*[8] have demonstrated that the rate of cumulative incidence of HCC was higher in HCV-antibody-positive alcoholic cirrhotics than in HCV-antibody-negative alcoholic cirrhotics or nondrinking type C cirrhotics, suggesting that alcohol intake, in conjunction with HCV, promotes the progression of HCC.

On the other hand, there is a study demonstrating that HCV patients transfused in the elder age exhibited a rapid progression to LC.[42] Therefore, we[43] also investigated whether habitual alcohol intake and the age of HCV infection can be factors that facilitate the development of chronic hepatitis C to LC and HCC in patients with hepatitis C and the history of blood transfusion.

Thirty LC and 85 HCC patients were enrolled and all had a history of a single blood transfusion, when HCV infection was assumed to be induced, more than 5 years ago. In patients with LC, no significant correlation was observed between the amount of alcohol intake and the period from transfusion to diagnosis. The period from transfusion to diagnosis in HCC patients with alcohol intake ≥46 g/day and <46 g/day for at least 10 years were 26 ± 6 and 31 ± 9 years, respectively, resulting in a significant difference ($P<0.05$). There was no difference in the age of transfusion between two groups and the age of diagnosis of HCC was significantly younger in ≥46 g/day than in <46 g/day ($P<0.05$); further, the proportion of chronic hepatitis or LC in the histology of noncancerous liver tissues was not significantly different between these two groups. The period from transfusion to diagnosis of LC and/or HCC showed significant inverse correlation with the age of transfusion (r = 0.82, $Y = -0.67X+48.0$, $P<0.01$; $r = 0.76$, $Y = -0.70X+54.1$, $P<0.001$, respec-

Table III. Comparison of Background, Laboratory Data, and the Period from Blood Transfusion to Diagnosis of HCC between HCV-Positive Light and Heavy Drinkers with HCC[a]

	Ethanol intake		
	<46 g/day (n = 67)	≥46 g/day (n = 18)	
Sex (M:F)	39:28	16:2	$P < 0.05$
HBsAg-positivity	1 (1%)	1 (5%)	NS
Age of diagnosis (yr)	65 ± 7	62 ± 4	$P < 0.05$
Age of blood transfusion (yr)	34 ± 10	35 ± 8	NS
Period from transfusion to diagnosis (yr)	31 ± 9	26 ± 6	$P < 0.05$
Histology of noncancerous lesion			
Chronic hepatitis	5 (7%)	0 (0%)	NS
Liver cirrhosis	18 (27%)	6 (33%)	NS
ND	44 (66%)	12 (67%)	NS
Liver function test at diagnosis			
ALT	110 ± 69	139 ± 102	NS
AST	89 ± 51	87 ± 40	NS
r-GTP	122 ± 118	205 ± 187	$P < 0.05$
Survivals	45 (67%)	11 (61%)	NS

[a]Data are expressed as mean ± SD; n, number of patients; NS, not significant; ND, not determined; r-GTP, r-glutamyltranspeptidase.

tively). This correlation was also observed in patients with HCC, regardless of the amount of alcohol intake (Table III). In conclusion, these data suggest that alcohol drinking might be an important factor that promotes an occurrence of HCC in patients with hepatitis C, and that HCV infection in the elderly promotes development of liver disease via LC to HCC. One interpretation for this finding is that alcohol promotes the progression to LC, and consequently enhances the process of carcinogenesis of the liver. Another interpretation is that alcohol directly promotes carcinogenesis by HCV infection. There has been no evidence showing the direct carcinogenetic effect of alcohol on the liver. In our study, no obvious relationship was observed between the amount of daily alcohol intake and the period from blood transfusion to diagnosis of LC, although the number of patients with LC who drank 46 g/day or more ethanol was limited. In patients with HCC, the proportion of chronic hepatitis and LC in the histology of noncancerous liver tissue was not different between patients of low and high alcohol intake. In addition, the multiplicity of tumors tended to be predominant in HCC patients who drank ethanol 46 g/day or more. Taken together, these data are consistent with the hypothesis that habitual alcohol intake might directly promote the hepatic carcinogenesis by persistent HCV infection.

Ikeda *et al.*[44] also showed that the risk factors for complication of HCC in HCV-positive patients with LC were the serum levels of α-fetoprotein, age, and the amount of alcohol intake, suggesting that alcohol promotes the development of HCC in patients with type C liver cirrhosis and that heavy drinkers with type C LC should be followed up as a high-risk group. There are a number of etiologic evidences indicating that the HCV infection is a cause of HCC.[45–47] However, little is known about the mechanism of hepatocarcinogenesis in patients with HCV. Because HCV is an RNA virus without reverse transcriptase activity, the integration of the HCV genome into hepatocyte DNA does not occur, as demonstrated in HBV.[48,49] One possible explanation for the high prevalence of HCV in HCC patients is that HCV is not oncogenic by itself, but may act as a cofactor by inducing necroinflammation, regeneration, and possibly malignant transformation to HCC.[50] Recently, evidences of multistep carcinogenesis in human HCC have been reported,[51] whereas it is not known how alcohol modifies the hepatocytes initiated by HCV and promotes carcinogenesis of the liver. Alcohol abusers with chronic hepatitis C exhibit a higher HCV-RNA level,[24,52] a higher degree of mutability in the HCV genome,[26] and a lower response to IFN therapy than nonabusers.[22,24,33] These alterations of HCV, both in quantity and in quality, by habitual alcohol intake might relate to the promoted carcinogenesis of the liver in drinkers with type C hepatitis. These possibilities should be clarified in future. Alternatively, chronic alcohol intake increases the conversion of procarcinogen to carcinogen via induction of cytochrome P450[30] and activates benzopyrene hydroxylase,[29] which enhances hepatocarcinogenesis by smoking. Alcohol also modifies dimethylnitrosamine,[31] a carcinogen, to a more bioactive form, which may result in mutagenicity of the host gene. In our study,[43] the tendency of a multiplicity of HCC was predominant in patients who drank ethanol, 46 g/day or more. There is a report that most habitual drinkers with HCC of <2 cm in diameter showed a histology of moderately or poorly differentiated HCC, frequently with intrahepatic metastasis or portal invasion.[53] These data also support a possibility that habitual alcohol intake might have some effect on the differentiation or proliferation of HCC.

In our study, the period from blood transfusion to diagnosis of LC had a significant inverse correlation with the age of transfusion. This correlation was also observed in patients with HCC, regardless of the amount of alcohol intake. Moreover, a Cox regression analysis showed that both the amount of alcohol intake and the age of blood transfusion were statistically significant factors for the development of HCC. These data suggest that HCV infection in the elder ages leads to a rapid progression to LC, and subsequently to a development of HCC.

Although some investigators reported older age at initial diagnosis as a risk factor for HCC,[44] little has been known about the relationship between the progression of liver disease and the age of acquiring HCV infection. It has been shown in the elderly that the clinical course of acute viral hepatitis prolongs and often leads to fulminant hepatitis, associated with poor prognosis.[54,55] Yano *et al.*[42] followed the histology of chronic hepatitis C for more than 10 years and demonstrated that progression of liver disease in the elderly was more rapid than in the young. In addition, there have been studies indicating that most patients showing rapid development of LC or HCC[45] were transfused in old age. The young seem to have an intense immunological response to HCV-infected liver cell compared with the elderly, which may result in less rapid C-type hepatitis-induced liver cell injury to LC in elderly patients. On the contrary, this might permit HCV to proliferate more in the elderly, associated with a higher level of HCV-RNA, which in turn might lead to a more rapid progression of liver injury to LC in the elderly than the young because of the direct cytotoxic effect of HCV. On the other hand, recent studies have documented the importance of apoptosis for the mechanism of liver cell injury by HCV infection.[56] The physiological decline of body cell mass with aging[54] is explained by a control of programmed cell death (apoptosis)[57] and by reduced cell regeneration. Taken together, these findings are consistent with the idea that the HCV-infected elderly reveal more rapid progression of C-type hepatitis-induced liver cell injury to LC–HCC than the young. Thus, the age of acquisition of HCV infection is presumably an important risk factor for developing HCC via LC.

Currently, the determining factor for the prognosis of cirrhotic patients is supposed to be the development of HCC; therefore, abstinence from alcohol may contribute to the prevention of hepatocarcinogenesis and improvement of the prognosis in patients with type C hepatitis. By contrast, a retrospective study by Lee[58] revealed an increase in the development of HCC after abstinence in patients with alcoholic LC; Lee's interpretation was that alcohol inhibits hepatocellular regeneration and the release of this inhibition by abstinence leads to an increase in hepatocarcinogenesis. Several similar studies in a prospective or retrospective manner supported the data presented by Lee; however, there are controversial reports at the same time. Indeed, lengthening the life span by abstinence may possibly be related to an increase in the development of HCC after abstinence in HCV-positive cirrhotics. Thus, more work will be required to elucidate the prognosis of patients with chronic viral liver disease following abstinence.

References

1. Choo QL, Kuo G, Weiner AJ, *et al:* Isolation of a cDNA clone derived from a blood-borne non-A, non-B viral hepatitis genome. *Science* 244:359–362, 1989.
2. Kuo G, Choo QL, Alter HJ, *et al:* An assay for circulating antibodies to a major etiologic virus of human non-A, non-B hepatitis. *Science* 244:362–364, 1989.
3. Garton JA, Tedder RS, Briggs M, *et al:* Detection of hepatitis C viral sequences in blood donations by nested polymerase chain reaction and prediction on infectivity. *Lancet* 335:1419–1422, 1990.
4. Weiner AJ, Kuo G, Bradley DW, *et al:* Detection of hepatitis C viral sequence in non-A, non-B hepatitis. *Lancet* 335:1–3, 1990.
5. Okamoto H, Munekata E, Tsuda F, *et al:* Enzyme-linked immunosorbent assay for antibodies against the capsid protein of hepatitis C virus with a synthetic oligopeptide. *Jpn J Exp Med* 60:223–233, 1990.

6. Shimizu S, Kiyosawa K, Sodeyama T, *et al:* High prevalence of antibody to hepatitis C in heavy drinkers with chronic liver disease in Japan. *J Gastroenterol Hepatol* 7:30–35, 1992.
7. Takase S, Takada N, Enomoto N, *et al:* Different types of chronic hepatitis in alcoholic patients: Does chronic hepatitis induced by alcohol exist? *Hepatology* 13:876–881, 1991.
8. Takase S, Takada S, Tsutsumi M: Alcohol and carcinogenesis, in Yirmiya R, Tayior AN (ed): *Alcohol, Immunity and Cancer.* Boca Raton, FL, CRC Press, 1993, pp 187–209.
9. Nalpas B, Driss F, Pol S, *et al:* Association between HCV and HBV infection in hepatocellular carcinoma and alcoholic liver disease. *J Hepatol* 12:70–74, 1991.
10. Orholm M, Andershvile J, Tage-Jensen V, *et al:* Prevalence of hepatitis B virus infection among alcoholic patients with liver disease. *J Clin Pathol* 34:1378–1380, 1981.
11. Ohnishi K, Iida S, Iwama S, *et al:* The effect of chronic habitual alcohol intake on the development of liver cirrhosis and hepatocellular carcinoma. Relation to hepatitis B surface antigen carriage. *Cancer* 49:672–677, 1982.
12. Hoofnagle JH, Mullen KD, Jones DB, *et al:* Treatment of chronic non-A, non-B hepatitis with recombinant human alpha interferon. *N Engl J Med* 315:1575–1578, 1986.
13. Okamoto H, Kurai K, Okada S, *et al:* Full-length sequence of a hepatitis C virus genome having poor homology to reported isolates: Comparative study of four distinct genotypes. *Virology* 188:331–341, 1992.
14. Weiner AJ, Geysen HM, Christopherson C, *et al:* Evidence for immune selection of hepatitis C virus (HCV) putative envelope glycoprotein variants: Potential role in chronic HCV infections. *Proc Natl Acad Sci USA* 89:3468–3472, 1992.
15. Nakase H, Yamada Y, Kimura A, *et al:* Sequence diversity of hypervariable region 1 in hepatitis C virus is the predictive factor for the efficacy of interferon therapy—Multivariate analysis. *Gastroenterology* 110:A1273, 1996.
16. Naito M, Hayashi N, Moribe T, *et al:* Hepatitis C viral quasi-species in hepatitis C virus carriers with normal liver enzymes and patients with type C chronic liver disease. *Hepatology* 22:407–412, 1995.
17. Yamada Y, Nakase H, Kimura A, *et al:* Sequence diversity of hypervariable region 1 in hepatitis C virus is a predictive factor for the efficacy of interferon therapy—Multivariate analysis (Abstract). 10th Asian-Pacific Congress of Gastroenterology, p 309, 1996.
18. Kimura A, Noda K, Yamaguchi Y, *et al:* Sequence diversity of hypervariable region 1 of hepatitis C virus in drinkers (Abstract). 10th Asian-Pacific Congress of Gastroenterology, p 301, 1996.
19. Hagiwara H, Hayashi N, Mita E, *et al:* Quantitative analysis of hepatitis C virus RNA in serum during interferon alpha therapy. *Gastroenterology* 104:877–883, 1993.
20. Okamoto H, Sugiyama Y, Okada S, *et al:* Typing hepatitis C virus by polymerase chain reaction with type-specific primers: Application to clinical surveys and tracing infectious sources. *J Gen Virol* 73:637–679, 1992.
21. Okamoto H, Kojima M, Okada S, *et al:* Genetic drift of hepatitis C virus during an 8.2 year infection in a chimpanzee: Variability and stability. *Virology* 190:894–899, 1992.
22. Ohnishi K, Matsuo S, Matsutari K, *et al:* Interferon therapy of chronic hepatitis C in frequent drinkers. *Am J Gastroenterol* 91:1374–1379, 1996.
23. Bagasura O, Howeedy A, Dorio R, *et al:* Functional analysis of T cell subsets in chronic alcoholism. *Immunology* 61:63–69, 1987.
24. Oshita M, Hayashi N, Kasahara A, *et al:* Increased serum hepatitis C virus RNA levels among alcoholic patients with chronic hepatitis C. *Hepatology* 20: 1115–1120, 1994.
25. Sawada M, Takada A, Takase S, *et al:* Effects of alcohol on the replication of hepatitis C virus. *Alcohol Alcohol Suppl* 28:85–90, 1993.
26. Finkelstein SD, Coelho-little E, Jeffers LJ, *et al:* HCV exhibits a higher degree of mutability in patients with a background of alcohol abuse. *Gastroenterology* 104:A903, 1993.
27. Dellarco VL: A mutagenicity assessment of acetaldehyde. *Mutation Res* 1995:1–20, 1988.
28. Yokoyama H, Nagata S, Moriya S, *et al:* Hepatitis C virus (HCV) infection enhances the formation of the circulating antibody (Ab) to the protein epitope related to a high acetaldehyde (Ach) concentration. *Hepatology* 22:223A, 1995.

29. Seiz HK, Garroo AJ, Lieber CS: Effect of chronic ethanol ingestion on intestinal metabolism of and mutagenicity of benzopyrene. *Biochem Biophys Res Commun* 85:1061–1066, 1978.
30. Lieber CS, Seiz HK, Garroo AJ, *et al:* Alcohol related disease and carcinogenesis. *Cancer Res* 39:2863–2886, 1979.
31. Garroo AJ, Seiz HK, Lieber CS: Enhancement of dimethylnitrosamine metabolism and activation to a mutagen following chronic alcohol consumption. *Cancer Res* 41:120–124, 1981.
32. Dreyer G, Dervan PB: Sequence-specific cleavage of single stranded DNA: Oligodeoxynucleotide-EDTA-FE(II). *Proc Natl Acad Sci USA* 82:968–972, 1985.
33. Okazaki T, Yoshihara H, Suzuki K, *et al:* Efficacy of interferon therapy in patients with chronic hepatitis C. Comparison between nondrinkers and drinkers. *Scand J Gastroenterol* 29:1039–1043, 1994.
34. Knodell RG, Ishak KG, Black WC, *et al:* Formulation and application of a numerical scoring system for assessing histological activity in asymptomatic chronic hepatitis. *Hepatology* 1:431–435, 1981.
35. Ulrich PP, Romeo JM, Lane PK, *et al:* Detection, semiquantitation and genetic variation in hepatitis C virus sequence amplified from the plasma of blood donors with elevated alanine aminotransferase. *J Clin Invest* 86:1609–1614, 1990.
36. Takase S, Matsuda Y, Sawada M, *et al:* Effect of alcohol abuse on HCV replication. *Gastroenterol Jpn* 28:322, 1993.
37. Takada N, Takase S, Enomoto N, *et al:* Clinical backgrounds of the patients having different types of hepatitis C virus genomes. *J Hepatol* 14:35–40, 1992.
38. Berenyi MR, Straus B, Avila L: T rosettes in alcoholic cirrhosis of the liver. *JAMA* 232:44–46, 1975.
39. Nei J, Matsuda Y, Takada A: Chronic hepatitis induced by alcohol. *Dig Dis Sci* 28:207–215, 1983.
40. Bruix J, Barrera JM, Calvet X, *et al:* Prevalence of antibodies to hepatitis C virus in Spanish patients with hepatocellular carcinoma and hepatic cirrhosis. *Lancet* 2:1004–1006, 1989.
41. Austin H, Delzell E, Grufferman S, *et al:* A case control study of hepatocellular carcinoma and the hepatitis B virus, cigarette smoking, and alcohol consumption. *Cancer Res* 46:962–966, 1986.
42. Yano M, Yatsuhashi H, Inoue O, *et al:* Epidemiology and long-term prognosis of hepatitis C virus infection in Japan. *Gut* 34 (Suppl):13–16, 1993.
43. Noda K, Yoshihara H, Suzuki K, *et al:* Progression of type C chronic hepatitis to liver cirrhosis and hepatocellular carcinoma—Its relationship to alcohol drinking and the age of transfusion. *Alcohol Clin Exp Res* 20:95–100, 1996.
44. Ikeda K, Saitoh S, Koida I, *et al:* A multivariate analysis of risk factors for hepatocellular carcinogenesis: A prospective observation of 795 patients with viral and alcoholic cirrhosis. *Hepatology* 18:47–53, 1993.
45. Kiyosawa K, Sodeyama T, Tanaka E, *et al:* Interrelationship of blood transfusion, non-A, non-B hepatitis and hepatocellular carcinoma: Analysis by detection of antibody to hepatitis C virus. *Hepatology* 12:671–675, 1990.
46. Garson JA, Wick AN, Ring CJA, *et al:* Detection of hepatitis C viremia in Caucasian patients with hepatocellular carcinoma. *J Med Virol* 38:152–156, 1992.
47. Simonetti RG, Camma C, Fiorello F, *et al:* Hepatitis C virus infection as a risk factor for hepatocellular carcinoma in patients with cirrhosis. *Ann Intern Med* 116:97–102, 1992.
48. Brechot C, Pourcel C, Louise A, *et al:* Presence of integrated hepatitis B virus DNA sequences in cellular DNA of human hepatocellular carcinoma. *Nature* 286:533–535, 1980.
49. Kim CM, Koike K, Saito I, *et al:* HBx gene of hepatitis B virus induces liver cancer in transgenic mice. *Nature* 351:317–320, 1991.
50. Kew MC: Hepatitis C virus and hepatocellular carcinoma. *FEM Microbiol Rev* 14:211–220, 1994.
51. Walker GJ, Hayward HK, Falvey S, *et al:* Loss of heterozygosity in hepatocellular carcinoma. *Cancer Res* 51:4367–4370, 1991.

52. Makoto S, Takada A, Takase S, *et al:* Effects of alcohol on the replication of hepatitis C virus. *Alcohol Alcohol* 28(S1B):85–90, 1993.
53. Kubo S, Kinoshita H: Effect of alcohol drinking on hepatocellular carcinoma at the time of operation. *Jpn J Gastroenterol* 91(Suppl):511, 1994.
54. Tanikawa K: Liver disease in the elderly. *Asian Med J* 31:173–178, 1988.
55. Fenster LF: Viral hepatitis in the elderly. An analysis of 23 patients over 65 years of age. *Gastroenterology* 49:262–271, 1965.
56. Kerr JFR, Cooksley WGE, Searle J, *et al:* The nature of piecemeal necrosis in chronic active hepatitis. *Lancet* 2:827–828, 1979.
57. Carson DA, Ribeiro JM: Apoptosis and disease. *Lancet* 341:1251–1254, 1993.
58. Lee FI: Cirrhosis and hepatoma in alcoholics. *Gut* 7:77–85, 1966.

Contents of Previous Volumes

Volume 2

II. Prostaglandins, Leukotrienes, and Alcohol *Richard A. Deitrich, Section Editor*

III. Cardiovascular Effects of Alcohol Abuse *David H. Van Thiel, Section Editor*

IV. Cerebral Functioning in Social Drinkers *Elizabeth Parker, Section Editor*

Volume 4

Volume 5

I. Alcohol and Memory *Henri Begleiter, Section Editor*

II. Alcohol Treatment and Society *Robin Room, Section Editor*

III. The Effects of Ethanol on Ion Channels *Richard A. Deitrich, Section Editor*

Volume 8

Volume 9

Volume 10

Index

ISBN 0-306-45747-4
90000
9 780306 457470